Fourth Canadian Edition

NURSING RESEARCH IN CANADA

Methods, Critical Appraisal, and Utilization

GERI LoBIONDO-WOOD, PhD, RN, FAAN

Professor and Coordinator, PhD in Nursing Program
University of Texas Health Science Center at Houston
School of Nursing
Houston, Texas

JUDITH HABER, PhD, APRN, BC, FAAN

The Ursula Springer Leadership Professor in Nursing
Associate Dean for Graduate Programs
New York University
College of Nursing
New York, New York

CHERYLYN CAMERON, RN, PhD

Dean, School of Community Studies and Creative
    Technologies
Bow Valley College
Calgary, Alberta

MINA D. SINGH, RN, PhD

Associate Director, Research
Associate Professor
School of Nursing
York University
Toronto, Ontario

ELSEVIER

ELSEVIER

Notices

The adaptation has been undertaken by Elsevier Canada Ltd., at its sole responsibility. Practitioners and researchers must always rely on their own experience and knowledge in evaluating and using any information, methods, compounds or experiments described herein. Because of rapid advances in the medical sciences, in particular, independent verification of diagnoses and drug dosages should be made. To the fullest extent of the law, no responsibility is assumed by Elsevier, authors, editors or contributors in relation to the adaptation or for any injury and/or damage to persons or property as a matter of products liability, negligence or otherwise, or from any use or operation of any methods, products, instructions, or ideas contained in the material herein.

Library and Archives Canada Cataloguing in Publication

LoBiondo-Wood, Geri, author

Nursing research in Canada : methods, critical appraisal, and utilization / Geri LoBiondo-Wood (PhD, RN, FAAN, Professor and Coordinator, PhD in Nursing Program, University of Texas Health Science Center at Houston, School of Nursing, Houston, Texas), Judith Haber (PhD, APRN, BC, FAAN, The Ursula Springer Leadership in Professional Nursing, Associate Dean for Graduate Programs, New York University, College of Nursing, New York, New York) ; Canadian editors: Cherylyn Cameron (RN, PhD, Dean, School of Community Studies and Creative Technologies, Bow Valley College, Calgary, Alberta), Mina D. Singh (RN, PhD, Associate Director, Research, Associate Professor, School of Nursing, York University, Toronto, Ontario). — Fourth Canadian edition.

Includes bibliographical references and index.
Has supplement: Study guide for Nursing research in Canada.
ISBN 978-1-77172-098-4 (softcover)

1. Nursing—Research—Canada—Textbooks. 2. Textbooks. I. Haber, Judith, author II. Cameron, Cherylyn, 1958-, editor III. Singh, Mina D., editor IV. Title.

RT81.5.L63 2017   610.73072'071   C2017-905204-7

Content Strategist: Roberta A. Spinosa-Millman
Senior Content Development Specialist: Heather Bays
Publishing Services Manager: Jeffrey Patterson
Senior Project Manager: Tracey Schriefer
Design Direction: Renee Duenow
Copyeditor: Jerri Hurlbutt
Proofreader: Claudia Forgas

Elsevier Canada
420 Main Street East, Suite 636, Milton, ON, Canada L9T 5G3
Phone: 416-644-7053

1 2 3 4 5 21 20 19 18 17

Ebook ISBN: 978-1-77172-095-3

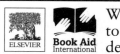

Working together to grow libraries in developing countries

www.elsevier.com • www.bookaid.org

Contents

Author Biographies

Geri LoBiondo-Wood, PhD, RN, FAAN, is Professor and Coordinator of the PhD in Nursing Program at the University of Texas Health Science Center at Houston, School of Nursing (UTHSC-Houston) and former Director of Research and Evidence-Based Practice Planning and Development at the MD Anderson Cancer Center, Houston, Texas. She received her Diploma in Nursing at St. Mary's Hospital School of Nursing in Rochester, New York; Bachelor's and Master's degrees from the University of Rochester; and a PhD in Nursing Theory and Research from New York University. Dr. LoBiondo-Wood teaches research and evidence-based practice principles to undergraduate, graduate, and doctoral students. At MD Anderson Cancer Center, she developed and implemented the Evidence-Based Resource Unit Nurse (EB-RUN) Program, a hospital-wide program that involves all levels of nurses in the application of research evidence to practice. She has extensive national and international experience guiding nurses and other health care professionals in the development and utilization of research. Dr. LoBiondo-Wood is an Editorial Board member of *Progress in Transplantation* and a reviewer for *Nursing Research, Oncology Nursing Forum, Oncology Nursing,* and *Nephrology Nursing Journal.* Her research and publications focus on chronic illness and oncology nursing.

Dr. LoBiondo-Wood has been active locally and nationally in many professional organizations, including the Oncology Nursing Society, Southern Nursing Research Society, the Midwest Nursing Research Society, and the North American Transplant Coordinators Organization. She has received local and national awards for teaching and contributions to nursing. In 1997, she received the Distinguished Alumnus Award from New York University, Division of Nursing Alumni Association. In 2001 she was inducted as a Fellow of the American Academy of Nursing and in 2007 as a Fellow of the University of Texas Academy of Health Science Education. In 2012 she was appointed as a Distinguished Teaching Professor of the University of Texas System.

Judith Haber, PhD, APRN, BC, FAAN, is the Ursula Springer Leadership Professor in Nursing and Associate Dean for Graduate Programs in the College of Nursing at New York University. She received her undergraduate nursing education at Adelphi University in New York, and she holds a Master's degree in Adult Psychiatric–Mental Health Nursing and a PhD in Nursing Theory and Research from New York University. Dr. Haber is internationally recognized as a clinician and educator in psychiatric–mental health nursing. She has extensive clinical experience in psychiatric nursing, having been an advanced practice psychiatric nurse in private practice for over 30 years, specializing in treatment of families coping with the psychosocial sequelae of acute and chronic catastrophic illness. Her NIH-funded program of research addressed physical and psychosocial adjustment to illness, focusing specifically on women with breast cancer and their partners and, more recently, breast cancer survivorship. Dr. Haber is also committed to an interprofessional program of clinical scholarship related to improving oral-systemic health outcomes and leads the *Oral Health Nursing Education and Practice (OHNEP)* program funded by the DentaQuest Foundation as well as the

HRSA-funded *Teaching Oral Systemic Health (TOSH)* program.

Dr. Haber has been active locally and nationally in many professional organizations, including the American Nurses Association, the American Psychiatric Nurses Association, and the American Academy of Nursing. She has received numerous local, state, and national awards for public policy, clinical practice, and research, including the APNA Psychiatric Nurse of the Year Award in 1998 and 2005 and the APNA Outstanding Research Award in 2005. She received the 2007 NYU College of Nursing Distinguished Alumnus Award, the 2011 NYU Distinguished Teaching Award, and the 2013 NYU Alumni Meritorious Service Award. In 1993, she was inducted as a Fellow of the American Academy of Nursing and in 2012 as a Fellow in the New York Academy of Medicine.

CANADIAN EDITORS

Cherylyn Cameron, RN, PhD, is the Dean of Community Studies and Creative Technologies at Bow Valley College in Calgary, Alberta. She received her Bachelor of Science in Nursing degree from the University of Alberta and a Master of Arts degree in education from Central Michigan University. She received her doctorate in theory and policy studies in education from the Ontario Institute for Studies in Education (OISE)/University of Toronto. Her dissertation, "The Lived Experience of Transfer Students from a Baccalaureate Nursing Program," won the Best Dissertation award from the Council for Study of Community Colleges in the United States. Her research interests include college–university relations, learner success, development of social emotional health in children, and leadership development in practical nurses. She is currently funded by the Social Science and Humanities Research Council to study the development of social emotional health in early childhood centres and to co-create of strategies and materials to empower Indigenous educators and communities to promote the social-emotional health of Indigenous children. Dr. Cameron also serves on the Board for the Health Information and Data Governance Committee at the Ministry of Health in Alberta.

Mina D. Singh, RN, PhD, is an Associate Professor at the School of Nursing, York University. At present, she is the Associate Director, Research. She has a long career in nursing, having worked in acute care, mental health, psychotherapy, and public health. Her expertise is as a research methodologist, statistician, and program evaluator. In addition, she is a psychotherapist. She won the 2012 National Nursing Research Scholar award and the 2014 Accreditation Reviewer Excellence award granted by the Canadian Association of Schools of Nursing (CASN). She has been an Accreditation Reviewer for CASN for over 16 years and has travelled internationally and nationally reviewing nursing education programs.

Contributors

Julie Barroso, PhD, ANP, APRN, BC, FAAN
Professor and Research Development Coordinator
Duke University School of Nursing
Durham, North Carolina

Joan L. Bottorff, PhD, RN, FCAHS, FAAN
Professor
School of Nursing
Faculty of Health and Social Development
University of British Columbia
Kelowna, British Columbia

Carol Bova, PhD, RN, ANP
Associate Professor of Nursing and Medicine
Graduate School of Nursing
University of Massachusetts–Worcester
Worcester, Massachusetts

Cherylyn Cameron, RN, PhD
Dean, School of Community Studies
    and Creative Technologies
Bow Valley College
Calgary, Alberta

Marsha Campbell-Yeo, PhD, NNP, BC RN
Assistant Professor
School of Nursing
Clinician Scientist
IWK Health Centre
Dalhousie University
Halifax, Nova Scotia

Nancy C. Edwards, RN, BScN, MSc, PhD
Full Professor
School of Nursing
University of Ottawa
Ottawa, Ontario

Stephanie Fulton, MSIS, AHIP
Executive Director, Research Medical Library
The University of Texas MD Anderson Cancer Center
Houston, Texas

Judith Haber, PhD, APRN, BC, FAAN
The Ursula Springer Leadership Professor in Nursing
Associate Dean for Graduate Programs
New York University
College of Nursing
New York, New York

Nancy E. Kline, PhD, RN, CPNP, FAAN
Director, Clinical Inquiry, Medicine
Patient Services
Boston Children's Hospital
Boston, Massachusetts;
Adjunct Clinical Assistant Professor
College of Nursing
New York University
New York, New York

Barbara Krainovich-Miller, EdD, RN, PMHCNS-BC, ANEF, FAAN
Professor and Associate Dean, Academic and Clinical
    Affairs
New York University College of Nursing
New York, New York

Geri LoBiondo-Wood, PhD, RN, FAAN
Professor and Coordinator, PhD in Nursing Program
University of Texas Health Science Center at Houston
School of Nursing
Houston, Texas

Christine Maheu, RN, PhD
Associate Professor
Ingram School of Nursing
McGill University
Montreal, Quebec

Gloria McInnis Perry, BScN, MScN, DNSc
Associate Professor
School of Nursing
University of Prince Edward Island
Charlottetown, Prince Edward Island

Louise Racine, RN, BScN, MScN, PhD
Associate Professor
College of Nursing
University of Saskatchewan
Saskatoon, Saskatchewan

Mina D. Singh, RN, PhD
Associate Director, Research
Associate Professor
School of Nursing
York University
Toronto, Ontario

Helen J. Streubert, EdD, RN, ANEF
President
College of Saint Elizabeth
Morristown, New Jersey

Susan Sullivan-Bolyai, DNSc, CNS, RN, FAAN
Associate Professor
Director, Florence S. Downs Doctoral Program in Research
    and Theory Development
College of Nursing
New York University
New York, New York

Sally Thorne, RN, PhD, FAAN, FCAHS
Professor
School of Nursing
University of British Columbia
Vancouver, British Columbia

Marita Titler, PhD, RN, FAAN
Professor and Chair, Division of Nursing Business and
    Health Systems
Rhetaugh G. Dumas Endowed Chair
Associate Dean, Office of Clinical Scholarship and Practice
    Development
Division of Nursing Business and Health Systems
University of Michigan School of Nursing
Ann Arbor, Michigan

Reviewers

Nora Ahmad, BNS, RN, DMedSci
Assistant Professor
Nursing
Brandon University
Brandon, Manitoba

Davina Banner-Lukaris, RN, PhD
Assistant Professor
School of Nursing
University of Northern British Columbia
Prince George, British Columbia

Mona Burrows, BScN, RN(EC), MScN, PHC-NP
Faculty
Collaborative BScN program
St. Lawrence College/Laurentian University
Cornwall, Ontario

Sara Craig, BA, BScN, RN, MN
Professor
Health Sciences
St. Lawrence College
Brockville, Ontario

Cheryl Forchuk, RN, PhD
Distinguished University Professor
Arthur Labatt Family School of Nursing
Western University
London, Ontario

Angela J. Gillis, RN, PhD
Professor
School of Nursing
Saint Francis Xavier University
Antigonish, Nova Scotia

Lisa Howard, BScN, RN, MN, PhD
Assistant Professor
Faculty of Health Sciences
University of Lethbridge
Lethbridge, Alberta

Lianne Jeffs, BScN, MSc, PhD
St. Michael's Hospital Volunteer Association Chair in
    Nursing Research
Keenan Research Centre of the Li Ka Shing Knowledge
    Institute
St. Michael's Hospital
Toronto, Ontario

Janet L. Kuhnke, BA, BScN, RN, MS, ET
Professor
School of Nursing
St. Lawrence College
Cornwall, Ontario

Madonna Susan Manuel, BN, MSN
Nurse Educator
Western Regional School of Nursing
Corner Brook, Newfoundland

Joyce O'Mahony, BN, RN, MN, PhD
Assistant Professor
School of Nursing
Thompson Rivers University
Kamloops, British Columbia

Louise Racine, BScN, RN, MScN, PhD
Associate Professor
College of Nursing
University of Saskatchewan
Saskatoon, Saskatchewan

Erna Snelgrove-Clarke, RN, MN, PhD
Assistant Professor
School of Nursing
Department of Obstetrics & Gynecology
Dalhousie University
Halifax, Nova Scotia

Acknowledgements

THIS MAJOR UNDERTAKING WAS ACCOMPLISHED WITH the help of many people, some of whom made direct contributions to the new edition and some of whom contributed indirectly. We acknowledge with deep appreciation and our warmest thanks the following people who made this fourth Canadian edition possible:

- Nursing educators across Canada who provided valuable and insightful comments that helped to direct the revisions featured in this edition and contributed to improving the content
- Our students, particularly the nursing students of Bow Valley College and York University programs, who inspired us with their feedback and willingness to use the information in this text by becoming research assistants
- Roberta A. Spinosa-Millman, Content Strategist, who got us started with encouragement, a sense of humour, and great insight
- Heather Bays, Developmental Editor, who encouraged us with positive feedback, made sense of the process, and extended deadlines graciously
- Jerri Hurlbutt, Copy Editor, and Tracey Schriefer, Senior Project Manager, whose attention to detail ensured that we had a very readable text for our students
- Renee Duenow, Design Manager, who redesigned this edition so that it is a pleasure to look at and read
- Our vignette contributors, whose willingness to share their wisdom and evidence of their innovative research made a unique contribution to this edition
- All of the reviewers, who provided thoughtful feedback not only on the first, second, and third editions but also on the fourth Canadian edition manuscript
- Our families, who supported us and picked up the "loose ends" while we wrote and revised.

To my husband John Cameron, who has always been there, loving, supporting, and encouraging me. Thanks for keeping our family and household together so that I could stay focused on this fourth edition.

Cherylyn Cameron

To my husband Neranjan, my daughter Sandhya, and my parents Ram and Betty Laljie, for their support and encouragement.

Mina D. Singh

Preface

THE FOUNDATION OF THE FOURTH CANADIAN edition of *Nursing Research in Canada: Methods, Critical Appraisal, and Utilization* continues to be the belief that nursing research is integral to all levels of nursing education and practice. Since the first edition of this textbook, we have seen the depth and breadth of nursing research grow. More nurses are conducting research and using research evidence to shape clinical practice, education, administration, and health policy.

The Canadian Nurses Association promotes the notion that nurses must provide care that is based on the best available scientific evidence. This is an exciting challenge to meet. Nurses are using the best available evidence, combined with their clinical judgement and patient preferences, to influence the nature and direction of health care delivery and to document outcomes related to the quality and cost-effectiveness of patient care. As nurses continue to develop a unique body of nursing knowledge through research, decisions about clinical nursing practice will be increasingly evidence informed.

As editors, we believe that all nurses not only need to understand the research process but also need to know how to critically read, evaluate, and apply research findings in practice. We realize that understanding research, as a component of evidence-informed practice, is a challenge for every student, but we believe that the challenge can be accomplished in a stimulating, lively, and learner-friendly manner.

Consistent with this perspective is a commitment to advancing implementation of the evidence-informed practice paradigm. Understanding and applying nursing research must be an integral dimension of nursing education, evident not only in the undergraduate nursing research course but also throughout the curriculum. The research role of nurses calls for evidence-informed practice competencies; central to this are critical appraisal skills—that is, nurses should be competent research consumers.

Preparing students for this role involves developing their critical thinking and reading skills, thereby enhancing their understanding of the research process, their appreciation of the role of the critiquer, and their ability to actually appraise research critically. An undergraduate course in nursing research should develop this basic level of competence, which is an essential requirement if students are to engage in evidence-informed clinical decision-making and practice. This is in contrast to a graduate-level research course, in which the emphasis is on carrying out research, as well as understanding and appraising it.

The primary audience for this textbook remains undergraduate students who are learning the steps of the research process, as well as how to develop clinical questions, critically appraise published research literature, and use research findings to inform evidence-informed clinical practice. This book is also a valuable resource for students at the master's and doctoral levels who want a concise review of the basic steps of the research process, the critical appraisal process, and the principles and tools for evidence-informed practice.

This text is also a key resource for doctoral students who are preparing to be experts at leading evidence-informed initiatives in clinical settings. Furthermore, it is an important resource for practising nurses who strive to use research evidence as the basis for clinical decision-making and development of evidence-informed policies, protocols, and standards, rather than rely on tradition, authority, or trial and error. It is an important resource for nurses who collaborate with nurse-scientists in the conduct of clinical research and evidence-informed practice.

Building on the success of the third edition, we maintain our commitment to introduce evidence-informed practice and research principles to baccalaureate students, thereby providing a cutting-edge research consumer foundation for their clinical practice.

Nursing Research in Canada: Methods, Critical Appraisal, and Utilization prepares nursing students and practising nurses to become knowledgeable nursing research consumers in the following ways:

- Addressing the evidence-informed practice role of the nurse, thereby embedding evidence-informed competence in the clinical practice of every baccalaureate graduate.
- Demystifying research, which is sometimes viewed as a complex process.
- Using an evidence-informed approach to teaching the fundamentals of the research process.
- Teaching the critical appraisal process in a user-friendly but logical and systematic progression.
- Promoting a lively spirit of inquiry that develops critical thinking and critical reading skills, facilitating mastery of the critical appraisal process.
- Developing information literacy, searching, and evidence-informed practice competencies that prepare students and nurses to effectively locate and evaluate the best available research evidence.
- Elevating the critical appraisal process and research appreciation to a position of importance comparable to that of producing research. Before students become research producers, they must become knowledgeable research consumers.
- Emphasizing the role of evidence-informed practice as the basis for informing clinical

decision-making and nursing interventions that support nursing practice, demonstrating quality and cost-effective outcomes of nursing care delivery.

- Presenting numerous examples of recently published research studies that illustrate and highlight each research concept in a manner that brings abstract ideas to life for students new to the research and critical appraisal process. These examples are a critical link for reinforcement of evidence-informed concepts and the related research and critiquing process.
- Showcasing, in **Research Vignettes,** the work of renowned nurse researchers whose careers exemplify the links among research, education, and practice.
- Providing numerous pedagogical chapter features, including **Learning Outcomes, Key Terms, Key Points,** new **Critical Thinking Challenges, Research Hints, Evidence-Informed Practice Tips,** new **Practical Applications**, and revised **Critical Thinking Decision Paths,** as well as numerous tables, boxes, and figures. At the end of each chapter that presents a step of the research process, we feature a section titled **Appraising the Evidence,** which reviews how each step of the research process should be evaluated from a consumer's perspective. This section is accompanied by an updated **Critiquing Criteria** box.
- Providing a **Study Guide** that promotes active learning and assimilation of nursing research content.
- Offering an Evolve site presenting free **Evolve Resources for Instructors** that includes a Test Bank, TEACH, PowerPoint slides, critiquing exercises, an Image Collection, and new critical appraisal activities. There are also Evolve resources for both the student and faculty that include an audio glossary.

The fourth Canadian edition of *Nursing Research in Canada: Methods, Critical Appraisal, and Utilization* is organized into six parts. Each part is preceded by an introductory section and opens with an exciting "Research Vignette" by a renowned nurse researcher.

Part One, Research Overview, contains six chapters. Chapter 1, "The Role of Research in Nursing," provides an excellent overview of research and evidence-informed practice processes that shape clinical practice. This chapter introduces the role that research plays in practice and education, the roles of nurses in research activities, a historical perspective, and future directions in nursing research. The style and content of this chapter are designed to make subsequent chapters more user-friendly. Chapter 2, "Theoretical Framework," focuses specifically on how theoretical frameworks guide and inform knowledge generation through the research process. Chapter 3, "Critical Reading Strategies: Overview of the Research Process," addresses students directly and highlights critical thinking and critical reading concepts and strategies, thereby facilitating students' understanding of the research process and its relationship to the critical appraisal process. This chapter introduces a model evidence hierarchy that is used throughout the text.

The next two chapters address foundational components of the research process. Chapter 4, "Developing Research Questions, Hypotheses, and Clinical Questions," focuses on how research questions, hypotheses, and evidence-informed practice questions are derived, operationalized, and critically appraised. Numerous clinical examples illustrating different types of research questions and hypotheses maximize student understanding. Students are also taught how to develop clinical questions that are used to guide evidence-informed inquiry. Chapter 5, "Finding and Appraising the Literature," showcases cutting-edge information literacy content, providing students and nurses with the tools necessary to effectively search, retrieve, manage, and evaluate research studies and their findings. This chapter also develops research consumer competencies that

prepare students and nurses to critically read, understand, and appraise a study's literature review and framework. The final chapter in this section, Chapter 6, "Legal and Ethical Issues," provides an overview of the increased emphasis on the legal and ethical issues facing researchers in Canada.

Part Two, Qualitative Research, contains two interrelated qualitative research chapters. Chapter 7, "Introduction to Qualitative Research," provides a framework for understanding qualitative research designs and literature, as well as the significant contribution of qualitative research to evidence-informed practice. Chapter 8, "Qualitative Approaches to Research," presents, illustrates, and, in examples from the literature, showcases major qualitative methods. This chapter highlights the questions most appropriately answered through the use of qualitative methods.

Part Three, Quantitative Research, contains Chapters 9 ("Introduction to Quantitative Research"), 10 ("Experimental and Quasiexperimental Designs"), and 11 ("Nonexperimental Designs"). These chapters delineate the essential steps of the quantitative research process, with published, current clinical research studies used to illustrate each step. Links between the steps and their relationship to the total research process are examined.

Part Four, Processes Related to Research, describes the specific steps of the research process for qualitative and quantitative studies. The chapters make the case for linking an evidence-informed approach with essential steps of the research process by teaching students how to critically appraise the strengths and weaknesses of each step of the research process. Students learn how to select participants (Chapter 12, "Sampling"), gather data (Chapter 13, "Data-Collection Methods"), analyze the results (Chapter 15, "Qualitative Data Analysis," and Chapter 16, "Quantitative Data Analysis"), and present their results (Chapter 17, "Presenting the Findings"). Chapter 14, "Rigour in Research," gives students the tools for assessing the quality and trustworthiness of a study.

Part Five, Critiquing Research, makes the case for linking an evidence-informed approach with essential steps of the research process by teaching students how to critically appraise the strengths and weaknesses of each step of the research process. Each chapter critiques two examples of actual published research. Chapter 18, "Critiquing Qualitative Research," focuses on qualitative research, whereas Chapter 19, "Critiquing Quantitative Research," is based on the quantitative research process.

Part Six, Application of Research: Evidence-Informed Practice, contains the final chapter in the book. Chapter 20, "Developing an Evidence-Informed Practice," provides a dynamic review of evidence-informed models. These models can be applied—step by step, at the organizational or individual patient level—as frameworks for implementing and evaluating the outcomes of evidence-informed health care.

The Evolve website that accompanies the fourth Canadian edition provides interactive learning activities that promote the development of critical thinking, critical reading, and information literacy skills designed to develop the competencies necessary to produce informed consumers of nursing research. Instructor resources are available at a passcode-protected website that gives faculty access to all instructor materials online, including the Instructor's Manual, Image Collection, PowerPoint Slides, a Test Bank that allows faculty to create examinations through the use of the ExamView test generator program, and more.

The development and refinement of an evidence-informed foundation for clinical nursing practice is an essential priority for the future of professional nursing practice. The fourth Canadian edition of *Nursing Research in Canada: Methods, Critical Appraisal, and Utilization* will help students develop a basic level of competence in understanding the steps of the research process that will enable them to critically analyze research studies, evaluate their merit, and judiciously apply evidence in clinical practice. To the extent that this goal is accomplished, the next generation of nursing professionals will include a cadre of clinicians who inform their practice by using theory and research evidence, combined with their clinical judgement, and specific to the health care needs of patients and their families in health and illness.

Cherylyn Cameron
ccameron@bowvalleycollege.ca

Mina D. Singh
minsingh@yorku.ca

To the Student

WE INVITE YOU TO JOIN US on an exciting nursing research adventure that begins as you turn the first page of the fourth Canadian edition of *Nursing Research in Canada: Methods, Critical Appraisal, and Utilization.* The adventure is one of discovery! You will discover that the nursing research literature sparkles with pride, dedication, and excitement about the research dimension of professional nursing practice. Whether you are a student or a practising nurse whose goal is to use research evidence as the foundation of your practice, you will discover that nursing research and a commitment to evidence-informed practice positions our profession at the forefront of change. You will discover that evidence-informed practice is integral to meeting the challenge of providing quality health care in partnership with patients and their families and significant others, as well as with the communities in which they live. Finally, you will discover the richness in the "who," "what," "where," "when," "why," and "how" of nursing research and evidence-informed practice, and you will develop a foundation of knowledge and skills that will equip you for clinical practice today and into the future.

We think you will enjoy reading this text. Your nursing research course will be short but filled with new and challenging learning experiences that will develop your evidence-informed practice skills. The fourth Canadian edition of *Nursing Research in Canada: Methods, Critical Appraisal, and Utilization* reflects cutting-edge trends for developing evidence-informed nursing practice. The six-part organization and special features in this text are designed to help you develop your skills in critical thinking, critical reading, information literacy, and evidence-informed clinical decision making, while providing a user-friendly approach to learning that expands your competence to deal with these new and challenging experiences. The companion *Study Guide,* with its chapter-by-chapter activities, will serve as a self-paced learning tool to reinforce the content of the text. The accompanying Evolve website offers "summative" review material to help you reinforce the concepts discussed throughout the book.

Remember that evidence-informed practice skills are used in every clinical setting and can be applied to every patient population or clinical practice issue. Whether your clinical practice involves primary care or specialty care and provides inpatient or outpatient treatment in a hospital, clinic, or home, you will be challenged to apply your evidence-informed practice skills and use nursing research as the foundation for your evidence-informed practice. The fourth Canadian edition of *Nursing Research in Canada: Methods Critical Appraisal, and Utilization* will guide you through this exciting adventure, where you will discover your ability to play a vital role in contributing to the building of an evidence-informed professional nursing practice.

Cherylyn Cameron
ccameron@bowvalleycollege.ca

Mina D. Singh
minsingh@yorku.ca

PART ONE

Research Overview

RESEARCH **VIGNETTE**

A Program of Research in Transcultural Nursing

Louise Racine, RN, MScN, PhD
Professor
University of Saskatchewan
Saskatoon, Saskatchewan

My interest in transcultural nursing developed during my years of practice as a bedside nurse at the Centre Hospitalier Universitaire de l'Université Laval (Hôtel-Dieu de Québec). I observed that patients from diverse ethnocultural backgrounds had different ways of understanding and coping with illness. These observations, arising from my clinical practice, triggered my interest in exploring cultural competency and safety. I was intrigued to know more about the process of becoming culturally competent. How do nurses become culturally competent in providing nursing care? These years of clinical practice revealed that culture influences patients' and families' conceptualizations of health and illness and that culture needs to be accounted for when caring for individuals and populations.

My thirst for knowledge and need to understand the complexity of culture within nursing practice inspired me to complete my bachelor's degree in nursing. My interest in the intersection of anthropology and health became greater while enrolled in an undergraduate nursing course called "Anthropology and Health," taught by Dr. Francine Saillant in the Faculty of Nursing at Université Laval.

Under Dr. Saillant's guidance, I got immersed in nursing research for two summer terms, working on historical research related to lay care practices that was archived in popular literature. Through this research assistantship, I discovered the critical role played by culture in shaping health and illness experiences. Under the mentoring of Dr. Saillant, I solidified my interests in anthropology, ethnography, and historical research. I conducted my master's thesis research on the delivery of home care services in a Montreal multicultural neighbourhood. Through interviewing both patients and nurses I discovered that professional nursing encounters could not be isolated from culture. I used Leininger's theory of cultural care diversity and universality (1991) to guide my research. This research was funded by a Fonds de la recherche en santé du Québec (FRSQ) Master Award. At that time, my understanding of culture was somewhat positivist and deterministic, yet I came to a better understanding of what Leininger meant by diversity and universality. In spite of cultural differences, humans share subjective, existential experiences when confronted with illness. Leininger understood that culture cannot be isolated from the environment and the social world. Culture is a construct that has to be examined within the historical, social, cultural, gendered, and economic contexts in which experiences of health and illness occur.

My master's study led me to further my quest for knowledge, and I decided to do doctoral studies. The doctoral program in the School of Nursing at the University of British Columbia (UBC) attracted me. There I wanted to study under the supervision and mentoring of Dr. Joan Anderson. I have been privileged to study at UBC and benefit from the mentoring of a great nurse scholar. In this program I was surrounded by stellar classmates and other outstanding professors of nursing; these giants in the field contributed to developing my thoughts regarding nursing research and science. As a doctoral student, I understood that culture is far from being a fixed concept; rather, it is a fluid and hybrid concept, open to change and adaptation. Humans are not determined or bounded by their culture as they have the possibilities of transcending the limitations of linear cultural experiences. To continue my doctoral education, I was privileged to receive doctoral awards from the FRSQ and the National Human Resource Development Plan (NHRDP).

I delved into study of the everyday life experiences of Haitian caregivers looking after aging relatives at home in the greater Montreal area. Heath care providers reported an underutilization of health and home care services among this immigrant community. The aim of my research was to shed light on the potential reasons for this underutilization. Was underutilization of services related to the home care programs per se? Was this underutilization related to the lack of cultural competency of health care practitioners? My doctoral research helped me understand how gender, ethnicity, culture, and social class intersect to influence Haitian caregivers' experiences with the health care system. Using a postcolonial feminist approach to guide the research, I gathered data which revealed that issues of power translate into gendering, ethnocentrism, and racism. Furthermore, the results indicated that ways of caring for aging relatives at home were enmeshed in a complex nexus of social relations where power, race, gender, and social class come into play to permeate each level of the caring commitment. Ways of caring were structured by Haitian values, gendering of caring activities, immigration, social "Othering," and cultural misunderstanding of mainstream health care practitioners. Many factors explained this underutilization of services, including the need to address racial, gendered, and social discrimination affecting the delivery of health services. In addition, my doctoral research was an eye-opener about the realities experienced by racialized individuals and populations. This research helped me understood what Bhabha (1994) refers to as "the location of culture." Culture cannot be subsumed under ethnicity or race because culture is influenced by racialization and "Othering." Drawing on the results of my dissertation, I published methodological and empirical articles

that provided an in-depth understanding of racialization through the lens of postcolonial feminism.

After completing my doctoral studies at UBC, I was hired in the College of Nursing at the University of Saskatchewan. As a newly minted assistant professor, I was able to secure a New Investigator Research Award from the Saskatchewan Health Research Foundation (SHRF). This grant represented the building block to develop my program of funded research on immigrants and refugees in Saskatchewan. At the time of my hiring, immigration was tenuous, but I remained confident in establishing a program of research. In contrast to Ontario, British Columbia, Alberta, and Quebec, it is not easy to get funding to study immigrants and refugees in Saskatchewan. However, I was able to start and establish my program of research in transcultural nursing. This SHRF New Investigator study explored the health needs of non-Western immigrants and refugees in Saskatchewan. Peer-reviewed articles and numerous regional, national, and international conferences resulted from this research. I then obtained peer-reviewed funds from the University of Saskatchewan President's Social Sciences and Humanities Research Council (SSHRC) and the University of Regina's Centre de Recherches sur les francophonies en milieu minoritaire to explore accessibility of health services in French for francophone populations living in demographic minority contexts. This line of investigation enabled interdisciplinary collaborations with Dr. Anne Leis, from the College

of Medicine at the University of Saskatchewan, as well as with other researchers, such as Dr. Margareth Zanchetta, from the Daphne Cockwell School of Nursing at Ryerson University; Dr. Christine Maheu, from Ingram School of Nursing at McGill University; and Dr. Margot Kaszap, from the Faculty of Education at Université Laval, to name a few. I am pursuing this line of research to explore the health needs of French-speaking African immigrants in Saskatchewan and Alberta with colleagues from the Faculty of Nursing at the University of Alberta.

While the delivery of culturally competent and safe care remains a central concept of my program of research, I have also examined the provision of end-of-life care to older non-Western immigrants and received a Catalyst Grant from the Canadian Institutes of Health Research (CIHR) to study this phenomenon. More specifically, it is important to know why some older non-Western immigrants seem to underutilize palliative care services in Saskatchewan. This study is captivating because the results indicate the pivotal role of culture in shaping ideas about end of life and how the word *end of life* may have different cultural meanings. Results underline that a change of vocabulary may be necessary to reach immigrants and refugees at the end of life.

With funding from the CIHR and SHRF, I am completing a study on internationally educated nurses (IENs) and their Canadian counterparts in Saskatchewan. This research stems from my interest in culture and seeks to reach a better understanding of how culture influences IENs' experiences of social and professional integration within nursing workplaces. My team is composed of nurse colleagues from the College of Nursing. This study on IENs shows that qualitative nursing research is doable in spite of the intense competition for Tri-Agency funds. This study is near completion. Our team expects that the results will shed light on IENs' experiences and help practising nurses and nurse administrators in managing a culturally diverse nursing workforce. As a co-principal investigator on an SSHRC grant with Dr. Linda Ferguson (PI),

we are exploring issues of social integration among immigrant and Indigenous students. We will be collecting data soon. In this era of globalization, migration is not about to cease, and nurses must be equipped to provide quality care to diverse clientele while being aware of issues of vulnerability, colonization, and racialization.

My program underlines the importance of research in nursing. As nurses, it is our responsibility to advance the scientific and social mandates of nursing. This book represents a precious resource that demonstrates the importance of applying evidence

in everyday nursing practice, whether qualitative or quantitative, while being cognizant of the limitations of strict empiricism in guiding nursing and health care. It is important to listen to the voices of patients, families, and communities for evidence to bring about changes and improve the quality of health and nursing care delivery. ■

REFERENCES

Bhabha, H. K. (1994). *The location of culture*. London: Routledge.

Leininger, M. M. (1991). *Culture care diversity & universality: A theory of nursing*. New York: National League for Nursing Press.

CHAPTER 1

The Role of Research in Nursing

Cherylyn Cameron

LEARNING OUTCOMES

After reading this chapter, you will be able to do the following:

- State the significance of research to the practice of nursing.
- Identify the role of the consumer of nursing research.
- Discuss the differences in trends in nursing research in Canada.
- Describe how research, education, and practice are related to each other.
- Evaluate the nurse's role in the research process as it relates to the nurse's level of education.
- Identify future trends in nursing research.
- Formulate the priorities for nursing research in the twenty-first century.

KEY TERMS

consumer	evidence-informed	phenomena
data	practice	research
evidence-based practice	generalizability	

STUDY RESOURCES

ⓔ Go to Evolve at http://evolve.elsevier.com/Canada/LoBiondo/Research for the Audio Glossary and Appendix Tables that provide supplemental information for Appendix E.

WE INVITE YOU TO JOIN US on an exciting nursing research adventure that begins as you read the first page of this chapter. The adventure is one of discovery! You will discover that the nursing research literature sparkles with pride in, dedication to, and excitement about this dimension of professional nursing practice. As you progress through your educational program you will be taught how to ensure quality and safety in practice through acquiring knowledge of the various sciences and health care principles. Another component critical for clinical knowledge is research knowledge as it applies to practising from an evidence-informed approach.

Whether you are a student or a practising nurse whose goal is to use research as the foundation of your professional practice, you will discover that nursing research and evidence-informed practice position the nursing profession at the cutting edge of change and improvement in patients' outcomes. You will also discover that nursing research is integral to achieving the goal of providing quality outcomes in partnership with patients, their families and significant others, and the communities in which they live. Finally, you will discover the "who, what, where, when, why, and how" of nursing research and develop a foundation of knowledge, evidence-informed practice, and competencies that will equip you for twenty-first century nursing practice.

Your nursing research adventure will be filled with new and challenging learning experiences that develop your evidence-informed practice skills. Your critical thinking, critical reading, and clinical decision-making skills will expand as you develop clinical questions, search the research literature, evaluate the research evidence found in the literature, and make clinical decisions about applying the best available evidence to your practice. For example, you will be encouraged to ask important clinical questions, such as the following:

- What makes an intervention effective with one group of patients who have a diagnosis of heart failure but not with another?
- What is the effect of using mobile applications to assist children in self-managing their asthma?
- What is the experience of men who undergo prostate surgery and therapy?
- What is the quality of studies on therapeutic touch?
- What nursing-delivered smoking cessation interventions are most effective?

This book will help you begin your adventure into evidence-informed nursing practice by giving you the tools to use research as a foundation for evidence-informed practice.

SIGNIFICANCE OF RESEARCH AND EVIDENCE-INFORMED PRACTICE IN THE FIELD OF NURSING

The health care environment is changing at an increasingly rapid pace. The challenges associated with these changes and with nursing's rapid pace of growth can best be met by integrating evidence-informed knowledge into nursing practice. Carper (1978) described four fundamental patterns of knowledge in nursing: (1) empirical knowledge ("empirics"), the science of nursing; (2) aesthetics, the art of nursing; (3) the component of personal knowing; and (4) ethics, the component of moral knowledge of nursing. Empirical knowledge, which is based on research findings, represents "one source of knowledge within a larger body of knowledge" (Tarlier, 2005, p. 126). Nursing research provides specialized scientific knowledge that empowers nurses to anticipate and meet these constantly shifting challenges and maintain the profession's societal relevance.

In learning about nursing research, it is important to differentiate between the terms *research, evidence-based practice,* and *evidence-informed practice.* **Research** is the systematic, rigorous, logical investigation with the aim of answering questions about nursing phenomena. **Phenomena** can be defined as occurrences, circumstances, or facts that are perceptible by the senses. Although the origin of the term *phenomena* refers to events that are observable and/or measurable, nurses are also interested in experiences that are not easily observed, such as the experiences of pain, loss, or anxiety.

Some of the first documentation discussing the importance of evidence-informed practice is from Florence Nightingale, who, in the 1850s, noted there was a connection between poor sanitary conditions and death rates among wounded soldiers (Nightingale, 1863). In the past 20 years, many health care disciplines have adopted the tenets of evidence-informed practice to provide the best health care possible for their patients. The roots of modern evidence-informed practice stem from Dr. Archie Cochrane's investigation of the efficacy of health care, particularly in the work of the medical profession. His work resulted in the establishment of the Cochrane Collaboration, which provides systematic reviews of health care interventions. In 1996, Sackett, Rosenberg, Gray, and colleagues defined "evidence-based medicines" as the "conscientious, explicit, and judicious use of current best evidence in making decisions about the care of individual patients" (p. 312). Since then, most health professions have adopted the tenets of **evidence-based practice.**

Much of the evidence used as a basis for practice is from research that has been completed, written about in papers, and then published. Published research studies are assessed so that decisions about application to clinical practice can be made, which results in practice that is evidence based. According to the Canadian Nurses Association (CNA), "Evidence-based nursing refers to the incorporation of evidence from research, clinical expertise, client preferences and other available resources to make decisions about clients" (CNA, 2002). Through research utilization efforts, knowledge obtained from research is transformed into clinical practice, which results in nursing practice that is evidence based.

Evidence-informed practice extends beyond the early definitions of evidence-based practice just described. Building on the foundation of evidence-based practice, evidence-informed practice also involves acknowledging and considering the myriad factors that constitute local ways of knowing, Indigenous knowledge, cultural and religious norms, and clinical judgement. Ways of knowing are ways in which we acquire knowledge about the world around us and figure out our relationship with it. Researchers must consider, for example, how Indigenous peoples' ways of knowing and being are based on relationships between mind, body, emotion, and spirit of community members and the natural world. Language and metaphors reflect how Indigenous peoples interpret, structure, and organize their world. Elders share their wisdom and experiences through storytelling to convey how to be in harmony with the world (University of Calgary, n.d.) This approach to the world is critical for researchers to understand, and when using specific research methodologies they must honour Indigenous ways of knowing.

With evidence-informed practice, the methods for gathering evidence (use of published research studies) are the same as the processes used for evidence-based practice; however, the evidence also incorporates expert opinion, clinical expertise, patient preference, and other resources (CNA, 2010b). It is important to remember that evidence-informed practice focuses on a more inclusive and interactive process:

> Evidence-informed decision-making is a continuous interactive process involving the explicit, conscientious and judicious consideration of the best available evidence to provide care. It is essential to optimize outcomes for individual clients, promote healthy communities and populations, improve clinical practice, achieve cost-effective nursing care and ensure accountability and transparency in decision making within the health-care system. (CNA, 2010b, p. 1)

For example, to understand the importance of evidence-informed practice, consider the work of Dr. Judith Ritchie, who won the Canadian Health Services Research Foundation's 2010 Excellence through Evidence Award for her work on the successful implementation of best practice guidelines to reduce falls, manage pain, and protect skin integrity among patients. It has been estimated that as a result of implementation of these best practices, the incidence of pressure ulcers was reduced from 21% to 10.6% in 5 years. Not only do these practices result in better outcomes for patients, but the potential cost savings are estimated at $2.9 million for every 1,000 people (CNA, 2008).

When you first read about the research and the evidence-informed practice processes, you will notice that both processes may seem similar. Each begins with a question. The difference is that in a research study, the question is tested with a design appropriate for the question and with specific methods (sample, instruments, procedures, and data analysis). In the evidence-informed practice process, a question is used to search the literature for studies already completed that you will critically appraise in order to answer your clinical question.

It has been proposed that all nurses share a commitment to the advancement of nursing science by conducting research and using research evidence in practice. Scientific investigation promotes accountability, which is one of the hallmarks of the nursing profession and is a fundamental competency for all nurses (CNA, 2010a). What does this mean for you? There is a consensus that effective use of research calls for the skills of critical appraisal; that is, you must be a knowledgeable consumer of research, whereby you can appraise research evidence and use existing standards to determine the merit and readiness of research for use in clinical practice: "Nurses support, use and engage in research and other activities that promote safe, competent, compassionate and ethical care, and they use guidelines for ethical research that are in keeping with nursing values" (CNA, 2017, p. 15). Therefore, to use research (evidence-informed practice), you may not necessarily be able to conduct research, but you can understand and appraise the steps of the research process in order to read the research literature critically and use it to inform your clinical decisions. Even as students you can participate by completing surveys, attending research conferences, and asking questions.

There are two types of research: quantitative and qualitative. Increasingly, many researchers use mixed methods—in other words, they utilize both types of research in one project. You will be introduced to these types of research in more depth in Chapter 2. The methods used by nurse researchers are the same methods used in other disciplines; the difference is that nurses study questions relevant to nursing practice. Nurse researchers also conduct research collaboratively with researchers from other disciplines. Through the conducting of research, they produce knowledge that is reliable and useful for clinical practice. The methods and findings of studies provide evidence that is evaluated, and their applicability to practice is used to inform clinical decisions.

Throughout this text, the steps of the research and evidence-informed practice processes are described. The steps are systematic and orderly and relate to the development of evidence-informed practice. Understanding the step-by-step process that researchers use will help you develop the assessment skills necessary to judge the soundness of research studies. Chapter 20 will describe how you can implement evidence into practice to improve patient outcomes.

This chapter provides an overview of the role that research plays in practice and education, the roles of nurses in research activities, a historical perspective, and future directions in nursing research.

RESEARCH: THE ELEMENT THAT LINKS THEORY, EDUCATION, AND PRACTICE

Research links theory, education, and practice. Theoretical formulations supported by research findings may become the foundations of theory-informed practice in nursing. Your educational setting, whether a nursing program or the health care organization where you are employed, provides an environment in which you, as a student or an employee, can learn about the research process. In the setting of a nursing program or a health care organization, you can also explore different theories and begin to evaluate them in light of research findings. See the Practical Application box for an example of applying theory to nursing practice.

> ### Practical Application
>
> Consider the research program that focused on building knowledge about improving the health and health care of women who experience intimate partner violence. This program continued for more than a decade and focused on the experiences of women who left abusive partners, the health of the women after leaving the relationships, and the degree of health care improvement for women after they left their abusive partners (Ford-Gilboe, Wuest, Varcoe, et al., 2006). The knowledge gained from this body of interrelated research led to the development of comprehensive interventions to support the health and quality of life of women who leave abusive partners. The findings of that 2006 study have had enormous implications both for nurses and for other health care professionals, who make up the interdisciplinary health care team that works with women who experience intimate partner violence. Meaningful intervention is crucial for these women because health problems persist after they leave their partners. Many of these women report continued abuse and harassment from their ex-partners and experience financial hardships. Although health care workers have an interest in improving health care for these women, most health care workers do not have the knowledge required to address their patients' needs in a meaningful and effective way. As the researchers noted, "the vast majority of health practitioners [are] unprepared to recognize and respond to [intimate partner violence] in ways that are sensitive to the complexity of women's experiences and respectful of women's safety and choices" (Ford-Gilboe et al., 2006, p. 148). Many other studies have since built on this body of work, including a study by Duffy (2015), who examined how women achieve a sustainable livelihood after leaving their abusive partners.

The example in the Practical Application box is an attempt to answer a question that you may have asked before taking this course: "How will the theory and research content of this course relate to my nursing practice?" More specifically, can I recognize and respond to intimate partner violence after becoming familiar with the research? The **data** from each study discussed thus far have clearly demonstrated implications for society and practice. In an era of continuing concern about health care costs, empirically supported programs that are cost-effective without compromising quality are essential. Many researchers directly evaluate the cost effectiveness of treatment models; for example, Forchuk, Martin, Chan, and colleagues (2005) found that a transition discharge model of care for patients experiencing chronic mental illness helped the patients achieve discharge from a psychiatric hospital early, by an average of 116 days, which resulted in considerable cost savings. Several studies have demonstrated that the use of research-based interventions is more likely to result in better outcomes than traditional or ritual-based nursing care (McGinty & Anderson, 2008; Williams, 2004).

At this point in your study of nursing research, you may be wondering how education in nursing research links theory and practice. The answer is twofold. First, learning about nursing research will provide you with an appreciation and understanding of the research process so that you can more easily become a participant in research activities. Second, learning the value of nursing research helps you to become an intelligent consumer of research. A **consumer** of research actively uses and applies research. To be a knowledgeable consumer, you must have knowledge about the relevant subject matter, the ability to discriminate and to evaluate information logically, and the ability to apply the knowledge gained. You need not actually conduct research to be able to appreciate and use research findings in practice. Rather, to be an intelligent consumer, you must understand the research process and develop the critical evaluation skills needed to judge the merit and relevance of evidence before applying it to practice. The success of evidence-informed practice depends on your ability, as a consumer of research, to understand the research process and to evaluate the evidence. Staff nurses who understand research and its contribution to knowledge are ideally suited to identify phenomenon and issues to be studied by asking relevant research questions. For example, how can we make injections less painful for children?

ROLES OF THE NURSE IN THE RESEARCH PROCESS

Every nurse practising in the twenty-first century has a role to play in the research process. The Canadian Association of Schools of Nursing (CASN) (n.d.) states that it "strongly supports nursing research and the training of nurse researchers across Canada [and] works to encourage and improve the quality of nursing research, as well as to promote research findings and support Canada's current and upcoming nursing research leaders." More specifically, CASN's objectives include the education of nurse scholars/researchers; securing of sufficient funding for nursing scholarship/research; enhancement of scholarship/research cooperation; dissemination of scholarship/research; and cooperation with other nursing and non-nursing organizations, at the provincial, national, and international level.

At a provincial level, each province in Canada has its own standards for entry into nursing practice, and many of these standards have specific related research competencies. For example, the College of Nurses of Ontario (2014, p. 7) outlined the following competencies in nursing that incorporate research:

- Proactively seeks new information, knowledge and best practices for use in the provision of nursing care. (Competency 33)
- Contributes to a culture that supports involvement in nursing or health research through collaboration with others in conducting, participating in and implementing research findings into practice. (Competency 34)
- Uses critical inquiry to support professional judgment and evidence-informed decision-making to develop health care plans. (Competency 45)

Nurses must also be intelligent consumers of research; that is, they must understand all steps of the research process and their interrelationships. The nurse interprets, evaluates, and determines the credibility of research findings. The nurse discriminates between interesting findings for which further investigation is required and those that are sufficiently supported by evidence before applying findings to practice. The nurse should then use these competencies to advance nursing or interdisciplinary evidence-informed practice projects (e.g., developing clinical standards, tracking quality improvement data, or coordinating implementation of a pilot project to test the efficacy of a new wound care protocol) of the workplace committees to which he or she belongs.

Nurses are also responsible for generating clinical questions to identify nursing issues that necessitate investigation and for participating in the implementation of scientific studies. Clinicians often generate research ideas or questions from hunches, gut-level feelings, intuition, or observations of patients or nursing care. These ideas often become the seeds of research investigations.

For example, a group of family practice nurses at Toronto's Women's College Hospital were concerned that their methods to reduce pain during immunizations in children were not effective. With a small research fund, a family practice nurse approached a nurse researcher and proposed a research study focusing on whether applying pressure to the site before injection would reduce the pain infants experience. The family practice nurses all agreed to participate in the research project. To prepare for the study, they evaluated their current injection practices against the most recent research. Many of the nurses were aspirating before injection, to check that they had not hit a blood vessel. The literature review revealed that there was no scientific basis to aspiration and, in fact, the practice caused more pain. The nurses also considered other practices, such as how to position a baby for immunization and the use of sugar water. Over a period of 18 months, 120 babies were recruited into the study, in which tactile stimulation was used as a distraction. Although the study did not demonstrate any difference in the amount of pain the infants experienced, other benefits, such as revisiting evidence-informed practices, a renewed commitment to reducing pain, and pride in the project, were reported. The team continues to review the research in their commitment to trying new practices. "We learned that by being on the front line of inquiry, we can identify and quickly implement practice changes that improve patient care. What's more, we find new satisfaction in our nursing practice" (Probst, 2014, p. 17).

Nurses may participate in research projects as members of interdisciplinary or intradisciplinary research teams in one or more phases of a project. For example, a staff nurse may work on a clinical research unit in which a particular type of nursing care is part of an established research protocol (e.g., for pain management, prevention of falls, or treatment of urinary incontinence). In situations such as these, the nurse administers care according to the format described in the protocol. The nurse may also be involved in collecting and recording data relevant to the administration of, and the patient's response to, nursing care.

As important as the generation of research is the sharing of research findings with colleagues. Examples of such sharing include developing an article or presentation for a research or clinical conference on the findings of a study and sharing the findings of a research report that was critiqued, found to have merit, and believed to have the potential for application to practice. In a more formal way, it may involve joining a health care agency's research committee or its quality assurance or quality improvement committee, in which research articles, integrative reviews of the literature, and clinical practice guidelines are evaluated for evidence-informed clinical decision making.

Nurses who have graduate degrees must also be sophisticated consumers of research and are specially prepared to conduct research as co-investigators or primary investigators. At the master's level, nurses are prepared to be active members of research teams. Nurses with master's-level training can assume the role of clinical expert, collaborating with an experienced researcher in proposal development, data collection, data analysis, and interpretation. Nurses with master's degrees enhance the quality and relevance of nursing research by providing not only clinical expertise but also evidence-informed knowledge about the way clinical services are delivered. Nurses with master's-level training also facilitate the investigation of clinical problems by enabling a climate that is open to nursing research and by engaging in evidence-informed practice projects. At the master's level, nurses conduct research investigations to monitor the quality of nursing in clinical settings and to help others apply scientific knowledge to nursing practice. A clinical nurse specialist prepared with a master's or doctoral degree in nursing who has clinical expertise in a specific practice area can be the primary researcher or act as a collaborator to "identify, conduct and support research that enhances or benefits nursing practice" ("The Pillars," 2014, p. 35). To achieve the greatest expertise in appraising, designing, and conducting research, nurses must complete PhDs. Nurses with doctoral degrees develop theoretical explanations for phenomena relevant to nursing, develop methods of scientific inquiry, and use a variety of methods to modify or extend existing knowledge so that it is relevant to nursing (or to other areas of health care). In addition to their role as researchers, nurses with doctoral-level training act as role models and mentors to guide, stimulate, and encourage other nurses who are developing their research skills. Nurses with doctoral degrees also collaborate and consult with social, educational, and health care institutions or governmental agencies in their respective research endeavours. These nurses then disseminate their research findings to the scientific community, clinicians, and—as appropriate—the general public through scientific journal articles and presentations for nursing research conferences.

Another essential responsibility of nurses, regardless of the level of education they achieve, is to pay special regard to the ethical principles of research, especially the protection of human participants. For example, nurses caring for patients who are participating in research on antinausea chemotherapy must ensure that patients have signed the informed consent form and that all their questions are answered by the research team before they begin participation. Furthermore, if patients have an adverse reaction to the medication, nurses must not administer more doses until they have notified an appropriate member of the research team. Not all nurses must or should conduct research, but all nurses must play some part in the research process. Nurses at all educational levels—whether they are consumers, researchers, or both—need to view the research process as integral to the growing professionalism in nursing.

Although historically nursing research has been conducted by academic researchers associated with universities, increasingly, Canadian hospitals are building research capacity to improve safety and high-quality patient care. Consider the program at St. Michael's Hospital in Toronto, Ontario, to "cultivate a culture of discovery" by building the capacity of professional nurses to participate in research. Seven strategies were implemented, including matching research mentors with 22 nurses to develop, implement, and evaluate a research project to advance safer patient care (Jeffs, Smith, Beswick, et al., 2013).

As a professional, you must take time to read research studies and evaluate them, using the standards congruent with scientific research. Also, you will need to use the critiquing process in order to identify the strengths and weaknesses of each study. Bearing in mind that each study has its limitations, you should consider whether sound and relevant evidence from one particular study can be used in other settings as well. Chapter 20 will expand on how to bring research into your nursing practice.

HISTORICAL PERSPECTIVE*

The groundwork for the research that exists today was laid in the late nineteenth century and throughout the twentieth century. Since the 1970s, nursing research has undergone many changes and developments. Box 1.1 shows the major milestones in the development of nursing research.

In the mid-nineteenth century, nursing as a formal discipline began to take root with the ideas and practices of Florence Nightingale. Her concepts have contributed to, and are congruent with, the current priorities of nursing research. Promotion of health, prevention of disease, and care of the sick were central ideas of her practice and publications. Nightingale believed that systematic collection and exploration of data were necessary for nursing. Her collection and analysis of data on the health status of British soldiers during the Crimean War led to a variety of reforms in health care. Nightingale (1863) also noted the need for measuring the outcomes of nursing and medical care and had expertise in statistics and epidemiology. Other than Nightingale's work, little research was conducted during the early years of development of the field of nursing. Schools of nursing had just begun to be established and were unequal in their ability to educate, whereas nursing leadership had just started to develop.

In the twentieth century, research focused mainly on nursing education, but some patient- and technique-oriented research was also evident (see Box 1.1). Changes in the educational system for nurses were crucial for the development of nursing research. A comprehensive study of nursing and nursing education was carried out by Dr. George Weir, sponsored jointly by the CNA and the Canadian Medical Association. The so-called Weir report (Weir, 1932) documented serious problems in

---

*This section (i.e., from pp. 12–15) is adapted with permission from Potter, P., Perry, A. G., Ross-Kerr, J., et al. (Eds.). (2014). *Canadian fundamentals of nursing* (5th ed., pp. 80–82). Toronto: Elsevier Canada.

BOX 1.1

HISTORICAL MILESTONES IN THE DEVELOPMENT OF NURSING RESEARCH

1858 and 1863	Florence Nightingale publishes *Notes on Matters Affecting the Health, Efficiency and Hospital Administration of the British Army* and *Notes on Hospitals.*
1932	The Weir report, sponsored by the Canadian Nurses Association and the Canadian Medical Association, calls for better nursing education and service.
1952	The American Nurses Association first publishes *Nursing Research.*
1959	The first Canadian nursing master's degree program is launched at the University of Western Ontario.
1964–1965	The first nursing research project is funded by a Canadian federal granting agency. *International Journal of Nursing Studies* and *International Nursing Index* are launched.
1969–1970	*Nursing Papers*, the forerunner of the *Canadian Journal of Nursing Research*, is published at McGill University.
1971	McGill University launches the Centre for Nursing Research, and the first national Canadian conference on nursing research is held; both are financed by the Department of National Health and Welfare.
1978	Heads of university nursing schools and deans of graduate studies attend the Kellogg National Seminar on Doctoral Education in Nursing.
1982	The Alberta Foundation for Nursing Research, the first funding agency for nursing research, is established. The Working Group on Nursing Research is established by the Medical Research Council of Canada (MRC).
1985	The report of the Working Group on Nursing Research is released by the MRC.
1988	The MRC and the National Health Research and Development Program establish a joint initiative to structure nursing research grants.
1990	Francine Ducharme is the first nurse to graduate with a PhD in nursing from a Canadian university, through a special case program at McGill University.
1991	The first fully funded Canadian nursing PhD programs are launched, first at the University of Alberta, then at the University of British Columbia, McGill University, and the University of Toronto.
1994	McMaster University launches its nursing PhD; MRC's mandate includes health research.
1999	The Nursing Research Fund is launched with a $25 million grant over 10 years; the Canadian Health Services Research Foundation (CHSRF) administers the funds. The PhD nursing program is launched at the University of Calgary.
2000	Five CHSRF/Canadian Institutes of Health Research (CIHR) Chair Awards are granted to nursing.
2004	A forum on doctoral education is held in Toronto, under the auspices of the Canadian Association of Schools of Nursing, to develop a national position paper on the PhD in nursing for Canada.
2007	Nursing Research in Canada: A status report, is published.
2008	Dr. Joy Johnson, the first nurse researcher, is appointed scientific director of the CIHR Institute of Gender and Health.
2003–2013	PhD programs in nursing are initiated at Dalhousie University, Queen's University, Université Laval, Université de Montréal, Université de Sherbrooke, University of Victoria, University of Western Ontario, University of Ontario, University of Saskatchewan, and Memorial University.

Adapted from Potter, P., Perry, A. G., Ross-Kerr, J., et al. (Eds.). (2014). *Canadian fundamentals of nursing* (5th ed., p. 72). Toronto: Elsevier Canada.

nursing education and drew attention to the need for changes to improve standards in education and practice. The Weir report's recommendation that authority and responsibility for schools of nursing be vested within provincial systems of education was revolutionary at the time, and more than half a century passed before it was fully implemented across the country.

The establishment of university nursing courses in 1918, followed by master's degree programs in the 1950s and 1960s and by doctoral programs in the 1990s and 2000s, was key to the development of nursing research.

The first nursing research journal, *Nursing Research,* was established in the United States in 1952. The first nursing research journal published in Canada, *Nursing Papers* (later called the *Canadian Journal of Nursing Research*), was established at McGill University in 1969. Other journals were later established; today, nurses publish their research, both within nursing and in interdisciplinary fields, in dozens of journals.

In 1971, McGill University established the Centre for Nursing Research. In the same year, the first National Conference on Nursing Research in Canada was held in Ottawa. These conferences were held annually or biennially for several years. Papers of the early conferences were published as monographs. The number of nursing research conferences increased and began to be sponsored by professional, research, and academic organizations. In addition, nurses began to participate in the research conferences of interdisciplinary groups, such as the Canadian Association on Gerontology.

Since the 1970s and 1980s, the two major factors in the development of nursing research have been the establishment of research training through doctoral programs and the establishment of funding to support nursing research. Throughout the 1970s and 1980s, university faculties and schools of nursing built their research resources so that they could mount doctoral programs. The first provincially approved doctoral nursing program was established at the University of Alberta Faculty of Nursing in 1991. The University of British Columbia School of Nursing was established later that year, and programs at McGill University and the University of Toronto followed in 1993. With the most recent program at Memorial University, established in 2013, the number of PhD nursing programs in Canada is now 16.

Growing awareness of the importance of nursing research, along with an increased number of doctorally prepared nurses, gradually led to the availability of research funds. The year 1964 marked the first time that a federal granting agency funded nursing research in Canada (Good, 1969). In 1999, in response to intensive lobbying by the CNA, the federal government established the Nursing Research Fund, budgeting $25 million for nursing research (i.e., $2.5 million over each of the following 10 years), with the Canadian Health Services Research Foundation (CHSRF) administering the funds. Unfortunately, the Nursing Research Fund expired in 2009. Although funding is still available from the federal government, the bulk of current funding for research-focused positions in universities and health organizations is provided by private organizations and individuals.

Increasingly, nursing research has focused on evidence-informed practice in response to demands to justify care practices and systems by improving patient outcomes and controlling costs. The scope of nursing research has also broadened to include historical and philosophical inquiry. The establishment of the Centre for Philosophical Nursing Research at the University of Alberta exemplifies this new direction. Training centres have also been funded by the CHSRF to increase training for graduate nursing students and to increase research capacity in nursing and related disciplines. For example, the Ontario Training Centre in Health Services and Policy Research comprises six Ontario universities for the purpose of enhancing health services and policy research. The centre's head-quarters are located at McMaster University and the program involves collaboration with the University of Toronto, York University, University of Ottawa, Laurentian University, and Lakehead University (website: http://www.fhs.mcmaster.ca/otc-hsr/).

Since the 1990s, some of the original nursing research pathfinders and many new ones have conducted research on a wide range of clinical topics, describing phenomena and testing interventions. The existence of the many nursing journals shows the growth in the variety, quality, and depth of research available for potential use in practice. In a report funded by the CHSRF, an analysis of the Canadian Institutes of Health Research (CIHR) database revealed a wide diversity of nursing research topics in Canada: 67% of studies were conducted in the areas of health issues, health service organizations, and health promotion. Not surprisingly, the research on health issues was dominant; the majority of studies focused on (1) chronic illness, (2) reproductive health, (3) pain, and (4) end-of-life and palliative care. While nurses have made significant research contributions to health care, they are far from finished with their quest for knowledge and research. The nursing leaders of the twentieth century have—by example—paved the way for those who are now emerging.

Nursing research capacity has expanded greatly in Canada, as evidenced by greater numbers of doctoral programs and graduates, increased funding, and the development of research teams and centres. However, the profession still faces many challenges. Despite the increased number of doctoral programs and graduate students, research-prepared faculty to supervise the research of graduate students are in short supply. In addition, the databases that researchers depend on for funding information are not coordinated, and many do not include classifications specifically for nursing (Jeans & Associates, 2008).

FUTURE DIRECTIONS

In the twenty-first century, the continuing expansion of nursing research provides numerous opportunities for nurses to study important research questions, promote health care, and ameliorate the adverse effects of illness and the consequences of treatment while also optimizing the health outcomes of patients and their families (Jennings & McClure, 2004). Villeneuve and MacDonald (2006), in *Toward 2020: Visions for Nursing* (p. 99), included the following prediction:

> . . . nurse researchers in 2020 [will] conduct studies that place less emphasis on nurses and nursing processes than was the case 20 years [earlier], focusing instead on health, the needs of clients and communities, and providing sound evidence to guide policy and practice. Research conducted by nurses [will be] interdisciplinary. Research to determine more cost-effective ways to provide safe, high-quality health and illness services [will be] led by nurse researchers.

Major shifts in the delivery of health care include the following:
- An emphasis on community-based care
- An emphasis on reducing disparities in health care
- A focus on health promotion and risk reduction
- An increase in severity of illness in inpatient settings
- An increased incidence of persons with co-morbid chronic conditions
- An expanding population of older adults
- An emphasis on provider accountability through a focus on quality and cost outcomes
- An increased emphasis on interdisciplinary collaborative practice
- The use of technology to serve human needs
- A focus on the needs of Indigenous peoples

In accordance with these trends, nurse researchers are beginning to focus on the development of quantitative and qualitative research programs and clinically based outcome studies. Strategies that enhance nurses' focus on outcomes management through evidence-informed quality improvement activities and the use of research findings for effective clinical decision making also are being refined and identified as priorities (see Chapter 20). Evidence-informed practice guidelines, standards, protocols, and critical pathways are becoming benchmarks for cost-effective, high-quality clinical practice. For example, the Registered Nurses' Association of Ontario (RNAO) (2016) has developed 50 best practice guidelines to support Ontario nurses in their efforts to provide the best possible patient care.

Nurse researchers and nurse leaders will become increasingly visible at the national level, functioning in policymaking roles, representing the field of nursing on expert panels, and lobbying for more funding dollars. In addition, the role of nurse scientists has become more firmly entrenched in research units and programs across Canada, increasingly in partnership with academic and health care organizations. For example, the RBC Professorship in Cardiac Nursing Research has been established at University Health Network and the Bloomberg School of Nursing at the University of Toronto. In this position the nurse scientist leads a research program focusing on cardiovascular health and provides mentorship to nurse researchers.

Promoting Depth In Nursing Research

Depth in nursing science becomes evident when research is replicated. Research programs that include a series of studies in a similar area, each of which builds on a prior investigation, promote depth in nursing science. Moreover, to maximize use of resources and to prevent duplication, researchers must develop intradisciplinary and interdisciplinary networks in similar areas of study. Researchers from a variety of health professions (e.g., medicine, nursing, and respiratory therapy) and other disciplines such as psychology, law, and business can come together to delineate common and unique aspects of patient care. Interdisciplinary health research may be seen as "a team of researchers who come together to research an important and challenging health issue" (Hall, Bainbridge, Buchan, et al., 2006, p. 764).

The work of Dr. Nancy Edwards, the director of the Community Health Research Unit, provides an excellent example of depth and interdisciplinary collaboration in nursing research. Working in partnership with Public Health and Long-Term Care–City of Ottawa, the University of Ottawa, and a large team of co-researchers, Dr. Edwards has enhanced the scientific and evidence-informed practice in public health. One of her areas of study is the incidence, causes, and prevention of falls among older adults. For example, in one study, investigators collected qualitative data on older adults' beliefs about falls and prevention behaviour; the key findings guided further study on the use of fall-prevention devices, such as grab bars in bathrooms (Community Health Research Unit, 2005). In another research study, Dr. Edwards and colleagues (2006) focused on the development and testing of tools to assess use of physical restraint. When Dr. Edwards became the scientific director of the Institute of Population and Public Health, Canadian Institutes of Health Research, her clinical and research interests focused on the fields of public and population health (http://cihr-irsc. gc.ca/e/12201.html). The health issues studied include preventing falls among older adults, maternal and child health care, heart health, tobacco cessation, and human immunodeficiency virus/ acquired immune deficiency syndrome (HIV/ AIDS). The research involves researchers from across Canada and internationally.

Dr. Edwards's work illustrates the value of building replication studies into research programs. Stone, Curran, and Bakken (2002) proposed that the adoption of research findings in practice, with their potential risks and benefits (including the cost of implementation), should be based on a series of replicated studies that provide a body of evidence, thereby increasing the degree to which the findings can be applied and generalized. When appropriate, a greater focus on **generalizability** is important if the evolving science is considered to be usable in health care settings and in health care policies. As such, future replication studies will yield more credible results and will play a crucial role in developing depth in nursing science (Fahs, Stewart, & Kalman, 2003).

Dr. Edwards's work also highlights why research training is likely to become an increasingly essential component of a research career plan. A larger cadre of nurse researchers who begin their research careers at a young age is important for the development of research programs like Dr. Edwards's. The goal is to increase the longevity of research careers, enhance the discipline's science development, promote mentoring opportunities, prepare the next generation of researchers, and provide leadership in health care for interdisciplinary health care debates.

An International Perspective

The continuing development of a national and international research environment is essential to the nursing profession's mission to "improve the health and well-being of all world citizens" (National Institute of Nursing Research, 2015, n.p.). The United Nations highlighted eight goals toward improving global health, known as the Millennium Development Goals, which act as a blueprint for the world community for 2000–2015. Many of the goals have important roles for nursing research, such as reducing child mortality. Moreover, nurses can educate and train health workers and contribute to finding solutions to common health problems (Grady, 2015). The CNA has been partnering with many international networks in more than 45 countries to strengthen the nursing profession's contribution to global health through study, research, and practice (CNA, 2012). Because of nursing's emphasis on the cultural aspects of care and the

influence of such factors on practice, international research is likely to increase. Access to multiple populations as a function of globalization allows the testing of nursing science from various perspectives. Interaction with colleagues from other countries provides a rich context for the generation and dissemination of research (Dickenson-Hazard, 2004; Ward, 2003).

International research projects are often focused on comparative research in which a phenomenon is studied in more than one country, usually by a single researcher conducting research in his or her home country and then travelling to the other international sites. Optimally, relationships are formed with researchers from the international sites, resulting in collaborative research projects. Despite the financial and logistical limitations to this method, the number of international collaborative research projects has increased. Nurse researchers participating in collaborative international research projects are well positioned to play a large role in improving health care globally (CNA, 2012; Chiang-Hanisko, Ratchneewan, Ludwick, et al., 2006; Grady, 2015).

International organizations committed to the goal of health care for all help create natural research partnerships. For example, the World Health Organization (WHO, n.d.) has established a series of collaboration centres in order to advance health care for the global community. One such centre works toward maximizing the contribution of nursing and midwifery and provides relevant research and clinical training to nurses worldwide.

Research Priorities

As the number of nurses with doctoral degrees has increased, and as nursing chairs have been created and funding expanded, a distinct set of Canadian nursing research priorities has emerged. Funding agencies often determine research priorities on the basis of their particular needs and interests. The Canadian Foundation for Healthcare Improvement (CFHI) supports new ways of spreading health care innovations throughout Canada by bringing together health care multidisciplinary professionals from across the country to solve persistent health care problems. Two projects of particular interest to nurses are reducing the use of antipsychotic medication in long-term care facilities and improving care for patients with chronic obstructive pulmonary disease (COPD) (CFHI, 2014).

The Canadian Institute for Health Research (CIHR) is one of the largest funders of health research, although the application process is highly competitive, with as few as 13% of applicants being successful in procuring funding (Semeniuk, 2016). Its priorities for 2014–2019 include the following:

- Enhanced patient experiences and outcomes through health innovation
- Health and wellness for Indigenous peoples
- A healthier future through preventive action
- Improved quality of life for persons living with chronic conditions

Reducing health disparities in underserviced communities and vulnerable populations is another major topic that will shape the focus of future nursing- and interdisciplinary-related research agendas, particularly among Indigenous peoples. For example, the health concerns of mothers and infants will continue to spur research that deals effectively with the maternal–neonatal mortality rate. Individuals of all ages who have sustained life-threatening illnesses will live with the help of new life-sustaining technology that will in turn create new demands for self-care and family support. Cancer, heart disease, arthritis, asthma, chronic pulmonary disease, diabetes, and Alzheimer's disease, prevalent during middle age and later life, will be responsible for expenditures of large proportions of the available health care resources. HIV/AIDS, a chronic illness that affects men, women, and children, will continue to have a significant effect on health care delivery.

Another vulnerable population, persons with mental health illness, will be served by a better understanding of mental disorders, which will emerge as a result of advancements in psychobiological knowledge and research initiatives. Mental health illnesses will continue to be a major public health issue; depression has been cited as the number one mental illness worldwide (WHO, 2001). Alcohol and drug abuse will continue to be responsible for significant health care expenses. Finally, as national initiatives are launched to improve end-of-life care, the shortage of nurses—as clinicians and investigators—will become a major problem worldwide (WHO, 2001).

In terms of the priority given to clinical research issues, the funding of investigations has increasingly emphasized populations of interest. For example, the historical exclusion of women as participants in clinical research is well documented; minority women in particular were even more likely to be excluded from research studies. As a result, research data on the health of minority women traditionally were extremely scarce. Nurse researchers such as Josephine Etowa in Canada are addressing this gap in research.

Along with national nursing research initiatives, specific nursing interest groups frequently establish their own research priorities specific to their specialty. Some associations provide funds to support research initiatives. The Canadian Association of Nephrology Nurses and Technologists (2016), for example, established a small research grant of $3,000 annually to support specific research activities in the area of nephrology nursing or technology.

International research priorities are influenced by social, political, and economic factors. Typically, international organizations such as the United Nations and the WHO prioritize health research that will affect the most marginalized of the world's population. As such, the goals identified by the United Nations Foundation (2016) focus on poverty, vulnerable populations (i.e., women and children), and specific health issues as follows:

- Preventing malaria deaths
- Eradicating polio
- Reducing measles mortality
- Mobile health for development
- Innovating health finance
- Improving health for every woman, every child

Other types of research investigations (e.g., those involving historical, feminist, or case study methods) embody the rich diversity of nursing research methods. The nursing profession must continue to value and promote creativity and diversity in research endeavours at all educational levels as a way of empowering nurses for the future. As opportunities are recognized and gaps in science are observed, nurses will conduct, critique, and use nursing research in ways that publicly demonstrate how nursing care makes a difference in patients' lives.

Nurse researchers will have an increasingly strong voice in shaping public policy relating to health care; Shaver (2004) has stated that disciplines such as nursing—because of its focus on treatment of chronic illness, health promotion, independence in health, and care of the acutely ill, all of which are heavily emphasized values for the future—will be central to the shaping of health care policy in the future. Research evidence that supports or refutes the merit of health care needs and programs focusing on these issues will be timely and relevant. Thus, nursing and its science base are strategically placed to shape health policy decisions (Fitzpatrick, 2004; Hinshaw & Grady, 2011). For example, O'Brien-Pallas and Hayes's (2008) research projects on health and human resource strategies have impacted related policy across Canada.

Communication of nursing research has also become increasingly important. Research findings continue to be disseminated in professional arenas (e.g., international, national, regional, and local electronic and print publications and conferences), as well as in consultations and staff development programs implemented on site through webinars and websites. Dissemination of research findings in the public sector has also gained importance.

Increasingly, nurse researchers are being asked to testify at governmental hearings and to serve on commissions and task forces related to health care. Nurses are quoted in the media when health care topics are addressed, and their visibility has expanded significantly. For example, Sue Johanson, RN, host of the *Sunday Night Sex Show,* brought more than 35 years of experience in sex education to the public discourse on sex. In addition to addressing all aspects of sex in a non-judgemental manner on her show, Ms. Johanson has written several books and wrote a weekly column on health for the *Toronto Star.* Although she retired in 2008, Ms. Johanson still lectures to a wide range of audiences. Dissemination of research through the public media provides excellent exposure of health-related information to thousands of potential viewers, listeners, and readers.

Nurses have a research heritage to be proud of. They also have a challenging and exciting future ahead of them. Both researchers and consumers of research need to engage in a united effort to gather and assess research findings that make a difference in the care that is provided and in the lives that are touched by their commitment to evidence-informed nursing practice.

CRITICAL THINKING CHALLENGES

- How can you access evidence-informed practice information when practising in the field?
- What assumption underlies the recommendation that the role of the nursing graduate in the research process be primarily that of a knowledgeable consumer?
- What effects will evidence-informed patient outcome studies have on the practice of nursing?

■ Discuss how research will contribute to the development of intradisciplinary and interdisciplinary networks.
■ How are research priorities established by organizations and professional bodies?

KEY POINTS

- Nursing research expands the unique body of scientific knowledge that forms the foundation of evidence-informed nursing practice. Research is the component that links education, theory, and practice.
- Nurses become knowledgeable consumers of research through educational processes and practical experience. As consumers of research, nurses must have a basic understanding of the research process and must demonstrate critical appraisal skills to evaluate the strengths and weaknesses of research before applying the research to clinical practice.
- Nursing research blossomed in the second half of the twentieth century: Graduate programs in nursing expanded, research journals began to be published, and funding for graduate education and nursing research increased dramatically.
- All nurses, whether they possess baccalaureate, master's, or doctoral degrees, have a responsibility to participate in the research process.
- The role of the baccalaureate graduate is to be a knowledgeable consumer of research. Nurses with master's and doctoral degrees are obliged to be researchers and sophisticated consumers of research studies.
- A collaborative research relationship within the nursing profession will extend and refine the scientific body of knowledge that provides the grounding for theory-informed practice.
- The future of nursing research will focus on the extension of scientific knowledge. Collaborative research relationships between education and practice will multiply. Programs of research studies and replication of studies will become increasingly valuable.

- Research studies will emphasize clinical issues, problems, and outcomes. Priority will be given to research studies that focus on health promotion, care for the health needs of vulnerable groups, and the development of cost-effective health care systems.
- Both consumers of research and nurse researchers will engage in a collaborative effort to further the growth of nursing research and accomplish the profession's research objectives.

FOR FURTHER STUDY

ⓔ Go to Evolve at http://evolve.elsevier.com/ Canada/LoBiondo/Research for the Audio Glossary and Appendix Tables that provide supplemental information for Appendix E.

REFERENCES

Canadian Association of Nephrology Nurses and Technologists. (2016). *Awards, bursaries and grants*. Retrieved from http://www.cannt.ca/en/resources/ cannt_awards_bursaries__grants/index.html.

Canadian Association of Schools of Nursing. (n.d.). *Standing Committee on Research and Scholarship*. Retrieved from http://www.casn.ca/standing-committee-research-scholarship/.

Canadian Foundation for Healthcare Improvement. (2014). *Spreading best practices across Canada*. Retrieved from http://www.cfhi-fcass.ca/sf-docs/ default-source/documents/2014-annual-report.pdf? sfvrsn=2.

Canadian Nurses Association. (2002). *Position statement: Evidence-based decision-making and nursing practice*. Retrieved from https://www.nurseone.ca/~/ media/nurseone/page-content/pdf-en/ps63_evidence_ based_decision_making_nursing_practice_e.pdf?la=en.

Canadian Nurses Association. (2008). *The health infrastructure advantage: Strengthening the health system and Canada's economy*. Retrieved from https://www. cna-aiic.ca/~/media/cna/page-content/pdf-fr/brief_ committee_finance_e.pdf?la=en.

Canadian Nurses Association. (2010a). *Canadian Registered Nurse Examination: Competencies*. Retrieved from http://www.cna-aiic.ca/CNA/nursing/rnexam/ competencies/default_e.aspx.

Canadian Nurses Association. (2010b). *Evidence-informed decision-making and nursing practice.* Retrieved from https://www.cna-aiic.ca/~/media/cna/page-content/pdf-en/ps113_evidence_informed_2010_e.pdf?la=en.

Canadian Nurses Association. (2012). *CNA global health partnerships retrospective.* Retrieved from https://nurseone.ca/~/media/cna/page-content/pdf-fr/global_health_partnership_program_2012_e.pdf?la=en.

Canadian Nurses Association. (2017). *Code of ethics for registered nurses.* Retrieved from https://www.cna-aiic.ca/html/en/Code-of-Ethics-2017-Edition/files/assets/basic-html/page-1.html.

Carper, B. A. (1978). Fundamental patterns of nursing. *Advanced Nursing Science, 1*(1), 13–24.

Chiang-Hanisko, L., Ratchneewan, R., Ludwick, R., et al. (2006). International collaborations in nursing research: Priorities, challenges and rewards. *Journal of Research in Nursing, 11*(4), 307–322.

College of Nurses of Ontario. (2014). *Competencies for entry-level registered nurse practice.* Toronto: Author. Retrieved from http://www.cno.org/globalassets/docs/reg/41037_entrytopracitic_final.pdf.

Community Health Research Unit. (2005). *Research projects funded in 2005.* Retrieved from http://aix1.uottawa.ca/~nedwards/chru/english/research2005.html.

Dickenson-Hazard, N. (2004). Global health issues and challenges. *Journal of Nursing Scholarship, 36*(1), 6–10.

Duffy, L. (2015). Achieving a sustainable livelihood after leaving intimate partner violence: Challenges and opportunities. *Journal of Family Violence, 30,* 403–417.

Edwards, N., Danseco, E., Heslin, K., et al. (2006). Development and testing of tools to assess physical restraint use. *Worldviews Evidence Based Nursing, 3*(2), 73–85.

Fahs, P. S., Stewart, L. L., & Kalman, M. (2003). A call for replication. *Journal of Nursing Scholarship, 35*(1), 67–72.

Fitzpatrick, J. J. (2004). Translating clinical research into research policy. *Applied Nursing Research, 17*(2), 71.

Forchuk, C., Martin, M. L., Chan, Y. L., et al. (2005). Therapeutic relationships: From psychiatric hospital to community. *Journal of Psychiatric and Mental Health Nursing, 12,* 556–564.

Ford-Gilboe, M., Wuest, J., Varcoe, C., et al. (2006). Developing an evidence-based health advocacy intervention for women who have left an abusive partner. *Canadian Journal of Nursing Research, 38,* 147–167.

Good, S. R. (1969). *Submission to the study of support of research in universities for the Science Secretariat of the Privy Council.* Ottawa: Canadian Nurses Association and Canadian Nurses Foundation.

Grady, P. (2015). Questions and answers. *Global Health Matters, 14*(1), 5.

Hall, J. G., Bainbridge, L., Buchan, A., et al. (2006). A meeting of the minds: Interdisciplinary research in the health sciences in Canada. *Canadian Medical Association Journal, 175*(7), 753–761.

Hinshaw, A. S., & Grady, P. A. (2011). *Shaping health policy through nursing research.* New York: Springer.

Jeans, M. E., & Associates. (2008). *Nursing research in Canada: A status report.* Retrieved from http://www.canr.ca/documents/NursingResCapFinalReport_ENG_Final.pdf.

Jeffs, L., Smith, O., Beswick, S., et al. (2013). Investing in nursing research in practice settings: A blueprint for building capacity. *Nursing Leadership, 26*(4), 44–59.

Jennings, B. M., & McClure, M. L. (2004). Strategies to advance health quality. *Nursing Outlook, 52,* 17–22.

McGinty, J., & Anderson, G. (2008). Predictors of physician compliance with American Heart Association guidelines for acute myocardial infarction. *Critical Care Nurse Quarterly, 31*(2), 161–172.

National Institute of Nursing Research. (2015). *Overview of global health research.* Retrieved from https://www.ninr.nih.gov/researchandfunding/globalhealth.

Nightingale, F. (1863). *Notes on hospitals.* London: Longman Group.

O'Brien-Pallas, L., & Hayes, L. (2008). Challenges in getting workforce research in nursing used for decision-making in policy and practice: A Canadian perspective. *Journal of Clinical Nursing, 17*(24), 3338–3346.

The pillars of CNS nursing practice. (2014). *Canadian Nurse, 110*(7), 32–35.

Potter, P., Perry, A. G., Ross-Kerr, J., et al. (Eds.). (2014). *Canadian fundamentals of nursing* (5th ed.). Toronto: Elsevier Canada.

Probst, J. (2014). The unexpected benefits of participating in research. *Canadian Nurse, 110*(6), 16–17.

Registered Nurses' Association of Ontario. (2016). *Best practice guidelines.* Retrieved from http://rnao.ca/bpg.

Sackett, D. L., Rosenberg, W., Gray, J. A., et al. (1996). Editorial: Evidence based medicine: What it is and what it isn't. *British Medical Journal, 312*(7023), 71.

Semeniuk, I. (2016, July 14). Pushback from scientists forces rethink of grant competition process. *The Globe and Mail.* Retrieved from http://www.theglobeandmail.com/news/national/pushback-from-scientists-forces-overhaul-of-funding-system/article30931215/.

Shaver, J. (2004). Improving the health of communities: The position. *Nursing Outlook, 52*, 116–117.

Stone, P. W., Curran, C. R., & Bakken, S. (2002). Economic evidence for evidence-based practice. *Journal of Nursing Scholarship, 34*(3), 277–282.

Tarlier, D. (2005). Mediating the meaning of evidence through epistemological diversity. *Nursing Inquiry, 12*, 126–134.

United Nations Foundation. (2016). *What we do: Globe and health*. Retrieved from http://www.unfoundation. org/what-we-do/issues/global-health/.

University of Calgary. (n.d.). *Indigenous ways of knowing and being*. Retrieved from http://www.ucalgary.ca/indigenous/research/knowing_being.

Villeneuve, M., & MacDonald, J. (2006). *Toward 2020: Visions for nursing*. Ottawa: Canadian Nurses Association.

Ward, L. S. (2003). Race as a cross-variable in research. *Nursing Outlook, 51*(3), 120–125.

Weir, G. M. (1932). *Survey of nursing education in Canada*. Toronto: Macmillan. [Note that this publication is often referred to as the Weir report or the Weir survey.]

Williams, D. O. (2004). Treatment delayed is treatment denied. *Circulation, 109*, 1806–1808.

World Health Organization. (n.d.). *Networks of WHO collaborating centres*. Retrieved from http://www. who.int/collaboratingcentres/networks/networksdetails/en/index1.html.

World Health Organization. (2001). *The World Health Report 2001—Mental health: New understanding, new hope*. Geneva, Switzerland: Author.

CHAPTER 2

Theoretical Framework

Cherylyn Cameron

LEARNING OUTCOMES

After reading this chapter, you will be able to do the following:

- Define key concepts in the philosophy of science.
- Identify and differentiate between theoretical/empirical, aesthetic, personal, sociopolitical, and ethical ways of knowing.
- Identify assumptions underlying the post-positivist, critical social, and interpretive/constructivist views of research.
- Compare inductive and deductive reasoning.
- Differentiate between conceptual and theoretical frameworks.
- Describe how a framework guides research.
- Differentiate between conceptual and operational definitions.
- Describe the relationships among theory, research, and practice.
- Discuss levels of abstraction related to frameworks guiding research.
- Describe the points of critical appraisal used to evaluate the appropriateness, cohesiveness, and consistency of a framework guiding research.

KEY TERMS

aim of inquiry
concept
conceptual definition
conceptual framework
constructivism
constructivist paradigm
context
critical social theory
critical social thought
deductive reasoning

epistemology
hypothesis
inductive reasoning
methodology
model
ontology
operational definition
paradigm
philosophical beliefs
positivism

post-positivism
qualitative research
quantitative research
text
theoretical framework
theory
values
variables
worldview

STUDY RESOURCES

ⓔ Go to Evolve at http://evolve.elsevier.com/Canada/LoBiondo/Research for the Audio Glossary and Appendix Tables that provide supplemental information for Appendix E.

THE NATURE OF KNOWLEDGE

ON A DAILY BASIS, NURSES DEVISE clinical questions that, if answered, improve upon the care they provide to individuals, families, and communities. A medical/surgical nurse may ask, "How do pediatric and adult patients experience surgical pain, and how, in turn, can we enhance pain management for both groups?" A mental health nurse may ask, "What is the relationship between the use of specific psychotropic medications and heart disease among schizophrenic patients?" A public health nurse might ask, "What factors contribute most significantly to the health of homeless youths living in a specific neighbourhood in Ontario, Canada?"

Each question requires that clinicians and nurse researchers engage in a knowledge development process (Figure 2.1). The process begins with the identification of *knowledge gaps:* the absence of theoretical or scientific knowledge relevant to the phenomenon of interest. *Knowledge generation* occurs next, with the conduct of

research that provides answers to well-thought-out research questions. This *knowledge* is then *distributed* through journal articles, textbooks, and public presentations to nurses. Next, the *knowledge* is *adopted,* as nurses alter their practice on the basis of published information or as health care organizations develop policies and protocols that are informed by newly generated knowledge. Finally, *knowledge is reviewed and revised* as new health issues arise, advances in clinical practice occur, or knowledge becomes outdated. In this chapter, we focus specifically on theoretical frameworks and how they guide and inform *knowledge generation.*

Figure 2.2 outlines the various ways by which nurses inform their practice. These include *theoretical/empirical, personal, experiential, ethical, aesthetic,* and *sociopolitical* ways of knowing (Chinn & Kramer, 2015; Zander, 2007). Theoretical/empirical knowledge is most commonly referred to as *scientific knowledge.* In comparison with all the other ways of knowing

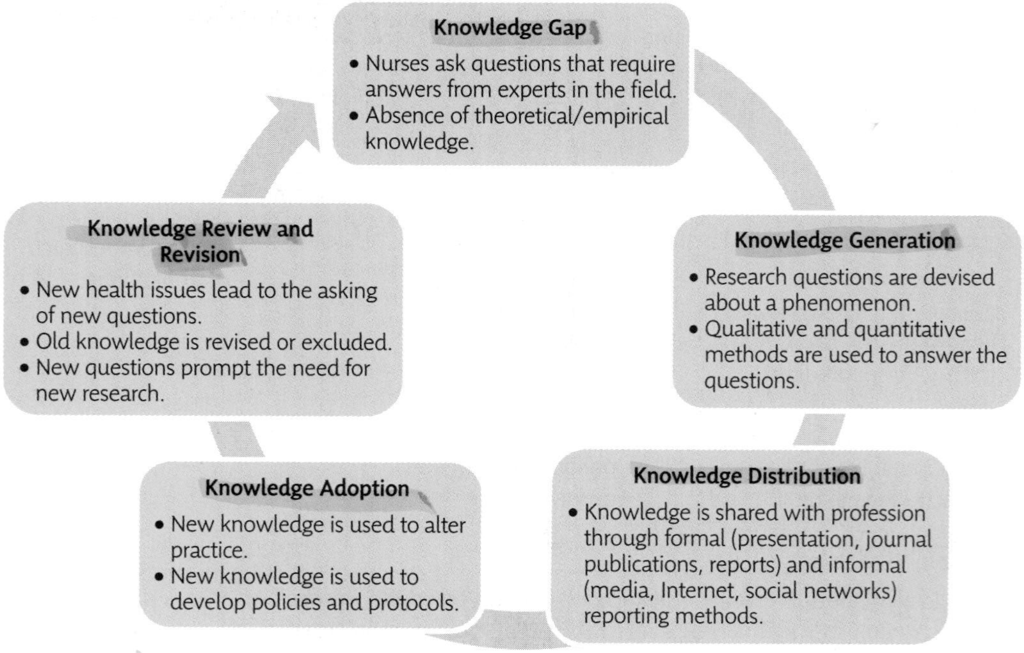

Knowledge Gap
- Nurses ask questions that require answers from experts in the field.
- Absence of theoretical/empirical knowledge.

Knowledge Generation
- Research questions are devised about a phenomenon.
- Qualitative and quantitative methods are used to answer the questions.

Knowledge Distribution
- Knowledge is shared with profession through formal (presentation, journal publications, reports) and informal (media, Internet, social networks) reporting methods.

Knowledge Adoption
- New knowledge is used to alter practice.
- New knowledge is used to develop policies and protocols.

Knowledge Review and Revision
- New health issues lead to the asking of new questions.
- Old knowledge is revised or excluded.
- New questions prompt the need for new research.

FIG. 2.1   Knowledge development process.

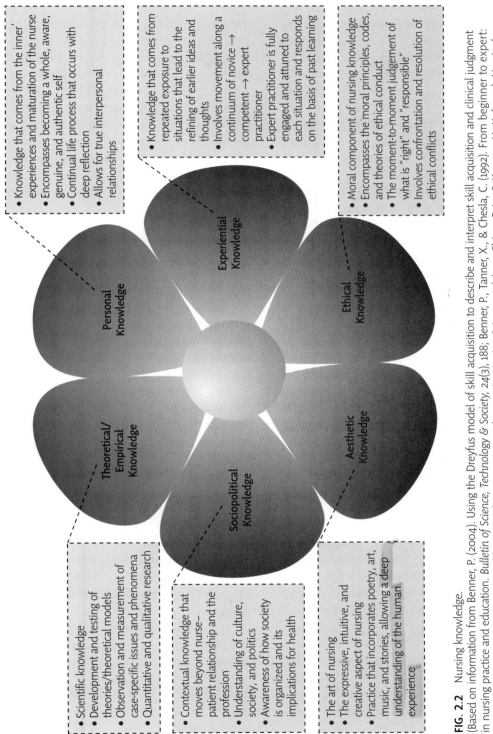

FIG. 2.2 Nursing knowledge.
(Based on information from Benner, P. (2004). Using the Dreyfus model of skill acquisition to describe and interpret skill acquisition and clinical judgment in nursing practice and education. *Bulletin of Science, Technology & Society, 24*(3), 188; Benner, P., Tanner, X., & Chesla, C. (1992). From beginner to expert: Gaining a differentiated clinical world in critical care nursing. *Advances in Nursing Science, 14*(3), 13; Chinn, P. L., & Kramer, M. K. (2010). Nursing's fundamental patterns of knowing. In P. Chinn & M. Kramer (Eds.), *Integrated knowledge development in nursing* (8th ed., pp. 1–17). St. Louis: Mosby; and Zander, P. E. (2007). Ways of knowing in nursing: The historical evolution of a concept. *Journal of Theory Construction and Testing, 11*(1), 7–11.)

The following text appears within the figure:

Personal Knowledge
- Knowledge that comes from the inner' experiences and maturation of the nurse
- Encompasses becoming a whole, aware, genuine, and authentic self
- Continual life process that occurs with deep reflection
- Allows for true interpersonal relationships

Experiential Knowledge
- Knowledge that comes from repeated exposure to situations that lead to the refining of earlier ideas and thoughts
- Involves movement along a continuum of novice → competent → expert practitioner
- Expert practitioner is fully engaged and attuned to each situation and responds on the basis of past learning

Ethical Knowledge
- Moral component of nursing knowledge
- Encompasses the moral principles, codes, and theories of ethical conduct
- The moment-to-moment judgement of what is "right" and "responsible"
- Involves confrontation and resolution of ethical conflicts

Theoretical/Empirical Knowledge
- Scientific knowledge
- Development and testing of theories/theoretical models
- Observation and measurement of case-specific issues and phenomena
- Quantitative and qualitative research

Sociopolitical Knowledge
- Contextual knowledge that moves beyond nurse–patient relationship and the profession
- Understanding of culture, society, and politics
- Awareness of how society is organized and its implications for health

Aesthetic Knowledge
- The art of nursing
- The expressive, intuitive, and creative aspect of nursing
- Practice that incorporates poetry, art, music, and stories, allowing a deep understanding of the human experience

outlined in Figure 2.2, theoretical/empirical knowledge has gained prominence in nursing and currently serves as the guide for evidence-informed practice. Theoretical and empirical knowledge really cannot be separated; however, theoretical knowing is concerned with developing or testing theories or ideas that nurse researchers have about how the world operates. Theoretical knowing is informed by empirical knowing, which involves observations of reality. Observations may include the following:

1. Speaking with people about their life experiences (e.g., living with Alzheimer's disease) and using their responses to specific and general questions to understand the phenomenon
2. Observing social or cultural interactions (e.g., homeless individuals interacting with service providers) as they naturally occur, interpreting what the interactions might mean for both parties, and using those interpretations to develop theories about health service delivery for that population
3. Delivering an intervention (e.g., a school health program for obese children) and assessing changes in health care–related behaviours (e.g., type of foods consumed, amount of daily exercise) after the delivery of the intervention
4. Using surveys or a questionnaire to ask a large group of men and women questions about experiences of violence and their current symptom levels with regard to pain, digestive problems, or depression.

Taking an example of published work, Erci, Sayan, Tortumuoglu, and colleagues (2003) hypothesized that nursing care guided by Jean Watson's theory of human caring would improve patient outcomes such as quality of life and blood pressure; this **hypothesis** is an example of *theoretical knowing*. However, it was only through developing an experiment that Erci and colleagues could observe these outcomes (e.g., blood pressure measured every 3 months) among patients who did and did not receive care guided by Watson's theory. These observations provided support for this hypothesis; this support is an example of *empirical knowing*.

PHILOSOPHIES OF RESEARCH

Thus far, we have used a number of terms that may be new to you. Every specialty has characteristic terminology for communicating important features of the work of that specialty. Learning new terminology is part of what nursing students do when they learn research methods and skills. Each research method and all philosophies of science have specialized language that nursing students will encounter in the literature. Thus, to help you comprehend the research you will read, it is important to clarify a few terms.

All research is based on **philosophical beliefs** about the world; these beliefs are the motivating values, concepts, principles, and the nature of human knowledge of an individual, group, or culture, and they are the basis of a **worldview,** or **paradigm.** *Paradigm* is from the Greek word *paradeigma,* meaning "pattern." Paradigms represent a "sets of beliefs and practices, shared by communities of researchers" that guide the knowledge development process (Weaver & Olson, 2006). Therefore, knowing and comprehending these beliefs and practices is important in understanding and using research findings. These beliefs are not right or wrong; rather, they represent different views of the world, and their use, the goals of the research.

Nursing research is guided by three research paradigms: positivism/post-positivism, constructivism, and critical theory. These three paradigms are compared in Table 2.1; however, first you need to understand the philosophical language used in the table. **Ontology** (from the Greek word *onto,* meaning "to be") is the science or study of being or existence and its relationship to nonexistence. Ontology addresses two primary questions: (1) What can be said to exist? and (2) Into what categories can existing things be sorted? **Epistemology** (from the Greek word *epistēmē,* meaning "knowledge") is the branch of philosophy that deals with what is known to be "truth." Epistemology addresses three central questions: (1) What is knowledge?; (2) How do we know what we know?; and (3) What is the scope or limitation of knowledge? **Methodology** refers to discipline-specific principles, rules, and procedures that guide the process through which knowledge is acquired. The **aim of inquiry** refers to the goals or specific objectives of the research. **Context** refers to the personal, social, and political environment in which a phenomenon of interest (that "thing of interest") occurs. The context of research studies can include physical settings, such as the hospital or home, or less concrete "environments," such as the context that cultural understandings and beliefs bring to an experience. **Values** are the personal beliefs of the researcher.

TABLE **2.1**

BASIC BELIEFS OF RESEARCH PARADIGMS

ITEM/QUESTIONS	POST-POSITIVISM	CRITICAL THEORY	CONSTRUCTIVISM
ONTOLOGY			
What can be said to exist? Into what categories can we sort existing things?	A material world exists. Not all things can be *understood, sensed,* or placed into a cause-and-effect relationship. The *senses* provide us with an imperfect understanding of the external/material world.	Reality is constructed by those with the most power at particular points in history. Reality is plastic and at all times imperfectly understood. Over time, reality is shaped by numerous social, political, economic, and cultural forces. Imperfectly shaped stories become accepted reality.	Reality is constructed by individual perception. There exists no absolute truth or validity. Truth is relative and subjective and based on perception or some particular frame of reference.
EPISTEMOLOGY			
What is knowledge? How is knowledge acquired? How do we know what we know?	Researchers are naturally biased. Objectivity (controlled bias) is the ultimate goal. Objectivity encourages triangulation and replication of findings across multiple perspectives. Objectivity encourages intense scrutiny of research findings from a larger community of scientists and the rejection of poorly conducted research.	Research is a transaction that occurs between the researcher and research participant. The perceptions (standpoint) of the researcher and the research participants naturally influence knowledge generation/creation. Perceptions (standpoints) are determined by context, and so contextual awareness and its relationship to the participant's understanding of reality is the focus of the research. Objectivity as outlined by the post-positivist is not a desired goal.	Research is a transaction that occurs between the researcher and research participant. The perceptions (standpoint) of the researcher and the research participants naturally influence knowledge generation/creation. Research emphasizes the meaning ascribed to human experiences. Context is not emphasized. Objectivity as outlined by the post-positivist is not a desired goal.
RESEARCHER'S VALUES			
How do the researcher's values influence the knowledge development process?	All attempts are made to exclude researcher bias. Influence is denied.	Researcher bias is recognized as potentially influential. Influence is limited with reflection and bracketing.	Researcher bias is recognized as potentially influential. Influence is limited with reflection and bracketing.

Continued

TABLE **2.1**

BASIC BELIEFS OF RESEARCH PARADIGMS—cont'd

ITEM/QUESTIONS	POST-POSITIVISM	CRITICAL THEORY	CONSTRUCTIVISM
METHODOLOGY			
Within a particular discipline, what principles, rules, and procedures guide the process through which knowledge is acquired?	Inquiry includes experimental, nonexperimental, and qualitative methods and is viewed as a series of logically related steps. Research questions/ hypotheses are proposed and subjected to empirical testing for the purpose of being proved incorrect rather than correct. Research is characterized by careful accounting for and control of factors that may influence research findings. Research entails the use of qualitative methods to develop hypotheses about people's social world and the meaning/purpose that people assign to their actions.	Inquiry requires dialogue between the investigator and research participant. Dialogue is *transformative* or consciousness raising. Dialogue brings to the forefront the historical context behind experiences of suffering, conflict, and collective struggles. Dialogue increases participants' awareness of actions required to incite change.	Inquiry requires dialogue between the investigator and research participant. Focus is on interpretation of written texts, art, pictures, and videos. Interpretation brings to the forefront the varying ways in which people construct their understanding of their social world and how their interpretation shifts as they interact with others.
AIM OF INQUIRY			
What is the goal of research?	Explanation, prediction, and control.	Critique, change and reconstructed reality, and emancipation.	Understanding and reconstructed reality.
CONTEXT			
What biographical, life, social, and political factors may influence the research findings?	Focus is on biographical context and its potential to influence research findings. Biographical context includes individual characteristics such as race, age, geographical location; it also accounts for past experiences in terms of both timing and content.	Focus is on historical, social, and political context. *Context* refers to the social and political climate in which an event or process occurred. Social context highlights how structural, economic, representational, and institutional factors of the past influence how people understand an issue today. Political context highlights how political dialogue and opinions, legal directives, and government policies of the past influence how people understand an issue.	Focus is on life context, including significant conditions and demands that provide greater understanding of the phenomena being studied; focus also emphasizes time and place.

From Denzin, Norman K.; Lincoln, Yvonna S. (2000). Handbook of Qualitative Research. SAGE Publications Inc.

Positivism is a philosophical orientation that suggests that a material world exists; that is, things can be *sensed* (i.e., seen, touched, heard, tasted). Furthermore, it is governed by the expressed belief that although not all things can be understood or explained, many things can be. In fact, our world can be observed, events and phenomena can be categorized, and we can create theories to explain why some things like *illness* and *health* occur or do not occur. Adherents to **post-positivism** emphasize that our observations cannot always be relied upon because they are subject to error and human bias—we all have different values, cultures, and life experiences. They believe that the best we can do is get to an approximation of reality by using a number of methods and observations.

Constructivism is a philosophical orientation that suggests reality and the way in which we understand our world are largely dependent on our perception. Truth is flawed because truth is never absolute. Truth and our understanding of the world are determined by our life experiences, which in turn inform how we view the world. Knowledge development, from the perspective of the constructivists, is not valuable if it is used simply to prove or disprove theories. Rather, the value of knowledge development lies in the ability to understand how people perceive their world. Knowledge development occurs through observation, dialogue with people, or both, and as a result of paying attention to the language people use to describe life experiences. Constructivists value subjectivity (personal knowing) over objectivity (quantified knowing), inasmuch as the aim of this form of research is to create an understanding of people and their life experiences from their point of view. Constructivism is often also referred to as *interpretivism*.

Another worldview is referred to as the *transformative approach* (Creswell, 2014). Although this worldview cannot be characterized as clearly as other worldviews, Creswell (2014) states that it arose "from individuals who felt that the post-positivist assumptions imposed structural laws and theories that did not fit marginalized individuals in our society or issues of power and justice, discrimination, and oppression that needed to be addressed" (p. 9). Several groups of researchers fall under this transformative worldview, including critical theorists, feminists, indigenous and postcolonial peoples, persons with disabilities, and members of lesbian, gay, bisexual, transsexual, and queer communities (Creswell, 2014). Many of their research projects contain an action agenda to reform or change the lives of participants in the study and to change oppressive structures affecting participants' lives (Creswell, 2014).

Critical social theorists' philosophical orientation suggests that reality and our understanding of reality are constructed by people with the most power at a particular point in history. Reality, and our understanding of the world, is always changing, and at all times we have an imperfect understanding of our world. **Critical social thought** places a strong emphasis on understanding health and illness within the context of history. This perspective supports the understanding that health and other aspects of reality are shaped by numerous social, political, economic, and cultural factors. Such factors include gender, social and economic status, minority versus majority status, and even a country's status as a developed or developing nation. A strong emphasis is placed on understanding how power imbalances associated with these factors influence health and well-being.

Feminist research, based on a transformative worldview, has been described as research that is done by, for, and about women, but, in fact, it is far more complex. Ollivier and Tremblay (2000) state that feminist research is informed by women's struggles against oppression, is grounded in feminist values and beliefs, and focuses on meanings that women give to their world. Current research informed by feminist theory challenges the way we think about how gender is expressed in society and how to achieve liberation of all humans. Collins and Bilge (2016) focus on the idea of *intersectionality*, where researchers examine how the experiences of women also interact with their experiences of class, race, and gender and sexual orientation.

 ### Research Hint

All research is based on a worldview or paradigm; however, the paradigm is rarely identified in a research report.

Table 2.1 provides an introduction to post-positivism, critical theory, and constructivism and how each might influence nursing research today. It is important to note that paradigms guide the development of the research question and the methods used to answer the questions. Some types of research are most congruent with the post-positivist paradigm; others are most congruent with the constructivist or social critical paradigm.

Consider the example of chemotherapy for cancer. A researcher who has a post-positivist orientation may be most interested in answering the question "How effective is tamoxifen in reducing breast cancer among at-risk women?" This nurse researcher may use an experiment to address this question. An experiment would involve putting together two groups of at-risk women and then giving one group tamoxifen and the other group a placebo (sugar pills) for a period of time (e.g., 2 years). After 2 years, the nurse researcher would measure how many people in each group developed breast cancer. This approach is guided by the belief that reality can be imperfectly understood through observation and measurement. The aim of the research is to understand exactly how the drug works and under what circumstances. In addition, the goal is to predict who (which type of patient) will benefit most from taking a specific drug such as tamoxifen. The post-positivist researcher recognizes that responses to tamoxifen will be influenced by the

biographical or personal context (e.g., age, gender, genetic background, and smoking history), and the researcher will attempt to account for the potential effect these influences might have on the research findings. Knowledge from this type of research will be used to promote evidence-informed practice, health public policy, and the actions of cancer care advocates.

A researcher with a constructivist orientation may be most interested in answering the question "What is the lived experience of women who are being treated for breast cancer?" Qualitative studies based on the **constructivist paradigm** are guided by the ontological view that multiple realities exist. As Olson (2006) stated, "Phenomena are studied through the eyes of people in their lived situations" (p. 461). For example, the meaning of cancer for a young mother is probably different from that for a grandmother. The meaning of cancer also may be different in Canada than in Japan.

Epistemology includes the view that truth varies and is subjective. Context is important, and description of the experience is vital. When seeking to understand patients' experiences of a treatment, nurse researchers would expect that what is important and "true" for one person may not be so for another. Some of the differences may result from context. The experience may well vary according to where the patient is treated and the patient's characteristics, such as age, gender, and ethnicity. The experience of having cancer may be different for a patient whose mother or father died a painful death from cancer than for a patient who knew people in whom cancer was cured. The values of everyone involved are acknowledged in qualitative research. Again, the finding from this research can be used to support evidence-informed practice and patient-centred care.

A researcher who shares a critical social orientation may be most interested in answering the questions "Does access to cancer treatment vary by racial/ethnic groups?" and "What steps must be taken to ensure equal access to cancer treatment such as tamoxifen?" Such a researcher may use a quantitative approach (e.g., mailing questionnaires to all people who received diagnoses of cancer in the previous 5 years and assessing whether race influenced access to early treatment) to address the first question and a qualitative approach, such as using focus groups (e.g., speaking with groups of five individuals from various racial/ethnic groups about equal access), to address the second question. This approach is guided by the ontological belief that "reality" is documented by individuals with the most power at particular points in history.

In addition, social critical researchers believe that reality and people's experiences are shaped by numerous social, political, economic, and cultural forces. The goal of critical research is to critique, change, and reconstruct reality (tell a different story) and to alleviate the experience of social injustices/inequalities. The research process creates change in study participants, the researcher, and society. This type of research, for example, would attempt to highlight from a historical perspective how the positions of various group (Indigenous peoples, Asians, Blacks) and the prestige (or lack thereof) granted to those groups influence their access to the appropriate treatments for breast cancer. Findings from these studies would support the researcher and the research participants in becoming "change agents" who advocate for transformations in service delivery practices and policies that intentionally or unintentionally support the unequal access to cancer treatment therapies.

 Research Hint_____

Values are involved in all research. For the post-positivist, it is vital that values not influence the results of the research. However, for the critical social and constructivist researcher, values and their potential influences on the research results are accepted as a natural part of the research process.

Another way of thinking about paradigms and linking them to research is illustrated in the

Critical Thinking Decision Path, on p. 32. This algorithm demonstrates that beliefs lead to different questions, which in turn lead to the selection of different research approaches. Qualitative and quantitative research methods are associated with different assumptions that are consistent with each method and are more specific than these global worldviews (post-positivism, critical theory, and constructivism). These beliefs and approaches lead to different research activities, as illustrated in the decision path.

RESEARCH METHODS: QUALITATIVE AND QUANTITATIVE

Research methods are the techniques, procedures, and processes used by researchers to organize a study in order for it to provide answers to the research question. Research methods can be classified into two major categories: qualitative and quantitative. A researcher chooses between these categories primarily on the basis of the question the researcher is asking. If a researcher wishes to test a cause-and-effect relationship, such as how social support (cause) leads to high blood pressure (effect), quantitative methods are most appropriate. If, however, a researcher wishes to discover and understand the meaning of an experience or process, such as death and dying, a qualitative approach would be appropriate. A researcher can also design a study that combines both categories; this mixed-methods approach is discussed later in this chapter.

Qualitative research is a systematic, interactive, and subjective research method used to describe and give meaning to life experiences. Figure 2.3 outlines the qualitative research process. A researcher would choose to conduct a qualitative research study if the question to be answered concerns understanding the meaning of a human experience, such as grief, hope, or loss.

A study completed by Pooler (2014) demonstrates the qualitative research process. She conducted a study to investigate individuals'

CRITICAL THINKING DECISION PATH

Selecting a Research Process

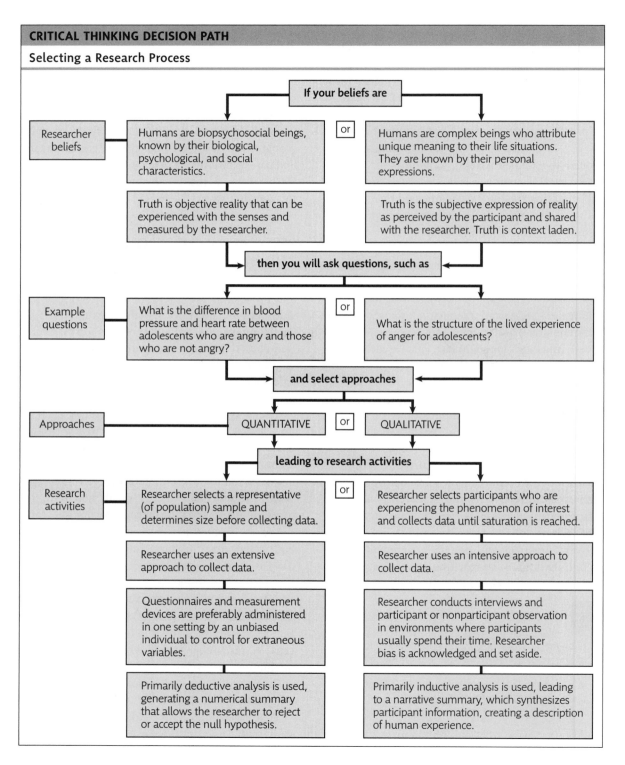

If your beliefs are

Researcher beliefs

Humans are biopsychosocial beings, known by their biological, psychological, and social characteristics.

or

Humans are complex beings who attribute unique meaning to their life situations. They are known by their personal expressions.

Truth is objective reality that can be experienced with the senses and measured by the researcher.

Truth is the subjective expression of reality as perceived by the participant and shared with the researcher. Truth is context laden.

then you will ask questions, such as

Example questions

What is the difference in blood pressure and heart rate between adolescents who are angry and those who are not angry?

or

What is the structure of the lived experience of anger for adolescents?

and select approaches

Approaches

QUANTITATIVE

or

QUALITATIVE

leading to research activities

Research activities

Researcher selects a representative (of population) sample and determines size before collecting data.

or

Researcher selects participants who are experiencing the phenomenon of interest and collects data until saturation is reached.

Researcher uses an extensive approach to collect data.

Researcher uses an intensive approach to collect data.

Questionnaires and measurement devices are preferably administered in one setting by an unbiased individual to control for extraneous variables.

Researcher conducts interviews and participant or nonparticipant observation in environments where participants usually spend their time. Researcher bias is acknowledged and set aside.

Primarily deductive analysis is used, generating a numerical summary that allows the researcher to reject or accept the null hypothesis.

Primarily inductive analysis is used, leading to a narrative summary, which synthesizes participant information, creating a description of human experience.

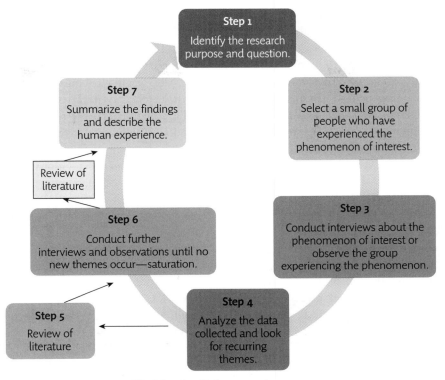

FIG. 2.3 Qualitative research process.

experiences of living with moderate to very severe chronic lower pulmonary disease, including asthma and chronic obstructive pulmonary disease (COPD). The research process as described in Figure 2.3 was used in this study as follows:

Step 1: Identified the research question as "What is it like to experience moderate to severe COPD or asthma?" (p. 3)

Step 2: A small sample of people (16) were selected to share their experiences; they were determined by pulmonary function tests to have moderate to very severe COPD or asthma and recruited from three pulmonary clinics.

Step 3: Eighteen interviews were conducted (two interviews were follow-up interviews) at participants' homes, and participants described their experiences in open-ended conversations.

Step 4: After the audiotapes from the interviews were transcribed, the data were analyzed to uncover themes or ideas.

Step 5: In this study, the author reviewed the literature after the interviews were complete and described the review in the discussion section.

Step 6: Analysis continued until no new ideas or themes emerged and there were sufficient data to richly describe the experiences of the participants.

Step 7: The findings were summarized under the emergent themes. Rich quotes from the participants illustrated each of the themes. One sentence summarized the findings as follows: "Impaired by their inability to breathe or distressed by severe shortness of breath, participants altered their mobility, tried to avoid triggers, slowed their speed, and limited their activities" (p. 9). The findings conveyed what it is like to live with moderate to severe COPD or asthma.

As this example demonstrates, qualitative methods emphasize understanding the meaning of an experience. The context of the experience also plays a role in qualitative research. As illustrated by this study, qualitative research is generally conducted in natural settings (in this case, the homes of participants), and data that are words **(text)**, rather than numerical data, are used to describe the experiences being studied. Qualitative data are also collected from a small number of participants, which allows an in-depth study of a particular phenomenon.

Although the methods of qualitative research are systematic, a subjective approach is used; that is, the emphasis is on capturing the personal perceptions of the study participants. Thus, data from qualitative studies help nurses understand experiences or phenomena that affect patients, and this information in turn leads to improved care and stimulates further research. Chapters 7

and 8 provide an in-depth overview of the underpinnings, designs, and methods of qualitative research.

Whereas the purpose of qualitative research is to create meaning about a phenomenon, that of **quantitative research** is to systematically describe a phenomenon. A researcher would choose to conduct a quantitative research study if the question to be answered concerned testing for the presence of specific relationships, assessing for group differences, clarifying cause-and-effect interactions, or explaining how effective a nursing intervention was. Quantitative methods entail the use of objective, precise, and highly controlled measurement techniques to gather information that can be analyzed and summarized statistically. Figure 2.4 outlines the quantitative research process. Like the qualitative research process, the quantitative research process begins with the development of a research question and a purpose

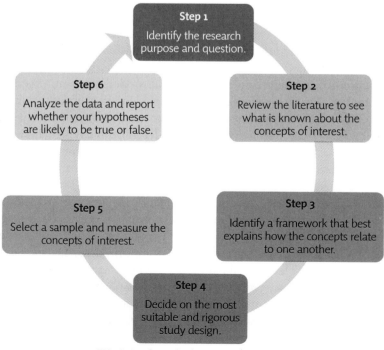

FIG. 2.4   Quantitative research process.

statement that highlight a relationship between two things.

A study completed by El-Masri, Fox-Wasylyshyn, Springer, and colleagues (2014) demonstrates the quantitative research process. They explored the impact of cancer radiation treatment on men with prostate cancer. The research process as described in Figure 2.4 was used in this study as follows:

Step 1: They defined the purpose of the study as being "to compare the effects of 3 types of radiation treatment on functions, bother, and well-being in men with prostate cancer at 1, 6, and 12 months after completion of treatment" (p. 42).

Step 2: Unlike the qualitative research process, in which researchers conduct their review of the literature after they have collected their data, the quantitative research process begins with a review of the literature, such as journal articles, books, government documents, and even Internet sources, to determine what is known about the phenomenon of interest and theories that explain the phenomenon. In their introduction and review of the literature, the authors noted that although there were several studies on urinary, sexual, and bowel function after treatment for prostate cancer, there was a dearth of studies that followed patients through the first year of recovery after the radiation treatments. They noted that studies focusing on the well-being and psychosocial impacts were inconsistent.

Step 3: The study was to compare the effect of three different types of radiation on the functions, bother, and well-being of men with prostate cancer.

Step 4: The researchers established a baseline survey prior to treatment, followed by a series of subsequent surveys to measure patients' self-perceived functions, bother, and well-being. The surveys, with the exception of the demographic data collected during the baseline survey (i.e., age), were identical. The authors described the survey tool in detail and provided rationale for the choice of the surveys, including reliability and validity.

Step 5: The researchers recruited participants during an orientation class that all patients attended before commencement of their radiation treatment. To be considered for inclusion, patients had to (1) have a confirmed case of localized prostate cancer; (2) be about to undergo radiation treatment (one of the three types identified); (3) be able to read and understand English; and (4) be able to provide consent.

Step 6: After conducting the statistical analysis, the authors concluded that there were "no differences among the three radiation treatments with regard to any of the outcome variables" (p. 50). They found that there was improvement over time in all of the variables measured; however, the researchers noted that although sexual function improved over time, sexual function continued to be a concern at 1 year post-treatment.

An important part of the quantitative research process is to decide which design is most appropriate for answering the research question. The numerous choices include descriptive, correlational, longitudinal, quasiexperimental, and experimental designs. El Masri and colleagues chose a repeated survey method to compare the function, bother, and well-being in men with prostrate cancer who had undergone three different radiation regimens.

As demonstrated in the article by El-Masri and colleagues (2014), quantitative research techniques are systematic, and the methodology emphasizes control of the research process, the environment in which the study is conducted, and how each variable is measured. In contrast to qualitative approaches—in which a question is asked and the participant is responsible for providing an in-depth response—quantitative responses are restricted to a preselected set of responses.

When you read research articles, remember that researchers may vary the steps slightly, depending on the nature of the research problem, but all of the steps should be addressed systematically.

INTRODUCTION TO FRAMEWORKS FOR RESEARCH

When research projects are conducted, particularly within the nursing discipline, great emphasis is placed on including a theoretical framework. For quantitative research projects, a theoretical framework offers researchers and consumers a way to understand how a phenomenon (that thing of interest) comes to exist. Frameworks can be abstract or concrete, but they provide a discipline-specific cause-and-effect explanation of the phenomenon. Furthermore, a framework guides the researcher in determining the questions to be asked and answered by the research project and in the development of the study hypotheses.

The social determinants of health perspective is one example of a theoretical framework that is often used in nursing (Chomik, 2001). This framework, developed by the Public Health Agency of Canada (2011), suggests that people's health and well-being are determined by 12 factors:

1. Income and Social Status
2. Social Support Networks
3. Education and Literacy
4. Employment/Working Conditions
5. Social Environments
6. Physical Environments
7. Personal Health Practices and Coping Skills
8. Healthy Child Development
9. Biology and Genetic Endowment
10. Health Services
11. Gender
12. Culture

The determinant of health framework guides the researcher in addressing the relationship between health and any of the 12 factors just listed. The researcher can determine how many factors to focus on and in what way the factors are related to each other and, in turn, to health. In some cases, the researcher may develop a diagram or a pictorial representation of these relationships.

Methodological frameworks serve as a guide for conducting qualitative research studies. Rather than explain how the phenomenon of interest comes to exist, the methodological framework identifies the principles, rules, and procedures that guide the process through which knowledge is acquired. The *human becoming basic research method* (Cody, 1995; Parse, 2005) has been used extensively to guide nursing research. In this method, hermeneutics are used to discover the meaning people assign to their lived experiences as expressed in text and art. The method consists of a dialogue between the researcher and text or art form to answer research questions such as "What does it mean to be human?" (Parse, 2001, p. 172). The analysis is completed in view of the principles of the theory of human becoming (Parse, 1987). Whereas the quantitative project begins with a theoretical framework, the findings of a qualitative study often lead to the creation of a theoretical framework that conveys an understanding of people's lived experiences.

As a follow-up exercise to this introduction to frameworks for research, read the following story and consider its message for the practising nurse who wishes to critique, understand, and conduct research.

Kate has worked in a coronary care unit (CCU) for nearly 3 years since graduating from nursing school. She has grown more comfortable with her job over time and now believes that she can readily manage the complexities of patient care in the CCU. Recently, she has observed the pattern of blood pressure change when health care providers enter a patient's room. This observation began when Kate noticed that one of her patients, a 62-year-old woman who had continuous arterial monitoring, showed dramatic increases in blood pressure, as much as 100%, each time the health care team made rounds in the CCU. Furthermore, this elevation in blood pressure persisted after the team left the patient's room, and then her blood pressure slowly decreased to preround levels within the following hour. Conversely, when the nurse manager visited the same patient on her usual daily rounds, the patient engaged calmly in conversation and was often left with lower blood pressure when the nurse manager moved on to the next patient. Kate thought about what was happening and adjusted her work so that she could closely observe the details of this phenomenon over several days.

Team rounds were led by the attending cardiologist and included nurses, pharmacists, social workers, medical students, and nursing students. The team discussed the patient, and, occasionally, she was asked to respond to a question about her history of heart disease or her current experience of chest discomfort. Participants took turns listening to her heart, and the students responded to questions related to her case. In contrast, the nurse manager's visit was a one-on-one meeting in which the patient was given the nurse's full attention. Kate noticed that the nurse manager was especially attentive to the patient's experience. In fact, the nurse manager usually sat and spent time talking to the patient about how her day was going, what she was thinking about while lying in bed, and what feelings were surfacing as she began to consider how life would be when she returned home.

Kate decided to talk to the nurse manager about her observations. The nurse manager, Alison, was pleased that Kate had noticed these blood pressure changes in association with interaction with health care providers. She told Kate that she, too, noticed these changes during her 8-year experience of working in the CCU. Her observation led her to the theory of attentively embracing story (Liehr & Smith, 2000; Smith & Liehr, 2003), which seemed applicable to the observation. Alison had learned the theory as a first-year master's degree student and now was applying it in practice and beginning plans to use the theory to guide her thesis research. The theory of attentively embracing story proposes that intentional nurse–patient dialogue (communication for a specific purpose), which engages the human story (encourages patients to discuss their experience), enables connecting with self-in-relation (self-reflection) to create ease (Figure 2.5). As depicted by the theory model, the central concept of the theory

is intentional dialogue (purposeful communication), which is what Kate first observed when she noticed Alison interacting with the patient.

Alison was fully attentive to the patient, following her lead in the conversation and pursuing what mattered most to the patient. Alison seemed to obtain a lot of information in a short time, and the patient seemed willing to share information that she was not sharing with other people. According to the theory of attentively embracing story, three concepts—intentional dialogue, connecting with self-in-relation, and creating ease—are intricately connected. Thus, when Kate observed intentional dialogue, she also observed connecting with self-in-relation as the patient reflected on her experience in the moment and creating ease when she saw the patient's blood pressure decrease after the nurse manager's visit. Alison and Kate shared an understanding that a relationship existed between the patient–health care provider interaction and the patient's blood pressure. They discussed several possible issues that might be affecting this relationship and made a list of research questions related to each issue (Table 2.2). Their list serves only as a reflection of the complexity of the relationship; other issues could generate a research question contributing to understanding of the relationship between the patient–health care provider interaction and the patient's blood pressure. The list developed by Kate and Alison highlights the fact that the relationship cannot be understood with one study; rather, a series of studies may enhance understanding and offer suggestions for change. For instance, a thorough understanding may lead to testing different approaches for conducting team rounds.

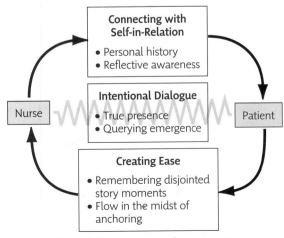

FIG. 2.5   Attentively embracing story.

TABLE **2.2**

| **ISSUES AFFECTING BLOOD PRESSURE CHANGE AND RELATED RESEARCH QUESTIONS** | |
ISSUES	**RESEARCH QUESTIONS**
Number of people in the patient's room	Is there a difference in BP for patients in the CCU when interacting with one person in comparison with interacting with two or more people?
Involvement of the patient	For the patient in the CCU, what is the relationship between BP and the amount of time spent listening to the health care team's discussion of personal qualities during routine rounds? What is the effect of the nurse–patient intentional dialogue on BP within the hour after the dialogue?
Continuing effect of experience on BP over the next hour	What is the BP pattern of patients in the CCU from the beginning of routine health care rounds until 1 hour after the completion of rounds?
Content of dialogue	What is the relationship between issues discussed during intentional dialogue and BP?
Meaning of experience for the patient	What is the patient's experience of being observed during routine health care rounds? What is the patient's experience of sharing personal matters with a nurse while in the CCU?

BP, blood pressure; *CCU*, coronary care unit.

LINKS CONNECTING PRACTICE, THEORY, AND RESEARCH

Several important aspects of frameworks for research are embedded in the story of Kate and Alison. First, it is important for you to notice the links between practice, theory, and research. Each is intricately connected with the other to create knowledge for the discipline of nursing (Figure 2.6). A **theory** is a set of interrelated concepts that provides a systematic view of a phenomenon. Theory guides practice and research; practice enables testing of theory and generates questions for research; and research contributes to theory building and establishing practice guidelines. Thus, what is learned through practice, theory, and research constitutes the knowledge of the discipline of nursing. From this perspective, each reader is in the process of contributing to the knowledge of the discipline. For example, if you are a practising nurse, you can use focused observation (Liehr, 1992), just as Kate did, to consider the nuances of situations

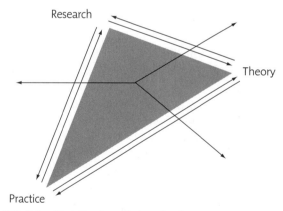

FIG. 2.6   Discipline knowledge: the theory–practice–research connection.

that matter to patient health. Kate noticed the changes in blood pressure occurring with interactions and systematically began to pay close attention to the effect of different interactions. This logical process often generates the questions that make the most sense for enhancing a patient's well-being.

Another major theme in the story of Kate and Alison can be found in each nurse's approach to the phenomenon of the relationship between the patient–health care provider interaction and blood pressure. Each nurse was using a different approach to look at the situation, but both were systematically evaluating what was observed. This approach is the essence of science: systematic collection, analysis, and interpretation of data. Kate was using **inductive reasoning,** a process of starting with the details of experience and moving to a general picture. Inductive reasoning involves the observation of a particular set of instances that belong to and can be identified as part of a larger set. Alison told Kate that she, too, had begun with inductive reasoning but now was using **deductive reasoning,** a process of starting with the general picture—in this case, the theory of attentively embracing story—and moving to a specific direction for practice and research. In deductive reasoning, the researcher uses two or more related concepts that, when combined, enable the researcher to suggest relationships between the concepts.

Inductive and deductive reasoning are basic in frameworks for research. Inductive reasoning is the pattern of "figuring out what is there" from the details of the nursing practice experience and is the foundation for most qualitative inquiry. Research questions related to the issue of the meaning of experience for the patient (see Table 2.2) can be addressed with the inductive reasoning of qualitative inquiry. Deductive reasoning begins with a structure that guides searching for "what is there." All but the last two research questions listed in Table 2.2 would be addressed with the deductive reasoning of quantitative inquiry.

In view of Alison's use of deductive reasoning guided by the theory of attentively embracing story, we can assume that she has read and critiqued the literature on theoretical frameworks and has chosen *attentively embracing story* to guide her master's thesis research. For Kate to move on in her thinking about research to study the way changes in blood pressure are related to the patient–health care provider interaction, she needs to become well-versed in the importance of theoretical frameworks. As she reads the literature and reviews research studies, she will critique the theoretical frameworks guiding those studies. By critiquing existing frameworks, she will develop the knowledge and understanding needed to choose an appropriate framework for research. As a beginning, Kate is reading this chapter, recognizing that she is critiquing nursing research.

Research Hint

Investigators may not always provide a detailed, explicit statement of the one or more observations that led them to their conclusions when using inductive reasoning. Likewise, you will not always find a clear explanation of the structure guiding a study in which deductive reasoning is used.

FRAMEWORKS AS STRUCTURES FOR RESEARCH

Whether you are evaluating a qualitative or a quantitative study, look for the framework that guided the study. In general, in an article in which the researcher is using qualitative inquiry and inductive reasoning methods, the framework is described at the end of the publication, in the discussion section. From the study's findings, the researcher builds a structure for moving forward. In an article by a researcher who uses quantitative inquiry and deductive reasoning methods, the framework is described at the beginning of the article, before a discussion of study methods.

A **model** is a symbolic representation of a set of concepts that is created to depict relationships. Figure 2.7 shows Stewart, Reutter, Letourneau, and colleagues' (2009) model of *social support*. It highlights the process through which support

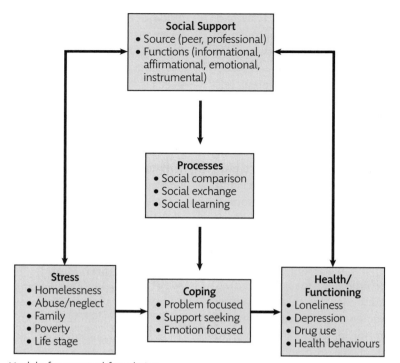

Social Support
- Source (peer, professional)
- Functions (informational, affirmational, emotional, instrumental)

Processes
- Social comparison
- Social exchange
- Social learning

Stress
- Homelessness
- Abuse/neglect
- Family
- Poverty
- Life stage

Coping
- Problem focused
- Support seeking
- Emotion focused

Health/ Functioning
- Loneliness
- Depression
- Drug use
- Health behaviours

FIG. 2.7 Model of conceptual foundation.
(From Stewart, M., Reutter, L., Letourneau, N., et al. (2009). A support intervention to promote health and coping among homeless youths. *Canadian Journal of Nursing Research, 41*(2), 54–77.) SAGE Publications Inc.

from peers and professionals influences the stressful life situations, coping behaviours, and health care–related behaviours of homeless youths. In this model, arrows are used to depict a process that explains how social support is related to the social network, stress, and health functioning. For example, the arrow from "social support" to "processes" suggests that social support has an effect on social network comparison, exchange, and learning. Whether this is positive or negative is unknown; however, the social network then influences coping behaviours (problem focused, support seeking, and emotion focused), which in turn influence health care–related functioning (loneliness, depression, drug use, and health behaviours). This model could be the basis for deductive reasoning. An example of a deductive

question that could be derived from the model is as follows:

> What is the difference in social comparison [an indicator of the quality of the social network] for homeless youths who participate in a supportive intervention, and how does this influence their problem-focused coping skills [one indicator of coping]?

The Ladder of Abstraction

The ladder of abstraction is a way for you to gain a perspective when reading and thinking about frameworks for research. When you critique the framework of a study, imagine a ladder (Figure 2.8). The highest level on the ladder, the worldview, includes beliefs and assumption or the paradigm to which the research belongs. The

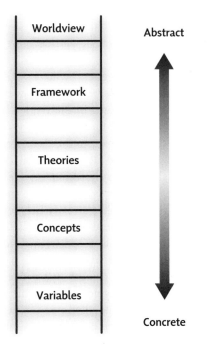

FIG. 2.8 Ladder of abstraction for evaluating research frameworks.

Research Hint_____
Some research reports embed conceptual definitions in the literature review. The reader should find the conceptual definitions so that the logical fit between the conceptual and the operational definitions can be determined.

Concepts

At the lower end of the ladder of abstraction is a **concept,** which is an image or symbolic representation of an abstract idea. Chinn and Kramer (2015, p. 160) define *concept* as a "complex mental formulation of experience." Concepts are the major components of theory and convey the abstract ideas within a theory. In this chapter, the concepts of the theory of attentively embracing story—intentional dialogue, connecting with self-in-relation, and creating ease—have been defined, and their relationships have been modelled. Each concept creates a mental image that is explained further through the conceptual definition. For example, the concept of pain creates a mental image that is based on experience. Its experiential meaning is different for a child who has just fallen off a bike, for an older adult with rheumatoid arthritis, and for a nurse with a doctoral degree who is studying pain mechanisms by using an animal model. These definitions and associated images of the concept of pain incorporate different experiential and knowledge components, all with the same label: *pain.* Therefore, it is important to know the meaning of the concept to the person. For a reader, it is important to know the meaning that the researcher gives to the concepts in a research study.

Theories

Next on the ladder, and as stated earlier, a *theory* is a set of interrelated concepts that serves the purpose of explaining or predicting phenomena. A theory is like a blueprint, a guide for modelling a structure. A blueprint depicts the elements of

middle portion of the ladder includes the framework, theories, and concepts that the researcher uses to articulate the problem, purpose, and structure for the research.

At the lowest level on the ladder of abstraction are variables. **Variables** are the elements that can be observed through the senses. The key empirical aspects of a study—its concepts and variables—are generally articulated through conceptual and operational definitions. A **conceptual definition** is much like a dictionary definition, conveying the general meaning of the concept. However, the conceptual definition goes beyond the general meaning found in the dictionary; the concept is defined as it is rooted in the theoretical literature. The **operational definition** specifies how the concept will be measured—that is, what instruments will be used to capture the essence of the variable.

a structure and the relationship of each element to the other, just as a theory depicts both the concepts that compose it and how they are related. Chinn and Kramer (2015) define *theory* as an "expression of knowledge . . . the creative and rigorous structuring of ideas that project a tentative, purposeful, and systematic view of phenomena" (p. 255). For example, consider the relationship between healthy child development, individual capacity and coping, and mental well-being. Several theories that account for the relationship between these variables have been developed by nurse researchers (e.g., Neuman's [1995] systems model). Such models address the ways in which stressful events deplete people's coping resources and, in turn, how both influence the mental health of people (children or adults).

Frameworks

Frameworks, such as the social determinants of health perspective, provide a general orientation to understanding a phenomenon of interest and identify what factors are most significant as we examine various aspects of health. As defined by the Canadian Public Health Association (n.d.), "Social determinants of health are the social and economic factors that can influence people's health" (n.p.) and include factors such as education, housing, gender, race, and Indigenous status. A framework does not necessarily reveal how every possible factor relates to one another; theories specify the relationship between the components of a framework.

The Critical Thinking Decision Path on p. 43 takes you through the thinking of a researcher who is about to begin conducting research. You can expect to find some, but not all, of the phases of decision making addressed in a research publication. Beginning with the worldview, the highest rung on the ladder of abstraction, the researcher is inclined to approach a research problem from the perspective of inductive or deductive reasoning. Researchers who pursue an inductive reasoning approach generally do not present a framework before beginning the discussion of methods. This is not to say that the literature will not be reviewed before the methods are introduced.

Conversely, researchers who use deductive reasoning must choose between a conceptual and a theoretical framework. In the theory literature, these terms are used interchangeably (Chinn & Kramer, 2015); however, in the case presented in the Critical Thinking Decision Path, each term is distinguished from the other on the basis of whether the researcher is creating the structure or whether the structure has already been created by someone else. In general, each of these terms refers to a structure that provides guidance for research. A **conceptual framework** is a structure of concepts, theories, or both that is used to construct a map for the study. It presents a theory, which explains why the phenomenon being studied exists. Generally, a conceptual framework is constructed from a review of the literature or is developed as part of a qualitative research project. A **theoretical framework** may also be defined as a structure of concepts, theories, or both that is used to construct a map for the study. However, it is based on a philosophical or theorized belief or understanding of why the phenomenon under study exists.

 Research Hint _____

When researchers have used conceptual frameworks to guide their studies, you can expect to find a system of ideas, synthesized for the purpose of organizing thinking and providing study direction.

From the perspective of the Critical Thinking Decision Path, whether the researcher is using a conceptual or a theoretical framework, conceptual and then operational definitions will emerge from the framework. The decision path moves down the ladder of abstraction from the philosophical to the empirical level, tracking thinking from the most abstract to the least abstract for the purposes of planning a research study and accruing evidence to guide nursing practice and research.

CRITICAL THINKING DECISION PATH

Choosing a Theoretical Path

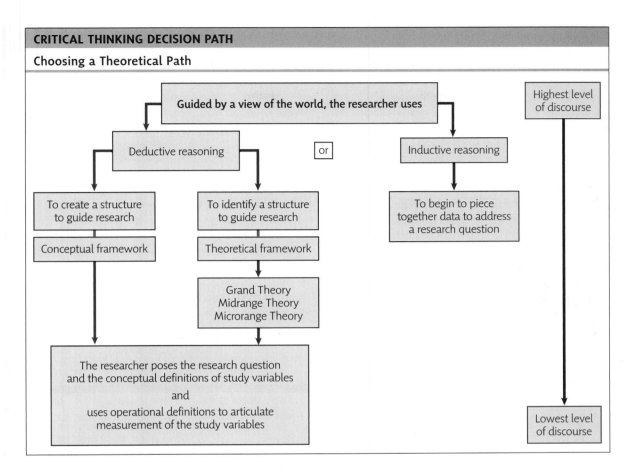

APPRAISING THE EVIDENCE

The Framework

The framework for research provides guidance for the researcher as study questions are fine-tuned, methods for measuring variables are selected, and analyses are planned. Once data are collected and analyzed, the framework is used as a basis for comparison. Did the findings coincide with the framework? If discrepancies exist, can they be explained by means of the framework? The reader of research needs to know how to critically appraise a framework for research (see the Critiquing Criteria box on p. 44).

The first question posed is whether a framework is presented. Sometimes, a structure may guide the research, but a diagrammed model is not included in the report. You must then look for the study structure in the description of the study concepts. When the framework is identified, consider its relevance for nursing. A nurse does not have to create the framework, but the importance of the study's content for nursing should be clear. The question of how the framework depicts a structure congruent with nursing should be addressed. Sometimes frameworks from very different disciplines, such as physics or art, may be relevant to nursing. The author must clearly articulate the meaning of the framework for the study and link the framework to nursing.

Once the meaning and relationship to nursing are articulated, you will be able to determine whether the framework is appropriate to guide the research. For instance, a

Continued

APPRAISING THE EVIDENCE—cont'd

The Framework

blatant mismatch occurs if a researcher is studying students' responses to the stress of being in the clinical setting for the first time but presents a framework of stress related to recovery from chronic illness. Such obvious mismatches do not generally arise; however, subtle versions of mismatch do occur. So you will need to look closely at the framework to determine whether it is appropriate and the "best fit" for the research question and proposed study design.

Next, focus on the concepts being studied. Do you know which concepts are being studied and how they are defined and translated into measurable variables? Does literature exist to support the choice of concepts? Concepts should clearly reflect the area of study; for example, if in a study the general concept of stress is used but the concept of anxiety is more appropriate to the research focus, difficulties will arise in defining variables and determining methods of measurement. These issues relate to the logical consistency within the framework, the concepts being studied, and the methods of measurement.

Throughout the entire critiquing process, from worldview to operational definitions, you are evaluating whether the theoretical framework is appropriate. At the end of a research article, you can expect to find a discussion of the findings as they relate to the model. This final point enables readers to evaluate the framework for use in further research. The discussion may suggest necessary changes to enhance the relevance of the framework for continuing study and thus focus the direction of future research.

Evaluating frameworks for research requires skill that can be acquired only through repeated critique and discussion with other nurses who have critiqued the same publication. The novice reader of research must be patient while developing these skills. With continuing education and a broader knowledge of potential frameworks, you will build a repertoire of knowledge to enable you to judge the foundation of a research study, the framework for research.

CRITIQUING CRITERIA

1. Is the framework for research clearly identified?
2. Is the framework consistent with a nursing perspective?
3. Is the framework appropriate to guide research on the subject of interest?
4. Are the concepts and variables clearly and appropriately defined?
5. Did the study present sufficient literature to support the selected concepts?
6. Is there a logical, consistent link between the framework, the concepts being studied, and the methods of measurement?
7. Are the study findings examined in relation to the framework?

CRITICAL THINKING CHALLENGES

- Explain the difference between research that is based on a constructivist paradigm and research that is based on a positivist paradigm.
- Discuss how a researcher's values can influence the results of a study. Include an example in your answer.
- You are taking an elective course in advanced pathophysiology. The professor compares the knowledge of various disciplines and states that nursing is an example of a nonscientific discipline, declaring in support of this position that

nursing's knowledge has been generated with unstructured methods, such as intuition, trial and error, tradition, and authority. What assumptions has this professor made? How would you counter or support this position?

- Nurse researchers contend that a theoretical framework is essential for systematically identifying the relationship between the chosen variables. If this is true, why do non-nursing research studies not identify theoretical frameworks?
- As a consumer of research, how would you use computer databases to verify tools for measuring operational definitions?

■ How would you argue against the following statement: "As a beginning consumer of research, it is ridiculous to expect me to determine whether a researcher's study has an appropriate theoretical framework; I've only had Nursing Theory 101."
■ Is it possible for a research study's theoretical framework and variables to be the same?

KEY POINTS

- The scientific approaches used to generate nursing knowledge reflect both inductive and deductive reasoning.
- The interaction among theory, practice, and research is central to knowledge development in the discipline of nursing.
- Conceptual frameworks are created by the researcher, whereas theoretical frameworks are identified in the literature.
- The use of a framework for research is important as a guide to systematically identify concepts and to link appropriate study variables with each concept.
- Conceptual and operational definitions are critical in the evolution of a study, regardless of whether they are explicitly stated.
- In developing or selecting a framework for research, knowledge may be acquired from other disciplines or directly from nursing. In either case, that knowledge is used to answer specific nursing questions.
- When you critique a framework for research, examine the logical, consistent link between the framework, the concepts for study, and the methods of data collection.

FOR FURTHER STUDY

ⓔ Go to Evolve at http://evolve.elsevier.com/ Canada/LoBiondo/Research for the Audio Glossary and Appendix Tables that provide supplemental information for Appendix E.

REFERENCES

Canadian Public Health Association. (n.d.). *What are the social determinants of health?* Retrieved from http://www.cpha.ca/en/programs/social-determinants/frontlinehealth/sdh.aspx.

Chinn, P. L., & Kramer, M. K. (2015). *Knowledge development in nursing. Theory and process* (9th ed.). St. Louis, MO: Elsevier.

Chomik, T. A. (2001). *The population health template: Key elements and actions that define a population health approach* (Discussion paper). Ottawa: Population and Public Health Branch.

Cody, W. K. (1995). Of life immense in passion, pulse, and power: Dialoguing with Whitman and Parse—A hermeneutic study. In R. R. Parse (Ed.), *Illuminations: The human becoming theory in practice and research* (pp. 269–307). New York: National League for Nursing Press.

Collins, P. H., & Bilge, S. (2016). *Intersectionality*. Toronto: Wiley.

Creswell, J. W. (2014). *Research design: Qualitative, quantitative, and mixed methods approaches* (4th ed.). Thousand Oaks, CA: Sage.

El-Masri, M. M., Fox-Wasylyshyn, S. M., Springer, C. D., et al. (2014). Exploring the impact of prostate cancer radiation treatment on functions, bother, and well-being. *Canadian Journal of Nursing Research*, *46*(2), 42–56.

Erci, I. B., Sayan, A., Tortumuoglu, G., et al. (2003). The effectiveness of Watson's caring model on the quality of life and blood pressure of patients with hypertension. *Journal of Advanced Nursing*, *41*(2), 130–139.

Liehr, P. (1992). Prelude to research. *Nursing Science Quarterly*, *5*, 102–103.

Liehr, P., & Smith, M. J. (2000). Using story to guide nursing practice. *International Journal of Human Caring*, *4*(2), 13–18.

Neuman, B. (Ed.). (1995). *The Neuman systems model* (3rd ed.). San Mateo, CA: Appleton & Lange.

Ollivier, M., & Tremblay, M. (2000). *Questionnements feministes et methodologie de la recherche*. Montreal: Harmattan.

Olson, J. (2006). Understanding paradigms used for nursing research. *Journal of Advanced Nursing*, *53*, 459–469.

Parse, R. R. (1987). *Nursing science: Major paradigms, theories, and critiques*. Philadelphia: W. B. Saunders.

Parse, R. R. (2001). *Qualitative inquiry: The path of sciencing*. Sudbury, MA: Jones & Bartlett.

Parse, R. R. (2005). The human becoming modes of inquiry: Emerging sciencing. *Nursing Science Quarterly*, *18*, 297–300.

Pooler, C. (2014). Living with chronic lower pulmonary disease: Disruptions of the embodied phenomenological self. *Global Qualitative Nursing Research*, 1–11.

Public Health Agency of Canada. (2011). *What determines health*? Retrieved from http://www.phac-aspc.gc.ca/ph-sp/determinants/index-eng.php.

Smith, M. J., & Liehr, P. (2003). *Middle range theory for nursing*. New York: Springer.

Stewart, M., Reutter, L., Letourneau, N., et al. (2009). A support intervention to promote health and coping among homeless youths. *Canadian Journal of Nursing Research*, *41*(2), 54–77.

Weaver, K., & Olson, J. K. (2006). Understanding paradigms used for nursing research. *Journal of Advanced Nursing*, *53*(4), 459–469.

Zander, P. E. (2007). Ways of knowing in nursing: The historical evolution of a concept. *Journal of Theory Construction and Testing*, *11*(1), 7–11.

CHAPTER 3

Critical Reading Strategies: Overview of the Research Process

Geri LoBiondo-Wood | Judith Haber | Cherylyn Cameron

LEARNING OUTCOMES

After reading this chapter, you will be able to do the following:

- Identify the steps that researchers use to conduct quantitative and qualitative research.
- Identify the importance of critical thinking and critical reading for the reading of research articles.
- Identify the steps associated with critical reading.
- Use the steps of critical reading to review research articles.
- Use identified strategies to critically read research articles.
- Use identified critical thinking and critical reading strategies to synthesize critiqued articles.
- Identify the format and style of research articles.

KEY TERMS

abstract	critical thinking	reliability
assumptions	critique	validity
critical reading	critiquing criteria	

STUDY RESOURCES

ⓔ Go to Evolve at http://evolve.elsevier.com/Canada/LoBiondo/Research for the Audio Glossary and Appendix Tables that provide supplemental information for Appendix E.

AS YOU READ THIS TEXT, YOU will learn how the steps of the research process unfold. The steps are systematic and orderly, and they relate to the development of nursing knowledge. Understanding the step-by-step process that researchers use will help you develop the critiquing skills necessary to judge the soundness of research studies you will encounter in the literature. Throughout the chapters in this book, research terms pertinent to each step are identified, defined, and illustrated with many examples from the research literature. Four published research studies are featured in the appendices (A–D), and they are used as examples to illustrate significant points in each chapter. Judging not only a study's soundness but also a study's applicability to practice is a key skill.

This chapter provides an overview of critical thinking, critical reading, and critiquing skills. The chapter also introduces the overall format of a research article and provides an overview of subsequent chapters in the book. These components of the chapter are designed to help you read research articles more effectively and with greater understanding. Throughout this text, as you encountered in Chapters 1 and 2, you will find special features that will help refine and develop your competence as a research consumer. A _critical thinking decision path_ related to each step of the research process will sharpen your decision-making skills as you critique research articles. Look for _Internet_ resources in chapters that will enhance your research consumer skills. _Critical thinking challenges_, which appear at the end of each chapter, are designed to reinforce your critical thinking and critical reading skills in relation to the steps of the research process. _Research hints_, designed to reinforce your understanding and critical thinking, appear at various points throughout the chapters. _Evidence-informed practice tips_, which will help you apply evidence-informed practice strategies in your clinical practice, are also provided in each chapter. Finally, _Practical Application boxes_ offer examples of translating principles and methods of nursing research into real-life nursing situations and interventions.

Before you can assess a study, however, you need to understand the differences between and among studies. As you read the chapters and the appendices, you will encounter many different study designs, as well as standards for critiquing the soundness of each step of a study and for judging both the strength of evidence provided by a study and its application to practice. The steps of the qualitative research process generally proceed in the order outlined in Table 3.1. Table 3.2 outlines the general steps associated with quantitative research. Remember that a researcher may vary the steps slightly, depending on the nature of the research problem, but all of the steps should be addressed systematically.

Once you complete a research critique or two, you will be ready to discuss your critique with your fellow students and professor. Best of all, you can enjoy discussing the points of your appraisal because your critique will be based on objective data, not just personal opinion. As you continue to use and perfect critical analysis skills by critiquing studies, remember that these very skills are an expected clinical competency for delivering evidence-informed nursing care.

CRITICAL THINKING AND CRITICAL READING SKILLS

To develop an expertise in evidence-informed practice, you need to be able to critically read all types of research literature. As you read articles, you may notice the difference in style or format between research articles and theoretical or clinical articles. The terms in a research article may be new to you, and the focus of its content is different. Reading research articles can be difficult and frustrating at first, but the best way to become a knowledgeable consumer of research is to use critical thinking and critical reading skills when you read research articles. As a student, you are not expected to completely understand a research article; you may also find it challenging to critique research articles until you obtain repeated experience doing so. Nor are you expected to develop critiquing skills on your own. A primary

TABLE **3.1**

STEPS OF THE RESEARCH PROCESS AND JOURNAL FORMAT: QUALITATIVE RESEARCH

RESEARCH PROCESS STEPS OR FORMAT ISSUES	USUAL LOCATION IN JOURNAL HEADING OR SUBHEADING
Identification of the phenomenon	In abstract, introduction, or both
Purpose of research study	In abstract, at beginning or end of introduction, or in more than one of these locations
Literature review	In introduction, discussion, or both
Design	In abstract, "Introduction" section, "Methods" subsection titled "Design," "Methods" section in general, or more than one of these locations
Sample	In "Methods" subsection titled "Sample," "Subjects," or "Participants"
Legal–ethical issues	In section on data collection, in "Procedures" section, or in description of sample
Data-collection procedure	In "Data Collection" or "Procedures" section
Data analysis	In "Methods" subsection titled "Data Analysis" or "Data Analysis and Interpretation"
Results	In abstract (briefly), in separate section titled "Results" or "Findings"
Discussion and recommendations	In separate "Discussion" or "Discussion and Implications" section
References	At end of article

TABLE **3.2**

STEPS OF THE RESEARCH PROCESS AND JOURNAL FORMAT: QUANTITATIVE RESEARCH

RESEARCH PROCESS STEPS OR FORMAT ISSUES	USUAL LOCATION IN JOURNAL HEADING OR SUBHEADING
Research problem	In abstract, introduction (not labelled as a research problem), or separate subsection titled "Problem"
Purpose	In abstract or introduction or both; at end of literature review or discussion of theoretical framework; or in separate section titled "Purpose"
Literature review	At end of introduction but not labelled as a literature review; in separate section titled "Literature Review," "Review of the Literature," or "Related Literature" Variables reviewed may appear as titles of sections or subsections
Theoretical framework, conceptual framework, or both	In "Literature Review" section (combined) or in separate sections titled "Theoretic Framework" and "Conceptual Framework"; or each concept or definition used in theoretical or conceptual framework may appear as title of separate section or subsection
Hypothesis/research questions	Stated or implied near end of "Introduction" section, which may be labelled; in separate sections or subsection titled "Hypothesis" or "Research Questions"; or, for first time, in "Results" section
Research design	In abstract or introduction (stated or implied) or in section titled "Methods" or "Methodology"
Sample: type and size	Size: may be stated in abstract, in "Methods" section, or in separate "Methods" subsection as "Sample," "Sample/Subjects," or "Participants" Type: may be implied or stated in any of previous headings described under size
Legal–ethical issues	In section titled "Methods," "Procedures," "Sample," "Subjects," or "Participants" (in all cases, stated or implied)

Continued

TABLE **3.2**

STEPS OF THE RESEARCH PROCESS AND JOURNAL FORMAT: QUANTITATIVE RESEARCH—cont'd

RESEARCH PROCESS STEPS OR FORMAT ISSUES	USUAL LOCATION IN JOURNAL HEADING OR SUBHEADING
Instruments (measurement tools)	In section titled "Methods," "Instruments," or "Measures"
Validity and reliability	In section titled "Methods," "Instruments," "Measures," or "Procedures" (specifically stated or implied)
Data-collection procedure	In "Methods" subsection titled "Procedure" or "Data Collection" or in separate section titled "Procedure"
Data analysis	In "Methods" subsection under subheading "Procedure" or "Data Analysis"
Results	In separate section titled "Results"
Discussion of findings and new findings	Combined with results or in separate section titled "Discussion"
Implications, limitations, and recommendations	Combined with discussion or presented in separate or combined major sections
References	At end of article
Communicating research results	In research articles, poster, and paper presentations

objective of this book is to help you acquire critical thinking and critical reading skills. No perfect critique exists; your interpretation will be based on your current knowledge, experience, and understanding. Remember that becoming a competent critical thinker and consumer of research, like learning the steps of the research process, takes time, patience, and experience.

Critical thinking is the rational examination of ideas, inferences, assumptions, principles, arguments, conclusions, issues, statements, beliefs, and actions (Paul & Elder, 2008). As applied to critically reading research, this means that you are engaged in the following:

- Systematic understanding of the research process
- Thinking that displays a mastery of the criteria for critiquing research and evidence-informed practice
- The art of being able to make your thinking better (i.e., clearer, more accurate, or more defensible) by clarifying what you understand and what you do not know

In other words, being a critical thinker means that you are consciously thinking about your own thoughts and what you say, write, read, or do, as well as what other people say, write, or do. While thinking about all of this, you are also questioning the appropriateness of the content, applying standards or criteria, and seeing how the information measures up.

Critical reading is "an active, intellectually engaging process in which the reader participates in an inner dialogue with the writer" (Paul & Elder, 2008, p. 461). A critical reader actively looks for **assumptions** (accepted truths), key concepts and ideas, reasons and justifications, supporting examples, parallel experiences, implications and consequences, and any other structured features of the text so as to interpret and assess the text accurately and fairly (Paul & Elder, 2008).

Critical reading is a process that involves the following levels of understanding and allows you to critically assess a study's validity:

- *Preliminary:* familiarizing yourself with the content (skimming the article)

- *Comprehensive:* understanding the researcher's purpose or intent
- *Analysis:* understanding the parts of the study
- *Synthesis:* understanding the whole article and each step of the research process in a study

Box 3.1 provides more in-depth strategies for attaining these levels of understanding.

Critical thinking and critical reading skills can be further developed by learning the research process. You will find that critical thinking and critical reading skills used in the nursing process can be transferred to understanding the research process and reading research articles. You will gradually be able to read an entire research article and reflect on it by identifying and challenging assumptions, identifying key concepts, questioning methods, and determining whether the conclusions are based on the study's findings. Once you have obtained this competency in critiquing research, you will be ready to synthesize the

findings of multiple research studies to use in developing evidence-informed practice.

Critiquing a research study requires several readings. At minimum, you should read it three or four times. The first strategy in this process is to keep your research textbook at your side as you read. Using this book while you read a study may help you do the following:

- Identify the steps of the research process and how the study was conducted
- Clarify unfamiliar concepts or terms
- Question assumptions and rationale
- Assess the study for validity

As you analyze and synthesize an article, you are ready to begin the appraisal process that will help determine a study's value. An illustration of how to use critical reading strategies is provided by the example in the Practical Application box, which contains excerpts from the abstract, introduction, literature review, theoretical framework

---

BOX **3.1**

HIGHLIGHTS OF CRITICAL READING PROCESS STRATEGIES

Photocopy or download and print out the article to be critiqued, and make notations directly on the copy.

STRATEGIES FOR PRELIMINARY UNDERSTANDING

- Keep a research textbook and a dictionary by your side.
- Review the chapters in the textbook on the various steps of the research process.
- Highlight or underline on your copy of the article any new terms, unfamiliar terms, and significant sentences.
- Look up the definitions of new terms, and write them on your copy of the article.
- Highlight or underline identified steps of the research process.

STRATEGIES FOR COMPREHENSIVE UNDERSTANDING

- Identify the main idea or theme of the article; state it in your own words in one or two sentences.
- Continue to clarify terms that may be unclear on subsequent readings.
- Before critiquing the article, make sure you understand the main points of each reported step of the research process that you identified.

STRATEGIES FOR ANALYSIS UNDERSTANDING

- Using the critiquing criteria, determine how well the study meets the criteria for each step of the process.
- Determine which level of evidence fits the study.
- Make notes about cues, relationships of concepts, and questions on your copy of the article.
- Ask fellow students to analyze the same study, using the same criteria, and then compare their results with yours.
- Consult faculty members about your evaluation of the study.

STRATEGIES FOR SYNTHESIS UNDERSTANDING

- Review your notes on the article, and determine how each step discussed in the article compares with the critiquing criteria.
- In your own words, compose a one-page summary of the reviewed study.
- Cite article references at the top according to the American Psychological Association (2010) style manual or another reference style.
- In your own words, and using the critiquing criteria, briefly summarize each reported research step.
- In your own words, briefly describe the study's strengths and weaknesses.

literature, and "Methods" and "Procedure" sections of the quantitative study by Laschinger (2014; see Appendix B). Note that this particular article contains both a literature review and a discussion of the theoretical framework that clearly supports the objectives and purpose of the study. Also note that in the Practical Application box, parts of the text of these sections from the article were deleted so that the examples could be as concise as possible.

Practical Application
EXAMPLE OF CRITICAL APPRAISAL READING STRATEGIES*

Introductory paragraphs, study's purpose and aims	"Workplace mistreatment is known to have detrimental effects on job performance and well-being. . . . It is reasonable to expect that work environments in which bullying or incivility are common are not conducive to a positive patient safety climate and may therefore be associated with higher patient risk. Indeed, research has linked workplace violence go caregiving errors and unsafe medication practices in nursing settings. However, we could find no studies linking more subtle forms of workplace mistreatment to patient safety risk and nurse-assessed patient care quality and patient adverse events. The purpose of this study was to investigate the impact of subtle forms of workplace mistreatment on Canadian nurses' perceptions of patient safety risk and, ultimately, nurse-assessed quality and prevalence of adverse events." (pp. 284–285)
Literature review: concepts	
Workplace mistreatment	"A growing body of knowledge in the management field has linked bullying and workplace incivility to numerous negative work outcomes, including increased turnover intentions, poor mental health, and absenteeism. . . . Hutchison and Jackson found that negative interpersonal [interactions] among nurses were associated with perceived threats to patient care quality as a result of decreased teamwork and poor morale, which ultimately hindered nurses' ability to provide high-quality patient care. . . . Bullying and incivility have also been linked to burnout, a phenomenon consistently associated with reduced performance and poor patient outcomes." (pp. 284–285)
Patient safety risk and adverse patient outcomes	"The patient safety literature has documented the importance of high-quality nursing environments to the provision of safe patient care. . . . Negative patient safety cultures have been linked to high medication error rates, increased work-related injuries, and reluctance to report errors. . . . Recent research has shown that nurses' assessments of patient care quality are valid indicators of actual quality." (p. 285)
Theoretical framework	"We used the concept of workplace bullying of Einarsen and Mikkelsen and the construct of workplace incivility of Andersson and Pearson to examine the influence of seemingly minor workplace mistreatment on nurses' assessment of patient safety risk and, ultimately, their rating of patient care quality and experiences of common adverse events." (p. 285)
Hypothesis	"We therefore expect that bullying and civility influence nurse-assessed quality outcomes through their effect on nurses' perceptions of patient safety risk in their work settings emanating from negative workplace interactions." (p. 285)
Design	"A random sample of nurses working in Ontario hospitals (N = 641) was obtained from the College of Nursing provincial registry list, who were invited to participate in this study. A total of 336 responded to a questionnaire that was mailed to their home address, for a response rate of 52%." (pp. 285–286)
Instrument	Five instruments were used to measure bullying behaviours, workplace incivility, patient safety risk, nurse-assessed adverse events, and perceptions of patient care quality (p. 286).

*For references cited in this box, please see Appendix B.
Adapted from Laschinger, H. K. S. (2014). Impact of workplace mistreatment on patient safety risk and nurse-assessed patient outcomes. *Journal of Nursing Administration*, 44(5), 284–290.

Research Hint_____

If you still have difficulty understanding a research study after using the strategies related to skimming and comprehensive reading, make another copy of your marked-up research article, include your specific questions or area of difficulty, and ask your professor to read this copy. Comprehensive understanding and synthesis are necessary for analyzing a research article. Understanding the author's purpose and methods for the study reflects critical thinking and facilitates evaluation of the study.

STRATEGIES FOR CRITIQUING RESEARCH STUDIES

The evaluation of a research article requires an appraisal or critique of the published study. The **critique** is the process of critical appraisal in which a person objectively and critically evaluates a research report's content for scientific validity or merit and application to practice. It requires some knowledge of the subject matter, as well as knowledge of how to read critically and use critiquing criteria. **Critiquing criteria** are the standards, appraisal guides, or questions used to judge (assess) an article. Guidelines for conducting a critique are presented in several of the following chapters of this book.

In analyzing a research report, you must evaluate each step of the research process and ask whether each step of the process meets the criteria. For instance, the critiquing criteria for assessing a literature review, discussed in Chapter 5 (p. 108), include whether the literature review identifies gaps and inconsistencies in the literature about a subject, concept, or problem; and whether all of the concepts and variables are included in the review. These two criteria relate to critiquing the research question and the literature review components of the research process. The Practical Application box shows several examples in which Laschinger (2014) identified gaps in the literature and how she intended to fill these gaps by conducting a study for the stated objective and purpose (see Appendix B for the complete study).

Remember that when you are doing a critique, you are pointing out strengths as well as weaknesses. To review the appraisal strategies that facilitate understanding when reading for analysis, see Box 3.1.

Critiquing can be thought of as looking at a completed jigsaw puzzle. Does it form a comprehensive picture, or is a piece out of place? What is the level of evidence provided by the study and its findings? What is the balance between the risks and benefits of the findings that contribute to clinical decisions? How can the evidence be applied in the treatment of a patient or a patient population or in a specific setting? In the case of reading several studies for synthesis, you need to consider how interrelated each of the studies are and determine the overall strength and quality of evidence and its applicability to practice. Reading for synthesis is essential in critiquing research studies.

EVIDENCE-INFORMED PRACTICE AND RESEARCH

Along with gaining confidence while reading and critiquing research studies, you need to undertake a final step of reading and appraising the research literature: deciding how, when, and whether to apply a study or studies to your practice so that your practice is evidence informed. Evidence-informed practice allows you to systematically use the best available evidence with the integration of individual clinical expertise, as well as the patient's values and preferences, in making clinical decisions (Sackett, Straus, Richardson, et al., 2000). Evidence-informed practice has processes and steps that are followed, as does the research process. These steps are presented throughout the text (see Chapter 20).

When you use evidence-informed practice strategies, the first step is to be able to read a research article and understand how each section is linked to each step of the research process. The following section introduces you to the steps of the research process as presented in published articles.

Once you read an article, you will need to decide which level of evidence a research article provides and how well the study was designed and executed. Figure 3.1 depicts a model for determining the levels of evidence associated with the design of a study, ranging from systematic reviews of randomized clinical trials to expert opinions. The rating system or evidence hierarchy model presented here is just one of many. Many hierarchies for assessing the relative worth of different types of research literature for both the qualitative and quantitative research literature are available.

You will note from Figure 3.1 that research evidence is traditionally categorized from weakest to strongest, with an emphasis on support for the effectiveness of interventions. The concept of levels of evidence tends to dominate the evidence-informed practice literature, rendering unclear the merit of qualitative studies. As suggested in Chapter 2, different research methods provide different types and levels of evidence, all of which inform practice. Although evidence provided by qualitative studies seems to rank lower in the hierarchy of evidence presented (i.e., levels V and VI), Sandelowski (2004) has noted that hierarchies are used under the assumption that randomized clinical trials are the "gold standard" of research; this assumption devalues qualitative

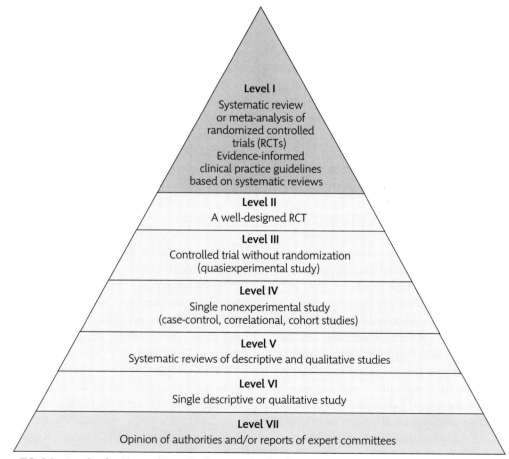

FIG. 3.1 Levels of evidence: hierarchy for rating levels of evidence, associated with a study's design. Evidence is assessed at a level according to its source.
(Based on Melynk, B. M., & Finoult-Overholt, E. (2011). *Evidence-based practice in nursing & literature: A guide to best practice* (2nd ed.). Philadelphia: Lippincott, Williams and Wilkins.)

research. However, qualitative research has increased and thrived over the years. Thousands of reports of well-conducted qualitative studies exist on topics such as (1) personal and cultural constructions of disease, prevention, treatment, and risk; (2) living with disease and managing the physical, psychological, and social effects of multiple diseases and their treatment; (3) decision-making experiences with beginning and end of life, as well as assistive and life-extending technological interventions; and (4) contextual factors favouring and mitigating against quality care, health promotion, prevention of disease, and reduction of health disparities (Sandelowski, 2004). The answers provided by qualitative data reflect important evidence that may offer valuable insights about a particular phenomenon, patient population, or clinical situation. It is important to remember that researchers, in choosing which research methodology to use, base their decision primarily on the question or questions they are trying to answer.

The meaningfulness of an evidence rating system will become clearer to you as you read the chapters on quantitative research. For example, the Laschinger (2014) study (see Appendix B) is level IV because of its descriptive design, whereas the study by MacDonald, Martin-Misener, Steenbeek, and colleagues (2015; see Appendix A) is level VI because of its qualitative design. Remember, as discussed earlier, the level by itself does not reveal the full worth of a study but is another tool that helps you think about the strengths and weaknesses of a study and the nature of the evidence provided in the findings and conclusions. The chapters on qualitative research provide an understanding of how qualitative studies can be assessed for use in practice. You will use the evidence hierarchy presented in Figure 3.1 throughout the book as you develop your research consumer skills, and so it is important to become familiar with its content.

This rating system represents an evidence hierarchy for judging the strength of a study's design, which is just one level of assessment that influences how confident the reader is about the conclusions drawn by the researcher. Assessing the strength of scientific evidence or potential research bias provides a vehicle to guide nurses in evaluating research studies for their applicability in clinical decision making. In addition to identifying the level of evidence needed to grade the strength of a body of evidence, it is important to consider the three domains of quality, quantity, and consistency (Agency for Healthcare Research and Quality, 2002):

- *Quality:* the extent to which a study's design, implementation, and analysis minimizes bias
- *Quantity:* the number of studies in which the research question has been evaluated, including overall sample size across studies, as well as the strength of the findings from the data analyses
- *Consistency:* the degree to which similar findings are reported from investigations of the same research question in studies that have similar and different designs

After the study's design has been assessed, specific processes and steps are followed to add to evidence-informed practice. The steps of the process are to ask, gather, assess and appraise, act, and evaluate (Figure 3.2). This is a circular

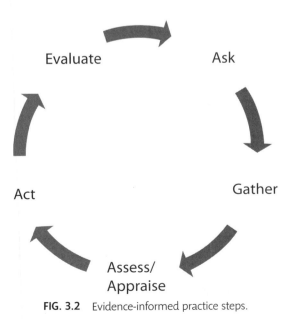

FIG. 3.2 Evidence-informed practice steps.

process in which evaluation may lead to questions. Chapter 20 provides an overview of evidence-informed practice and introduces you to the steps and strategies associated with evidence-informed practice.

RESEARCH ARTICLES: FORMAT AND STYLE

Before you consider reading research articles, it is important to have a sense of their organization and format. Many journals publish either only research articles or research in addition to clinical or theoretical articles. Although many journals have some common features, they also have unique characteristics. All journals have guidelines for manuscript preparation and submission; these guidelines are published by each journal. A review of these guidelines will give you an idea of the format of articles that appear in specific journals.

It is important to remember that even though each step of the research process is discussed at length in this text, you may find only a short paragraph or a sentence in the research article that gives the details of the step in a specific study. Because of the journal's publishing guidelines, the published study that appears in a journal is a shortened version of the complete work carried out by the researcher or researchers. You will also find that some researchers devote more space in an article to the results, whereas others present a longer discussion of the methods and procedures. Since the 1990s, most authors have given more emphasis to the method, results, and discussion of implications than to the details of assumptions, hypotheses, or definitions of terms. Decisions about the amount of material presented for each step of the research process are constrained by the following:

- A journal's space limitations
- A journal's author guidelines
- The type or nature of the study
- An individual researcher's evaluation of what is the most important component of the study

The following discussion provides a brief overview of each step of the research process

and how it might appear in an article (refer to Tables 3.1 and 3.2). It is important to remember that the format of a quantitative research article will differ from that of a qualitative research article.

Abstract

An **abstract** is a short, comprehensive synopsis or summary of a study at the beginning of an article. An abstract quickly focuses the reader on the main points of a study. A well-presented abstract is accurate, self-contained, concise, specific, nonevaluative, coherent, and readable.

Abstracts vary in length from 50 to 250 words. The length and format of an abstract are dictated by the journal's style. Both quantitative and qualitative research studies have abstracts that provide a succinct overview of the study. An example of an abstract can be found at the beginning of the study by Laschinger (2014; see Appendix B). That abstract follows an outline format that highlights the major steps of the study. Rather than a narrative of approximately 100 words, a common format for many journals, the format lists the objective, background, methods, results, and conclusions. It reads in part as follows:

> **Conclusions:** Bullying and workplace incivility have unfavorable effects on nurse-assessed patient quality through their effect on perceptions of patient safety risk. (p. 284)

All of the other studies in the appendices have narrative abstracts.

 Research Hint

A journal abstract is usually a single paragraph that provides a general reference to the research purpose, research questions, or hypothesis, or a combination of these aspects, and highlights the methodology and results, as well as the implications for future practice or research.

Introduction

Early in a research article, in a section that may or may not be titled "Introduction," the researcher presents a background picture of the area researched and its significance to practice. In the study by Pauly, McCall, Browne, and colleagues (2015; see Appendix C) on nurse and patient perceptions of illicit substance use in a hospitalized setting, the reader can find the basis of the research question early in the report:

> While stigma and discrimination associated with illicit substance use have repeatedly been identified as concerns in health care practice, few models for health care have been developed to address these issues. (p. 121)

Another example is found in the study by Héon, Goulet, Garofalo, et al. (2016; see Appendix D):

> Few breastfeeding education and support interventions for mothers of preterm infants can be identified in the scientific literature.

Definition of the Purpose

The purpose of the study is defined either at the end of the researcher's initial introduction or at the end of the "Literature Review" or "Conceptual Framework" section. The study's purpose may or may not be labelled as such, or it may be referred to as the study's aim or objective. Pauly and colleagues (2015; see Appendix C) described the goal of the study in the last paragraph in the introductory paragraphs:

> Our goal was to generate knowledge to foster an understanding of the meaning and context of cultural safety in acute care settings for people who use, have used in the past, or are suspected of using illicit substances and are affected by poverty and/or homelessness. (p. 122)

Héon and colleagues (2016; see Appendix D) stated in the introductory paragraphs:

> The objective of this article is to present the estimation of the intervention effects on breast milk production outcomes. (p. 531)

Literature Review and Theoretical Framework

Authors of studies and journal articles present the literature review and theoretical framework in different ways. In many research articles, the literature review is merged with the discussion of the theoretical framework. The resulting section includes the main concepts investigated and may be titled "Review of the Literature," "Literature Review," "Theoretical Framework," "Related Literature," "Background," or "Conceptual Framework"; or it may not be a separate section at all. In reviewing Appendices A through D, you will find differences in the headings used. For example, MacDonald et al. (2015) have a general introduction that includes a brief literature review and a "Theoretical and Methodological Perspectives" section (see Appendix A). Alternately, Laschinger (2014) reviewed the literature in two sections titled "Workplace Mistreatment" and "Patient Safety Risk and Adverse Patient Outcomes" and described the theoretical model in a section entitled "Hypothesized Model" (see Appendix B). Héon et al. (2016) presented the theoretical framework as the section named as such (see Appendix D). One style is not better than another; all of the studies in the appendices contain all of the critical elements but present the elements differently.

Hypothesis or Research Question

A study's research questions or hypotheses can also be presented in different ways. Research reports in journals often do not have separate headings for reporting the hypotheses or research question. They are often embedded in the "Introduction" or "Background" section or not labelled at all (e.g., as in the studies in the appendices). Quantitative research studies have hypotheses or research questions. If a researcher uses hypotheses in a study, the researcher may report whether the hypotheses were or were not supported; such reporting occurs toward the end of the article, in the "Results" or "Findings" section. Laschinger (2014) (Appendix B) states the hypothesis in the section titled "Hypothesized Model," whereas Héon et al. (2016) pose their hypothesis in the introductory section. Qualitative research studies do not have hypotheses but do have research questions and purposes. MacDonald et al. (2015) (Appendix A) and Pauly et al. (2015) (Appendix C) both pose their research questions in the introduction.

Research Design

The type of research design can be found in the abstract, within the purpose statement, or in the introduction to the "Procedures" or "Methods" section, or it may not be stated at all. For example, the studies in Appendices A, B, C, and D all identify the design type in both the abstract and the body of the study report.

One of your first objectives is to determine whether the study is qualitative or quantitative, so that the appropriate criteria are used. Although the rigour of the critiquing criteria addressed does not substantially change, some of the terminology of the questions differs for qualitative and quantitative studies. For instance, in the study by Héon et al. (2016; see Appendix D), you might ask whether the hypotheses were generated from the theoretical framework or the literature review and whether the design chosen was appropriate and consistent with the study's questions and purpose. With a qualitative study such as that by Pauly et al. (2015; see Appendix C), however, you might be asking whether the researchers conducted the study in a manner consistent with the principles of qualitative research and therefore focused on the identification of the themes of knowledge and choice.

Do not get discouraged if you cannot easily determine the design. More often than not, the specific design is not stated, or, if an advanced design is used, the details are not spelled out. One of the best strategies is to review the chapters in this text that address designs and to ask your professors for assistance. The following tips will help you determine whether the study you are reading employs a quantitative design:

- Hypotheses are stated or implied.
- The terms *control* and *treatment group* appear.
- The term *survey, correlational,* or *ex post facto* is used.
- The term *random* or *convenience* is mentioned in relation to the sample.
- Variables are measured by instruments or scales.
- Reliability and validity of instruments are discussed.
- Statistical analyses are used.

In contrast, qualitative studies do not usually focus on "numbers." In some articles about qualitative studies, standard quantitative terms (e.g., *subjects*) may be used rather than qualitative terms (e.g., *informants* or *participants*). Deciding on the type of qualitative design can be confusing; one of the best strategies is to review this text's chapters on qualitative design, as well as to critique qualitative studies. Begin trying to link the study's design with the level of evidence associated with that design as illustrated in Figure 3.1. This will give you a context for evaluating the strength and consistency of the findings and their applicability to practice. Although many studies may not specify the particular design used, all studies inform the reader of the specific methodology used, which can help you decide the type of design used to guide the study.

Sampling

The population from which the sample was drawn is discussed in the section titled "Methods" or "Methodology" under the subheadings of "Subjects," "Participants," or "Sample." For example, MacDonald et al. (2015) discuss the sample in a section titled "Recruitment of Mi'kmaq Women" under the larger heading of "The Study" (see Appendix A). However, Laschinger (2014) presents the sample selection criteria in a section titled "Design and Sample" under the general heading of "Methods" (see Appendix B). Researchers should describe both the population from which the sample was chosen and the number of participants who took part in the study, and they should also mention whether participants dropped out of the study and if they did, how many. The authors of all of the studies in the appendices discuss their samples in enough detail so that who the participants were and how they were selected are quite clear.

Reliability and Validity

The discussion related to instruments used to measure the variables of a study is usually included in a "Methods" subsection titled "Instruments" or "Measures." The researcher usually describes the particular measure (i.e., instrument or scale) used by discussing its reliability and validity. **Reliability** refers to the consistency or constancy of the measuring tool, whereas **validity** describes whether the measuring tool actually measures the correct phenomenon. Laschinger (2014; see Appendix B) describes the reliability of each of the five instruments used to measure bullying behaviours, workplace incivility, patient safety risk, nurse-assessed adverse events, and perception of patient care quality in a "Methods" subsection titled "Measures."

 Research Hint_____

Remember that not all research articles include headings related to each step or component of the research process, but each step is presented at some point in the article.

In some cases, researchers do not report the reliability and validity of commonly used, established instruments in an article and may refer you to other references. Ask for assistance from your instructor if you are in doubt about the validity or reliability of a study's instruments. Qualitative researchers typically report on the validity of the findings and on how potential biases are acknowledged and worked with (see Chapter 7). For example, Pauly et al. (2015; see Appendix C) describe how they met the standards for rigour in qualitative research in a section called "Research Design and Sample."

Procedures and Data-Collection Methods

The procedures used to collect data or the step-by-step way in which the researcher used the measures (instruments or scales) is generally described in the "Procedures" section. In each of the studies in Appendices A through D, the researchers indicated how they conducted the study in detail in sections and subsections as follows:

Appendix A: "The Study" with subsections of "Qualitative Participatory Action Research Design" and "In-depth Interviews"
Appendix B: "Methods" with subsections of "Design and Sample" and "Measures"
Appendix C: "Research Design and Sample"
Appendix D: "Method" with subsection of "Data Collection"

Notice that the researchers in each study in Appendices A through D also state that the studies were approved by an institutional review board (see Chapter 6), thereby ensuring that each met ethical standards.

Data Analysis/Results

The data analysis procedures (i.e., the statistical tests used and the results of descriptive and inferential tests applied in quantitative studies) are presented in the section titled "Results" or "Findings." Although qualitative studies do not involve the use of statistical tests, the procedures for analyzing the themes, concepts, and observational or print data are usually described in the "Methods" or "Data Collection" section and reported in the "Results," "Findings," or "Data Analysis" section. MacDonald et al. (2015) reported on the methods of qualitative data analysis in their "Data Analysis" subsection and the results of their analysis in their "Findings and Discussion" section (see Appendix A). The article by Laschinger (2014) has several sections: the subsection "Data Analysis" describes how the data were analyzed, and two subsections under "Results" describe the results of the hypotheses tested (see Appendix B).

Discussion

The last part of an article about a research study is the "Discussion" section. In this section, the researchers explain how all of the parts of the study are related and analyze the study as a whole. The researchers refer to the literature reviewed and discuss how their study is similar to or different from other studies. Researchers may report the results and discussion in one section but usually report them in separate "Results" and "Discussion" sections (see Appendices A, B, C, and D). One way is not better than the other. Journal and space limitations determine how these sections are handled. Any new findings or unexpected findings are usually described in the "Discussion" section.

Recommendations and Implications

In some articles, a separate section titled "Conclusions" describes the implications of the findings for practice and education, as well as related limitations based on the findings, and future studies may be recommended (see Appendices A, B, and D); in other articles, this information appears in several sections with titles such as "Discussion," "Limitations," "Nursing Implications," "Implications for Research and Practice," and "Summary." Some authors may include the "Limitations" and other sections discussed above in the section "Discussion." Again, one way is not better than another, only different.

References

All of the references cited in a research article are included at the end of the article. The main purpose of the reference list is to support the material presented by identifying the sources in a manner that allows for easy retrieval by the reader. Journals have various referencing styles to organize references. American Psychological Association (APA) style is commonly used in the health sciences, thus a journal entry would be formatted as follows:

Author, A. A. (Year). Title of article. *Title of Periodical, volume number*(issue number), pp.–pp.

References and citations in this text follow APA style.

Communicating Results

Communicating the results of a study can take the form of a research article, poster, or paper presentation. All are valid ways of providing nurses with the data and the ability to provide high-quality patient care that is based on research findings. Evidence-informed nursing care plans and practice protocols, guidelines, or standards are outcome measures that effectively indicate communicated research.

As you develop critical thinking and reading skills by using the strategies presented in this chapter, you will become more familiar with the research and appraisal processes. Your ability to read and critique research articles will gradually improve. You will be well on your way to becoming a knowledgeable user of research from nursing and other scientific disciplines for application in nursing practice.

 Research Hint_____

When writing a paper on a specific concept or topic that requires you to critique and synthesize the findings from several studies, you might find it useful to create an evidence table of the data. Include the following information: author, date, type of study, design, level of evidence, sample, data analysis, findings, and implications.

SYSTEMATIC REVIEWS: META-ANALYSES, INTEGRATIVE REVIEWS, AND META-SYNTHESES

Another variety of articles that is appearing more frequently in the literature and is very important for understanding evidence-informed practice are systematic reviews. "The systematic review is essentially an analysis of the available literature (that is, evidence) and a judgement of the effectiveness or otherwise of a practice, involving a series of complex steps" (Joanna Briggs Institute, 2016, n.p.). Systematic reviews include meta-analyses, integrative reviews, and meta-syntheses. The authors of these articles investigate a number of studies related to a specific clinical question and, using a specific set of criteria and methods, evaluate those articles as a whole.

The methods detailed here are not prescriptive but serve as a general outline of how you will find these articles formatted. Overall, although they vary somewhat in their approach, these reviews are intended, in essence, to better inform practice and develop evidence-informed practice.

The components of these types of articles are as follows:

- *Background:* The introduction covers content related to the background of the clinical question and clarifies the specific question that the review answers. The article's authors clarify the definitions of the concepts in the question so that the reader understands the concepts that were used in assessment.
- *Method:* The methods used for searching the literature are detailed. The exact electronic databases, the dates, and the keywords used to conduct the search are provided. In addition, the article details the inclusion and exclusion criteria by which the literature was chosen to review and critique. If a number of articles were found and not used, the authors detail why articles were excluded from the review.
- *Appraisal of the literature:* The articles that are included in the literature review are discussed in the body of the article, and an evidence table is used to present the highlights of each article. The author uses the evidence table to compare and contrast the articles, critique them for scientific validity, and discuss how well they answer the clinical question. If the author uses a meta-analysis format, a summary of the data is presented.

- *Conclusions/summary:* In the conclusions or summary, the strength, quality, and consistency of the data are described as they apply to practice. This section contains recommendations about which aspects of practice are supported by the data in the articles and for which aspects further research is needed to more fully answer the question posed in the review.

For example, Bottorff, Poole, Kelly, et al. (2014) set out to conduct a scoping review of the literature to learn about tobacco and alcohol use during pregnancy and the postpartum period by initially identifying studies focused on adolescent pregnancy and substance use from January 1990 to 2012. The review team then refined their inclusion criteria and extracted the following information from 40 articles: methodology, sample, purpose/focus of study, and the findings. They identified gaps in the research, including a lack of intervention-based research and qualitative studies to develop appropriate interventions.

CLINICAL GUIDELINES

Clinical guidelines are systematically developed statements or recommendations that serve as a guide for practitioners. Guidelines have been developed to assist in bridging practice and research. Guidelines are developed by professional organizations, government agencies, institutions, and convened expert panels. Guidelines provide clinicians with an algorithm for clinical management or for decision making with regard to specific diseases (e.g., colon cancer) or treatments (e.g., pain management). For example, the Canadian Diabetes Association (2013) has posted clinical practice guidelines on its website that are intended to help health care providers administer the "very best patient-centered diabetes care and chronic disease management for their patients." One of the guidelines includes an algorithm for calculating the vascular risk of patients with diabetes—a higher score will determine if vascular protective medicine is required.

Not all guidelines are well developed and, like research, must be assessed before implementation. Clinical guidelines, although they are systematically developed and make explicit recommendations for practice, may be formatted differently. Guidelines should clearly present scope and purpose of the practice, detail who contributed to the development of the guidelines, demonstrate scientific rigour, demonstrate clinical applicability, and demonstrate editorial independence. The Appraisal of Guidelines for Research and Evaluation (AGREE; http://www.agreetrust.org/about-the-agree-enterprise/agree-research-teams/agree-collaboration/) Enterprise has developed an instrument, AGREE II, for assessing the quality of clinical guidelines (AGREE Enterprise, 2010). The guideline, last updated in 2013, includes the following areas as part of the appraisal:

- Overall quality of guideline development methods
- Overall quality of guideline presentation
- Completeness of reporting
- Overall quality of guideline recommendations
- Overall quality of the guideline

As you venture through this textbook, you will be challenged to think about not only reading and understanding research studies but also applying the findings to your practice. Nursing has a rich legacy of research that has grown in depth and breadth. Producers of research and clinicians must engage in a joint effort to translate findings into practice that will make a difference in the care of patients and families.

CRITICAL THINKING CHALLENGES

- The critical reading of research articles may require a minimum of three or four readings. Is this always the case? What assumptions underlie this claim?
- Why is it necessary to reach an analysis stage of critical reading before you can critique a study?
- To synthesize a research article, what questions must you first be able to answer?

- If nurses are not expected to conduct research, how can nursing students be expected to critique each step of the nursing process, an entire study, or several studies?
- Discuss several strategies that might motivate practising nurses to critically appraise research articles.
- What level of evidence is presented in each of the articles that appear in Appendices A, B, C, and D? Justify your answers.

KEY POINTS

- Critical thinking and critical reading skills will enable you to question the appropriateness of the content of a research article, apply standards or critiquing criteria to assess the study's scientific merit for use in practice, and consider alternative ways of handling the same topic.
- Critical reading involves active interpretation and objective assessment of an article and searching for key concepts, ideas, and justifications.
- Critical reading requires four stages of understanding: preliminary (skimming), comprehensive, analysis, and synthesis. Each stage is characterized by specific strategies to increase your critical reading skills.
- Critically reading for preliminary understanding is accomplished by skimming or quickly and lightly reading an article in order to familiarize yourself with its content and to provide you with a general sense of the material.
- Critically reading for a comprehensive understanding is designed to increase your understanding both of the concepts and research terms in relation to the context and of the parts of the study in relation to the whole study, as presented in the article.
- Critically reading for analysis understanding is designed to divide the content into parts so that each part of the study is understood. The critiquing process begins at this stage.
- Critical reading to reach the goal of synthesis understanding combines the parts of a research study into a whole. During this final stage, the reader determines how each step of the research process relates to all the other steps,

how well the study meets the critiquing criteria, and the usefulness of the study for practice.

- Critiquing is the process of objectively and critically evaluating the strengths and weaknesses of a research article for scientific merit and application to practice, theory, and education. The need for more research on the topic or clinical problem is also addressed at this stage.
- Each article should be reviewed for level of evidence as a means of judging the application of the findings to practice.
- Research articles have different formats and styles, depending on journal manuscript requirements and whether they are quantitative or qualitative studies.
- The basic steps of the research process are presented in journal articles in various ways. Detailed examples of such variations can be found in chapters throughout this text.
- Evidence-informed practice begins with the careful reading and understanding of research articles.

FOR FURTHER STUDY

(e) Go to Evolve at http://evolve.elsevier.com/ Canada/LoBiondo/Research for the Audio Glossary and Appendix Tables that provide supplemental information for Appendix E.

REFERENCES

Agency for Healthcare Research and Quality. (2002). *Systems to rate the strength of scientific evidence* (File inventory, Evidence Report/Technology Assessment No. 47, AHRQ Publication No. 02-E016). Rockville, MD: Author.

AGREE Enterprise. (2010). *The AGREE II Instrument* [Electronic version]. Retrieved from http://www. agreetrust.org.

American Psychological Association. (2010). *Publication manual of the American Psychological Association* (6th ed.). Washington, DC: Author.

Bottorff, J. L., Poole, P., Kelly, M. T., et al. (2014). Tobacco and alcohol use in the context of adolescent pregnancy and postpartum: A scoping review of the literature. *Health and Social Care in the Community*, *22*(6), 561–574.

Canadian Diabetes Association. (2013). *Reducing vascular risk*. Retrieved from http://guidelines.diabetes.ca/ vascularprotection/riskassessment.

Héon, M., Goulet, C., Garofalo, C., et al. (2016). An intervention to promote breast milk production in mothers of preterm infants. *Western Journal of Nursing Research*, *38*(5), 529–552.

Joanna Briggs Institute. (2016). *Critical appraisal tools*. http://www.joannabriggs.org/research/critical-appraisal-tools.html.

Laschinger, H. K. S. (2014). Impact of workplace mistreatment on patient safety risk and nurse-assessed patient outcomes. *Journal of Nursing Administration*, *44*(5), 284–290.

MacDonald, C., Martin-Misener, R., Steenbeek, A., et al. (2015). Honouring stories: Mi'kmaq women's experiences with Pap screening in Eastern Canada. *Canadian Journal of Nursing Research*, *47*(1), 72–96.

Paul, R., & Elder, L. (2008). *The miniature guide to critical thinking concepts and tools*. Dillon Beach, CA: Foundation for Critical Thinking Press.

Pauly, B., McCall, J., Browne, A. J., et al. (2015). Toward cultural safety: Nurse and patient perceptions of illicit substance use in a hospitalized setting. *Advances in Nursing Science*, *38*(2), 121–135.

Sackett, D. L., Straus, S. E., Richardson, W. S., et al. (2000). *Evidence-based medicine: How to practise and teach EBM*. London: Churchill Livingstone.

Sandelowski, M. (2004). Using qualitative research. *Qualitative Health Research*, *14*(10), 1366–1386.

CHAPTER 4

Developing Research Questions, Hypotheses, and Clinical Questions

Judith Haber | Cherylyn Cameron

LEARNING OUTCOMES

After reading this chapter, you will be able to do the following:

- Discuss the purpose of developing a research question.
- Describe how the research question and hypothesis are related to the other components of the research process.
- Describe the process of identifying and refining a research question.
- Identify the criteria for determining the significance of a research question.
- Discuss the appropriate use of the purpose, aim, or objective of a research study.
- Discuss how the purpose, research question, and hypothesis suggest which level of evidence is to be obtained from the findings of a research study.
- Identify the characteristics of research questions and hypotheses.
- Describe the advantages and disadvantages of directional and nondirectional hypotheses.
- Compare the use of statistical hypotheses with that of research hypotheses.
- Discuss the appropriate use of research questions versus hypotheses in a research study.
- Discuss the differences between a research question and a clinical question in relation to evidence-informed practice.
- Identify the criteria used for critiquing a research question and a hypothesis.
- Apply the critiquing criteria to the evaluation of a research question and a hypothesis in a research report.

KEY TERMS

clinical question	nondirectional hypothesis	research question
dependent variable	population	statistical hypothesis
directional hypothesis	problem statement	testability
hypothesis	purpose	testable
independent variable	research hypothesis	variable

STUDY RESOURCES

ⓔ Go to Evolve at http://evolve.elsevier.com/Canada/LoBiondo/Research for the Audio Glossary and Appendix Tables that provide supplemental information for Appendix E.

AS YOU READ EACH CHAPTER, REMEMBER that each step of the research process is defined and discussed as to how that particular step relates to evidence-informed practice. At the beginning of this chapter, you will learn how to generate your own clinical questions that you will use to guide the development of evidence-informed practice projects. Then you will learn about research questions and hypotheses from the perspective of the researcher. From a clinician's perspective, you must understand how the research question and hypothesis align with the rest of the study.

The first step in developing evidence-informed practice is also to ask a question, referred to as a *clinical question*. After posing the clinical question, a quest begins to find the best evidence to answer the question and to apply it to clinical practice. For a clinician making an evidence-informed decision about a patient care issue, a clinical question would guide the nurse in searching for and retrieving the best available evidence. For example, is chlorhexidine or povidone-iodine more effective in preventing infections in central catheters? Finding the evidence, combined with clinical expertise and patient preferences, would provide an answer on which to base the most effective decision about which antiseptic is most effective.

If there is no clear satisfactory answer to the clinical question, a specific research question or hypothesis may be developed to lead a study. All research studies begin with questions and/or hypotheses.

When nurses ask certain questions, they are often well on their way to developing a research question or hypothesis. Such questions include "What is happening in this situation?"; "What are the patient's experiences?"; "Why are things being done this way?"; "I wonder what would happen if . . . ?"; "What characteristics are associated with . . . ?"; and "What is the effect of . . . on patient outcomes?" Research questions are usually generated from situations or problems that emerge from practice. These are often articulated in a **problem statement** such as the following, posed by Laschinger (2014): "Workplace mistreatment is known to have detrimental effects on job performance and in nursing may threaten patient care quality" (p. 284). (See Appendix B.)

For an investigator conducting a study, the research question or the hypothesis is a key preliminary step in the research process. The **research question** presents the idea that is to be examined in the study and is the foundation of the research study. Once the research question is clear, the researcher selects the most appropriate research design. If the research question is primarily explorative, descriptive, or theory generating, the researcher opts for qualitative methods. In these studies, a hypothesis is not formulated. For studies in which the researcher is seeking a specific answer to a research question, however, a hypothesis is generated and tested.

Hypotheses can be considered intelligent hunches, guesses, or predictions that help researchers seek the solution or answer to the research question. Hypotheses are a vehicle for testing the validity of the theoretical framework assumptions and provide a bridge between theory and actuality. In the scientific world, researchers derive hypotheses from theories and subject them to empirical testing. A theory's validity is not directly examined. Instead, through testing hypotheses, researchers can evaluate the merit of a theory.

Research questions or hypotheses often appear at the beginning of research articles. However, because of space constraints or stylistic considerations in journal publications, the research question or hypothesis may be embedded in the purpose, aims, goals, or even the results section of the research report. Both the consumer and the producer of research need to understand the importance of research questions and hypotheses as the foundational elements of a research study.

DEVELOPING AND REFINING A CLINICAL QUESTION

Practising nurses, as well as students, are challenged to keep their practice up to date by searching for, retrieving, and critiquing research articles that apply to practice issues that they encounter in their clinical setting (Cullum, 2000). As Melnyk and Fineout-Overholt (2011) commented, "without current best evidence, practice is rapidly outdated, often to the detriment of clients" (p. 8).

Practitioners strive to use the current best evidence from research in making clinical and health care decisions. Although they may not be conducting research studies, their search for information from practice is also converted into focused, structured clinical questions that are the foundation of evidence-informed practice. Clinical questions often arise from clinical situations for which there are no ready answers. You have probably had the experience of asking, "What is the most effective treatment for . . . ?" or "Why do we still do it this way?"

Focused clinical questions are used as a basis for searching the literature to identify supporting evidence from research. A **clinical question** has five components:

1. Population
2. Intervention
3. Comparison
4. Outcome
5. Time

The five components, known as PICOT, constitute a format that is effective in helping nurses develop searchable clinical questions (Melnyk & Fineout-Overholt, 2011). Box 4.1 presents each component of the clinical question. An additional method is to utilize the SPIDER tool, which also has five components for searching the literature (Cooke, Smith, & Booth, 2012). (See the Practical Application box in Chapter 5, p. 92, for examples of PICOT and SPIDER.) The SPIDER tool has terminology that is more suited to qualitative-based questions (Figure 4.1):

1. Sample
2. Phenomenon of Interest
3. Design
4. Evaluation
5. Research type

The significance of the clinical question becomes obvious as the research evidence from the literature is critiqued. The research evidence is used side by side with clinical expertise and the patient's perspective to develop or revise nursing standards, protocols, and policies that are used

---

BOX **4.1**

PICOT COMPONENTS OF A CLINICAL QUESTION

Population: The individual patient or group of patients with a particular condition or health care problem (e.g., adolescents aged 13 to 18 with type 1 insulin-dependent diabetes)

Intervention: The particular aspect of health care that is of interest to the nurse or the health team—for example, a therapeutic intervention (inhaler or nebulizer for treatment of asthma), a preventive intervention (pneumonia vaccine), a diagnostic intervention (measurement of blood pressure), or an organizational intervention (implementation of a bar coding system to reduce medication errors)

Comparison intervention: Standard care or no intervention (e.g., antibiotic or ibuprofen for children with otitis media); a comparison of two treatment settings (e.g., rehabilitation centre or home care)

Outcome: Improved outcome (e.g., improved glycemic control, decreased hospitalizations, decreased medication errors)

Time: Time involved to demonstrate an outcome (e.g., weight loss maintained over a period of 2 years)

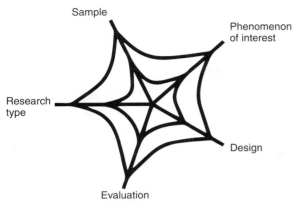

Sample

Phenomenon of interest

Research type

Design

Evaluation

FIG. 4.1 Elements of the SPIDER research tool. (From Cooke, A., Smith, S., & Booth, A. (2012). Beyond PICO: The SPIDER tool for qualitative evidence synthesis. *Qualitative Health Research, 22*(10), 1435–1443.) SAGE Publications Inc.

to plan and implement patient care (Cullum, 2000; Melnyk & Fineout-Overholt, 2011; Sackett, Straus, Richardson, et al., 2000; Thompson, Cullum, McCaughan, et al., 2004). Issues or questions can arise from multiple clinical and managerial situations (see the Practical Application box).

Sometimes it is helpful for nurses who develop clinical questions from a consumer's perspective to consider three elements—(1) the situation, (2) the intervention, and (3) the outcome—as they frame their focused question:

- The situation is the patient or problem being addressed. This can be a single patient or a group of patients with a particular health problem (palliative care of patients with cancer).
- The intervention is the dimension of health care interest, and the question is often about whether a particular intervention (in this case, pain diaries) is a useful treatment.
- The outcome encompasses the effect of the treatment (intervention) for this patient or the patient population in terms of quality (e.g., decreased pain perception) and cost (low cost). It essentially answers whether the intervention makes a difference for the patient population.

The individual parts of the question are vital pieces of information to remember when you search for evidence in the literature. One of the easiest ways to do this is to use a table, such as Table 4.1. Examples of clinical questions are highlighted in Box 4.2. Chapter 5 provides examples of how to effectively search the literature to find answers to questions posed by researchers and research consumers.

Practical Application _____

With regard to the example of pain, a nurse working in a palliative care setting wondered whether completing pain diaries was useful for patients with advanced cancer who were receiving palliative care. She wondered whether they were spending time developing something that had previously been shown to be useless or even harmful—it is conceivable that monitoring one's pain in a diary actually heightens one's awareness and experience of pain. To focus her search of the literature, the nurse developed the following question: "Does the use of pain diaries in the palliative care of patients with cancer lead to improved pain control?"

Evidence-Informed Practice Tip ____

You should formulate clinical questions that arise from your clinical practice. Once you have developed a focused clinical question by using the PICOT format, search the literature for the best available evidence to answer your clinical question.

TABLE **4.1**			
ELEMENTS OF A CLINICAL QUESTION			
POPULATION	**INTERVENTION**	**COMPARISON INTERVENTION**	**OUTCOME**
People with advanced cancer	Pain diaries	No pain diaries	Increased pain control

BOX **4.2**

EXAMPLES OF CLINICAL QUESTIONS

- Do children younger than 12 years pose a higher infection potential for immunosuppressed patients than visitors older than 12 years? (Falk, Wongsa, Dang, et al., 2012)
- In a population of hospitalized older adults, is the onset of new urinary incontinence associated with the use of continence products (incontinence pads, urinary catheters, or independent toileting)? (Zisberg, Gary, Gur-Yaish, et al., 2011)
- In patients with chronic diseases like type 2 diabetes, can nurse practitioners trained in diabetes management deliver care similar to that of primary care physicians? (Houweling, Kleefstra, van Hateren, et al., 2011)
- Does use of effective home safety devices reduce home injuries in children younger than 3 years? (Phelan, Khoury, & Xu, 2011)
- Does an immunization navigator program for urban adolescents increase immunization rates? (Szilagyi, Humiston, Gallivan, et al., 2011)
- Do residents, family members, and clinicians find a sensor data interface used to monitor activity levels of older adults useful in independent living settings? (Alexander, Wakefield, Rantz, et al., 2011)

DEVELOPING AND REFINING A RESEARCH QUESTION

A researcher spends a great deal of time refining a research idea or problem into a research question. Unfortunately, the evaluator of a research study is not privy to this creative process because it occurs during the study's conceptualization. The final research question usually does not appear in the research article unless the study is qualitative rather than quantitative. Although this section does not teach you how to formulate a research question, it does provide an important glimpse into the researcher's process of developing a research question.

Research questions or topics do not arise spontaneously. As shown in Table 4.2, research questions should indicate that practical experience, critical appraisal of the scientific literature, or interest in an untested theory was the basis for the generation of a research idea. The research question should reflect a refinement of the researcher's initial thinking. The evaluator of a nursing research study should be able to discern that the researcher has done the following:

1. Defined a specific topic area
2. Reviewed the relevant scientific literature
3. Examined the question's potential significance in nursing
4. Pragmatically examined the feasibility of studying the research question

Defining the Research Question

Brainstorming with teachers, advisers, or colleagues may provide valuable feedback to help the researcher focus on a specific question area. For example, suppose a researcher told a colleague that an area of interest was whether men and women recovered differently after cardiac surgery. The colleague may have said, "What is it about the topic that specifically interests you?" Such a conversation may have initiated a train of thought that resulted in a decision to explore the recovery processes and gender differences. Box 4.3 illustrates how a broad area of interest was narrowed to a specific research topic.

Evidence-Informed Practice Tip ____

A well-developed research question guides a focused search for scientific evidence about assessing, diagnosing, treating, or assisting patients with understanding their prognosis with regard to a specific health problem.

Beginning the Literature Review

The literature review should reveal a collection of relevant individual studies and systematic reviews that have been critically examined (see Chapter 5). Concluding sections in such articles—that is, the recommendations and implications for practice—often identify remaining gaps in the literature, the need for replication, or the need for extension of the knowledge base about a particular research focus.

TABLE **4.2**

HOW PRACTICAL EXPERIENCE, SCIENTIFIC LITERATURE, AND UNTESTED THEORY INFLUENCE DEVELOPMENT OF A RESEARCH IDEA

AREA	INFLUENCE	EXAMPLE
Practical experience	Clinical practice provides a wealth of experience from which research problems can be derived. The nurse may observe the occurrence of a particular event or pattern and become curious about why it occurs, as well as its relationship to other factors in the patient's environment.	Of the 98,500 emergency visits by children, 25% are for the treatment of lacerations and open wounds. Although the treatment is relatively painless with the use of topical anaesthesia, the fear, anxiety, and distress associated with the experience are significant. Several techniques, such as distraction, have proved to have a positive effect on procedural distress. Can music be a useful tool to distract the child and involve the parent in positive behaviour (Sobieraj, Bhatt, LeMay, et al., 2009)?
Critical appraisal of the scientific literature	The critical appraisal of research studies that appear in journals may indirectly suggest a problem area by stimulating the reader's thinking. Nurses may observe the outcome data from a single study or a group of related studies that provide the basis for developing a pilot study or quality improvement project to determine the effectiveness of this intervention in their own practice.	Several studies have been conducted on the needs of family members of patients in the ICU. A subset focused on the informational needs of families. Families benefitted from informational interventions, as evidenced by improved comprehension, decreased anxiety, and increased satisfaction. The researchers recognized a need for better understanding of the family members' (1) perception of informational support, (2) anxiety levels, and (3) satisfaction with care and the relationships between these. The overall objective was to further refine the informational program and to initiate a formal evaluation program (Bailey, Sabbagh, Loiselle, et al., 2010).
	A research idea may also be suggested by a critical appraisal of the literature that identifies gaps and suggests areas for future study. Research ideas also can be generated by research reports that suggest the value of replicating a particular study to extend or refine the existing body of scientific knowledge.	Workplace bullying is prevalent in Canada, affecting millions of women every year. Being bullied at work is a devastating life experience with many negative consequences particularly related to physical, emotional, social, and economic well-being. Although many of the consequences have been studied extensively, absence because of sickness has not been extensively explored (O'Donnell, MacIntosh, & Wuest, 2010).
	Verification of an untested nursing theory provides relatively uncharted territory from which research questions can be derived. Inasmuch as theories themselves are not tested, a researcher may think about investigating a particular concept or set of concepts related to a particular nursing theory. The deductive process would be used to generate the research question. The researcher would pose questions such as "If this theory is correct, what kind of behaviour will I expect to observe in particular patients and under which conditions?" or "If this theory is valid, what kind of supporting evidence will I find?"	Health care structuring in Canada has resulted in considerable role changes for senior nurse leaders (SNLs), providing the opportunity for nurse leaders to leverage their leadership skills and play a greater role in decision making at the senior level. Little is known about the patterns of SNL decision making. Using an adapted theoretical framework on health care providers' participation in strategic decision making in health care organizations, Wong, Laschinger, Cummings, and associates (2010) described the scope and degree of involvement of SNLs in executive-level decisions in acute care organizations across Canada.

ICU, intensive care unit.

BOX **4.3**

DEVELOPMENT OF A RESEARCH QUESTION

IDEA EMERGES

- Senior nurse leaders' (SNLs') work post-restructuring

BRAINSTORMING

- Do the changes subsequent to the health care restructuring provide new opportunities for leadership and greater roles in decision making?
- Do the changes result in diminished authority and a decrease in representation at the policymaking level?
- What do nursing leaders perceive about their decision making?
- What are the organizational outcomes?

LITERATURE REVIEW

- In many cases the restructuring resulted in opportunities to provide leadership and to play a greater role in decision making.
- However, in other organizations without discipline-based nursing service, SNLs reported decreased direct supervision of nurses.
- Decision-making involvement can be measured, and there is a connection between involvement in decision activities, perceived influence over decisions, and organizational outcomes.
- The scope and intensity of SNL involvement in strategic decision-making is related to their perceptions of influence in the organization.

VARIABLES

- Independent (predictor) variable
  - Scope (timing and breadth) and intensity of participation (number of decision activities)
- Dependent variable
  - Decision-making influence

RESEARCH QUESTION

- Does the scope and intensity of SNL participation in executive decision-making processes predict the degree of SNL decision influence?

From Wong, C. A., Laschinger, H., Cummings, G. G., et al. (2010). Decisional involvement of senior nurse leaders in Canadian acute care hospitals. *Journal of Nursing Management, 18*, 122–133.

Qualitative and quantitative researchers conduct literature reviews differently. For qualitative researchers, the value of the literature review is controversial. Many researchers believe that an extensive literature review causes investigators to develop biases or beliefs that limit their openness to exploring the phenomenon under study. As a general rule, qualitative researchers usually start with a very cursory or general review of the literature to help focus the study, whereas quantitative researchers begin their study with an extensive review of the literature on their research questions and related topics (Streubert & Carpenter, 2011). The literature review also helps researchers determine whether their study can contribute to the field of nursing.

Qualitative researchers conduct a literature review during the data analysis or discussion of the findings to "tell the reader how the findings fit into what is already known about the phenomenon" (Streubert & Carpenter, 2011, p. 26).

The databases that researchers use for the literature review—for example, Cumulative Index to Nursing and Allied Health Literature (CINAHL), PsycINFO, MEDLINE, and PubMed—contain relevant articles that have been critically examined. Concluding sections in such articles (i.e., the recommendations and implications for practice) often identify remaining gaps in the literature, the need for replication, or the need for extension of the knowledge gleaned on a particular research focus.

In the example about decision making among senior nurse leaders (SNLs; see Box 4.3), the researchers may have conducted a preliminary review of books and journals for theories and research studies on the changes in the health care system, governance structures, and organizational models and factors related to decision making. These factors, termed *variables* in the language of research, should be potentially relevant, of interest, and measurable.

The search for relevant factors to SNL decision making that are mentioned in the literature might begin with an exploration of the scope and degree of SNLs' contributions to executive-level decisions in acute care organizations across Canada. Wong, Laschinger, Cummings, and associates (2010) investigated participation in strategic organizational decision making as a theoretical framework for describing such participation with the use of information processing and complexity science theories. The researcher can then use this information to further define the research question, to address a gap in the literature, and to extend the body of knowledge related to decision making among SNLs. At this point, the researcher could write the following tentative research question: "What is the scope and degree of SNL involvement after restructuring in acute care organizations across Canada?" After reading this question, you should be able to envision the interrelatedness of the initial definition of the research question, the literature review, and the refined research question. Readers of research reports examine the end product of this process in the form of a research question, hypothesis, or both. Thus, readers need an appreciation of how the researcher formulates the final research question directing the study.

 Research Hint _____

Reading the literature review or theoretical framework section of a research article helps you trace the development of the implied research question, hypothesis, or both.

Examining Significance

When considering a research question, it is crucial that the researcher has examined the question's potential significance to nursing. The research question should have the potential to contribute to and extend the scientific body of nursing knowledge. Guidelines for selecting research questions should meet the following criteria:

- Patients, nurses, the medical community in general, and society will potentially benefit from the knowledge derived from the study.
- The results will be applicable for nursing practice, education, or administration.
- The results will be theoretically relevant.
- The findings will lend support to untested theoretical assumptions, extend or challenge an existing theory, or clarify a conflict in the literature.
- The findings could lead to improved patient outcomes.
- The findings will potentially enable professionals to formulate or alter nursing practices or policies.

If the research question has not met any of these criteria, the researcher needs to extensively revise the question or discard it. For example, in the research question "Does the scope and intensity of SNL participation in executive decision-making processes predict the degree of SNL decision influence?" (see Box 4.3), the significance of the question includes the following facts:

- Health care restructuring has contributed to significant changes in SNLs' roles.
- New governance structures and organizational models have radically changed nursing leadership structures.
- SNLs' participation in decision making is important for an organization's strategic decisions.
- Participation in organizations' strategic decisions is associated with reductions in hospital costs and improvement in patient outcomes.

Evidence-Informed Practice Tip ____

Without a well-developed research question, the researcher may search for incorrect, irrelevant, or unnecessary information. Such information is a barrier to identifying the potential significance of the study.

Determining Feasibility

The feasibility of a research question must be examined pragmatically. Regardless of how significant or researchable a question may be, pragmatic considerations—such as time; availability of participants, facilities, equipment, and money; experience of the researcher; and any ethical considerations—may render the question inappropriate because it lacks feasibility. One of the most frequent issues is whether a sufficient number of participants can be recruited. If potential issues emerge affecting the feasibility of the study, the researcher may need to reconsider the research question and/or design.

THE FULLY DEVELOPED RESEARCH QUESTION

As discussed previously, qualitative researchers develop and refine a research question that outlines a general topic area. Examples include the following:

- What is the impact of an education program about acquired immune deficiency syndrome (AIDS) on the lives of a group of Ugandan nurses and nurse-midwives (Harrowing & Mill, 2010)?
- What is the effect of a brief, focused educational intervention on the quality of verbal interactions between nursing staff and patients in a chronic care facility (Boscart, 2009)?
- What is it about immunizing children who strongly resist needle injection that is a problem for public health nurses (Ives & Melrose, 2010)?

As a quantitative researcher finalizes a research question, the following three characteristics should be evident:

1. The *variables* under consideration are clearly identified.

2. The *population* being investigated is specified.
3. The possibility of empirical *testing* is implied.

Because each of these elements is crucial in the formulation of a satisfactory research question, the criteria are discussed in greater detail in the following sections. These elements can often be found in the introduction of the published article; however, they are not always stated in an explicit manner.

Research Hint _____

Remember that research questions are used to guide all types of research studies

Evidence-Informed Practice Tip ____

The answers to questions generated by qualitative data reflect evidence that may provide the first insights about a phenomenon that has not been studied previously.

Variables

Researchers call the properties that they study *variables*. Such properties take on different values. Thus, a **variable** is, as the name suggests, something that varies. Properties that differ from each other, such as age, weight, height, religion, and ethnicity, are examples of variables. Researchers attempt to understand how and why differences in one variable relate to differences in another variable. For example, a researcher may be concerned about the rate of pneumonia in postoperative patients on ventilators in critical care units. This rate is a variable because not all critically ill postoperative patients on ventilators have pneumonia. A researcher may also be interested in what other factors can be linked to ventilator-acquired pneumonia (VAP). Clinical evidence suggests that elevation of the head of the bed is also associated with VAP. You can see that these factors are also variables that need to be considered in relation to the development of VAP in postoperative patients.

When speaking of variables, the researcher is essentially asking, "Is X related to Y? What is the effect of X on Y? How are X_1 and X_2 related to Y?"* The researcher is asking a question about the relationship between one or more independent variables (X) and a dependent variable (Y).

An **independent variable,** usually symbolized by X, is the variable that has the presumed effect on the dependent variable. In experimental research studies, the researcher manipulates the independent variable. For example, a nurse may study how different methods of administering pain medication affect the patient's perception of pain intensity. The researcher may manipulate the independent variable (i.e., the method of administering pain medication) by using nurse- versus patient-controlled administration of analgesics. In nonexperimental research, the independent variable is not manipulated and is assumed to have occurred naturally before or during the study. For example, the researcher may be studying the relationship between gender and the perception of pain intensity. The independent variable—gender—is not manipulated; it is presumed to exist and is observed and measured in relation to pain intensity.

The **dependent variable,** represented by Y, is often referred to as the consequence or the presumed effect that varies with a change in the independent variable. The dependent variable is not manipulated. It is observed and assumed to vary with changes in the independent variable. Predictions are based on how changes to the independent variable will affect the dependent variable. The researcher is interested in understanding, explaining, or predicting the response of the dependent variable. For example, a researcher might assume that the perception of pain (i.e., the dependent variable) will vary according to the person's gender (i.e., the independent variable). In this case, the researcher is trying to

explain the perception of pain in relation to the gender: that is, male or female. Although variability in the dependent variable is assumed to depend on changes in the independent variable, this assumption does not imply that a causal relationship exists between X and Y or that changes in X cause Y to change.

In a study about nurses' attitudes toward patients with hepatitis C, the researcher discovered that older nurses had a more negative attitude about such patients than did younger nurses. The researcher did not conclude that the nurses' attitudes toward patients with hepatitis C were negative because of their age; however, it is apparent that there was a directional relationship between age and negative attitudes about patients with hepatitis C—that is, the older the nurses were, the more negative were their attitudes about patients with hepatitis C. This example highlights the fact that causal relationships are not necessarily implied by the independent and dependent variables; rather, only a relational statement with possible directionality is proposed.

Table 4.3 presents a number of examples to help you learn how to write research questions. Practise substituting other variables for the examples in the table. You will be surprised at the skill you develop in writing and critiquing research questions.

Although one independent variable and one dependent variable were used in the examples just given, there is no restriction on the number of variables that can be included in a research question. Remember, however, that questions should not be unnecessarily complex or unwieldy, particularly in beginning research efforts. Research questions that include more than one independent or dependent variable may be divided into more concise subquestions.

Finally, note that variables are not inherently independent or dependent. A variable that is classified as independent in one study may be considered dependent in another study. For example, a nurse may review an article about sexual behaviours

---

*Note: In cases in which multiple independent or dependent variables are present, subscripts are used to indicate the number of variables under consideration.

TABLE **4.3**

RESEARCH QUESTION FORMAT		
TYPE	FORMAT	EXAMPLE
QUANTITATIVE		
Correlational	Is there a relationship between X (independent variable) and Y (dependent variable) in the specified population?	Is there a relationship between the effectiveness of pain management strategies and quality of life?
Comparative	Is there a difference in Y (dependent variable) between people who have characteristic X (independent variable) and those who do not have characteristic X?	Is there a difference in prevention of osteoporosis in at-risk survivors of breast cancer who receive a combination of long-term progressive strength training exercises, alendronate, calcium, and vitamin D, in comparison with those who do not receive this treatment?
Experimental	Is there a difference in Y (dependent variable) between Group A, which received X (independent variable), and Group B, which did not receive X?	What is the difference in physical, social, and emotional adjustment in women with breast cancer (and their partners) who have received phase-specific standardized education by video versus phase-specific telephone counselling?
QUALITATIVE		
Phenomenological	What is or was it like to have X?	How do older adults learn to live with early-stage dementia?
Ethnographic	What is the experience of a select culture group with a specific phenomenon?	"What constitutes culturally safe care for people who use(d) illicit drugs and are affected by social disadvantages such as poverty and homelessness?" (Pauly, McCall, Browne, et al., 2015, p. 122) (Appendix C)

that are predictive of the risk for HIV infection or AIDS. In this case, HIV/AIDS is the dependent variable. In another article in which the relationship between HIV/AIDS and maternal parenting practices is considered, HIV/AIDS status is the independent variable. Whether a variable is independent or dependent depends on the role it plays in a particular study.

Population

The **population** (a well-defined set that has certain properties) is either specified or implied in the research question. If the scope of the question has been narrowed to a specific focus and the variables have been clearly identified, the nature of the population is evident to the reader of the research report. For example, a research question may be "Is there a relationship between the type of discharge planning for older adults hospitalized with heart failure and the outcomes for participating patients and their caregivers?" This question suggests that the population under consideration includes older adults hospitalized for heart failure and their caregivers. The question also implies that some of the older adults and their caregivers were involved in a provider–patient partnership model of discharge planning, in contrast to other older adults who received the usual discharge planning. The researcher or reader will have an initial idea of the composition of the study population from the outset.

Evidence-Informed Practice Tip

Make sure that the population of interest and the setting have been clearly described so that if you plan to replicate the study, you will know exactly who the study population needs to be.

Testability

The research question must be phrased in such a way that there is a specific issue that needs to be answered. In many cases, the question is **testable**—that is, measurable by quantitative methods. For example, the research question "Should postoperative patients control how much pain medication they receive?" is stated incorrectly, for a variety of reasons. One reason is that the question is not testable; it represents a value statement rather than a relational problem statement. A scientific or relational question must propose a relationship between an independent variable and a dependent variable in such a way that the variables can be measured. Many interesting and important questions are not valid research questions because they are not amenable to testing.

The question "Should postoperative patients control how much pain medication they receive?" could be revised from a philosophical question to a research question that implies testability. Examples of the revised research question are as follows:

- Is there a relationship between patient-controlled analgesia versus nurse-administered analgesia and the perception of postoperative pain?
- What is the effect of patient-controlled analgesia on pain ratings provided by postoperative patients?

These examples illustrate the relationship between the variables, identify the independent and dependent variables, and imply the testability of the research question.

Now that the elements of the formal research question have been presented in greater detail, this information can be integrated by formulating a formal research question. Earlier in this chapter, the following unrefined research question was formulated: "What is the scope and degree of SNL involvement after restructuring in acute care organizations across Canada?"

This research question was originally derived from a general area of interest: understanding the new role of SNLs in acute care organizations. The topic was more specifically defined by delineating a particular research question. The question crystallized further after a preliminary literature review and emerged in the unrefined form just given. It is now possible to propose a refined research question in which the problem is stated specifically in question form and the relationship of the key variables in the study, the population being studied, and the empirical testability of the question are specified: "Does the scope and intensity of SNL participation in executive decision-making processes predict the degree of SNL decision influence?"

As another example, Table 4.4 lists the components of the research question regarding variance in the perception of pain in relation to a person's age and gender.

 Research Hint _____

Remember that research questions are often not explicitly stated. The reader must infer the research question from the report's title, the abstract, the introduction, or the purpose.

TABLE **4.4**

COMPONENTS OF THE RESEARCH QUESTION AND RELATED CRITERIA

Testability	Differential effect of pain intensity and number of painful sites on functional disability (physical and social functioning)
Population	Adolescent males and females
Variables	**Independent Variables:** Pain intensity Pain sites Gender Health (number of limiting diagnoses) **Dependent Variables:** Management effectiveness Functional status

STUDY PURPOSE, AIMS, OR OBJECTIVES

Once the research question is developed and the literature review is critiqued in terms of the level, strength, and quality of evidence available for the particular research question, the purpose, aims, or objectives of the study become focused. The researcher can then decide whether a hypothesis should be tested or a research question answered.

The **purpose** of the study encompasses the aims or objectives the investigator hopes to achieve with the research, not the question to be answered. For example, a nurse working with patients with bladder dysfunction who are in rehabilitation may be disturbed by the high incidence of urinary tract infections. The nurse may propose the following research question: "What is the optimum frequency of changing urinary drainage bags in patients with bladder dysfunction to reduce the incidence of urinary tract infection?" If this nurse were to design a study, its purpose might be to determine the differential effect of 1-week and 4-week schedules of changing urinary drainage bags on the incidence of urinary tract infections in patients with bladder dysfunction.

The purpose communicates more than just the nature of the question. Through the researcher's selection of verbs, the purpose statement suggests the manner in which the researcher sought to study the question. Verbs such as *discover, explore,* or *describe* suggest an investigation of a relatively underresearched topic that might be more appropriately guided by research questions than by hypotheses. In contrast, verbs such as *test* (testing the effectiveness of an intervention) or *compare* (comparing two alternative nursing strategies) suggest a study with a better-established body of knowledge that is hypothesis testing in nature. Box 4.4 provides other examples of purpose statements.

 Evidence-Informed Practice Tip

The purpose, aims, or objectives often provide the most information about the intent of the research question and hypotheses and suggest the level of evidence to be obtained from the findings of the study.

DEVELOPING THE RESEARCH HYPOTHESIS

Like the research question, hypotheses are often not stated explicitly in a research article. The hypotheses are often embedded in the data analysis, results, or discussion section of the research report. You then need to discern the nature of the hypotheses being tested. Similarly, the population may not be explicitly described but is identified in the background, significance,

---

BOX 4.4

EXAMPLES OF PURPOSE STATEMENTS

"The aim of this study was to investigate the impact of subtle forms of workplace mistreatment (bullying and incivility) on Canadian nurses' perception of patient safety risk and, ultimately, nurse-assessed quality and prevalence of adverse events" (Laschinger, 2014, p. 284) (Appendix B).

"The purpose of this article is to report on findings from a community-based participatory study conducted in partnership with two Mi'kmaq communities in eastern Canada focused on cervical cancer screening" (MacDonald, Martin-Misener, Steenbeek, et al., 2015, p. 75) (Appendix A).

"Our goal was to generate knowledge to foster an understanding of the meaning and context of cultural safety in acute care settings for people who use, have used in the past, or are suspected of using illicit substances and are affected by poverty and/or homelessness" (Pauly et al., 2015, p. 122) (Appendix C).

"The purpose of this study was to design an approach to supporting the development of gender- and Aboriginal-specific messages regarding the link between tobacco exposure and breast cancer, drawing on youth perspectives" (Bottorff, Haines-Saah, Oliffe, et al., 2014, p. 66).

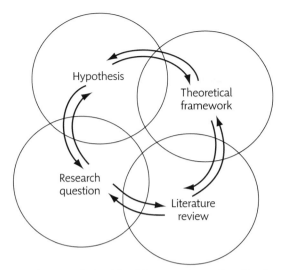

FIG. 4.2 Interrelationship of the research question, literature review, theoretical framework, and hypothesis.

and literature review. It is then up to you to discern the nature of the hypotheses and population being tested.

Hypotheses flow from the research question, literature review, and theoretical framework. Figure 4.2 illustrates this flow. A **hypothesis** is a statement about the relationship between two or more variables that suggests an answer to the research question. A hypothesis converts the question posed by the research question into a declarative statement that predicts an expected outcome. It explains or predicts the relationship or differences between two or more variables in terms of the expected results or outcomes of a study. Hypotheses are formulated before the study is actually conducted; they provide direction for the collection, analysis, and interpretation of data.

 Research Hint_____

When hypotheses are not explicitly stated by the author at the end of the "Introduction" section or before the "Methods" section, they are embedded or implied in the "Results" or "Discussion" section of a research article.

Characteristics

Nurses who are conducting research or critiquing published research studies must have a working knowledge of what constitutes a "good" hypothesis. Such knowledge provides a standard for evaluating their own work and the work of others. The following discussion about the characteristics of hypotheses presents criteria to be used when a hypothesis is formulated or evaluated.

Relationship Statement

The first characteristic of a hypothesis is that it is a declarative statement identifying the predicted relationship between two or more variables. This implies a systematic relationship between an independent variable *(X)* and a dependent variable *(Y)*. The direction of the predicted relationship is also specified in this statement. Phrases such as "greater than"; "less than"; "positively related," "negatively related," or "curvilinearly related"; and "difference in" connote the directionality that is proposed in the hypothesis. The following is an example of a directional hypothesis: "The rate of continuous smoking abstinence [dependent variable] at 6 months postpartum, according to self-report and biochemical validation, will be significantly higher in the treatment group [receiving postpartum counselling intervention] than in the control group [independent variable]." The dependent and independent variables are explicitly identified, and the relational aspect of the prediction in the hypothesis is contained in the phrase "significantly higher than."

The nature of the relationship, either causal or associative, is also implied by the hypothesis. A causal relationship is one in which the researcher can predict that the independent variable *(X)* causes a change in the dependent variable *(Y)*. In research, it is rare that a definitive stand can be assumed about a cause-and-effect relationship. For example, a researcher might hypothesize that relaxation training would have a significant effect on the physical and psychological health status of patients who have suffered myocardial infarction.

The researcher would have difficulty predicting a strong cause-and-effect relationship, however, because the multiple intervening variables (e.g., age, medication, and lifestyle changes) might also influence the participant's health status.

Variables are more commonly related in non-causal ways; that is, the variables are related but in an associative way. This means that variables change in relation to each other. For example, because strong evidence exists that asbestos exposure is related to lung cancer, a researcher may be tempted to state a causal relationship between asbestos exposure and lung cancer. However, not all individuals exposed to asbestos develop lung cancer and, conversely, not all individuals who have lung cancer have been exposed to asbestos. Thus, a position advocating a causal relationship between these two variables would be scientifically unsound. Instead, only an associative relationship exists between the variables of asbestos exposure and lung cancer, with a strong systematic association between the two phenomena.

Testability

The second characteristic of a hypothesis is its **testability.** The variables of the study must lend themselves to observation, measurement, and analysis. The hypothesis is either supported or not supported after the data have been collected and analyzed. The predicted outcome proposed by the hypothesis is or is not congruent with the actual outcome when the hypothesis is tested. Hypotheses advance scientific knowledge by confirming or refuting theories.

A hypothesis may fail to meet the criteria of testability because the researcher has not made a prediction about the anticipated outcome, because the variables are not observable or measurable, or because the hypothesis is couched in terms that are value laden.

Research Hint

When a hypothesis is complex (i.e., contains more than one independent or dependent variable), it is difficult for the findings to indicate unequivocally that the

hypothesis is supported or not supported. In such cases, the reader must infer which relationships are significant from the "Findings" or "Discussion" section.

Theory Base

A sound hypothesis is consistent with an existing body of theory and research findings. Whether a researcher arrives at a hypothesis inductively or deductively, the hypothesis must be based on a sound scientific rationale. Readers should be able to identify the flow of ideas from the research question to the literature review, to the theoretical framework, and to the hypotheses.

Wording the Hypothesis

As you become more familiar with the scientific literature, you will observe that a hypothesis can be worded in various ways. Regardless of the specific format used to state the hypothesis, the statement should be worded in clear, simple, and concise terms. If this criterion is met, the reader will understand the following:

- The variables of the hypothesis
- The population being studied
- The predicted outcome of the hypothesis

Information about hypotheses may be further clarified in the "Instruments," "Sample," or "Methods" section of a research report.

Statistical versus Research Hypotheses

Readers of research reports may observe that a hypothesis is further categorized as either a research or statistical hypothesis. A **research hypothesis,** also known as a *scientific hypothesis,* consists of a statement about the expected relationship of the variables. A research hypothesis indicates what the outcome of the study is expected to be. A research hypothesis is also either directional or nondirectional. If the researcher obtains statistically significant findings for a research hypothesis, the hypothesis is supported. The examples in Table 4.5 represent research hypotheses.

TABLE **4.5**

EXAMPLES OF HOW TO WORD A HYPOTHESIS

VARIABLES	HYPOTHESIS	TYPE OF DESIGN; LEVEL OF EVIDENCE SUGGESTED
1. There are significant differences in self-reported cancer pain, symptoms accompanying pain, and functional status according to gender.		
Independent Gender	Nondirectional, research	Nonexperimental; level IV
Dependent Self-reported cancer pain Symptoms accompanying pain Functional status		
2. Individuals who participate in usual care plus blood pressure telemonitoring will have a greater reduction in blood pressure from baseline to 12-month follow-up than will individuals who receive only usual care.		
Independent Telemonitoring Usual care	Directional, research	Experimental; level II
Dependent Blood pressure		
3. There will be a greater decrease in state anxiety scores for patients receiving structured informational videos before abdominal or chest tube removal than for patients receiving standard information.		
Independent Preprocedure structured video information Standard information	Directional, research	Experimental; level II
Dependent State anxiety		
4. The incidence and degree of severity of participants' discomfort will be lower after administration of medications by the Z-track intramuscular injection technique than after administration of medications by the standard intramuscular injection technique.		
Independent Z-track intramuscular injection technique Standard intramuscular injection technique	Directional, research	Experimental; level II
Dependent Participant discomfort		
5. Nurses with high levels of social support from co-workers have low perceived job stress.		
Independent Social support	Directional, research	Nonexperimental; level IV
Dependent Perceived job stress		
6. There will be no difference in rates of complications from anaesthetics between hospitals in which anaesthetics are administered primarily by certified registered nurse anaesthetists (CRNAs) and hospitals in which anaesthetics are administered primarily by anaesthesiologists (MDs).		
Independent Type of anaesthesia provider (CRNA or MD)	Nondirectional; null	Nonexperimental; level IV
Dependent Anaesthesia complication rate		

Continued

TABLE **4.5**

EXAMPLES OF HOW TO WORD A HYPOTHESIS—cont'd

VARIABLES	HYPOTHESIS	TYPE OF DESIGN; LEVEL OF EVIDENCE SUGGESTED
7. There will be no significant difference in the duration of patency of a 24-gauge intravenous lock in a neonatal patient when flushed with 0.5 mL of heparinized saline (2 U/mL), standard practice, in comparison with 0.5 mL of 0.9% normal saline.		
Independent Heparinized saline Normal saline	Nondirectional; null	Experimental; level II
Dependent Duration of patency of intravenous lock		

According to a **statistical hypothesis** (also known as a *null hypothesis*), there is no relationship between the independent and dependent variables. The examples in Table 4.6 illustrate statistical hypotheses. If, in the data analysis, a statistically significant relationship emerges between the variables at a specified level of significance, the statistical hypothesis is rejected. Rejection of the statistical hypothesis is equivalent to acceptance of the research hypothesis. For example, Simonson, Ahern, and Hendryx (2007) sought to identify differences in the rates of anaesthetic complications in hospitals whose obstetrical anaesthesia is provided solely by certified registered nurse anaesthetists (CRNAs) in comparison with hospitals with only anaesthesiologists. The statistical hypothesis—that there would be no differences in anaesthetic complication rates between the hospitals that relied on different anaesthesia providers—was supported. Because the difference in outcomes was not greater than that expected by chance, the statistical hypothesis was accepted. To further differentiate between a statistical hypothesis and a research hypothesis, consider the following hypotheses:

Research hypothesis: Hospitals with higher nurse-to-patient ratios will have fewer adverse patient events.

Statistical (null) hypothesis: There is no difference in the number of adverse patient events in hospitals with higher nurse-to-patient ratios.

Some researchers refer to the statistical hypothesis as a statistical contrivance that obscures a straightforward prediction of the outcome.

TABLE **4.6**

EXAMPLES OF STATISTICAL (NULL) HYPOTHESES

HYPOTHESIS	VARIABLES	TYPE OF DESIGN SUGGESTED
Oxygen inhalation by nasal cannula of up to 6 L/min does not affect oral temperature measurement taken with an electronic thermometer.	Independent: Oxygen inhalation by nasal cannula Dependent: Oral temperature	Experimental
There will be no difference in performance accuracy between adult nurse practitioners (ANPs) and family nurse practitioners (FNPs) in formulating accurate diagnoses and acceptable interventions for suspected cases of domestic violence.	Independent: Nurse practitioner (ANP or FNP) category Dependent: Diagnosis and intervention performance accuracy	Nonexperimental

Others state that it is more exact and conservative statistically and that failure to reject the statistical hypothesis implies that the evidence to support the idea of a real difference is insufficient. You will note that research hypotheses are generally used more often than statistical hypotheses because they are more desirable for stating the researcher's expectation. Readers then have a more precise idea of the proposed outcome. In any study that involves statistical analysis, the underlying statistical hypothesis is usually assumed without being explicitly stated.

Directional versus Nondirectional Hypotheses

Hypotheses can be formulated directionally or nondirectionally. A **directional hypothesis** specifies the expected direction of the relationship between the independent and dependent variables. The reader of a directional hypothesis may observe not only that a relationship is proposed but also the nature or direction of that relationship. The following is an example of a directional hypothesis: "The scope (timing and breadth) and intensity (number of decision-making processes) *positively* predicts the degree of SNL decision influence" (Wong et al., 2010, p. 125). Examples of directional hypotheses can also be found in examples 2 to 7 of Table 4.5.

Whereas a **nondirectional hypothesis** indicates the existence of a relationship between the variables, it does not specify the anticipated direction of the relationship. The following is an example of a nondirectional hypothesis ". . . bullying and civility influence nurse-assessed quality outcomes through their effect at nurses' perceptions of patient safety risk in their work settings emanating from negative workplace interactions" (Laschinger, 2014, p. 285).

Nurses who are learning to critique research studies should be aware that both the directional and nondirectional forms of hypothesis statements are acceptable. There are definite advantages and disadvantages that pertain to each form.

Proponents of the directional hypothesis argue that researchers naturally have hunches, guesses, or expectations about the outcome of their research. It is the hunch, the curiosity, or the guess that initially leads them to speculate about the question. The literature review and the conceptual framework provide the theoretical foundation for deriving the hypothesis. For example, the theory (e.g., self-efficacy theory) provides a critical rationale for proposing that relationships between variables have particular outcomes. When there is no theory or related research on which to base a rationale, or when findings in previous research studies are ambivalent, a nondirectional hypothesis may be appropriate. As you read research articles, you will note that directional hypotheses are much more commonly used than nondirectional hypotheses.

In summary, when you evaluate a hypothesis, note that directional hypotheses have several advantages that make them appropriate for use in most studies:

- Directional hypotheses indicate that a theory base was used to derive the hypotheses and that the phenomena under investigation have been critically examined and interrelated. You should note that nondirectional hypotheses may also be deduced from a theory base. Because of the exploratory nature of many studies for which the hypotheses are nondirectional, in contrast, the theory base may not be as developed.
- Directional hypotheses provide a specific theoretical frame of reference within which the study is being conducted.
- They suggest that the researcher believes that the evidence is indicative of a particular outcome, and as a result, the analyses of data can be accomplished in a statistically more sensitive way.

The important point about the directionality of the hypotheses is whether the rationale for the choice the researcher has proposed is sound.

RELATIONSHIP AMONG THE HYPOTHESIS, THE RESEARCH QUESTION, AND THE RESEARCH DESIGN

Regardless of whether the researcher uses a statistical or research hypothesis, there is a suggested relationship among the hypothesis, the research question, the research design of the study, and the level of evidence provided by the results of the study. The type of design, experimental or nonexperimental, influences the wording of the hypothesis. For example, when an experimental design is used, the research consumer would expect to see hypotheses that reflect relationship statements, such as the following:

- X_1 is more effective than X_2 on Y.
- The effect of X_1 on Y is greater than that of X_2 on Y.
- The incidence of Y will not differ in participants receiving X_1 and X_2 treatments.
- The incidence of Y will be greater in participants after X_1 than after X_2.

Such hypotheses indicate that an experimental treatment (i.e., independent variable X) will be used and that two groups of participants, experimental and control groups, are being used to test whether the difference in the outcome (i.e., dependent variable Y) predicted by the hypothesis exists. Hypotheses reflecting experimental designs also concern the effect of the experimental treatment (i.e., independent variable X) on the outcome (i.e., dependent variable Y).

In contrast, hypotheses related to nonexperimental designs reflect associative relationship statements such as the following:

- X will be negatively related to Y.
- A positive relationship will exist between X and Y.

Thus, in a study in which the hypotheses were associative relationship statements, the evidence provided by the results of that investigation have level IV strength (nonexperimental design).

The Critical Thinking Decision Path will help you determine both the type of hypothesis

presented in a study and the study's readiness for a hypothesis-testing design.

Evidence-Informed Practice Tip ____

Think about the relationship between the wording of the hypothesis, the type of research design suggested, and the level of evidence provided by the findings of a study with each kind of hypothesis. The research consumer may want to consider which type of hypothesis potentially will yield the strongest results applicable to practice.

CRITIQUING THE RESEARCH QUESTION

The Critiquing Criteria box on p. 86 provides several criteria for evaluating this initial phase of the research process: the research question. Because the research question represents the basis for the study, it is usually introduced at the beginning of the research report to indicate the focus and direction of the study. Readers are then in a position to evaluate whether the rest of the study logically pertains to this basis. The author often begins by identifying the background and significance of the issue that led to crystallizing development of the unanswered question. The clinical and scientific background, significance, or both are summarized, and the purpose, aim, or objective of the study is identified. Finally, the research question and any related subquestions are proposed before or after the literature review.

The purpose of the introductory summary of the theoretical and scientific background is to provide the reader with a contextual glimpse of how the author critically thought about the development of the research question. The introduction to the research question places the study within an appropriate theoretical framework and begins the description of the study. This introductory section should also include the significance of the study (i.e., why the investigator is conducting the study). For example, the significance may be to answer a question encountered in the clinical area and thereby improve patient care, to resolve a conflict in the literature regarding a clinical issue, or to provide data

CRITICAL THINKING DECISION PATH

Determining the Type of Hypothesis or Readiness for Hypothesis Testing

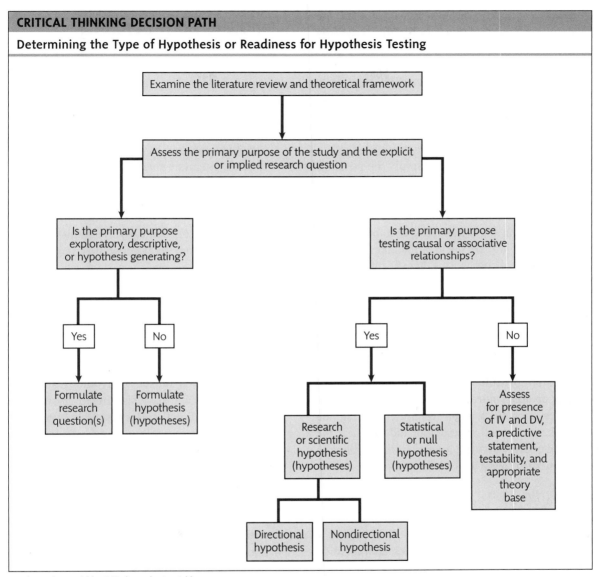

DV, dependent variable; IV, independent variable.

supporting an innovative form of nursing intervention that is more effective and is also cost-effective.

Sometimes readers find that the research question is not clearly stated at the conclusion of the introduction. In some cases, the author only hints at the research question, and the reader is challenged to identify it. In other cases, the author embeds the research question in the introductory text or purpose statement. To some extent, where or whether the author states the research question depends on the style of the journal. Nevertheless, the evaluator must remember that the main research question should be implied if it is not clearly identified in the introductory section—even if the subquestions are not stated or implied.

When critiquing the research question, the reader looks for the presence of the three key elements, described on p. 72:

- Does the research question express a relationship between two or more variables or, at least, between an independent variable and a dependent variable?
- Does the research question specify the nature of the population being studied?
- Does the research question imply the possibility of empirical testing?

You will use these three elements as criteria for judging the soundness of a stated research question. If the variables, the population, and the implications for testability are unclear, then the remainder of the study will probably falter. For example, a research study on anxiety during the perioperative period contained introductory material on anxiety in general, anxiety as it relates to the perioperative period, and the potentially beneficial influence of nursing care in relation to anxiety reduction. The author concluded that the purpose of the study was to determine whether selected measures of patient anxiety could be shown to vary when different approaches to nursing care were used during the perioperative period. The author did not state the research questions. A restatement of the problem in question form might be as follows:

> What is the difference in patient anxiety level in relation to different approaches to nursing care during the perioperative period?

If this process of developing a research question is clarified at the outset of a research study, the report that follows can develop logically. Readers will have a clear idea of what the report should convey and can knowledgeably evaluate the material that is presented. When you critically appraise clinical questions, remember that they should be focused and specify the patient or problem being addressed, the intervention, and the outcome for a particular patient population. The author should provide evidence that the clinical question guided the literature search and that the question suggests the design and level of evidence to be obtained from the study findings.

CRITIQUING THE HYPOTHESES

As illustrated in the Critiquing Criteria box, several criteria for critiquing the hypotheses should be used as a standard for evaluating the strengths and weaknesses of the hypotheses in a research report:

1. When reading a research study, you may find the hypotheses clearly delineated in a separate hypothesis section of the research article (i.e., after the literature review or theoretical framework section or sections). In many cases, the hypotheses are not explicitly stated and are only implied in the results or discussion section of the article. In such cases, you must infer the hypotheses from the purpose statement and the type of analysis used. You should not assume that if hypotheses do not appear at the beginning of the article, they do not exist in the particular study. Even when hypotheses are stated at the beginning of an article, they are re-examined in the results or discussion section as the findings are presented and discussed.

2. If a hypothesis or set of hypotheses is presented, the data analysis should answer the hypotheses directly. Because the hypothesis should reflect the culmination and expression of this conceptual process, its placement in the research report logically follows the literature review and the theoretical framework discussion. It should be consistent with both the literature review and the theoretical framework.

3. Although a hypothesis can legitimately be nondirectional, it is preferable and more common for the researcher to indicate the direction of the relationship between the variables in the hypothesis. You will find that when data for the literature review are unavailable (i.e., the researcher has chosen to study a relatively undefined area of interest), a nondirectional hypothesis may be appropriate. Enough information simply may not be available for making a sound judgement about the direction of the proposed relationship. All that can be proposed is that there will be a relationship between two variables. Essentially, you will want

to determine the appropriateness of the researcher's choice regarding directionality of the hypothesis.

4. The notion of testability is central to the soundness of a hypothesis. One criterion related to testability is that the hypothesis should be stated in such a way that it can be clearly supported or dismissed. Although this criterion is very important to keep in mind, you should also understand that, ultimately, theories or hypotheses are never proved beyond a doubt through hypothesis testing. Claims that certain data have "proved" the validity of their hypothesis should be regarded with grave reservation. At best, findings that support a hypothesis are considered tentative. If repeated replication of a study yields the same results, more confidence can be placed in the conclusions advanced by the researchers. It is important to remember about testability that although hypotheses are more likely to be accepted with increasing evidence, they are ultimately never proved.

5. Another point about testability to consider is that the hypothesis should be objectively stated and devoid of any value-laden words. Value-laden hypotheses are not empirically testable. Quantifiable phrases—such as "greater than"; "less than"; "decrease"; "increase"; "positively related"; "negatively related"; and "related"—convey the idea of objectivity and testability. You should immediately be suspicious of hypotheses that are not stated objectively.

6. You should recognize that how the proposed relationship of the hypothesis is phrased suggests the type of research design that is appropriate for the study, as well as the level of evidence to be derived from the findings. For example, if a hypothesis proposes that treatment X_1 will have a greater effect on Y than treatment X_2, an experimental (level II evidence) or quasiexperimental design (level III evidence) is suggested. If a hypothesis proposes that there will be a positive relationship between variables X and Y, a nonexperimental design (level IV evidence) is suggested. Table 4.5 contains additional examples of hypotheses, the type of research design, and the level of evidence that is suggested by each hypothesis. The design and level of evidence have important implications for the remainder of the study in terms of the appropriateness of sample selection, data collection, data analysis, interpretation of findings, and—ultimately—the conclusions advanced by the researcher.

7. If the research report contains research questions rather than hypotheses, you will want to evaluate whether this is appropriate for the study. One criterion for making this decision, as presented earlier in this chapter, is whether the study is of an exploratory, a descriptive, or a qualitative nature. If it is, then it is appropriate to have research questions rather than hypotheses.

APPRAISING THE EVIDENCE

The Research Question and Hypotheses

The care taken by a researcher when developing the research question or hypothesis is often representative of the overall conceptualization and design of the study. A methodically formulated research question provides the basis for hypothesis development. In a quantitative research study, the remainder of the study revolves around testing the hypothesis or, in some cases, the research question. In a qualitative research study, the objective is to answer the research question. This task may be a time-consuming, sometimes frustrating endeavour for the researcher, but in the final analysis, the outcome, as evaluated by the consumer, is most often worth the struggle. Because this text focuses on the nurse as a critical consumer of research, the sections in this chapter pertain primarily to the evaluation of research questions and hypotheses in published research reports.

CRITIQUING CRITERIA

THE RESEARCH QUESTION

1. Was the research question introduced promptly?
2. Is the question stated clearly and unambiguously in declarative or question form?
3. Does the research question express a relationship between two or more variables or at least between an independent variable and a dependent variable, thereby implying its empirical testability?
4. Does the research question specify the nature of the population being studied?
5. Has the research question been substantiated by adequate experiential and scientific background material?
6. Has the research question been placed within the context of an appropriate theoretical framework?
7. Has the significance of the research question been identified?
8. Have pragmatic issues, such as feasibility, been addressed?
9. Have the purpose, aims, or goals of the study been identified?
10. Are research questions appropriately used (i.e., for an exploratory, descriptive, or qualitative study or in relation to ancillary data analyses)?

THE HYPOTHESES

1. Is the hypothesis related directly to the research question?
2. Is the hypothesis stated concisely in a declarative form?
3. Are the independent and dependent variables identified in the statement of the hypothesis?
4. Are the variables measurable or potentially measurable?
5. Is each of the hypotheses specific to one relationship so that each hypothesis can be either supported or not supported?
6. Is the hypothesis stated in such a way that it is testable?
7. Is the hypothesis stated objectively, without value-laden words?
8. Is the direction of the relationship in each hypothesis clearly stated?
9. Is each hypothesis consistent with the literature review?
10. Is the theoretical rationale for the hypothesis explicit?

CRITICAL THINKING CHALLENGES

- Drawing from your nursing experience, develop some research questions using both the PICOT and SPIDER tools. How do the questions differ?
- Discuss how the wording of a research question or hypothesis suggests the type of research design and level of evidence that will be provided.
- A nurse is caring for patients in a clinical situation that produces a clinical question that has no ready answer. The nurse wants to develop and refine this clinical question by using the PICOT approach so that it becomes the basis for an evidence-informed practice project. How can the nurse accomplish that objective?

KEY POINTS

- Focused clinical questions arise from clinical practice and guide the literature search for the best available evidence to answer the clinical question.
- Formulation of the research question and stating the hypothesis are key preliminary steps in the research process.
- The research question is refined through a process that proceeds from the identification of a general idea of interest to the definition of a more specific and circumscribed topic.
- A preliminary literature review reveals related factors that appear to be critical for the research topic of interest and helps further define the research questions.
- The significance of the research question must be identified in terms of its potential contribution to patients, nurses, the medical community in general, and society. The applicability of the question for nursing practice and its theoretical relevance must be established. The findings should also have the potential for formulating or altering nursing practices or policies.
- The feasibility of a research question must be examined in light of pragmatic considerations: for example, time; the availability of participants, money, facilities, and equipment; the nurse's experience; and ethical issues.

- The final research question consists of a statement about the relationship of two or more variables. The question clearly identifies the relationship between the independent variables and dependent variables, specifies the nature of the population being studied, and implies the possibility of empirical testing.
- A hypothesis is an attempt to answer the research question. When the validity of the assumptions of the theoretical framework is tested, the hypothesis connects the theory and reality.
- A hypothesis is a declarative statement about the relationship between two or more variables in which an expected outcome is predicted. The characteristics of a hypothesis include a relationship statement, implications regarding testability, and consistency with a defined theory base.
- Hypotheses can be formulated directionally or nondirectionally. Hypotheses can be further categorized as either research or statistical (null) hypotheses.
- Research questions may be used instead of hypotheses in exploratory, descriptive, or qualitative research studies. Research questions may also be formulated in addition to hypotheses to answer questions related to ancillary data.
- The purpose, research question, or hypothesis provides information about the intent of the research question and hypothesis and suggests the level of evidence to be obtained from the study findings.
- The critiquing criteria are a set of guidelines for evaluating the strengths and weaknesses of the research question and hypotheses as they appear in a research report.
- In critiquing, the reader assesses the clarity of the research question and the related subquestions, the specificity of the population, and the implications for testability.
- The interrelatedness of the research question, the literature review, the theoretical framework, and the hypotheses should be apparent.

- The appropriateness of the research design suggested by the research question is also evaluated.
- The purpose of the study (i.e., why the researcher is conducting the study) should be differentiated from the research question.
- The reader evaluates the wording of the hypothesis in terms of the clarity of the relational statement, its implications for testability, and its congruence with theory. The appropriateness of the hypothesis in relation to the type of research design is also examined. In addition, the appropriate use of research questions is evaluated in relation to the type of study conducted.

FOR FURTHER STUDY

(e) Go to Evolve at http://evolve.elsevier.com/ Canada/LoBiondo/Research for the Audio Glossary and Appendix Tables that provide supplemental information for Appendix E.

REFERENCES

Alexander, G. L., Wakefield, B. J., Rantz, M., et al. (2011). Passive sensor technology interface to assess elder activity in independent living. *Nursing Research*, *60*(5), 114–122.

Bailey, J. J., Sabbagh, M., Loiselle, C. G., et al. (2010). Supporting families in the ICU: A descriptive correlational study of informational support, anxiety, and satisfaction with care. *Intensive & Critical Care Nursing*, *26*(2), 114–122.

Boscart, V. M. (2009). A communication intervention for nursing staff in chronic care. *Journal of Advanced Nursing*, *65*(9), 1823–1832.

Bottorff, J. L., Haines-Saah, R., Oliffe, J. L., et al. (2014). Designing tailored messages about smoking and breast cancer: A focus group study with youth. *Canadian Journal of Nursing Research*, *46*(1), 66–86.

Cooke, A., Smith, S., & Booth, A. (2012). Beyond PICO: The SPIDER tool for qualitative evidence synthesis. *Qualitative Health Research*, *22*(10), 1435–1443.

Cullum, N. (2000). User's guides to the nursing literature: An introduction. *Evidence-Based Nursing, 3*(2), 71–72.

Falk, J., Wongsa, S., Dang, J., et al. (2012). Using an evidence-based practice process to change child visitation guidelines. *Clinical Journal of Oncology Nursing, 16*(1), 21–23.

Harrowing, J. N., & Mill, J. (2010). Moral distress among Ugandan nurses providing HIV care: A critical ethnography. *International Journal of Nursing Studies, 47*, 723–731.

Houweling, S. T., Kleefstra, N., van Hateren, K. J., et al. (2011). Can diabetes management be safely transferred to nurses in a primary care setting: A randomized controlled trial. *Journal of Clinical Nursing, 20*, 1264–1272.

Ives, M., & Melrose, S. (2010). Immunizing children who fear and resist needles: Is it a problem for nurses? *Nursing Forum, 45*(1), 29–39.

Laschinger, H. K. S. (2014). Impact of workplace mistreatment on patient safety risk and nurse-assessed patient outcomes. *Journal of Nursing Administration, 44*(5), 284–290.

MacDonald, C., Martin-Misener, R., Steenbeek, A., et al. (2015). Honouring stories: Mi'kmaq women's experiences with Pap screening in Eastern Canada. *Canadian Journal of Nursing Research, 47*(1), 72–96.

Melnyk, B. M., & Fineout-Overholt, E. (2011). *Evidence-based practice in nursing and healthcare: A guide to best practice* (2nd ed.). New York: Wolters Kluwer.

O'Donnell, S., MacIntosh, J., & Wuest, J. (2010). A theoretical understanding of sickness absences among women who have experienced workplace bullying. *Qualitative Health Research, 20*(4), 439–452.

Pauly, B., McCall, J., Browne, A. J., et al. (2015). Toward cultural safety: Nurse and patient perceptions of illicit substance use in a hospitalized setting. *Advances in Nursing Science, 38*(2), 121–135.

Phelan, K. J., Khoury, J., & Xu, Y. (2011). A randomized controlled trial of home injury hazard reduction the HOME injury study. *Archives of Pediatric Adolescent Medicine, 165*, 339–345.

Sackett, D. L., Straus, S. E., Richardson, W. S., et al. (2000). *Evidence-based medicine: How to practise and teach EBM*. London: Churchill Livingstone.

Simonson, D. C., Ahern, M. M., & Hendryx, M. S. (2007). Anesthesia staffing and anesthetic complications during cesarean delivery: A retrospective analysis. *Nursing Research, 56*(1), 9–17.

Sobieraj, G., Bhatt, M., LeMay, S., et al. (2009). The effect of music on parental participation during pediatric laceration repair. *Canadian Journal of Nursing Research, 41*(4), 68–82.

Streubert, H. J., & Carpenter, D. R. (2011). *Qualitative research in nursing: Advancing the humanistic imperative* (5th ed.). Philadelphia: Wolters Kluwer.

Szilagyi, P. G., Humiston, S. G., Gallivan, S., et al. (2011). Effectiveness of a citywide patient immunization navigator program on improving adolescent immunizations and preventive care visit rates. *Archives of Pediatric Adolescent Medicine, 165*, 547–553.

Thompson, C., Cullum, N., McCaughan, D., et al. (2004). Nurses, information use, and clinical decision making: The real world potential for evidence-based decisions in nursing. *Evidence-Based Nursing, 7*(3), 68–72.

Wong, C. A., Laschinger, H., Cummings, G. G., et al. (2010). Decisional involvement of senior nurse leaders in Canadian acute care hospitals. *Journal of Nursing Management, 18*, 122–133.

Zisberg, A., Gary, S., Gur-Yaish, N., et al. (2011). In-hospital use of continence aids and new-onset urinary incontinence in adults aged 70 and older. *Journal of the American Geriatric Society, 59*, 1099–1104.

CHAPTER 5

Finding and Appraising the Literature

Stephanie Fulton | Barbara Krainovich-Miller | Cherylyn Cameron

LEARNING OUTCOMES

After reading this chapter, you will be able to do the following:

- Discuss the relationship of the literature review to nursing theory, research, education, and practice.
- Discuss the purposes of the literature review research projects and for evidence-informed projects.
- Differentiate between primary and secondary sources.
- Compare the advantages and disadvantages of the most commonly used online databases for conducting a literature review.
- Identify the characteristics of an effective electronic search of the literature.
- Critically read, appraise, and synthesize primary and secondary sources used for the development of a literature review.
- Apply critiquing criteria to the evaluation of literature reviews in selected research studies.

KEY TERMS

Boolean operator	literature review	refereed (peer-reviewed)
citation management	online database	journal
software	primary sources	secondary sources
controlled vocabulary	print indexes	web browser

STUDY RESOURCES

(e) Go to Evolve at http://evolve.elsevier.com/Canada/LoBiondo/Research for the Audio Glossary and Appendix Tables that provide supplemental information for Appendix E.

YOU MAY WONDER WHY AN ENTIRE chapter of a research text is devoted to finding and appraising the literature. The main reason is that searching for, retrieving, and critically appraising the literature is a key step in the research process for researchers and for nurses implementing evidence-informed practice. A more personal question you might ask is "Will knowing more about how to critically appraise and gather the literature really help me as a student or later as a practising nurse?" The answer is that it most certainly will! Your ability to locate and retrieve research studies, critically appraise them, and decide that you have the best available evidence to inform your clinical decision making is a skill essential for your current role as a student and your future role as a nurse who is a competent research consumer.

Your critical appraisal, also called a *critique of the literature,* is an organized systematic approach to evaluating a research study or group of research studies. It involves the use of a set of established critical appraisal criteria to objectively determine the strength, quality, and consistency of evidence; these characteristics help you determine the applicability of the evidence to research, education, or practice. As a research consumer, you will become skilled at critically appraising research studies, combining the evidence with your clinical experience and the patient population who you are caring for, to make an evidence-informed decision about the applicability of a particular nursing intervention for your patient or for the patient population in your practice setting.

The section of a published research report titled "Literature Review" generally appears near the beginning of the report. It provides an abbreviated version of the complete literature review conducted by a researcher and represents the foundation for the study. Therefore, the **literature review,** a systematic and critical appraisal of the most important literature on a topic, is a key step in the research process that provides the basis of a research study.

The conceptual framework, or theoretical framework, of a research report is a structure of concepts or theories pulled together as a map for the study; this map provides rationale for the development of research questions or hypotheses. This section of a research report is often a titled subsection of the literature review and may be accompanied by a diagram illustrating the proposed relationships between and among the concepts. Alternatively, the conceptual/theoretical framework may not be separately identified; it may be embedded in the literature review section of an article or simply not included. The links between theory, research, education, and practice are intricately connected; together they create the knowledge base for the nursing discipline, as shown in Figure 5.1.

The purpose of this chapter is to introduce you to the literature review as it is used in research and evidence-informed practice projects. It provides you with the systematic tools to (1) consider how the theoretical or conceptual framework guides development of a research study; (2) critically appraise a research study or group of research studies; (3) locate, search for, and retrieve research studies, systematic reviews, documents, and statistical reports; and (4) differentiate between a research article and a conceptual article or book. This set of tools will help you

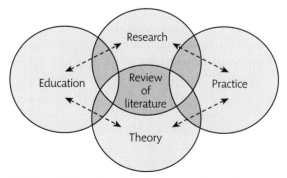

FIG. 5.1 Relationship of the literature review to theory, research, education, and practice.

develop your research consumer competencies and prepare your academic papers and evidence-informed practice projects.

REVIEW OF THE LITERATURE

The Literature Review: Evidence-Informed Project

From the perspective of a clinical practitioner, you review a number of studies to answer a clinical question or to solve a clinical problem. Therefore, you search the literature widely and gather multiple resources to answer your question by using an evidence-informed practice approach. This process includes (1) asking clinical questions; (2) identifying and gathering the evidence; (3) critically appraising and synthesizing the evidence or literature; (4) acting to change practice by using the best available evidence, coupled with your clinical experience and patient preferences (values, setting, and resources); and (5) evaluating the use of the research evidence found to assess applicability of the research findings to the practice change. In Box 5.1, objectives 1 through 3 reflect the purposes of a literature review for nurses involved in evidence-informed practice projects.

As a student or practising nurse, you may be asked to generate a clinical question for an evidence-informed practice project. For this you need to search for, retrieve, review, and critically appraise the literature to identify the "best available evidence" that provides the answer to a clinical question. A clear and precise articulation of a question is crucial for finding the best evidence. Evidence-informed questions may sound like research questions, but they are questions used to search the existing literature for answers. The evidence-informed practice process follows the PICOT format to generate clinical questions. For example, students in an adult health course were asked to generate a clinical question related to health care promotion for older women by

---

BOX 5.1

OVERALL PURPOSES OF A LITERATURE REVIEW

MAJOR GOAL
To develop a strong knowledge base to carry out a research study or an evidence-informed practice project

OBJECTIVES
A review of the literature helps you do the following:
1. Uncover one or more new practice interventions or obtain supporting evidence for revising or maintaining current interventions, protocols, and policies
2. Promote evidence-informed revision and development of new practice protocols, policies, and projects or activities related to nursing practice
3. Generate clinical questions that guide development of evidence-iznformed practice projects
4. Determine what is known and unknown about a subject, concept, or problem
5. Determine gaps, consistencies, and inconsistencies in the literature about a subject, concept, or problem
6. Discover conceptual traditions used to examine problems
7. Generate useful research questions and hypotheses
8. Determine an appropriate research design, methodology, and analysis for answering the research questions or hypotheses on the basis of an assessment of the strengths and weaknesses of earlier works
9. Determine the need for replication of a study or refinement of a study
10. Synthesize the strengths and weaknesses and findings of available studies on a topic or problem

---

using the PICOT format. As discussed in Chapter 4, The PICOT format is as follows:

P: Problem/patient population; specifically defined group

I: Intervention; what intervention or event will be studied

C: Comparison intervention; with what the intervention will be compared

O: Outcome; the effect of the intervention

T: Time; the time frame

An example of its use is given in the following Practical Application box. You may also utilize the SPIDER tool, as described in Chapter 4, Figure 4.1 (p. 67).

> ### Practical Application
>
> One group of students was interested in whether regular exercise prevented osteoporosis for postmenopausal women who had osteopenia. The PICOT format for the clinical question that guided their search was as follows:
>
> **P:** Postmenopausal women with osteopenia
> **I:** Regular exercise program
> **C:** No regular exercise program
> **O:** Prevention of osteoporosis
> **T:** After 1 year
>
> Another set of students was interested in whether regular exercise improved the quality of life for postmenopausal women who had osteopenia. The SPIDER format that guided their search was as follows:
>
> **S:** Postmenopausal women with osteopenia
> **PI:** Quality of life of postmenopausal women with osteopenia who regularly exercised
> **D:** Exploratory studies, lived experience, survey, focus group, case study
> **E:** Quality of life, well-being, attitude, experience
> **R:** Qualitative, mixed-research, quantitative
>
> Their assignment required that the students do the following:
> - Search the literature by using electronic databases (e.g., Cumulative Index to Nursing and Allied Health Literature [CINAHL] via EBSCO; MEDLINE; Scopus; and Cochrane Database of Systematic Reviews) for the background information that enabled them to identify the significance of osteopenia and osteoporosis as a health problem in women.
> - Identify systematic reviews, practice guidelines, and individual research studies that provided the "best available evidence" related to the effectiveness and experiences of regular exercise programs on prevention of osteoporosis.
> - Critically appraise systematic reviews, practice guidelines, and research studies in accordance with standardized critical appraisal criteria (see Chapter 20).
> - Synthesize the overall strengths and weaknesses of the evidence provided by the literature.
> - Establish a conclusion about the strength, quality, and consistency of the evidence.
> - Make recommendations on the applicability of the evidence to clinical nursing practice that guides development of a health promotion project about osteoporosis risk reduction for postmenopausal women with osteopenia.

As a practising nurse, you may be called on to revise or continue current evidence-informed practice protocols, practice standards, or policies in your health care organization or to develop new ones. This requires that you know how to retrieve and critically appraise research articles, systematic reviews, and practice guidelines to determine the degree of support or lack of support found in the literature. A critical appraisal of the literature related to a specific clinical question uncovers data that contribute evidence to support current practice and clinical decision making, as well as for making changes in practice.

The Literature Review: Research Study

The overall purpose of the literature review in a research study is to present a strong knowledge base for the conduct of the research study.

Objectives 4 through 10 listed in Box 5.1 reflect the purposes of a literature review for conducting quantitative research and most qualitative research. It is important to understand when you read a research article that the researcher's main goal when developing the literature review was to develop the knowledge foundation for a sound study and to generate research questions and hypotheses.

An extensive literature review is essential for all steps of the quantitative research process and for some qualitative methods. From this perspective, the review is broad and systematic, as well as in-depth. It is a critical collection and evaluation of the important published literature in journals, monographs, books, and book chapters, as well as unpublished research print and online materials (e.g., doctoral dissertations and masters' theses), audiovisual materials (e.g., audio

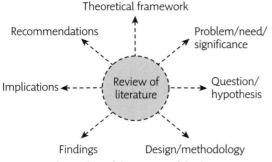

Theoretical framework

Recommendations

Problem/need/ significance

Implications ← Review of literature → Question/ hypothesis

Findings

Design/methodology

FIG. 5.2 Relationship of the review of the literature to the steps of the research process.

and video recordings), and sometimes personal communications (e.g., conference presentations and one-on-one interviews).

From a researcher's perspective, the objectives in Box 5.1 direct the questions the researcher asks while reading the literature to determine one or more useful research questions or hypotheses and how best to design a particular study.

The following brief overview about the use of the literature review in relation to the steps of the research process will help you to understand the researcher's focus (Figure 5.2). A critical review of relevant literature affects the steps of the quantitative research process as follows:

- *Theoretical or conceptual framework:* A literature review reveals conceptual traditions, concepts, theories, or conceptual models from nursing and other related disciplines that can be used to examine problems. This framework presents the context for studying the problem and can be viewed as a map for understanding the relationships between or among the variables in research studies. The literature review provides rationale for the variables and explains concepts, definitions, and relationships between or among the independent and dependent variables used in the theoretical framework of the study. However, in many research articles the literature review may not be labelled.

- *Primary and secondary sources:* The author of a literature review should use mainly **primary sources**—that is, articles and books by the original author. Sometimes it is appropriate to use **secondary sources,** which are published articles or books that are written by persons other than the individual who developed the theory or conducted the research study. The studies selected for the literature review should offer the strongest and most consistent level of evidence available on the topic (Table 5.1 lists examples).

- *Research question and hypothesis:* The literature review helps you determine what is known and not known; uncover gaps, consistencies, or inconsistencies; or to disclose unanswered questions in the literature about a subject, concept, theory, or problem that generate or allow for refinement of research questions, hypotheses, or both.

- *Design and method:* The literature review exposes the strengths and weaknesses of previous studies in terms of designs and methods and helps the researcher choose an appropriate new, replicated, or refined design, including data-collection method, sampling strategy and size, valid and reliable measurement instruments, an effective data analysis method, and appropriate informed consent forms. Often, because of journal space limitations, researchers only include abbreviated information about these aspects in their journal article.

- *Outcome of the analysis (i.e., findings, discussion, implications, and recommendations):* The literature review is used to help the researcher accurately interpret and discuss the results or findings of a study. In the discussion section of a research article, the researcher refers to the research studies and theoretical articles or books described earlier in the article in the literature review and uses this conceptual and research literature to interpret and explain the study's findings.

TABLE **5.1**

PRIMARY AND SECONDARY SOURCES

PRIMARY: ESSENTIAL	SECONDARY: USEFUL
Material written by the original person who conducted the study, developed the theory (model), or prepared the scholarly discussion on a concept, topic, or issue of interest (i.e., the original author).	Material written by one or more individuals other than the person who conducted the research study or developed a theory; the author is someone other than the original author who writes about or presents the original author's work. The material is usually in the form of a summary or critique (i.e., analysis and synthesis) of someone else's scholarly work or body of literature.
Primary sources can be published or unpublished.	Secondary sources can be published or unpublished.
Research example: An investigator's report of his or her research study (e.g., articles in Appendices A through D).	Secondary source examples are the following: response, commentary, or critique articles of a research study, a theory or model, or a professional view of an issue; review of literature article published in a refereed scholarly journal; abstracts of a published work written by someone other than the original author; examples: a biography or a systematic review.
Theoretical example: Senior nurse leaders' participation in organizational decision making is the theoretical framework used by Wong, Laschinger, Cummings, et al. (2010) in their study of the scope and degree of senior nurse leaders' contributions to executive-level decisions. The theoretical framework used in this study was adapted from the work of Ashmos, Huonker, and McDaniel (1998) and Anderson and McDaniel (1998) and cited as such in the research report. Other primary source examples include autobiographies, diaries, films, letters, artifacts, periodicals, and tapes.	*Hint:* Use secondary sources sparingly; however, secondary sources—especially of studies that include a research critique—are a valuable learning tool for a beginning research consumer.
Hint: Critical evaluation of mainly primary sources is essential in a thorough and relevant review of the literature.	

Differences and Similarities in Literature Reviews for Evidence-Informed Projects and Research Studies

How does the literature review differ when it is used for evidenced-informed research purposes from when it is used for a research study? The literature review in a research study is used to develop a sound research proposal for a research study that will generate knowledge. From a broader perspective, the major focus of reviewing the literature for a research-informed project is to uncover multiple sources of evidence on a given topic that have been generated by researchers in their research studies that can potentially be used to improve clinical practice and patient outcomes.

 Research Hint _____

Remember that the findings of one study on a topic do not usually provide sufficient evidence to support a change in practice; be cautious when a nurse colleague tells you to change your practice on the basis of the results of one study.

From a student perspective, the ability to critically appraise the literature is essential to acquiring a skill set for successfully completing scholarly papers, presentations, debates, and evidence-informed practice projects. Both types of literature reviews are similar in that both should be framed in the context of previous research and theoretical literature and pertinent to the objectives presented in Box 5.1.

Evidence-Informed Practice Tip ___

For a research consumer, formulating a clinical question provides a focus that guides the literature review.

SEARCHING FOR EVIDENCE

In your student role, when you are preparing an academic paper, you read the required course materials, as well as additional literature retrieved from the library. Students often state, "I know how to do research." Perhaps you have thought the same thing because you "researched" a topic for a paper in the library. In that situation, however, it would be more accurate for you to say that you have been "searching" the literature to uncover research and conceptual information to prepare an academic term paper on a certain topic. You search for primary sources, which are articles, books, or other documents written by the person who conducted the study, developed the theory, or prepared the scholarly discussion on a concept, topic, problem, or issue of interest. You also search for secondary sources, which are materials written by persons other than the individuals who conducted a research study or developed a particular theory. Table 5.1 provides more extensive definitions and examples of primary and secondary sources.

Although reviewing the literature for research purposes and research consumer activities requires the same critical thinking and reading skills, a literature review for a research proposal is usually much more extensive and comprehensive, and the critiquing process is more in-depth. From an academic standpoint, requirements for a literature review for a particular assignment differ, depending on the level and type of course, as well as the specific objective of the assignment. These factors determine whether a student's literature search requires a limited, selective review or a major or extensive review. Regardless of extent, discovering knowledge is the goal of any search; therefore, a consumer of research must know how to search the literature. Reference librarians and technicians can provide excellent help in searching for various sources of scholarly literature. If you are unfamiliar with the process of conducting a scholarly computer search, your reference librarian can help. Table 5.2 provides you with steps and strategies for conducting a literature search.

Prioritizing the Search for Evidence

In Chapter 3, an evidence hierarchy is presented for grading the strength and quality of evidence provided by individual studies or resources located

TABLE **5.2**	
STEPS AND STRATEGIES FOR CONDUCTING A LITERATURE SEARCH	
STEPS OF LITERATURE REVIEW	**STRATEGY**
Step 1: Determine the clinical question or research topic.	Keep focused on the characteristics of patients you deal with in your work setting. You know what works and does not work in the delivery of nursing care. In your student role, keep focused on the assignment's objective; use the literature to support opinions or develop a concept under discussion.
Step 2: Identify the key variables/terms.	Ask your reference librarian for help, and read research guidebooks, which are usually found near the computers that are used for student searches; include "research" as one of your variables.
Step 3: Conduct a computer search by using at least two recognized online databases.	Conduct the search yourself or with the help of your librarian; it is essential to use at least two health-related databases, such as CINAHL via EBSCO, MEDLINE, PsycINFO, or ERIC.
Step 4: Review abstracts online and disregard irrelevant articles.	Scan through your search, read the abstracts provided, and make a note of only those that fit your topic; select "references," as well as "search history" and "full-text articles" if available, before printing, saving, or emailing your search.

Continued

TABLE **5.2**

STEPS AND STRATEGIES FOR CONDUCTING A LITERATURE SEARCH—cont'd

STEPS OF LITERATURE REVIEW	STRATEGY
Step 5: Retrieve relevant sources.	Organize by article type or study design and year and reread the abstracts to determine whether the articles chosen are relevant and worth retrieving.
Step 6: Print or download articles; if you are unable to print directly from the database, you can order them through interlibrary loan.	Save yourself time and money: Buy a library copying card ahead of time so that you avoid wasting time midway to secure change; you can also bring a thumb drive to download PDF versions of your articles.
Step 7: Conduct preliminary reading and disregard irrelevant sources.	Review critical reading strategies (see Chapter 3; e.g., read the abstract at the beginning of the articles, and see the example in this chapter).
Step 8: Critically read each source (summarize and critique each source).	Use the critical appraisal strategies from Chapter 1 (e.g., use a standardized critiquing tool), take time to type up each summary and critical appraisal (no more than one page long), include the references in APA style at the top or bottom of each abstract, and attach the original article. Invest time in learning a citation management software tool. This will save you the hassle of formatting all of your citations.
Step 9: Synthesize critical summaries of each article.	Decide how you will present your synthesis of overall strengths and weaknesses of the reviewed articles (e.g., chronologically or according to type: research or conceptual) and type up the synthesized material and a reference list.

APA, American Psychological Association; *CINAHL,* Cumulative Index to Nursing and Allied Health Literature; *ERIC,* Education Resources Information Center.

during a search. In this chapter, an evidence-informed model, called the "6S" pyramid, is used to help you identify the highest-level information resource to facilitate your search for the best evidence about your clinical question or problem (DiCenso, Bayley, & Haynes, 2009). This model, as illustrated in Figure 5.3, a suggests that when searching the literature, consider prioritizing your search strategy and begin by looking for the highest-level information resource available. For example, individual original studies such as those found in MEDLINE or CINAHL (e.g., a randomized clinical trial) are at the lowest level of the information resource pyramid. The next information resource levels of the 6S pyramid are *synopses of studies* (e.g., a brief summary of a high-quality study), then *syntheses* (e.g., Cochrane Library), followed by *synopses of syntheses* (a comprehensive summary of all the research related to a clinical question), and *summaries* (e.g., evidence-informed clinical practice guidelines and textbooks).

The highest information resource level portrayed in the 6S levels of organization (see Figure 5.3)

pertains to computerized decision support systems, a resource built into an electronic medical record that links your patient's distinctive needs with current evidence-informed practice guidelines. These computerized systems are under development, but this does not mean that the information found within the other information resource levels is not useful or appropriate. The 6S model is a tool that can help guide your search for the strongest and most relevant evidence-informed information; however, it does not replace the importance of critically reading each piece of evidence and assessing its quality and applicability for current practice.

 Research Hint _____

- Make an appointment with your educational institution's reference librarian so you can take advantage of his or her expertise in accessing electronic databases.
- Take the time to set up your computer for electronic library access.
- If the full text of an article is unavailable through your electronic search, read the abstract to determine whether you want to order the article through interlibrary loan.

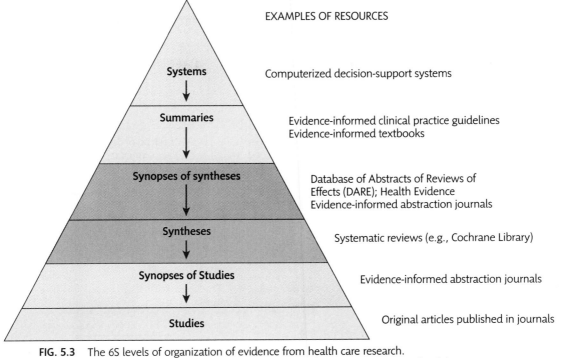

FIG. 5.3 The 6S levels of organization of evidence from health care research. (Adapted from *Evidence Based Nursing*, Alba DiCenso, Liz Bayley, R Brian Haynes, Vol. 12(4), pages 99-101, © 2009, BMJ Publishing Group Ltd and the RCN Publishing Company Ltd. with permission from BMJ Publishing Group Ltd.)

Performing an Online Database Search

Why Use an Online Database?

Perhaps you are still not convinced that online database searches are the best way to acquire information for a review of the literature. Maybe you have searched by using Google or Yahoo and found relevant information. This is an understandable temptation, especially if your assignment requires you to use only five articles. Try to think about it from another perspective, and ask yourself the following question: "Is this the most appropriate and efficient way to find out what is the latest and strongest research on a topic that affects patient care?" If you take the time to learn how to perform a sound database search, you will have the essential competency needed for your career in nursing. Duncan and Holtslander (2012) looked at the information-seeking behaviours of senior nursing students and found that more time is needed to teach nursing students to use electronic resources, including CINAHL. This study specifically highlighted that students were frustrated with their ability to locate appropriate terms to use in their search. A way to decrease your frustration is to take the time to learn how to do a sound database search. Following the strategies and hints provided in this chapter will help you gain the essential competencies needed for your course assignments and career in nursing. The Critical Thinking Decision Path illustrates a method for locating evidence to support your research or clinical question.

CRITICAL THINKING DECISION PATH

Search for Evidence Thought Flow

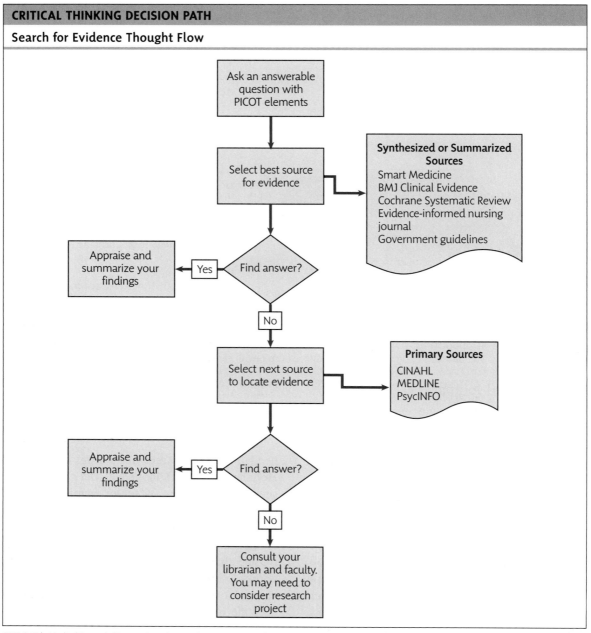

BMJ, British Medical Journal; CINAHL, Cumulative Index to Nursing and Allied Health Literature; *PICOT,* population, intervention, comparison, outcome, time. Based on Kendall, S. American College of Physicians (ACP). (2008). Evidence-based resources simplified. *Canadian Family Physician,* 54(2), 241 -243. ©2001, 2003, 2004 Sandra Kendall (Mount Sinai Hospital), reprinted with permission.

TYPES OF RESOURCES

Print: Books, Journals, and Indexes

Most college and university libraries have an online card catalogue to find print and online books, journals (titles only), videos and other media items, scripts, monographs, conference proceedings, masters' theses, dissertations, archival materials, and more.

Before the 1980s, a search was usually done manually with **print indexes,** which were listings of published material. This was a tedious and time-consuming process. The print indexes are useful today for finding sources that have not been entered into electronic (online) databases. Some of your professors might talk about the "Red Books" in referring to print versions of what is now CINAHL. The print index started in 1956 but is no longer produced. Print resources are still necessary if a search requires materials not entered into an electronic database before a certain year.

Print: Refereed Journals

A major portion of most literature reviews consists of journal articles. In contrast to books and textbooks, which take much longer to publish, journals are a ready source of up-to-date information on almost any subject. Therefore, journals are the preferred mode of communicating the most recent theory or results of a research study. For you as a beginning research consumer, refereed journals should be your first choice when looking for theoretical, clinical, or research articles. A **refereed (peer-reviewed) journal** has a panel of internal and external reviewers who review submitted manuscripts for possible publication. The external reviewers are drawn from a pool of nurse scholars, and possibly scholars from other related disciplines, who are experts in various specialties. In most cases, the reviews are "blind"; that is, the reviewers do not know who the authors of manuscript are. The reviewers use a set of scholarly criteria to judge whether a manuscript meets the publication standards of the journal. These criteria are similar to those that you use when you are critically appraising the strengths and weaknesses of a study. The credibility of a published theoretical or research article is strengthened by the peer review process. Most refereed journals are available in print and accessible electronically through your library's online resources. If you cannot access some research articles from your library, consider the use of Google Scholar as a search engine to locate them.

Internet: Online Bibliographic and Abstract Databases

An **online database** is used to find journal sources (periodicals) of research and conceptual articles on a variety of topics (e.g., doctoral dissertations), as well as the publications of professional organizations and various governmental agencies. These sources contain bibliographic citation information such as the author, title, journal, date, and indexed terms for each record. Some also include the abstract. Box 5.2 lists examples of the more commonly used online databases.

Your college or university probably enables you to access such databases from your residence, whether it is or is not on campus. The most relevant and frequently used source for nursing literature remains CINAHL. Full text has been added to this database; thus, in many cases you can find the full article. Another premier resource is MEDLINE, which is produced by the National Library of Medicine. MEDLINE focuses on the life sciences, and its sources date back to the early 1950s.

Internet: Online Secondary or Summary Databases

Some databases contain more than just journal article information. These online resources contain either summaries or synopses of studies, overviews of diseases or conditions, or a summary of

BOX **5.2**

ONLINE DATABASES

COCHRANE LIBRARY

- Collection of databases that contain high-quality evidence
- Includes the Cochrane Database of Systematic Reviews
- Full Cochrane Library available from Wiley Online Library; other databases that make up the Cochrane Library available from other vendors, including Ovid Technologies
- Cochrane systematic reviews are indexed and searchable in both CINAHL and MEDLINE

CUMULATIVE INDEX TO NURSING AND ALLIED HEALTH LITERATURE (CINAHL)

- Initially called Cumulative Index to Nursing Literature
- Produced by CINAHL
- Electronic version available as part of the EBSCO online service
- Over 1,800 journals indexed for inclusion in database
- Citations in CINAHL are assigned index terms from a controlled vocabulary

EDUCATION RESOURCE INFORMATION CENTER (ERIC)

- Sponsored by the Institute of Education and the U.S. Department of Education
- Focuses on education research and information
- Currently indexes more than 600 journals and also includes references to books, conference papers, and technical reports
- References date from 1966
- Available from the ERIC website and by subscription from EBSCO, OCLC, and Ovid Technologies

EXCERPTA MEDICA

- Biomedical database
- More than 24 million indexed records
- Approximately 7,500 current, mostly peer-reviewed journals

MEDLINE (MEDICAL LITERATURE ANALYSIS AND RETRIEVAL SYSTEM ONLINE)

- Produced by the National Library of Medicine
- Premier bibliographic database for journal articles in life sciences
- References date from 1950, and approximately 5,200 worldwide journals are indexed
- Indexed with MeSH (Medical Subject Headings)
- MEDLINE is available for free through PubMed (tutorial available; National Library of Medicine, 2016) and by subscription from EBSCO, OCLC, and Ovid Technologies

PROQUEST DISSERTATIONS AND THESES

- Produced by ProQuest
- PDF downloads available for over 1 million dissertations
- Available from ProQuest (n.d.)

PSYCINFO

- Produced by the American Psychological Association (APA, n.d.)
- An abstract database of the psychosocial literature beginning with citations dating back to 1800
- Covers more than 2,150 journals
- Of the journals covered, 98% are peer reviewed
- Also includes book chapters and dissertations
- Indexed with the Thesaurus of Psychological Index Terms
- Available through APA PsycNET, EBSCO, Ovid Technologies, and ProQuest

SCOPUS

- Largest abstract and citation database of peer-reviewed science literature and quality Web sources
- Provides 100% MEDLINE coverage
- Offers sophisticated tools to track, analyze, and visualize research

OCLC (ONLINE COMPUTER LIBRARY CENTER)

- A global library network representing 100 countries
- Provides shared technology services and original research
- Provides an comprehensive database of information about library collections
- OCLC also conducts research

THE JOANNA BRIGGS INSTITUTE

A not-for-profit research and development centre within the Faculty of Health Sciences at the University of Adelaide, South Australia that promotes and supports the synthesis, transfer, and utilization of evidence through identifying feasible, appropriate, meaningful, and effective health care practices to assist in the improvement of health care outcomes globally.

The free JBI COnNECT+ provides easy access to evidence-based resources such as the following:

- JBI databases (including the JBI Library of Systematic Reviews, Best Practice Information Sheets, Evidence Summaries, and Evidence Based Recommended Practices)
- JBI Library of Systematic Reviews
- External databases (including the Cochrane Library, PubMed)

the most recent evidence to support a particular treatment. For example, the Cochrane Library is an online resource that consists of six databases, including the Cochrane Database of Systematic Reviews. Using at least two electronic health-related databases, such as CINAHL and MEDLINE (see Box 5.2), is recommended.

Internet: Online Search Engines

You are probably familiar with accessing a **web browser** (a software program used to connect to or search the World Wide Web—e.g., Internet Explorer, Mozilla Firefox, or Safari) to conduct searches for music or other entities and using search engines such as Google or Google Scholar to find information or articles. However, "surfing" the Web is not a good use of your time for scholarly literature searches. There are a number of concerns with only using or heavily depending on general Internet searches:

- Many academic articles are not available.
- Information is not stable on the Internet—the information may be deleted, moved, or altered.
- You do not know whether the information has come from a credible source and therefore you cannot depend on accuracy, currency, or reliability of the information.

Table 5.3 lists sources of free online information. Review the table carefully to determine whether it is a good source of primary research studies. Note that some sites are sources of health information and others are clinical guidelines based on systematic reviews of the literature, but

TABLE **5.3**

SELECTED EXAMPLES OF WEBSITES AND OUTCOMES FOR LITERATURE SEARCHES

WEBSITE	SCOPE	NOTES
Canadian Nurses Association (CNA): http://www.nurseone.ca	This site gives CNA members access to online libraries including electronic books, full-text journals, and evidence-informed resources in EBSCO databases (including CINAHL and MEDLINE), Cochrane Collaboration, e-CPS (Electronic drug manual), e-Therapeutics, STAT!Ref Electronic Health Library, and much more.	This site is managed by the CNA and can only be accessed by members.
Cochrane Collaboration: http://www.cochrane.org	Provides free access to abstracts from the Cochrane Database of Systematic Reviews. Full text of reviews and access to the databases that are part of the Cochrane Library—Database of Abstracts of Reviews of Effectiveness, Cochrane Controlled Trials Register, Cochrane Methodology Register, Health Technology Assessment database (HTA), and National Health Service (NHS) Economic Evaluation Database (EED)—are accessible through Wiley Online library.	Abstracts of Cochrane Reviews are available without charge and can be browsed or searched; many databases are used in its reviews, including CINAHL via EBSCO and MEDLINE; some are primary sources (e.g., systematic reviews/meta-analyses); others (if commentaries of single studies) are a secondary source. Important source for clinical evidence but limited as a provider of primary documents for literature reviews.
National Guideline Clearinghouse: https://www.guideline.gov	Public resource for evidence-informed clinical practice guidelines. It contains more than 1,900 guidelines, including non–U.S. publications.	Offers a useful online feature of side-by-side comparison of guidelines.

Continued

TABLE **5.3**

SELECTED EXAMPLES OF WEBSITES AND OUTCOMES FOR LITERATURE SEARCHES—cont'd

WEBSITE	SCOPE	NOTES
National Institute of Nursing Research: https://www.ninr.nih.gov	Promotes science for nursing practice, funding for nursing and interdisciplinary research, and nurse scientist training programs. Provides links to many nursing organizations and search sites. Excellent site for graduate students.	Able to link to Computer Retrieval of Information on Scientific Projects (CRISP) and PubMed (search service of the National Library of Medicine), which accesses literature via MEDLINE and PreMEDLINE and other related material from online journals; however, this site has limited utility for the beginning consumer of research for conducting scholarly review of nursing research literature because MEDLINE alone does not include all nursing literature; searching CINAHL and MEDLINE on your own would be your first choice. Useful site for graduate students in addition to CINAHL and MEDLINE and as third database related to topic.
Statistics Canada: http://www.statcan.gc.ca	Collects data on the Canadian population that are related to demographic trends, labour, health, trade, and education. Data on health trends are useful in identifying populations at risk and suggest associations among health determinants, health status, and population characteristics. Research papers on a variety of topics are also published.	Free source of primary data essential for comprehensive demographic data and socioeconomic trends; updated daily.
Turning Research into Practice (Trip): http://www.tripdatabase.com	Content from a wide variety of free online resources, including synopses, guidelines, medical images, electronic textbooks, and systematic reviews; accessed together by the Trip search engine (Trip, 2016).	Provides a wide sampling of available evidence.
Virginia Henderson Global Nursing e-Repository: https://www.nursinglibrary.org/vhl/	Open access to the Registry of Nursing Research database, which contains nearly 30,000 abstracts of research studies and conference papers.	Service offered without charge; locate conference abstracts and research study abstracts. This library is supported by Sigma Theta Tau International, honour society of nursing.

most websites are not a primary source of research studies. Less common and less used sources of scholarly material are audiotapes and other audio recordings, videos, personal communications (e.g., letters or telephone or in-person interviews), unpublished doctoral dissertations, master's theses, and conference proceedings.

Most searches with electronic databases include not only citation information but also the abstract of the article and options for obtaining the full text. When possible, print or copy the full text, which of course will include the abstract and the complete references. If the text is not available, choose the option "complete reference," which will include the abstract. Reading the abstract is critical for determining whether you need to retrieve the article through another mechanism. Both the CINAHL and MEDLINE electronic databases will facilitate all steps of critically reviewing the literature, especially the gaps.

 Evidence-Informed Practice Tip ____

Reading systematic reviews, if they are available, on your clinical question or topic will enhance your ability to implement evidence-informed nursing practice because they generally offer the strongest and most consistent level of evidence.

HOW FAR BACK MUST THE SEARCH GO?

Students often ask questions such as the following: "How many articles do I need?"; "How much is enough?"; and "How far back in the literature do I need to go?" When conducting a search, you should use a rigorous focusing process; otherwise, you may end up with hundreds or thousands of citations. Retrieving too many citations is usually a sign that there was something wrong with your search technique or that you may have not sufficiently narrowed your clinical question.

Each online database offers an explanation of each feature; it is worth your time to click on each icon and explore the explanations offered because this will increase your confidence. Also keep in mind the types of articles you are retrieving. Many online resources allow you to limit your search to randomized controlled trials or systematic reviews. In CINAHL, there is a limit for "Research" that will restrict the number of citations you retrieve to research articles. A general timeline for most academic or evidence-informed practice papers and projects is to go back in the literature at least 3 years, but preferably 5 years, although some research projects may warrant going back 10 years or more until the researcher is satisfied that he or she has found literature that accurately represents the body of knowledge. In some cases, seminal research or research that has had a huge effect in the field

should be reviewed regardless of publication date. For example, conducting a literature review on the effects of stress would not be complete without reading Hans Selye's (1955) pioneering work on stress. Extensive literature reviews on particular topics or a concept clarification methodology study helps you limit the length of your search.

 Research Hint _____

Ask your instructor for guidance if you are uncertain how far back you need to conduct your search. If you come across a systematic review on your specific clinical topic, scan it to see what years the review covers; then begin your search from the last year to the present.

As you scroll through and mark the citations you wish to include in your downloaded or printed search, make sure you include all relevant fields when you save or print the publications. If you are writing a paper and need to produce a bibliography, you can export your citations to **citation management software,** which is a software program that formats and stores your citations so that they are available for electronic retrieval when they must be inserted in a paper you are writing. Quite a few of these programs are available; some, such as Zotero, are free, and others, including EndNote and RefWorks, must be purchased, by either you or your institution. Microsoft Word also has a reference tab that allows you to manage your citations and references.

What Do I Need to Know?

Each database usually has a specific search guide that provides information on the organization of the entries and the terminology used. The following suggestions and strategies, as listed in Box 5.3, incorporate general search strategies, as well as those related to CINAHL and MEDLINE. Finding the right terms to "plug in" as keywords for a computer search is an important aspect of conducting a search. When it is possible, you

TIPS: USING CINAHL VIA EBSCO

- Locate CINAHL from your library's home page. It may be located under databases, online resources, or nursing resources.
- In the "Advanced" tab, type in your keyword or key phrase (e.g., prenatal bonding). Do not use complete sentences. (Ask your librarian for the manual guide for each database or use the guide in the database.)
- Before you choose "Search," make sure you mark "Research Articles" to ensure that you have retrieved only articles that are actually about research. See the results in Figure 5.4.
- Note that in the "Limit Your Results" section, you can limit by year, age group, clinical queries, and other specific characteristics.
- To narrow your search, use the Boolean connector "and" between each of the keywords you wish to use and between additional variables. To broaden your search, use the Boolean connector "or."
- Note in Figure 5.4 that you can set up an RSS feed so that you are notified whenever new citations are added to the CINAHL database.
- Once the search results appear and you determine that they are manageable, you can decide whether to review them online; print, save, or export them; or email them to yourself.

CINAHL, Cumulative Index to Nursing and Allied Health Literature; *RSS,* Really Simple Syndication (syndicates content from the Internet and sends it out [feeds] it to a subscriber).

want to match the words that you use to describe your question with the terms that indexers have assigned to the articles. In many online databases, you can browse the **controlled vocabulary** terms and search. Used to conduct searches in databases, controlled vocabulary terms are carefully selected words and phrases that are applied to similar pieces of information units. If you are still having difficulty, ask your reference librarian for help.

Figure 5.4 is a screenshot of CINAHL in the EBSCO interface. As noted, you have the option of a search using the controlled vocabulary of CINAHL or a keyword search. If you wanted to locate articles about maternal-fetal attachment as they relate to the health practices or health behaviours of low-income mothers, you would first want to construct your PICOT:

P: Maternal-fetal attachment in low-income mothers (specifically defined group)
I: Health behaviours or health practices (event to be studied)
C: None (comparison intervention)
O: Neonatal outcomes (outcome)
T: 1997–2012

In this example, the two main concepts are maternal-fetal attachment and health practices and how these impact neonatal outcomes. Many times when conducting a search, you only enter in keywords or controlled vocabulary for the first two elements of your PICOT—in this case, maternal-fetal attachment and health practices or behaviours. The other elements can be added if your list of results is overwhelming, but often you can pick from the results you have by just combining the first two. Figure 5.5 shows a Venn diagram of this approach.

Maternal-fetal attachment should be part of your search as a keyword search, but "prenatal bonding" is the appropriate CINAHL subject heading. To be comprehensive, you should use "OR" to link these terms together. The second concept, health practices OR health behaviours, is accomplished in a similar manner. The subject heading or controlled vocabulary assigned by the indexers could be added in for completeness. (See Figure 5.4 for screenshots from CINAHL on how to build a multi-line search using both keywords and subject headings.)

Note that these two concepts are connected with the **Boolean operator,** which defines the relationships between words or groups of words in your literature search. Boolean operators dictate the relationship between words and concepts. "AND," "OR," "NOT" are Boolean operators. "AND" requires that both concepts be located within the results that are returned. "OR" allows you to group together like terms or synonyms, and "NOT" eliminates terms from your search.

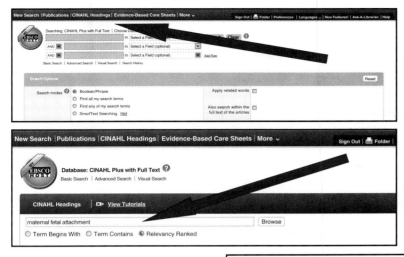

Start your search by selecting CINAHL Headings to locate subject heading terms.

Enter in your term to see if it is part of the controlled vocabulary.

In this case, prenatal bonding is the controlled CINAHL subject heading for maternal-fetal attachment.

It is suggested to use a combination of both controlled vocabulary terms, in this case prenatal bonding, in conjunction with words or phrases searched in the title or abstract. Combine with Boolean "OR."

You would then repeat steps 1 to 4 for the next concept of health behaviours.

Here is a final search strategy that combines both of these concepts and applies the "Research Article" limit. Note that the Alhusen article is first on the list!

FIG. 5.4 Example from CINAHL to locate articles on maternal-fetal attachment and health practices.

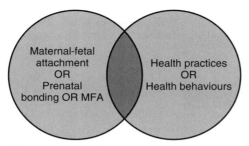

FIG. 5.5 Venn diagram illustrating Boolean search for articles on maternal-fetal attachment (MFA) and health behaviours.

To restrict our retrieval to research, the "Research Article" limit has been applied. Searching is an iterative process and takes some trial and error to use the correct terms to locate the articles you will find useful for your search question.

Research Hint _____

Look for useful tools within the search interfaces of online databases to make your searching more efficient. For example, when you search for a particular age group, use the built-in limits of the database instead of relying on a keyword search. Other shortcuts include the "Clinical Queries" in CINAHL and MEDLINE that retrieve articles about therapy or diagnosis.

How Do I Complete the Search?

Now the truly important aspect of your searching begins: your critical reading of the retrieved materials. Critically reading scholarly material, especially research articles, requires several readings and the use of critiquing criteria. Do not be discouraged if not all of the retrieved articles are as useful as you first thought; this happens with the most experienced reviewers of literature. If most of the articles are not useful, be prepared to perform another search, but discuss with your instructor, the reference librarian, or both the search terms that you will use next time; you may want to add a third database. In the previous example of a search to locate articles on maternal-fetal attachment, the third database of choice may be PsycINFO (see Box 5.2). Remind yourself how quickly you will be able to perform the search, now that you have experience with searching.

Research Hint _____

Read the abstract carefully (review the discussion on critical reading strategies in Chapter 3) to determine whether the article is about research. It is also a good idea to review the references of the articles; if any seem relevant, you can retrieve them.

LITERATURE REVIEW FORMAT: WHAT TO EXPECT

Familiarity with the format of the literature review helps research consumers use critiquing criteria to evaluate the review. To decide which style you will use so that your review is presented in a logical and organized manner, you must consider the following:

- The research or clinical question or topic
- The number of retrieved sources reviewed
- The number and type of research materials versus conceptual materials

Some reviews are written according to the variables being studied and presented chronologically in the discussion of each variable. In others, the entire material is presented chronologically, and subcategories or variables are discussed within each time period. In still others, the variables are presented and the subcategories are related to the study's type or designs or related variables.

For example, as you will remember in Chapter 4, Laschinger's (2014) hypothesis stated that bullying and incivility influences nurse-assessed quality outcomes. The preliminary literature review was divided into two separate categories. The first section, titled "Workplace Mistreatment," explored workplace mistreatment and the research linking bullying and negative work outcomes. A separate section, titled "Patient Safety Risk and Adverse Patient Outcomes," described the research on the importance of high-quality nursing environments to the provision of patient care (see Appendix B). Review the literature reviews in Appendices A–D to appreciate the different styles.

In contrast to the styles of previous quantitative studies, the literature reviews of qualitative studies are usually handled in a different manner. Often, little is known about the topic under study. The literature review may be conducted at the beginning of the study or after the data analysis is completed.

The researchers always compare the literature review with their findings. In some cases, the reviewed literature is used during the analysis process as well. In a study by Seneviratne, Mather, and Then (2009), on understanding nursing on an acute stroke unit, the background section included a literature review that focused on the role of nurses in stroke rehabilitation, attitudes and perceptions of their role in stroke care, and observations of nurses in acute and rehabilitative care settings. After the data analysis, Seneviratne and associates returned to the literature to help explain and discuss the findings. For example, they

compared the literature on space limitations and time constraints to further explore the challenges faced by nurses in the study.

Evidence-Informed Practice Tip _____

Sort the research articles you retrieve according to the model of levels of evidence in Chapter 3. Remember that articles that are systematic reviews, especially meta-analyses, generally provide the strongest and most consistent evidence to include in a literature review.

Research Hint _____

When you write up your literature review, include enough information so that your professor or fellow students could re-create your search path and come up with the same results. This means specifying the databases searched, the date you searched, years of coverage, terms used, and any limits or restrictions that you used.

APPRAISING THE EVIDENCE

Review of the Literature

Whether you are a researcher writing the literature review for the research study you are planning to conduct or a nurse writing a literature review for an evidence-informed practice project, you need to critically appraise individual research reports by using appropriate criteria. If you are appraising an individual research study that is to be included in a literature review, it must be evaluated in terms of critical appraisal criteria that are related to each step of the research process so that the strengths and weaknesses of each study can be identified. Standardized critical appraisal tools (e.g., Critical Appraisal Skills Programme [CASP] Tools and Appraisal of Guidelines for Research and Evaluation [AGREE] Guidelines) available for specific types of research designs (e.g., clinical trials, cohort studies, systematic reviews) can also be used to critically appraise an individual research study.

Critiquing the literature review of research or conceptual reports is a challenging task for seasoned consumers of research, so do not be surprised if you feel a little intimidated by the prospect of critiquing the published research. The important issue is to determine the overall value of the literature review, including both the research and theoretical materials. The purposes of a literature

review (see Box 5.1) and the characteristics of a well-written literature review (Box 5.4) provide the framework for developing the evaluation criteria for a literature review.

The literature review should be presented in an organized manner. The theoretical and research literature can be presented chronologically from earliest studies to most recent; sometimes the theoretical literature that provided the foundation for the existing research is presented first, followed by the research studies that were derived from this theoretical base. Other times, the literature can be clustered by concept, grouped according to supportive or nonsupportive positions, or categorized by evidence that highlights differences in theoretical and/or research findings. The overall question to be answered is "Does the review of the literature develop and present a knowledge base for a research study or an evidence-informed practice project that builds on previous research, identifies a conflict or gap in the literature, or proposes to extend the current knowledge base?" (see Box 5.1).

Regardless of how the literature review is organized, it should provide a strong knowledge base for carrying out the research, educational, or clinical practice project. Questions related to the logical organization and presentation of the reviewed studies are somewhat more

Continued

Review of the Literature

challenging for beginning research consumers. The more you read research studies, the more competent you will become at differentiating a well-organized literature review from one that has no organizing framework.

Whenever possible, read both qualitative (meta-syntheses) and quantitative (meta-analyses) systematic reviews that pertain to a clinical question and provide level I evidence. Systematic reviews are considered examples of secondary sources because they represent a body of completed research studies that have been critically appraised and synthesized by a team other than the original researchers; however, they often represent the best available evidence on a particular clinical issue. The article by Cummings, MacGregor, Davey, and associates (2010) is an example of a quantitative systematic review in which the authors critically appraised and synthesized the evidence from research studies related to the leadership behaviours and outcomes for nurses and organizations. After reviewing and synthesizing 53 studies, Cummings and associates concluded that "transformational and relational leadership are needed to enhance nurse satisfaction, recruitment, retention and health work environments" (p. 363). In her article "Becoming a Nurse: A Meta-study of Early Professional Socialization and Career Choice in Nursing," Price (2009) gathered 10 primary qualitative studies on professional socialization in nursing and nurses' career choice decisions. After synthesizing the studies, Price reported "that nursing socialization is strongly associated with a person's preconceived notions and expectations of nursing" (p. 14).

The Critiquing Criteria box summarizes general critiquing criteria for a review of the literature. In other sets of critiquing criteria, these questions may be phrased differently or more broadly. For instance, questions may be the following: "Does the literature search seem adequate?" and "Does the report demonstrate scholarly writing?" You may have difficulty answering these questions; you may begin, however, by determining whether the source is a refereed journal. It is reasonable to assume that the manuscripts published in a scholarly refereed journal are adequately searched, are based mainly on primary sources, and are written in a scholarly manner. This does not mean, however, that every study reported in a refereed journal meets all the critiquing criteria for a literature review and other components of the study in an equal manner. Because of style differences and space constraints, each citation summarized is often very brief, or related citations may be summarized as a group and lack a critique. You still must answer the critiquing questions. Consultation with a faculty adviser may be necessary to develop skill in answering the two questions.

The key to a strong literature review is a careful search of the published and unpublished literature. Whether you write or critically appraise a literature review written for a published research study, it should reflect a synthesis or compilation of the main points or value of all of the sources reviewed in relation to the study's research question or hypothesis (see Box 5.1). The relationship between and among these studies must be explained. The synthesis of a written review of the literature usually appears at the end of the review section before the section about the research question or hypothesis.

Searching the literature, like critiquing the literature, is an acquired skill. Practising your search and critical appraisal skills on a regular basis will make a huge difference. Seeking guidance from faculty is essential for developing critical appraisal skills. Synthesizing the body of literature you have critiqued is even more challenging. Critiquing the literature will help you apply new knowledge to practice. This process is vital to the "survival and growth of the nursing profession and is essential to evidence-based practice" (Pravikoff & Donaldson, 2001).

CRITIQUING CRITERIA

1. Are all the relevant concepts and variables included in the review?
2. Does the search strategy include an appropriate and adequate number of databases and other resources to identify key published and unpublished research and theoretical sources?
3. Are both theoretical literature and research literature included?
4. Does an appropriate theoretical or conceptual framework guide the development of the research study?
5. Are mainly primary sources used?
6. What gaps or inconsistencies in knowledge does the literature review uncover?
7. Does the literature review build on the findings of earlier studies?

CRITIQUING CRITERIA—cont'd

8. Does the summary of each reviewed study reflect the essential components of the study design (e.g., type and size of sample, reliability and validity of instruments, consistency of data-collection procedures, appropriate data analysis, identification of limitations)?

9. Does the critique of each reviewed study mention strengths, weaknesses, or limitations of the design; conflicts; and gaps in information related to the area of interest?

10. Does the synthesis summary follow a logical sequence in which the overall strengths and weaknesses of the reviewed studies are presented and a logical conclusion is established?

11. Is the literature review presented in an organized format that flows logically (e.g., chronologically, clustered by concept or variables), enhancing the reader's ability to evaluate the need for the particular research study or evidence-informed practice project?

12. Does the literature review follow the proposed purpose of the research study or evidence-informed practice project?

13. Does the literature review generate research questions or hypotheses or answer a clinical question?

Research Hint

- Use standardized critical appraisal criteria to evaluate your research articles.
- Make a table to represent the components of your study, and fill in your evaluation to help you see the "big picture" of your analysis.
- Synthesize the results of your analysis to try to determine what was similar or different among and between these studies in relation to your topic or clinical question, and then draw a conclusion.

BOX 5.4

CHARACTERISTICS OF A WELL-WRITTEN REVIEW OF THE LITERATURE

Each reviewed source of information reflects critical thinking and scholarly writing and is relevant to the study, topic, or project, and the content satisfies the following criteria:

- The literature review is organized in a systematic approach.
- Each research or conceptual article is summarized succinctly and with appropriate references.
- Established critical appraisal criteria are used for specific study designs to evaluate the study for strengths, weaknesses, or limitations, as well as for conflicts or gaps in information that relate directly or indirectly to the area of interest.
- Evidence of a synthesis of the critiques is provided to highlight the overall strengths and weaknesses of the studies reviewed.
- The review consists of mainly primary sources; there are a sufficient number of research sources.
- The review concludes with a synthesis of the reviewed material that reflects why the study or project should be implemented.
- Research questions and hypotheses are identified, or clinical questions are answered.

CRITICAL THINKING CHALLENGES

- Using the PICOT format, generate a clinical question related to health promotion for children in elementary school.
- How does a research article's theoretical or conceptual framework interrelate concepts, theories, conceptual definitions, and operational definitions?
- A general guideline for a literature search is to use a timeline of 3 to 5 years. When would a nurse researcher need to search beyond this timeline?
- What is the relationship of the research article's literature review to the theoretical or conceptual framework?

KEY POINTS

- The review of the literature is defined as a broad, comprehensive, in-depth, systematic critique and synthesis of scholarly publications, unpublished scholarly print and online materials, audiovisual materials, and personal communications.
- The review of the literature is used for development of research studies, as well as other activities for consumers of research, such as development of evidence-informed practice projects.
- With regard to conducting and writing a literature review, the main objectives for the consumer of research are to acquire the abilities to accomplish the following: (1) conduct an appropriate search of electronic or print

research on a topic; (2) efficiently retrieve a sufficient amount of materials for a literature review in relation to the topic and scope of project; (3) critically appraise (i.e., critique) research and theoretical material in accordance with accepted critiquing criteria; (4) critically evaluate published reviews of the literature in accordance with accepted standardized critiquing criteria; (5) synthesize the findings of the critiqued materials for relevance to the purpose of the selected scholarly project; and (6) determine applicability of the findings to practice.

- Primary research and theoretical resources are essential for literature reviews.
- The use of secondary sources, such as commentaries on research articles from peer-reviewed journals, is part of a learning strategy for developing critical critiquing skills.
- It is more efficient to use electronic rather than print databases for retrieving scholarly materials.
- Strategies for efficiently retrieving scholarly nursing literature include consulting the reference librarian and using at least two online sources (e.g., CINAHL and MEDLINE).
- Literature reviews are usually organized according to variables, as well as chronologically.
- Critiquing and synthesizing a number of research articles, including systematic reviews, is essential for implementing evidence-informed nursing practice.

FOR FURTHER STUDY

(e) Go to Evolve at http://evolve.elsevier.com/ Canada/LoBiondo/Research for the Audio Glossary and Appendix Tables that provide supplemental information for Appendix E.

REFERENCES

American Psychological Association. (n.d.). *PsycINFO*. Retrieved from http://www.apa.org/pubs/databases/psycinfo/index.aspx.

Anderson, R. A., & McDaniel, R. R. (1998). Intensity of registered nurse participation in nursing home decision-making. *The Gerontologist*, *38*(1), 90–100.

Ashmos, D. P., Huonker, J. W., & McDaniel, R. R. (1998). Participation as a complicating mechanism: The effect of clinical professional and middle manager participation on hospital performance. *Health Care Management Review*, *23*(4), 7–20.

Cummings, G. G., MacGregor, T., Davey, M., et al. (2010). Leadership styles and outcome patterns for the nursing workforce and work environment: A systematic review. *International Journal of Nursing Studies*, *47*, 363–385.

DiCenso, A., Bayley, L., & Haynes, R. B. (2009). Accessing pre-appraised evidence: Fine-tuning the 5S model into a 6S model. *Evidence Based Nursing*, *12*(4), 99–101.

Duncan, V., & Holtslander, L. (2012). Utilizing grounded theory to explore the information-seeking behavior of senior nursing students. *Journal of the Medical Library Association*, *100*(1), 20–27.

Laschinger, H. K. S. (2014). Impact of workplace mistreatment n patient safety risk and nurse-assessed patient outcomes. *Journal of Nursing Administration*, *44*(5), 284–290.

National Library of Medicine. (2016). *PubMed tutorial*. Retrieved from http://www.nlm.nih.gov/bsd/disted/pubmedtutorial/010_050.html.

Pravikoff, D., & Donaldson, N. (2001). Special section: Online journal publication. *Online Journal of Issues in Nursing*, *6*(2). Retrieved from http://www.nursingworld.org/MainMenuCategories/ANAMarketplace/ANAPeriodicals/OJIN/TableofContents/Volume62001/No2May01/ArticlePreviousTopic/ClinicalInnovations.aspx.

Price, S. L. (2009). Becoming a nurse: A meta-study of early professional socialization and career choice in nursing. *Journal of Advanced Nursing*, *65*(1), 11–19.

ProQuest. (n.d.). *ProQuest dissertations and theses global: Fast facts*. Retrieved from http://www.proquest.com/products-services/pqdtglobal.html.

Selye, H. (1955). Stress and disease. *Science*, *122*, 625–631.

Seneviratne, C. C., Mather, C. M., & Then, K. L. (2009). Understanding nursing on an acute stroke unit: Perceptions of space, time and interprofessional practice. *Journal of Advanced Nursing*, *65*(9), 1872–1881.

Turning Research into Practice [Trip]. (2016). *What is Trip?* Retrieved from http://www.tripdatabase.com/about.

Wong, C. A., Laschinger, H., Cummings, G. G., et al. (2010). Decisional involvement of senior nurse leaders in Canadian acute care hospitals. *Journal of Nursing Management*, *18*, 122–133.

CHAPTER 6

Legal and Ethical Issues

Judith Haber | Mina D. Singh

LEARNING OUTCOMES

After reading this chapter, you will be able to do the following:

- Describe the historical background that led to the development of ethical guidelines for the use of human participants in research.
- Identify the essential elements of an informed consent form.
- Evaluate the adequacy of an informed consent form.
- Describe the role of the research ethics board in the research review process.
- Identify populations of participants who require special legal and ethical research considerations.
- Appreciate the nurse researcher's obligations to conduct and report research in an ethical manner.
- Describe the nurse's role as patient advocate in research situations.
- Discuss the nurse's role in ensuring that Health Canada guidelines for testing of medical devices are followed.
- Discuss animal rights in research situations.
- Critique the ethical aspects of a research study.

KEY TERMS

animal rights	consent	research ethics board (REB)
anonymity	ethics	respect for persons
assent	informed consent	risk–benefit ratio
beneficence	justice	risks
benefits	process consent	
confidentiality	product testing	

STUDY RESOURCES

ⓔ Go to Evolve at http://evolve.elsevier.com/Canada/LoBiondo/Research for the Audio Glossary and Appendix Tables that provide supplemental information for Appendix E.

NURSES ARE IN AN IDEAL POSITION to promote the public's awareness of the role played by research in the advancement of science and improvement in patient care. In Canada, the professional code of ethics (Canadian Nurses Association [CNA], 2008) outlines the ethical standards for practice, which can include research and patients' rights with regard to research. Not only do the standards represent rules and regulations regarding practice, but when research becomes the domain of a nurse, these standards can be applied to the participation of human research participants to ensure that nursing research is conducted legally and ethically. The Code states that nurses must strive to uphold human rights and call attention to any violations of these rights. The *Code of Ethics for Registered Nurses,* originally published in 1985, was revised in 2008 and 2017. The revised 2017 CNA code includes new content addressing medical assistance in dying and advocating for quality work environments that support the delivery of safe, compassionate, competent and ethical care. There are seven primary values within this Code. Under the first value of Providing Safe, Compassionate, Competent and Ethical Care, there are ethical responsibilities related to research (p.9) These responsibilities also translate to patients' or participants' rights in research around "informed consent, the risk-benefit balance, the privacy and confidentiality of data and the monitoring of research" (p.9). Nurses need to be advocates in this context to ensure that ethical concepts in nursing research are upheld.

Researchers and caregivers of patients who are research participants must be fully committed to the tenets of informed consent and patients' rights. The principle "the ends justify the means" must never be tolerated. Researchers and caregivers of research participants must take every precaution to protect the people being studied from physical or mental harm or discomfort (although it is not always clear what constitutes harm or discomfort).

The focus of this chapter is on the legal and ethical considerations that need to be addressed before, during, and after the conducting of research to ensure that the research does not harm the patient. Informed consent, research ethics boards (REBs), and research involving vulnerable populations—older adults, pregnant women, children, prisoners, Indigenous people, and persons with acquired immune deficiency syndrome (AIDS) or other serious illnesses, as well as animals—are discussed. The nurse's role as patient advocate, whether functioning as researcher, caregiver, or research consumer, is addressed.

ETHICAL AND LEGAL CONSIDERATIONS IN RESEARCH: A HISTORICAL PERSPECTIVE

Past Ethical Dilemmas in Research

Ethical and legal considerations regarding medical research first arose in the United States and received focused attention after World War II. Lawyers defending war criminals intended to justify the atrocities committed by Nazi physicians by claiming their actions were in the name of "medical research." On learning of this defense, the U.S. Secretary of State and the Secretary of War asked the American Medical Association to appoint a group to develop a code of ethics for research to serve as a standard for judging the medical experiments committed by physicians on concentration camp prisoners.

The Code of Ethics, developed as 10 rules, became known as the *Nuremberg Code* (Box 6.1). The Nuremberg Code's definitions of the terms *voluntary, legal capacity, sufficient understanding,* and *enlightened decision* have been the subject of numerous court cases and U.S. presidential commissions involved in setting ethical standards in research (Amdur & Bankert, 2011). The Code that was developed requires informed consent in all cases but makes no provisions for any special treatment of children, older adults, or people who are mentally incompetent. Several other international standards have followed; the most notable is the Declaration of Helsinki, adopted in 1964 by the World Medical Assembly and revised in 1975 (Levine, 1979).

> **BOX 6.1**
>
> ## ARTICLES OF THE NUREMBERG CODE
>
> 1. The voluntary consent of the human subject is absolutely essential.
> 2. The study should be conducted so as to yield fruitful results for the good of society, unprocurable by other means of study, and not random and unnecessary in nature.
> 3. The experiment should be so designed and based on the results of animal experimentation and knowledge of the natural history of the disease or other problems under study that the anticipated results will justify the performance of the experiment.
> 4. The experiment should be conducted to avoid all unnecessary physical and mental suffering and injury.
> 5. No experiment should be conducted where there is an a priori reason to believe that death or disabling injury will occur. . . .
> 6. The degree of risk to be taken should never exceed that determined by the humanitarian importance of the problem to be solved by the experiment.
> 7. Proper preparations should be made and adequate facilities provided to protect the subject against even remote possibilities of injury, disability, or death.
> 8. The experiment should be conducted only by scientifically qualified persons. . . .
> 9. . . . The human subject should be at liberty to bring the experiment to an end. . . .
> 10. During the course of the experiment the scientist in charge must be prepared to terminate the experiment at any stage, if he [or she] has probable cause to believe . . . that a continuation of the experiment is likely to result in injury, disability, or death to the experimental subject.
>
> From United States Government Printing Office. (2008). The medical case. In *Trials of war criminals before the Nuremberg Military Tribunals under Control Council Law No. 10* (Vol. 2, pp. 181–182). Washington, DC: Author, 1949. Retrieved from http://www.loc.gov/rr/frd/Military_Law/pdf/NT_war-criminals_Vol-II.pdf.

The research heritage in the United States and Canada is well documented and is used here to illustrate the human consequences of not adhering to ethical standards when conducting research. Some examples are highlighted in Table 6.1 and incorporated into Table 6.2 to show the violation of human rights that occurred in these studies.

In the United States, under the National Research Act of 1974 (Public Law 93-348), the National Commission for the Protection of Human Subjects of Biomedical and Behavioral Research was created. A major charge of the commission was to identify the basic principles that should underlie the conduct of biomedical and behavioural research involving human participants and to develop guidelines to ensure that research is conducted in accordance with those principles (Levine, 1986). Three ethical principles (Box 6.2) were identified as relevant to the conduct of research involving human participants:

- **respect for persons** (the idea that people have the freedom to participate or not participate in research),
- **beneficence** (the obligation to do no harm and maximize possible benefits), and
- **justice** (the principle that human subjects should be treated fairly).

These three principles have formed the basis of many ethical guidelines in Canada.

In Canada, for the protection of human participants in all types of research, Health Canada has adopted the *Good Clinical Practice: Consolidated Guidelines* (Health Canada, 1997/2004). The collaboration of the three major funding agencies—the Canadian Institutes of Health Research (CIHR), the Natural Sciences and Engineering Research Council of Canada (NSERC), and the Social Sciences and Humanities Research Council of Canada (SSHRC)—has led to a joint statement for the protection of human participants. The revision of this document, the *Tri-Council Policy Statement: Ethical Conduct for Research Involving Humans* (CIHR et al., 2014), offers a more inclusive approach to delineating current trends in ethical issues. This revised document, sometimes called the Tri-Council Policy Statement-2, is henceforth referred to as TCPS 2.

The original statement listed eight guiding principles, which are now subsumed under the three core principles "respect for person," "concern

TABLE 6.1

HIGHLIGHTS OF UNETHICAL RESEARCH STUDIES CONDUCTED IN THE UNITED STATES AND CANADA

RESEARCH STUDY	DATE OF STUDY	FOCUS OF STUDY	ETHICAL PRINCIPLE VIOLATED
Tuskegee syphilis study, Tuskegee, Alabama	1932–1973	For 40 years, the U.S. Public Health Service conducted a study using two groups of poor Black male sharecroppers. One group consisted of men with untreated syphilis; the other group was judged to be free of the disease. Treatment was withheld from the group with syphilis even after penicillin became generally available and accepted as effective treatment for syphilis in the 1950s. Steps were even taken to prevent the research participants from obtaining penicillin. The researcher wanted to study the untreated disease.	Many of the research participants who consented to participate in the study were not informed about the purpose and procedures of the research. Others were unaware that they were participants. The degree of risk outweighed the potential benefit. Withholding of known effective treatment violates the participants' right to fair treatment and protection from harm (Levine, 1986).
Sterilization experiments in Auschwitz concentration camp, Germany	1940–1944	Sterilization experiments	Basic human rights and rights to fair and ethical treatment were violated, and the research participants did not give informed consent. Nurses who were prisoners were forced to participate in the experiments, which was against their prima facie duty to protect (Benedict & Georges, 2006).
Dr. Ewen Cameron's psychiatric experiments, Allan Memorial Psychiatric Institute, Montreal, Quebec	1950s–1960s	The U.S. Central Intelligence Agency (CIA) funded psychic driving, or brainwashing, experiments on patients with psychiatric illnesses (Collins, 1988, as cited in Charron, 2000). Psychic driving is a psychiatric procedure pioneered by Dr. Cameron in which electroconvulsive therapy (ECT) and psychedelic drugs, such as lysergic acid (LSD), are used in an attempt at mind control. To develop the psychic driving, increasingly higher levels of ECT were applied to patients as often as three times a day. This treatment would continue for 30 days. Considerable damage was done to patients after such severe treatment. Patients were unable to walk or feed themselves and were incontinent (Gillmor, 1987, as cited in Charron, 2000).	The ethical principles of respect for persons and beneficence were severely violated. Dr. Cameron used patients with diminished autonomy (patients with psychiatric illnesses), even though, as a physician, he was obliged to protect them. The ECT treatments did more harm than good.
Hyman v. Jewish Chronic Disease Hospital, Jewish Chronic Disease study, New York City	1965	Doctors injected aged, senile patients with cancer cells to study the patients' response to injection of the cells.	Informed consent was not obtained, and no indication was given that the study had been reviewed and approved by an ethics committee. The two physicians involved claimed that they did not wish to evoke emotional reactions or New York City refusals to participate by informing the research participants of the nature of the study (Hershey & Miller, 1976).

TABLE **6.1**

HIGHLIGHTS OF UNETHICAL RESEARCH STUDIES CONDUCTED IN THE UNITED STATES AND CANADA—cont'd

RESEARCH STUDY	DATE OF STUDY	FOCUS OF STUDY	ETHICAL PRINCIPLE VIOLATED
Milledgeville, Georgia, study	1969	Researchers administered investigational drugs to mentally disabled children without first obtaining the opinion of a psychiatrist.	The study protocol or institutional approval of the program was not reviewed before implementation (Levine, 1986).
San Antonio contraceptive study, San Antonio, Texas	1969	In a study of the adverse effects of oral contraceptives, 76 impoverished Mexican American women were randomly assigned to an experimental group receiving birth control pills or a control group receiving placebos. Research participants were not informed about the placebo and the attendant risk of pregnancy. Of the participants, 11 became pregnant; 10 of these women were in the placebo control group.	Principles of informed consent were violated; full disclosure of the potential risk, harm, results, and adverse effects was not evident in the informed consent document. The potential risk outweighed the benefits of the study. The participants' right to fair treatment and protection from harm was violated (Levine, 1986).
Willowbrook Hospital study, New York State	1972	Children with mental incompetence ($N = 350$) were not admitted to Willowbrook Hospital, a residential treatment facility, unless parents consented to their children's being research participants in a study of the natural history of infectious hepatitis and the effect of γ-globulin. The children were deliberately infected with the hepatitis virus under various conditions; some received γ-globulin, whereas others did not.	The principle of voluntary consent was violated. Parents were coerced into consenting to their children's participation for the research. Participants or their guardians have a right to self-determination; in other words, they should be free of constraint, coercion, and undue influence of any kind. Many participants feel pressured to participate in studies if they are in powerless, dependent positions (Rothman, 1982).
Schizophrenia medication study, University of California, Los Angeles	1983	In a study of the effects of withdrawing psychotropic medications in 50 patients receiving treatment for schizophrenia, 23 research participants suffered severe relapses after their medication was stopped. The goal of the study was to determine whether some patients with schizophrenia might do better without medications that had deleterious adverse effects.	Although all participants signed informed consent documents, they were not informed about how severe their relapses might be or that they could suffer worsening symptoms with each recurrence. Principles of informed consent were violated; full disclosure of the potential risk, harm, results, and adverse effects was not evident in the informed consent document. The potential risk outweighed the benefits of the study. The participants' right to fair treatment and protection from harm was violated (Hilts, 1995).
Côte d'Ivoire, Africa, AIDS/AZT case	1994	In research supported by the U.S. government and conducted in the Côte d'Ivoire, Dominican Republic, and Thailand, some pregnant women infected with HIV were given placebo pills rather than AZT, a drug known to prevent passing of the virus from mothers to their babies. Babies born to these mothers were in danger of contracting a fatal disease.	Research participants who consented to participate and who were randomly assigned to the control group were denied access to a medication regimen with a known benefit. This denial violates the participants' right to fair treatment and protection (French, 1997; Wheeler, 1997).

AIDS, acquired immune deficiency syndrome; *AZT*, azidothymidine; *HIV*, human immunodeficiency virus.

TABLE **6.2**

PROTECTION OF HUMAN RIGHTS

BASIC HUMAN RIGHT	DEFINITION
Right to self-determination	This right is based on the ethical principle of respect for persons; people should be treated as autonomous agents who have the freedom to choose without external controls. An autonomous agent is one who is informed about a proposed study and is allowed to choose to participate or not to participate (Brink, 1992). Moreover, research participants have the right to withdraw from a study without penalty.
Right to privacy and dignity	This right is based on the ethical principle of respect for persons; privacy is the freedom of a person to determine the time, extent, and circumstances under which private information is shared or withheld from other people.
Right to anonymity and confidentiality	This right is based on the ethical principle of respect for persons; anonymity exists when the participant's identity cannot be discerned, even by the researcher, from his or her individual responses (American Nurses Association, 1985).
	Confidentiality means that the individual identities of participants will not be linked to the information they provide and will not be publicly divulged.

VIOLATION OF BASIC HUMAN RIGHT	EXAMPLE
A participant's right to self-determination is violated through the use of coercion, deception, and covert data collection. • In coercion, an overt threat of harm or excessive reward is presented to ensure participants' compliance. • In deception, participants are misinformed about the purpose of the research. • In covert data collection, people become research participants and are exposed to research treatments without knowing it. • The potential for violation of the right to self-determination is greater for research participants with diminished autonomy, who have decreased ability to give informed consent and are vulnerable.	Participants may believe that their care will be adversely affected if they refuse to participate in research. The Willowbrook Hospital Study (see Table 6.1) is an example of how coercion was used to obtain the consent of parents of vulnerable children with mental retardation, who would not be admitted to the institution unless they participated in a study in which they were deliberately injected with the hepatitis virus. The Jewish Chronic Disease Hospital Study (see Table 6.1) is an example of a study in which patients and their personal physicians did not know that cancer cells were being injected. In Milgram's (1963) study, research participants were deceived when asked to administer electric shocks to another person, who was an actor pretending to suffer from the shocks. Participants administering the shocks were very distressed by participating in this study, although they were not administering shocks at all. This study is an example of deception.
The U.S. Privacy Act of 1974 was instituted to protect participants from privacy violations. These violations occur most frequently during data collection, when responses to invasive questions might result in the loss of a job, friendships, or dignity or might create embarrassment and mental distress. These violations also may occur when participants are unaware that information is being shared with other people.	Research participants may be asked personal questions such as "Were you sexually abused as a child?"; "Do you use drugs?"; and "What are your sexual preferences?" When questions are asked in the presence of hidden microphones or hidden recording devices, the participants' privacy is invaded because they have no knowledge that the data are being shared with other people. Participants' right to control access of other people to their records is also violated.
Anonymity is violated when the participants' responses can be linked to their identity.	Researchers who choose to identify data by using the participant's name are breaching the basic human right of anonymity. Instead, researchers should assign participants a code number that is used for identification purposes. Research participants' names are never used in the reporting of findings.

TABLE **6.2**

PROTECTION OF HUMAN RIGHTS—cont'd

VIOLATION OF BASIC HUMAN RIGHT	EXAMPLE
Confidentiality is breached when a researcher, by accident or direct action, allows an unauthorized person to gain access to study data that contain information about the participant's identity or responses, which creates a potentially harmful situation for the participant.	Breaches of confidentiality with regard to sexual preference, income, drug use, prejudice, or personality variables can be harmful to research participants. Data should be analyzed as group data so that participants cannot be identified by their responses.

BASIC HUMAN RIGHT	DEFINITION
Right to fair treatment	This right is based on the ethical principle of justice; people should be treated fairly and should receive what they are due or owed. "Fair treatment" refers to the equitable selection of research participants and their treatment during the research study. This treatment includes selection of participants for reasons directly related to the problem studied, as opposed to selection of participants because of convenience, the compromised position of the participants, or their vulnerability. Fair treatment also extends to the treatment of participants during the study, including fair distribution of risks and benefits of the research regardless of age, race, or socioeconomic status.
Right to protection from discomfort and harm	This right is based on the ethical principle of beneficence; people must take an active role in promoting good and preventing harm both in the world around them and in research studies. Discomfort and harm can be physical, psychological, social, or economic in nature. The five levels of harm and discomfort are as follows: 1. No anticipated effects 2. Temporary discomfort 3. Unusual level of temporary discomfort 4. Risk of permanent damage 5. Certainty of permanent damage Participants with diminished autonomy are entitled to protection. They are more vulnerable because of age, legal or mental incompetence, terminal illness, or confinement to an institution. A justification for the use of vulnerable participants must be provided.

VIOLATION OF BASIC HUMAN RIGHT	EXAMPLE
Injustices with regard to participant selection have occurred as a result of social, cultural, racial, and gender biases in society.	The Tuskegee Syphilis Study that ended in 1973 (Levine, 1986), the Jewish Chronic Disease Study of 1965 (Hershey & Miller, 1976), the San Antonio Contraceptive Study of 1969 (Levine, 1986), and the Willowbrook Hospital Study of 1972 (Rothman, 1982) (see Table 6.1) all are examples of unfair participant selection and the use of vulnerable populations.
Historically, research participants were often recruited from groups of people who were regarded as having less "social value," such as people living in poverty, prisoners, slaves, people who are mentally incompetent, and people who are dying. Participants were often treated carelessly, without consideration of physical or psychological harm.	Investigators should not be late for data-collection appointments, should terminate data collection on time, should not change agreed-upon procedures or activities without consent, and should provide agreed-upon benefits, such as a copy of the study findings or a participation fee.

Continued

TABLE **6.2**

PROTECTION OF HUMAN RIGHTS—cont'd

VIOLATION OF BASIC HUMAN RIGHT	EXAMPLE
Research participants' right to be protected is violated when discomfort or disabling injury will occur and, thus, the benefits do not outweigh the risks.	Temporary physical discomfort involving minimal risk includes fatigue or headache; emotional discomfort includes the expense involved in travelling to and from the data-collection site. Studies of sensitive issues (such as rape, incest, or spouse abuse) might cause unusual levels of temporary discomfort by increasing participants' awareness of current or past traumatic experiences. In these situations, researchers assess distress levels and provide debriefing sessions, during which the participant may express feelings and ask questions. The researcher has the opportunity to make referrals for professional intervention. Studies with the potential to cause permanent damage are more likely to be medical in nature rather than nursing in nature, inasmuch as physiological damage may be permanent. One clinical trial of a new drug, a recombinant activated protein C (Zovan) for treatment of sepsis, was halted when interim findings from the phase III clinical trials revealed that the rate of mortality among the patients receiving treatment was lower than that among those receiving the placebo. Evaluation of the data led to termination of the trial to make a known beneficial treatment available more quickly to all patients. In some research, such as the Tuskegee Syphilis Study or Nazi medical experiments, participants experienced permanent damage or died. In Dr. Cameron's study (see Table 6.1), the continued electroconvulsive therapy increased the damage.

BOX **6.2**

BASIC ETHICAL PRINCIPLES RELEVANT TO THE CONDUCTING OF RESEARCH

RESPECT FOR PERSONS

People have the right to self-determination and to treatment as autonomous agents. Thus they have the freedom to participate or not participate in research. Persons with diminished autonomy are entitled to protection.

BENEFICENCE

Beneficence is an obligation to do no harm and maximize possible benefits. Persons are treated in an ethical manner when their decisions are respected, they are protected from harm, and efforts are made to secure their well-being.

JUSTICE

Human subjects should be treated fairly. An injustice occurs when benefit to which a person is entitled is denied without good reason or when a burden is imposed unduly.

From Elder, G. (1981). Social history & life experience. In D. H. Eichorn, J. A. Clausen, N. Haan, et al. (Eds.), *Present and past in middle life* (pp. 3–31). New York: Academic Press. Copyright 1981 Academic Press.

for welfare," and "justice." Of the others, "respect for human dignity" is articulated through these three core principles; "respect for free and informed consent" and "respect for vulnerable persons" are now reflected in the principle of "respect for persons," and "respect for vulnerable persons" is also reflected in the principle of "justice"; "respect for privacy and confidentiality" is part of "concern for welfare"; and "respect for justice and inclusiveness" is in the core principle of "justice." The core principle "concern for welfare" now also includes "balancing harms and benefits," "minimizing harm," and "maximizing benefit."

 Research Hint _____

The qualitative researcher must be especially diligent in protecting the privacy and confidentiality of participants. When the participants' verbatim quotations are used in the "Results" or "Findings" section of the research report to highlight the findings, the smallness of the sample size may make it easy to identify an individual participant. Moreover, when researchers and REBs are engaging in naturalistic observation, the TCPS 2 indicates that these boards "and researchers need to consider the methodological requirements of the proposed research project and the ethical implications associated with observational approaches, such as the possible infringement of privacy. They should pay close attention to the ethical implications of such factors as the nature of the activities to be observed, the environment in which the activities are to be observed, whether the activities are staged for the purpose of the research, the expectations of privacy that prospective participants might have, the means of recording the observations, whether the research records or published reports involve identification of the participants, and any means by which those participants may give permission to be identified" (CIHR et al., 2014, p. 142).

The Evolution of Ethics in Nursing Research

The evolution of ethics in nursing research can be traced back to 1897 and the constitution of the Nurses' Associated Alumnae Organization in the United States. One of the first purposes of this organization was to establish a code of ethics for the nursing profession. In 1900, Isabel Hampton Robb wrote *Nursing Ethics: For Hospital and Private Use*. In describing the moral laws by which people must abide, she stated the following:

> Etiquette, speaking broadly, means a form of behavior or manners expressly or tacitly required on particular occasions. It makes up the code of polite life and includes forms of ceremony to be observed, so that we invariably find in societies that certain etiquette is required and observed either tacitly or by expressed agreement.

Although Robb's comments reflect the norms of Victorian society, they also highlight a historical concern for ethical actions by nurses as health care providers (Robb, 1900). In 1953, the International Council of Nurses (ICN) adopted the Code of Ethics for Nurses, and it is used as the standard for nurses worldwide.

The Code is regularly reviewed and revised, most recently in 2017, in response to the changing trends and realities in nursing. The Code guides nurses and nursing to demonstrate respect for human rights, the right to life and to dignity, and the right to be treated with respect. The ICN code of ethics also supports a nurse's right to refuse to participate in activities that conflict with caring and healing (ICN, 2012).

In Canada, most disciplines have developed their own code of ethics with guidelines for research. The CNA's first document on ethical principles related to nursing research, *Ethical Guidelines for Nurses in Research Involving Human Participants*, was released in 1983. It was revised in 1994 and 2002 and is now titled *Ethical Research Guidelines for Registered Nurses* (CNA, 2002).

Clearly, ignorance and naïveté regarding ethical and legal guidelines for conducting research is never an excuse for a nurse's failure to be familiar with such guidelines and to act on behalf of patients, whose human rights must be safeguarded at all times. Nurse researchers are often among the most responsible and conscientious investigators in respecting the rights of human participants. All nurses should be aware that, in addition to the ethical research guidelines of the CNA, universities and hospitals may also have supplemental sets of ethical guidelines to follow.

Current and Future Ethical Dilemmas in Research

Ethics is the theory or discipline dealing with principles of moral values and moral conduct. The ethical dilemmas in research for the twenty-first century concern biotechnology, the use of animals for research, and the creation of an organizational culture that values and nurtures research ethics and the rights of people who engage in research either as investigators or as participants. For example, in only 12 years, the Human Genome Project, an international research project launched in 1988 by investigators in the United States, provided a vast amount of data on DNA, including the molecular details about the DNA of more than 26 organisms. To engage in genome research, genetic engineering and genetic information are required (Carroll & Ciaffa, 2003), which can raise ethical concerns about the purpose of the engineering. If the purpose is to treat a disease, then the research is ethically acceptable, but the existence of germline intervention raises "more significant ethical concerns, because risks will extend across generations, magnifying the impact of unforeseen consequences" (Carroll & Ciaffa, 2003). Ethical concerns also arise with regard to the privacy of genetic information, mandatory testing of newborns, and mandatory genetic screening.

Other areas of research that engender much discussion and controversy are fetal tissue research and the use of women who are of child-bearing potential as participants in drug or therapeutic studies. The Tri-Council (i.e., the CIHR, the NSERC, and the SSHRC) worked over a period of several years to make stem cell research a reality in Canada, with the appropriate ethical guidelines for the use of embryos, fetuses, gametes, and pluripotent stems cells. These guidelines are detailed in the TCPS 2 (CIHR et al., 2014).

Of note is the following information:
Researchers conducting genetic research shall:

(a) in their research proposal, develop a plan for managing information that may be revealed through their genetic research;
(b) submit their plan to the REB; and
(c) advise prospective participants of the plan for managing information revealed through the research. (CIHR et al., 2014, p. 194, Article 13.2)

In the past, women of child-bearing potential were denied participation in studies of a drug or potential therapy because of the unknown, potentially teratogenic effects of drugs and other therapies that were in various stages of testing. Guidelines related to the inclusion of pregnant women as research participants have been even more stringent than previous guidelines; as a result, women have been excluded from many important drug and research studies over the years.

The TCPS 2 also has a well-articulated policy on the ethical guidelines for research with Indigenous populations to ensure protection of the rights of those communities (CIHR et al., 2014). This guideline includes the need for research when benefit is mutual, incorporating the role of community elders in consent and the responsibilities of the researcher to understand and protect sacred knowledge. The inclusion of a separate chapter (Chapter 9, p. 109) in TCPS 2 outlining how to engage with and honour Indigenous communities reflects the work that was accomplished over several years to advance the need for equitable partnerships and to provide safeguards with these communities. It is noted that "Aboriginal entities at local, regional and national levels have published and implemented principles and codes governing research practice—including ethical protections—that emphasize collective rights, interests and responsibilities" (CIHR et al., 2014, p. 110).

PROTECTION OF HUMAN RIGHTS

Human rights are the claims and demands that have been justified according to an individual or by a group of individuals. The term *human rights* is applied to the following five rights outlined in the CNA's (2002) guidelines and linked to the Tri-Council's principles of respect for research participants:

1. Right to self-determination
2. Right to privacy and dignity
3. Right to anonymity and confidentiality
4. Right to fair treatment
5. Right to protection from discomfort and harm

These rights apply to everyone involved in a research project, including research team members involved in data collection, practising nurses involved in the research setting, and people participating in the study. As consumers of research read a research article, they must realize that any issues highlighted in Table 6.2 should have been addressed and resolved before a research study is approved for implementation.

Procedures for Protecting Basic Human Rights

Informed Consent

Informed consent, illustrated by the ethical principles of respect and the related right to self-determination, is outlined in Box 6.3. Nurses need to understand the elements of informed consent to be knowledgeable participants when either obtaining informed consent from patients or critiquing this process as it is presented in research articles.

BOX **6.3**

ELEMENTS OF INFORMED CONSENT

1. A statement that the study involves research
2. An explanation of the purposes of the research, delineating the expected duration of the subject's participation
3. A description of the procedures to be followed and identification of any procedures that are experimental
4. A description of any reasonably foreseeable risks or discomforts to the subject
5. A description of any benefits to the subject or to others that may reasonably be expected from the research
6. A disclosure of appropriate alternative procedures or course of treatment, if any, that might be advantageous to the subject
7. A statement describing the extent to which the anonymity and confidentiality of the records identifying the subject will be maintained
8. For research involving more than minimal risk, an explanation as to whether any medical treatments are available if injury occurs and, if so, what they consist of or where further information may be obtained
9. An explanation about whom to contact for answers to questions about the research and researcher subjects' rights and whom to contact in the event of a research-related injury to the subject
10. A statement that participation is voluntary, that refusal to participate will not involve any penalty or less benefit to which the subject is otherwise entitled, and that the subject may discontinue participation at any time without penalty or loss of otherwise entitled benefits

From Code of Federal Regulations: Protection of human subjects, 45 CFR 46, *OPRR Reports*, revised March 8, 1983.

Informed consent is the legal principle that requires a researcher to inform individuals about the potential benefits and risks of a study before the individuals can participate voluntarily. In theory, this principle governs the patient's ability to accept or reject individual medical interventions designed to diagnose or treat an illness. According to the TCPS 2 (CIHR et al., 2014), free and informed consent is at the heart of ethical research and is a process of dialogue and information sharing to allow participants the choice to participate in research. Free and informed consent must be given without manipulation, undue influence, or coercion.

For example, Baumann, Idriss-Wheeler, Blythe, et al. (2015) conducted an evaluation to determine the usability of an employment website for internationally educated nurses. Approval for the use of human participants was obtained from appropriate ethics review boards before the data collection. The study rationale was explained to all participants prior to obtaining informed consent, and confidentiality was assured and maintained. Another example involves a pilot study conducted to estimate the effects of a breast milk expression education and support on breast milk production. Héon, Goulet, Garofalo, and associates (2016) (Appendix D) obtained ethical approval from the hospital's REB, and the "principal investigator approached eligible mothers within 24 hr after birth, explained the study, and obtained their informed written consent" (p. 533).

No investigator may involve a human being as a research participant until the legally effective informed consent has been obtained from either the participant or a legally authorized representative of the participant, and prospective participants must have time to decide whether to take part in a study. The researcher must not coerce the participant into taking part in the study, nor may researchers collect data on participants who have explicitly refused to take part in a study.

An ethical violation of this principle is illustrated by the case of *Halushka v. University of Saskatchewan et al.* (1965). In this landmark case, a university student volunteered for a study testing a new anaesthetic, for which he would be paid $50.00. He consented to be in the study, based on the following information disclosed to him: the test would last a few hours, the test was safe and had been conducted many times before, and the student had nothing to worry about. He was informed that the procedure would include placement of electrodes on his arms, legs, and head and insertion of a catheter into a vein in his arm. He signed a consent form releasing the physicians and the university from liability for any untoward effects or accidents, which were explained to him as "falling down at home after the test" (McLean, 1996, p. 49). The test proceeded with administration of an *untested* anaesthetic, and the student suffered a cardiac arrest. He was unconscious for 4 days in the hospital and left with a residual inability to concentrate. The physicians and the university were found negligent for failing to "disclose that there was risk involved with the use of an anaesthetic and that this particular drug had not been previously tested by them" (McLean, 1996, p. 49).

When composing an informed consent form, researchers must ensure that the language is understandable. For example, the level of language used should be appropriate to the age and comprehension/reading level of the participant population, generally at approximately a grade 6–8 reading level (Health Canada, 2014). The elements that need to be contained in an informed consent form are listed in Box 6.3. Note that many institutions require additional elements. Figure 6.1 is an example of an informed consent form for a quantitative study; Figure 6.2 is an example of an informed consent form for a qualitative study. Note that in each consent form, the elements of participation, risk and benefits, withdrawal, confidentiality, and whom to contact for further queries are clearly outlined.

 Research Hint_____

Remember that research reports rarely provide readers with detailed information regarding the degree to which the researcher adhered to ethical principles, such as informed consent; this is because of space limitations in journals, which make it impossible to describe all aspects of a study. Failure to mention procedures to safeguard participants' rights does not necessarily mean that such precautions were not taken.

Most investigators obtain **consent** (agreement to participate in a study) through personal discussion with potential participants. This process allows the person who is the potential participant to obtain immediate answers to questions. Consent forms, written in narrative or outline form, highlight elements that both inform and remind participants of the nature of the study and their participation When one participant is scheduled to participate in many interviews, the participant must give **process consent** (voluntary continued participation in a study, which can be verbal) for each data-collection point.

Assurance of anonymity and confidentiality (defined in Table 6.2), which is conveyed in writing, is sometimes difficult in unique research situations that capture the public's attention. For example, when physicians at Loma Linda University Hospital in California transplanted a baboon's heart into a 2-week-old infant, her identity was hidden **(anonymity)**—she was known only as Baby Fae—and **confidentiality** was ensured in that the reports could not be linked to her and her family. Maintaining anonymity and confidentiality is particularly important for qualitative researchers because the researcher often functions as the data-collection "instrument" and meets the participant. The consent form must be signed and dated by the participant. The presence of witnesses is not always necessary but does constitute evidence that the participant concerned actually signed the form. In cases in which the participant is a minor or is physically or mentally incapable of signing the consent, the signature must be obtained from a legal guardian or representative.

CONSENT TO PARTICIPATE IN A RESEARCH STUDY

Title
VISUAL DIFFERENTIATION IN LOOK-ALIKE MEDICATION NAMES

University Health Network Principal Investigator
Tasmine Halevy, Clinical Director of Pharmacy, UHN, 416-XXX-XXXX

Study Principal Investigator
Monica Blum, Associate Professor, Reed University, 416-XXX-XXXX

Co-Investigators
Joyce Davis, Vice President, ISMP Canada
Dr. Mina D. Singh, Associate Professor, York University, Faculty of Health, School of Nursing
Ravinder Sharma, Human Factors Engineer, Red Forest Consulting
Dr. Irmgard Mirren, Psychiatrist, Child and Parent Resource Institute
Evan Ross, Chief Pharmacist, Child and Parent Resource Institute

Collaborator
Jude Hartman

Sponsors
Canadian Patient Safety Institute, ISMP Canada; Red Forest Consulting; Child and Parent Resource Institute; York University Faculty of Graduate Studies, Department of Design and Faculty of Health

Introduction
You are being asked to take part in a research study. Please read this explanation about the study and its risks and benefits before you decide if you would like to take part. You should take as much time as you need to make your decision. You should ask the Principal Investigator or Research Assistants to explain anything that you do not understand and make sure that all of your questions have been answered before signing this consent form. Before you make your decision, feel free to talk about this study with anyone you wish. Participation in this study is voluntary.

Background and Purpose
This study will look at the visual display of look-alike medication names. It is hoped that this research will contribute to the design of shelf labelling, packaging, and computer displays to help reduce instances of medication errors due to look-alike medication names. The results from this research are intended to support health care workers in the safe delivery of health care. You have been asked to take part in this research study because you have or may come into contact with look-alike medications. A total of 130 to 135 nursing staff and 10 pharmacy staff from Princess Margaret Hospital, Toronto General Hospital and Toronto Western Hospital will participate in this study.

Study Design
You will help us evaluate the best ways to display look-alike names for ease and accuracy in recognition and selection of medications. If you choose to participate in this study, you will be asked to answer a short questionnaire to establish your demographic information and to ask you your opinion of current practices related to the display of look-alike medication names. You will participate in three experiments that emulate the selection of medications. The first two experiments are screen based, and you will be asked to identify look-alike names on a laptop display. For the third experiment, you will be asked to select medications from a series of baskets. The tasks will be explained thoroughly before each experiment. Your commitment for this study will be one session lasting approximately 45 to 60 minutes.

FIG. 6.1 Example of an informed consent form for a quantitative study. *ISMP,* Institute for Safe Medication Practices; *UHN,* University Health Network.

Continued

CONSENT TO PARTICIPATE IN A RESEARCH STUDY—cont'd

Risks Related to Being in the Study

There are no known risks if you take part in this study, but you may refuse to answer questions or stop the experiments at any time if there is any discomfort. Your responses to the questionnaires will not have an impact on your employment, nor will they be shared with your supervisors or managers.

Benefits to Being in the Study

You will not receive any direct benefit from being in this study. Information learned from this study may help in the safe delivery of health care.

Voluntary Participation

Your participation in this study is voluntary. You may decide not to be in this study, or to be in the study now and then change your mind later. You may leave the study at any time without affecting your employment status. You may refuse to answer any question you do not want to answer on the questionnaire by writing "pass," or stop participating in the experiment at any time.

Confidentiality

The information that is collected for the study will be kept in a locked and secure area at York University by the study Principal Investigator for 10 years. Only the study team and the people or groups listed below will be allowed to look at the data. All information collected during this study will be kept confidential and will not be shared with anyone outside the study unless required by law. Any information about you that is collected for the study will have a code and will not show your name or address, or any information that directly identifies you. You will not be named in any reports, publications, or presentations that may come from this study. If you decide to leave the study, the information about you that was collected before you left the study will still be used. No new information will be collected without your permission. Representatives of the University Health Network Research Ethics Board may look at the study records to check that the information collected for the study is correct and to make sure the study followed proper laws and guidelines.

Questions about the Study

If you have any questions or concerns, or would like to speak to the study team for any reason, please call: Tasmine Halevy, University Health Network, at **416-XXX- XXXX** or Monica Blum, Reed University, **416-XXX-XXXX**.

The research has been reviewed and approved by the University Health Network Research Ethics Board (REB) and the Human Participants Review Committee (HPRC) at Reed University for compliance with senate ethics policy. If you have any questions about your rights as a research participant or have concerns about this study, call the Chair of the UHN (REB) or the Research Ethics office number at 416-XXX-XXXX or Manager, Research Ethics—Alicia Collins-Walker: 309 Elsevier Lanes, Reed University, 416-XXX-XXXX. The HPRC and REB are groups of people who oversee the ethical conduct of research studies. These people are not part of the study team. Everything that you discuss will be kept confidential.

Consent

This study has been explained to me and any questions I had have been answered. I know that I may leave the study at any time. I agree to take part in this study.

Print Study Participant's Name   Signature   Date

(You will be given a signed copy of this consent form.)

My signature means that I have explained the study to the participant named above. I have answered all questions.

Print Name of Person Obtaining Consent   Signature   Date

FIG. 6.1, cont'd

INFORMATION AND INFORMED CONSENT STATEMENT: INTERVIEW

Title
BETTER UNDERSTANDING HOW COUPLES COPE WITH A CHILD'S LIFE-THREATENING ILLNESS

Principal Investigator
Dr. Susan Cadell, Associate Professor; Director, Manulife Centre for Healthy Living; Lyle S. Hallman Faculty of Social Work, Wilfrid Laurier University, 519-XXX-XXXX

Co-Investigators
Dr. Rosemary Stiles, School of Nursing, York University
Dr. Anna DeLaurentis, The Centre for Health and Coping Studies, University of British Columbia

Research Assistants
Matilde Negrini, Faculty of Social Work, Wilfrid Laurier University
Julian Millman, Faculty of Social Work, Wilfrid Laurier University
Nella Leone, Faculty of Social Work, Wilfrid Laurier University

Contact Person
Matthew Philips, Research Coordinator: 1-800-XXX-XXXX

We are inviting couples to participate in the next phase of this research study. The purpose of this study is to discover the experience of spouses/partners who are together caring for a child with a life-limiting illness. This study is being conducted by Dr. Susan Cadell, Associate Professor and Director of the Manulife Centre for Healthy Living at Wilfrid Laurier University, and Co-Investigator on the Canadian Institutes for Health Research's New Emerging Team (NET): *Transitions in Pediatric Palliative and End-of-Life Care.*

Information
During the interview, you and your spouse/partner will be interviewed together. You will be asked questions about your personal experience of caring for a child with a life-limiting condition, as well as questions about the role that each spouse/partner plays in the coping of the other. The interview will take approximately 1.5 to 2 hours. The interview will be conducted by a trained, sensitive interviewer and will take place at a location convenient to you. In order to make sure that we have an accurate record of what you have shared during the interview, your interview will be recorded and transcribed. All identifying information will be removed from the transcripts and only the investigators and research staff will have access to them. The recordings and transcripts will be identified only by code number and stored in a locked filing cabinet or secured information system. They will be stored for 5 years after the publication of the results from this study. After 5 years, the recordings and the transcripts will be destroyed. The recordings will not be used for any other purposes without your additional permission.

Phase Two of this study will involve the participation of approximately 15 to 20 couples who are together caring for their child. Due to the nature of this study, it is possible that quotes from your interview may be used in publication. To maintain confidentiality, all identifying information will be removed from the quotations. If a specific family or disease characteristic is rare and could potentially be identifying, the information will be changed in the quote. Please indicate your preference below regarding the use of your quotations.

Name: _____   Name: _____
□ Yes – I can be quoted with no identifying information.   □ Yes – I can be quoted with no identifying information.
□ No – Please do not use quotes.   □ No – Please do not use quotes.

FIG. 6.2 Example of an informed consent form for a qualitative study.

Continued

INFORMATION AND INFORMED CONSENT STATEMENT: INTERVIEW—cont'd

Risk

This research project deals with a sensitive topic. The interviewer will monitor your distress level and will stop the interviewing process if you become upset. The interviewer will then ensure that you are aware of your right not to answer any questions asked and your right to terminate the interview at any time. If necessary, the interviewer will refer you to appropriate services and resources to ensure your support needs are met.

Benefits

You may benefit from the ability to communicate your experiences of pediatric palliative care in a safe, nonjudgemental setting. In addition, your participation may benefit other families, researchers, and policy makers in pediatric palliative care by providing a better understanding of the caregiver experience.

Confidentiality

Confidentiality will be provided to the fullest extent possible by law. Your identity and the identity of all family members will be kept strictly confidential. All identifying information will be removed from the data. All documents and recordings will be identified only by code number and the information will be retained in a secured information system and locked filing cabinet. All identifying information will be kept separate from the data. All documents that are kept on a computer will be password protected. Identifying information will not be emailed to anyone at any time. You will not be identified by name in any reports of the completed study. Only study personnel will have access to the study data.

Compensation

For participating in this study, you and your spouse/partner will each receive $30 at the beginning of the interview. If you withdraw from the study after this point, you will still receive the full amount.

Participation

Your participation in this study is voluntary; you may decline to participate without penalty. If you decide to participate, you may withdraw from the study at any time without penalty and without loss of benefits to which you are otherwise entitled. If you withdraw from the study before data collection is completed, your data will be destroyed. You have the right to omit any question(s)/procedure(s) you choose.

Feedback and Publication

It is expected that the results of this study will be presented and published as a journal article. If you would like to be notified of the results of the study, please indicate below.

Name: _____   Name: _____

☐ Yes – I would like to be notified of results.   ☐ Yes – I would like to be notified of results.

Contact

If you have questions at any time about the study or the procedures, or if you experience adverse effects as a result of participating in this study, you may contact the Research Coordinator, Matthew Philips, at 1-800-XXX-XXXX. This project has been reviewed and approved by the University Research Ethics Board at Wilfrid Laurier University. If you feel you have not been treated according to the descriptions in this form, or your rights as a participant in research have been violated during the course of this project, you may contact Dr. Mark Billingsley, Chair, University Research Ethics Board, Wilfrid Laurier University, 519-XXX-XXXX.

Consent

I have read and understand the above information. I have received a copy of this form. I agree to participate in this study.

_____   _____
Participant's signature   Date

_____   _____
Participant's signature   Date

_____   _____
Investigator's signature   Date

FIG. 6.2, cont'd

The investigator also signs the form to indicate commitment to the agreement of anonymity and confidentiality.

In studies in which the researcher suspected child abuse or neglect, the participants need to be clearly informed that the researcher has a legal responsibility to report any suspicions to the child welfare agency, even though, the participants' anonymity and confidentiality were guaranteed. Another strategy that can be used to ensure confidentiality is to ask the transcribers, who are not part of the research team, in a qualitative study to sign a confidentiality agreement.

In general, the signed informed consent form is given to the participant. The researcher should also keep a copy. Some research, such as a retrospective chart audit, may require only institutional approval, not informed consent. In some cases, when minimal risk is involved, the investigator may have to provide the participant only with an information sheet and a verbal explanation. In other cases, such as a volunteer convenience sample, completion and return of research instruments constitute evidence of consent. The REB advises on exceptions to these guidelines, as in cases in which the REB might grant waivers or amend its guidelines in other ways. The REB makes the final determination regarding the most appropriate documentation format. Research consumers should note whether and what kind of evidence of informed consent has been provided in a research article.

 Research Hint_____

Note that researchers often do not obtain written informed consent when the major means of data collection is through self-administered questionnaires. Implied consent is usually assumed in such cases; in other words, the return of the completed questionnaire reflects the respondent's voluntary consent to participate.

Research Ethics Boards

Research ethics boards (REBs) are panels that review research projects to assess whether ethical standards are met in relation to the protection of the rights of human participants. Such boards are established in agencies to review biomedical and behavioural research involving human subjects within the agency or in programs sponsored by the agency. Universities, hospitals, and other health agencies applying for a grant or contract for any project or program that involves the conduct of biomedical or behavioural research with human participants are required by the Tri-Council and most funding agencies to submit with their application assurances that they have established an REB that reviews the research projects and protects the rights of the human participants (CIHR et al., 2014). The Panel on Research Ethics has an online applied course with 10 modules for researchers and members of REBs, which can be found at http://www.pre.ethics.gc.ca/eng/education/tutorial-didacticiel/. Students engaged in research are encouraged to complete this tutorial.

The Tri-Council also requires that the REB have at least five members, including both men and women. Membership must include at least two professionals who have expertise in relevant research disciplines, fields, and methodologies covered by the REB; at least one who is knowledgeable in ethics; at least one who is knowledgeable in the relevant law (but that member should not be the institution's legal counsel or risk manager); and at least one who is a community member and has no affiliation with the institution but is recruited from the community served by the institution (CIHR et al., 2014).

The REB is responsible for protecting participants from undue risk and loss of personal rights and dignity. For a research proposal to be eligible for consideration by an REB, it must already have been approved by a departmental review group, such as a nursing research committee, that attests to the proposal's scientific merit and congruence with institutional policies, procedures, and mission. The REB reviews the study's protocol to ensure that it meets the requirements of ethical research. Most boards provide guidelines or instructions for researchers that include steps to be taken to receive REB approval. For example, guidelines for writing a standard consent form or criteria for qualifying for an expedited rather than a full REB review may be available. The REB has the authority to approve research, require modifications, or disapprove a research study, on the basis of the guidelines outlined in Box 6.4. A researcher must receive REB approval before beginning to conduct research. For instance, REB approval was obtained from York University and from Mackenzie Health for a study to evaluate a Knowledge Transfer Team approach to implementing a stroke best practice guideline (Singh, Hynie, Rivera, et al., 2015). REBs have the authority to suspend or terminate approval of research that is not conducted in accordance with REB requirements or that has been associated with unexpected serious harm to participants.

REBs in Canada also provide for reviewing research in an expedited manner when the risk to research participants is minimal. An expedited review usually shortens the length of the review

process but does not automatically exempt the researcher from obtaining informed consent.

Not all research requires an ethical review. To follow protocol, researchers can submit a proposal to their own REB; however, according to the TCPS 2 (CIHR et al., 2014), this step is not necessary when the research relies exclusively on information that is legally accessible to the public and appropriately protected by law or that is publicly accessible and there is no reasonable expectation of privacy. Legally accessible information includes registries of deaths, court judgements, and public archives and publicly available statistics (e.g., Statistics Canada public use files).

REB review is also not required when researchers use exclusively publicly available information that may contain identifiable information and for which there is no reasonable expectation of privacy. For example, identifiable information may be disseminated in the public domain through print or electronic publications; film, audio, or digital recordings; press accounts; official publications of private or public institutions; artistic installations, exhibitions, or literary events freely open to the public; or publications accessible in public libraries. Research that is nonintrusive and does not involve direct interaction between the researcher and individuals through the Internet also does not require REB review. Online material such as documents, records, performances, online archival materials, or published third-party interviews to which the public is given uncontrolled access on the Internet and for which there is no expectation of privacy is considered to be publicly available information.[1]

> **BOX 6.4**
>
> **PARTIAL GUIDELINES FOR RESEARCH ETHICS BOARD APPROVAL OF RESEARCH STUDIES**
>
> To approve research, the REB must determine that the following guidelines have been satisfied:
> 1. There is an analysis of balance and distribution of harms and benefits.
> 2. There is a proportionate approach based on the general principle that the level of review is determined by the level of risk presented by the research: the lower the level of risk, the lower the level of scrutiny (delegated review); the higher the level of risk, the higher the level of scrutiny (full board review).
> 3. There is a formal informed consent process.
>
> ---
> *REB*, research ethics board.
> From Canadian Institutes of Health Research, Natural Sciences and Engineering Research Council of Canada, & Social Sciences and Humanities Research Council of Canada. (2014, December). *Tri-Council policy statement: Ethical conduct for research involving humans.* Retrieved from http://www.pre.ethics.gc.ca/eng/policy-politique/initiatives/tcps2-eptc2/Default/.

---

[1]Adapted from Canadian Institutes of Health Research, Natural Sciences and Engineering Research Council of Canada, & Social Sciences and Humanities Research Council of Canada. (2014, December). *Tri-Council policy statement: Ethical conduct for research involving humans.* Chapter 2, "Scope and approach." Retrieved from http://www.pre.ethics.gc.ca/eng/policy-politique/initiatives/tcps2-eptc2/Default/.

CRITICAL THINKING DECISION PATH

Evaluating the Risk–Benefit Ratio of a Research Study

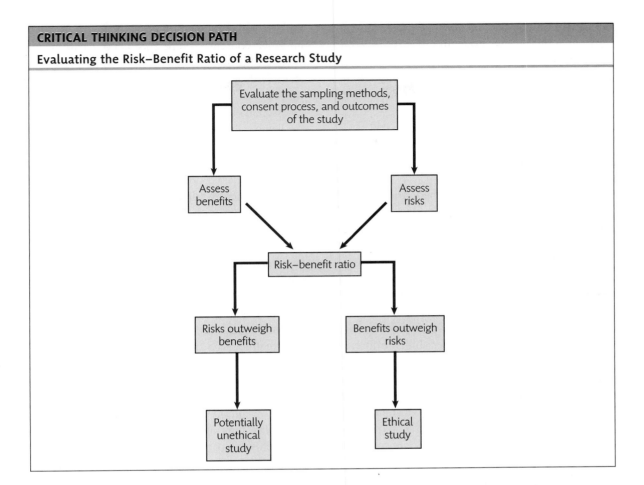

The TCPS 2 exempts quality assurance studies, quality improvement studies, performance reviews, or testing within normal educational requirements from REB reviews. However, performance reviews or studies that contain an element of research in addition to assessment may need ethics review (CIHR et al., 2014, Article 2.5).

The Critical Thinking Decision Path illustrates the ethical decision-making process an REB might use in evaluating the risk–benefit ratio of a research study.

Protecting the Basic Human Rights of Vulnerable Groups

Researchers are advised to consult their agency's REB for the most recent guidelines when considering research involving vulnerable groups, such as older adults, children, pregnant women, unborn children, persons who are emotionally or physically disabled, prisoners, deceased persons, students, and persons with AIDS or other serious illnesses. In addition, researchers should consult the REB before planning research that potentially involves an oversubscribed research population, such as patients who have undergone organ transplantation, patients with AIDS, or "captive" and convenient research populations, such as prisoners. The use of special populations does not preclude undertaking research; safeguards must be undertaken, however, to protect the rights of these participants (CIHR et al., 2014).

Pediatric research can be particularly problematic. Mitchell (1984) discussed the U.S. National Commission's concept of assent versus consent in regard to pediatric research. **Assent**—an aspect of informed consent that pertains to protecting the rights of children as research subjects—is composed of the following three fundamental elements:

1. A basic understanding by the child of what the child will be expected to do and what will be done to the child
2. A comprehension by the child of the basic purpose of the research
3. An ability of the child to express a preference regarding participation

An example of research in a pediatric group in which assent was used is the study of Stewart, King, Blood, and colleagues (2013). These researchers were interested in understanding the health equities of Indigenous children with respiratory conditions. The children gave assent verbally or in writing, and their parents provided written consent for their children to participate.

In contrast to assent, *consent* requires a relatively advanced level of cognitive ability. Informed consent reflects competency standards requiring abstract appreciation of and reasoning about the information provided. According to Health Canada (2014), "a child under 16 years of age should provide his/her assent and may refuse to participate even if the parent has provided their consent. The age of consent to participate in research in Quebec is 18 years of age, and the assent form for the involvement of minors in research should be used for any individuals under the age of 18" (p. 1).

If the research involves more than minimal risk and does not offer a direct benefit to the individual child, then both parents must grant permission. When children reach maturity, usually at 18 years of age in the case of research, they may render their own consent. They may do so at a younger age if they have been legally declared emancipated minors. Questions regarding assent, consent, and the age of the individual should be addressed by the REB or research administration office and not left to the discretion of the researcher to answer.

Special ethical considerations also exist when research is conducted with older adults. The issue of the legal competence of older adults is often raised (Flaskerud & Winslow, 1998), but no issue exists if the potential participant can supply legally effective informed consent. Competence is not clearly measurable. The complexity of the study may affect an individual's ability to consent to participate. The capacity to give informed consent should be assessed in each individual for each research protocol being considered. For example, an older person may be able to consent to participate in a simple observation study but not in a clinical drug trial.

No vulnerable population may be singled out for study merely for convenience. For example, neither people with mental illness nor prisoners may be studied simply because they are available and their presence is convenient. Prisoners may be studied if the study pertains to them—for example, studies concerning the effects and processes of incarceration. Similarly, people with mental illness may participate in studies that focus on expanding knowledge about psychiatric disorders and treatments. Students also are often a conveniently available group. They must not, however, be singled out as research participants because of convenience; the research questions must have some bearing on their status as students.

Researchers and patient caregivers involved in research with vulnerable people are well advised to seek advice from appropriate REBs, clinicians, lawyers, ethicists, and other professionals. In all cases, the burden should be on the investigator to show the REB that it is appropriate to involve vulnerable participants in research.

 Research Hint_____

Keep in mind that researchers rarely mention explicitly that the study participants were vulnerable participants or that special precautions were taken to appropriately safeguard the human rights of this vulnerable group. Research consumers need to be attentive to the special needs of individuals who may be unable to act as their own advocates or are unable to adequately assess the risk–benefit ratio of a research study.

RESEARCH INVOLVING INDIGENOUS PEOPLE

When developing ethical guidelines, attention is paid to the culture and traditions of Indigenous people in Canada. To this end, the Tri-Council (CIHR et al., 2014) developed the following "good practices" for researchers and REBs to consider when engaged in research (CIHR et al., 2014, Chapter 9):

- To respect the culture, traditions, and knowledge of the Indigenous group
- To conceptualize and conduct research with the Indigenous group as a partnership
- To consult members of the group who have relevant expertise
- To involve the group in the design of the project
- To examine how the research may be shaped to address the needs and concerns of the group
- To make best efforts to ensure that the emphasis of the research, and the ways chosen to conduct it, respect the many viewpoints of different segments of the group in question
- To provide the group with information respecting the following:
  - Protection of the Indigenous group's cultural estate and other property
  - The availability of a preliminary report for comment
  - The potential employment by researchers of members of the community appropriate and without prejudice
  - Researchers' willingness to cooperate with community institutions
  - Researchers' willingness to deposit data, working papers, and related materials in an agreed-upon repository
- To acknowledge in the publication of the research results the various viewpoints of the community on the topics researched
- To afford the community an opportunity to react and respond to the research findings before the completion of the final report, in the final report, or even in all relevant publications

Stewart and colleagues (2013), in using a participatory action research approach, were able to acknowledge many of these considerations by involving leaders of the community and other key informants in the research design through forming a Community Advisory Committee. The community provided guidance on the development, implementation, and evaluation of the study to understand the health inequities experienced by Indigenous children with respiratory problems and their parents. In addition, the Committee reviewed the process of informed assent and consent for cultural and linguistic appropriateness. To understand the evidence being collected, and to make informed choices about what First Nations leaders need in order to improve the social and economic conditions of their people, an ethical framework, "Ownership, Control, Access, and Possession" (OCAP), was developed by the First Nations Statistics Initiative. This initiative is important because a perceived mistrust exists between First Nations people and researchers, and researchers tend to choose participants and studies on the basis of their own interests rather than the needs of the participants (First Nations Information Governance Centre, 2014).

In a qualitative research study of the experiences of Mi'kmaq women's experiences with Pap screening (see Appendix A), MacDonald, Martin-Misener, Steenbeek, and associates (2015) obtained ethics approval from Dalhousie University's REB, the Mi'kmaq Ethics Watch at Cape Breton University, and Mi'kmaq community leaders. The 2007 CIHR's guidelines of OCAP were respected by "informing the women about the entire study prior to their participation, discussing anonymity and confidentiality with them, ensuring that each informed consent form was signed and a copy given to the participant, and engaging participants in discussions about the findings and their dissemination" (p. 77).

SCIENTIFIC FRAUD AND MISCONDUCT

Fraud

Periodically, articles reporting the unethical actions of researchers appear in the professional and lay literature. Data may have been falsified or fabricated, or participants may have been coerced into participating in a research study (Fanelli, 2009; Office of Research Integrity, U.S. Department of Health and Human Services, 2016; Tilden, 2000). In a climate of "publish or perish" in academic and scientific settings and declining research dollars, academics and scientists are under increasing pressure to produce significant research findings. Job security and professional recognition are coveted, essential, and often predicated on being a productive scientist and a prolific writer. These pressures have been known to overpower some people, who then take shortcuts, fabricate data, and falsify findings to advance their positions.

The risks of engaging in fraudulent research are many, including harming research participants or basing clinical practice on false data. As advocates of patient welfare and professional practice, nurses should be aware that sometimes they might observe or suspect a researcher's misconduct. In such cases, nurses must contact the appropriate group, such as the REB, to ensure that this matter receives appropriate attention and review.

Misconduct

Of equal importance is the issue of basing nursing practice on reports that appear in journals when subsequent research and reports on those participants change the scientific basis for practice. Corrections or further research in follow-up reports may be buried, obscure, or underreported. As patient advocates and research consumers, nurses must keep up to date on scientific reports related to nursing practice and must adjust their practice as directed by ever-evolving, evidence-informed research findings. In addition, researchers have a responsibility to keep current with federal compliance regulations on prevention, detection, investigation, and adjudication of scientific misconduct.

Unauthorized Research

At times, ad hoc or informal and unauthorized research is conducted, including **product testing** (the testing of medical devices). Although the testing may seem harmless, it is, again, not the purview of the investigator to make that determination. Nurses must carefully avoid being involved in unauthorized research, for a number of reasons, including the following (Raybuck, 1997):

- These treatments or methods of care are usually not monitored as closely for untoward effects; hence, the patient may be exposed to unwarranted risk.
- Patients' rights to informed consent in clinical trials are not protected.
- The success or failure of these unrecorded trials contributes nothing to the organized scientific knowledge of the efficacy or complications of the treatment.
- The lack of independent quality supervision allows deviations from the adopted experimental program that may eliminate the program's effectiveness.

Product Testing

Nurses are often approached by manufacturers to test products on patients. Often, nurses assume the role of research coordinator in clinical drug or product trials (Raybuck, 1997). Consequently, nurses should be aware of the Health Products and Food Branch Inspectorate guidelines (see Health Canada, 2017) and regulations for testing of medical devices before they initiate any form of clinical testing. Medical devices are classified according to the extent of control necessary to ensure the safety and effectiveness of each device.

LEGAL AND ETHICAL ASPECTS OF ANIMAL EXPERIMENTATION

The laws that have been written regarding **animal rights**—guidelines used to protect the rights of animals in the conduct of research—in research emanate from an interesting history of attitudes toward animals and the value that people place on them. In 1963, the Medical Research Council of Canada (now CIHR) requested that a committee be established to investigate the care and use of experimental animals. The Canadian Council on

Animal Care (CCAC) was formed and became a nonprofit, autonomous, and independent body in 1982 (CCAC, 2016). It is now funded by the CIHR and the NSERC and conducts assessment visits to each institution every 3 years, often unannounced. The CCAC requires that institutions conducting animal-based research, teaching, or testing establish an animal care committee and that this committee be functionally active. The CCAC has a detailed guide regarding developing terms of reference for animal care committees (CCAC, 2006).

The CIHR scrutinized the proposed amendments to the Cruelty to Animal Provisions of the *Criminal Code of Canada,* Bill-C15. The objective of these changes is to strengthen but simplify the existing penal code and "to enhance the effectiveness of the offence provisions for clearly abusive, brutal and cruel treatment of animals." The CIHR supported this objective in principle and, with the NSERC, prepared a joint submission to the House of Commons Standing Committee on Justice and Human Rights in the fall of 2001, recommending amendments to clarify certain provisions of the bill with regard to their application to health research.

This section serves only as an introduction to the concept of legal and ethical issues related to animal experimentation. Principles of protection of animal rights in research have evolved over time. Animals, unlike humans, cannot give informed consent, but other conditions related to their welfare must not be ignored. Nurses who encounter the use of animals in research should be alert to their rights.

RESEARCH INVOLVING HUMAN GAMETES, EMBRYOS, OR FETUSES

Research on the human genome and other reproductive issues have caused much ethical debate and concern; thus, the Tri-Council (CIHR et al., 2014) developed pertinent guidelines, as demonstrated by these examples:

- Materials related to human reproduction for research use shall not be obtained through commercial transaction, including exchange for services (Article 12.6).
- Research on in vitro embryos already created and intended for implantation to achieve pregnancy is acceptable if:
  - The research is intended to benefit the embryo
  - Research interventions will not compromise the care of the woman or the subsequent fetus
  - Researchers closely monitor the safety and comfort of the woman and the safety of the embryo
  - Consent was provided by the gamete donors (Article 12.7)
- Research involving embryos that have been created for reproductive or other purposes permitted in Canada under the Assisted Human Reproduction Act (CIHR et al., 2014, Article 12.8), but are no longer required for these purposes, may be ethically acceptable if:
  - The ova and sperm from which they are formed were obtained in accordance with Article 12.7
  - Consent was provided by the gamete donors
  - Embryos exposed to manipulations not directed specifically to their ongoing normal development will not be transferred for continuing pregnancy
  - Research involving embryos will take place only during the first 14 days after their formation by combination of the gametes, excluding any time during which embryonic development has been suspended (Article 12.8)
- Research involving a fetus or fetal tissue (CIHR, 2014 et al., Article 12.9):
  - Requires the consent of the woman
  - Should not compromise the woman's ability to decide whether to continue her pregnancy

Nurses working in labour rooms, especially those being required to assist with embryonic research, should be aware of these ethical issues.

APPRAISING THE EVIDENCE:

The Legal and Ethical Aspects of a Research Study

Research articles and reports often do not contain detailed information regarding either the degree to which or all of the ways in which the investigator adhered to the legal and ethical principles presented in this chapter. Space considerations in articles preclude extensive documentation of all legal and ethical aspects of a research study. Lack of written evidence regarding the protection of human rights does not imply that appropriate steps were not taken.

The Critiquing Criteria box provides guidelines for evaluating the legal and ethical aspects of a research report. Although research consumers reading a research report will not see all areas explicitly addressed in the research article, they should be aware of them and should determine that the researcher has addressed them before gaining REB approval to conduct the study.

A nurse who is asked to serve as a member of an REB will find the critiquing criteria useful in evaluating the legal and ethical aspects of the research proposal.

Information about the legal and ethical considerations of a study is usually presented in the "Methods" section of a research report, probably in the subsection on the sample or data-collection methods. The author most often indicates in a few sentences that informed consent was obtained and that approval from an REB or similar committee was granted. A manuscript without such a discussion will probably not be accepted for publication; thus, it is almost impossible for unauthorized research to be published. Therefore, when a research article provides evidence of having been approved by an external review committee, the reader can feel confident that the ethical issues raised by the study have been thoroughly reviewed and resolved.

CRITIQUING CRITERIA

1. Was the study approved by an REB or other agency committee members?
2. Is there evidence that informed consent was obtained from all participants or their representatives? How was it obtained?
3. Were the participants protected from physical or emotional harm?

4. Were the participants or their representatives informed about the purpose and nature of the study?
5. Were the participants or their representatives informed about any potential risks that might result from participation in the study?
6. Was the research study designed to maximize the benefit or benefits and to minimize the risks to human participants?

7. Were participants coerced or unduly influenced to participate in this study? Did they have the right to refuse to participate or withdraw without penalty? Were vulnerable participants used?
8. Were appropriate steps taken to safeguard the privacy of participants? How have data been kept anonymous or confidential?

To protect participant and institutional privacy, the locale of the study frequently is described in general terms in the report's subsection on the sample. For example, the article might state that data were collected at a 500-bed tertiary care centre in Ontario, without mentioning the centre's name. Protection of participant privacy may be explicitly addressed by statements indicating that the anonymity or confidentiality of the data was maintained or that grouped data were used in the data analysis.

Determining whether participants were subjected to physical or emotional risk is often accomplished indirectly by evaluating the study's "Methods" section. The reader evaluates the **risk–benefit ratio:** that is, the extent to which the **benefits** of the study—the potential positive outcomes of participation in a research study—are maximized and the **risks**—the potential negative outcomes of participation in a research study—are minimized, so that participants are protected from harm during the study. The Practical Application boxes list examples of how researchers attempt to protect study participants from harm.

Practical Application

Chalmers, Sequire, and Brown (2002) reported the attitudes, beliefs, and personal behaviours of baccalaureate students in regard to tobacco use. The researchers adhered to the principles of informed consent and confidentiality and ensured that the team remained sensitive to the issues of power differences between the students and the faculty engaged in the study. In addition, the students were reassured that their participation or nonparticipation in the study would not affect their education.

Practical Application

Dupuis, Kontos, Mitchell, and associates (2016) described a community-based, critical arts-based project to construct an alternative discourse of dementia. Approval was granted by the local REB, and all members of the project—persons with dementia, family members, visual and performance artists—were approached for consent to participate in audio-taped or video-recorded focus groups.

The obligation to balance the risks and benefits of a study is the responsibility of the researcher. However, the research consumer reading a research report also should be confident that participants have been protected from harm.

When considering the special needs of vulnerable participants, research consumers should be sensitive to whether the investigators have addressed the special needs of individuals who are unable to act on their own behalf. For example, has the right of self-determination been addressed by the informed consent protocol identified in the research report? Schell, Brienning, Lebet, and associates (2010) conducted a study to compare upper arm and calf automatic blood pressures in a convenience sample of 221 children, aged 1 to 8 years, admitted to a pediatric intensive care unit of a 180-bed teaching hospital. Informed consent was obtained from the parent or guardian for all enrolled participants. Informed assent was obtained from children aged 7 and 8 years, if appropriate.

When qualitative studies are reported, verbatim quotations from informants often are incorporated into the "Findings" section of the article. In such

cases, the reader can evaluate how effectively the author protected the informant's identity, either by using a fictitious name or by withholding information such as age, gender, occupation, or other potentially identifying data.

Although the need for guidelines for the use of human and animal participants in research is evident and the principles themselves are clear, many instances arise in which nurses must use their best judgement, as both patient advocates and researchers, when evaluating the ethical nature of a research project. In any research situation, the basic guiding principle of protecting the patient's human rights must always apply. When conflicts arise, nurses must feel free to raise suitable questions with appropriate resources and personnel. In an institution, raising questions may include contacting the researcher first; then, if there is no resolution, the matter must be raised with the director of nursing research and the chairperson of the REB. In cases in which ethical considerations in a research article are in question, clarification from a colleague, agency, or the researcher's REB is indicated. Nurses should pursue their concerns until they are satisfied that the patient's rights and their rights as professionals are protected.

CRITICAL THINKING CHALLENGES

- As part of a needs assessment for future health care delivery planning, the Ministry of Health is interested in determining the number of babies infected with the human immunodeficiency virus (HIV). A province-wide study is funded that will include the testing of all newborns for HIV, but the mothers will not be told that the test is being done, nor will they be told the results. Using the basic ethical principles found in Box 6.2, defend or refute this practice.
- The REB of your health care agency does not include a nurse, and you think it should. You discuss this matter with your supervisor, who states that including a nurse is not necessary because the REB uses strict guidelines. What essential arguments

and explanations should your proposal address for including a nurse on your institution's REB?

- A qualitative researcher intends to conduct a phenomenological study on caring and to recruit informants who are severely and persistently mentally ill and attend an outpatient clinic. The REB denies the study, indicating that informed consent cannot be obtained and that these patients will not be able to tolerate an interview. What assumptions have the members of this REB made? If you were the researcher and you were given the opportunity to address their concerns, what would you say? Include information from Table 6.2.

- How do you see electronic databases and websites assisting researchers in conducting ethical studies? Do you think that REBs can use this technology to assist them in their goals?

KEY POINTS

- Ethical and legal considerations in research first received attention after World War II, during the Nuremberg trials, which resulted in the development of the Nuremberg Code. This code became the standard for research guidelines protecting the human rights of research participants.
- The U.S. National Research Act, passed in 1974, created the National Commission for the Protection of Human Subjects of Biomedical and Behavioral Research. The findings, contained in the Belmont Report (National Commission for the Protection of Human Subjects of Biomedical and Behavioral Research, 1978), are discussed with regard to the three basic ethical principles of respect for persons, beneficence, and justice that underlie the conduct of research involving human participants. U.S. federal regulations developed in response to the Commission's report provide guidelines for informed consent and REB protocols.
- Protection of human rights includes the rights to (1) self-determination, (2) privacy and dignity, (3) anonymity and confidentiality, (4) fair treatment, and (5) protection from discomfort and harm.

- Procedures for protecting basic human rights include obtaining informed consent, which illustrates the ethical principle of respect, and obtaining REB approval, which illustrates the ethical principles of respect, beneficence, and justice.
- Special consideration of ethics should be addressed in studies involving vulnerable populations, such as children, older adults, prisoners, and those who are mentally or physically disabled.
- Scientific fraud or misconduct represents unethical conduct, and professional responsibility must include monitoring for such conduct. Informal, ad hoc, or unauthorized research may expose patients to unwarranted risk and may not protect participants' rights adequately.
- Nurses who are asked to be involved in product testing should be aware of Health Canada guidelines and regulations for testing medical devices before becoming involved in product testing and, perhaps, violating guidelines for ethical research.
- Animal rights need to be protected, and regulations for animal research have evolved over time. Nurses who encounter the use of animals in research should be alert to their rights.
- As consumers of research, nurses must be knowledgeable about the legal and ethical components of a research study so that they can evaluate whether a researcher has ensured appropriate protection of human or animal rights.

FOR FURTHER STUDY

ⓔ Go to Evolve at http://evolve.elsevier.com/ Canada/LoBiondo/Research for the Audio Glossary and Appendix Tables that provide supplemental information for Appendix E.

REFERENCES

Amdur, R., & Bankert, E. A. (2011). *Institutional review board: Member handbook* (3rd ed.). Boston: Jones & Bartlett.

American Nurses Association. (1985). *Code for nurses with interpretive statements*. Kansas City, MO: Author.

Baumann, A., Idriss-Wheeler, D., Blythe, J., et al. (2015). Developing a website: A strategy for employment integration of internationally educated nurses. *Canadian Journal of Nursing Research, 47*(4), 7–20.

Benedict, S., & Georges, J. M. (2006). Nurses and the sterilization experiments of Auschwitz: A postmodernist perspective. *Nursing Inquiry, 13*, 277–288.

Brink, P. J. (1992). Autonomy versus do no harm. *Western Journal of Nursing Research, 14*, 264–266.

Canadian Council on Animal Care. (2006). *Terms of reference for animal care committees*. Retrieved from http://www.ccac.ca/Documents/Standards/Policies/Terms_of_reference_for_ACC.pdf.

Canadian Council on Animal Care. (2016). *About the Canadian Council on Animal Care*. Retrieved from http://ccac.ca/en_/about.

Canadian Institutes of Health Research, Natural Sciences and Engineering Research Council of Canada, & Social Sciences and Humanities Research Council of Canada. (2014). *Tri-Council policy statement: Ethical conduct for research involving humans*. Retrieved from http://www.pre.ethics.gc.ca/eng/policy-politique/initiatives/tcps2-eptc2/Default/.

Canadian Nurses Association. (1983). *Ethical guidelines for nurses in research involving human participants*. Ottawa: Author.

Canadian Nurses Association. (2002). *Ethical research guidelines for registered nurses*. Ottawa: Author.

Canadian Nurses Association. (2017). *Code of ethics for registered nurses: 2017 edition*. Ottawa: Author. Retrieved from https://www.cna-aiic.ca/html/en/Code-of-Ethics-2017-Edition/files/assets/basic-html/page-14.html.

Carroll, M. L., & Ciaffa, J. (2003). *The human genome project: A scientific and ethical overview*. Retrieved from http://www.actionbioscience.org/genomics/carroll_ciaffa.html.

Chalmers, K., Sequire, M., & Brown, J. (2002). Tobacco use and baccalaureate nursing students: A study of their attitudes, beliefs and personal behaviours. *Journal of Advanced Nursing, 40*(1), 17–24.

Charron, M. (2000). *Ewen Cameron and the Allan Memorial Psychiatric Institute: A study in research and treatment ethics*. Retrieved from http://www.illuminati-news.com/ewen-cameron.htm.

Collins, A. (1988). *In the sleep room: The story of the CIA brainwashing experiments in Canada*. Toronto: Lester & Orpen Dennys.

Dupuis, S. L., Kontos, P., Mitchell, G., et al. (2016). Re-claiming citizenship through the arts. *Dementia, 13*(3), 358–380.

Fanelli, D. (2009). How many scientists fabricate and falsify research? A systematic review and meta-analysis of survey data. *PLoS ONE, 4*(5), e5738. Retrieved from http://journals.plos.org/plosone/article?id=10.1371/journal.pone.0005738.

First Nations Information Governance Centre. (2014, May). *Ownership, Control, Access and Possession (OCAP™): The path to First Nations information governance*. Ottawa: Author. Retrieved from http://fnigc.ca/sites/default/files/docs/ocap_path_to_fn_information_governance_en_final.pdf.

Flaskerud, J. H., & Winslow, B. J. (1998). Conceptualizing vulnerable populations' health-related research. *Nursing Research, 47*, 69–78.

French, H. W. (1997, October 9). AIDS research in Africa: Juggling risks and hopes. *New York Times*, pp. A1, A12.

Gillmor, D. (1987). *I swear by Apollo: Dr. Ewen Cameron and the CIA-brainwashing experiments*. Montreal: Eden Press.

Halushka v. University of Saskatchewan, et al. (1965). 53 D.L.R. (2nd) 436, 52 W.W.R. 608 (Sask. CA).

Health Canada. (1997, revised 2004). *ICH Guidance E6: Good clinical practice: Consolidated guideline*. Ottawa: Health Products and Food Branch. Retrieved from http://www.hc-sc.gc.ca/dhp-mps/prodpharma/applic-demande/guide-ld/ich/efficac/e6-eng.php.

Health Canada. (2014). *Requirements for informed consent documents*. Retrieved from http://www.hc-sc.gc.ca/sr-sr/advice-avis/reb-cer/consent/index-eng.php.

Health Canada. (2017). *Drugs and health products: Medical devices*. Retrieved from http://www.hc-sc.gc.ca/dhp-mps/compli-conform/info-prod/md-im/index-eng.php.

Héon, M., Goulet, C., Garofalo, C., et al. (2016). An intervention to promote breast milk production in mothers of preterm infants. *Western Journal of Nursing Research, 38*(5), 529–552.

Hershey, N., & Miller, R. D. (1976). *Human experimentation and the law*. Germantown, MD: Aspen.

Hilts, P. J. (1995, March 9). Agency faults a UCLA study for suffering of mental patients. *New York Times*, pp. A1, A11.

International Council of Nurses. (2012). *ICN Code of Ethics for Nurses*. Retrieved from http://www.icn.ch/images/stories/documents/about/icncode_english.pdf.

Levine, R. J. (1979). Clarifying the concepts of research ethics. *Hastings Center Report, 93*(3), 21–26.

Levine, R. J. (1986). *Ethics and regulation of clinical research* (2nd ed.). Baltimore: Urban and Schwartzenberg.

MacDonald, C., Martin-Misener, R., Steenbeek, A., et al. (2015). Honouring stories: Mi'kmaq women's experiences with Pap screening in Eastern Canada. *Canadian Journal of Nursing Research, 47*(1), 72–96.

McLean, P. (1996, November). Biomedical research and the law of informed consent. *Canadian Nurse, 92,* 49–50.

Milgram, S. (1963). Behavioral study of obedience. *Journal of Abnormal and Social Psychology, 67,* 371–378.

Mitchell, K. (1984). Protecting children's rights during research. *Pediatric Nursing, 10,* 9–10.

National Commission for the Protection of Human Subjects of Biomedical and Behavioral Research. (1978). *Belmont report: Ethical principles and guidelines for research involving human subjects (DHEW Pub. No. [OS] 78-0012).* Washington, DC: U.S. Government Printing Office.

Office of Research Integrity, U.S. Department of Health and Human Services. (2016). *Case summaries.* Retrieved from http://www.ori.dhhs.gov/misconduct/cases/.

Raybuck, J. A. (1997). The clinical nurse specialist as research coordinator in clinical drug trials. *Clinical Nurse Specialist, 11*(1), 15–19.

Robb, I. H. (1900). *Nursing ethics: For hospital and private use.* Milwaukee, WI: GN Gaspar.

Rothman, D. J. (1982). Were Tuskegee and Willowbrook studies in nature? *Hastings Centre Report, 12*(2), 5–7.

Schell, K., Brienning, E., Lebet, R., et al. (2010). Comparison of arm and calf automatic non-invasive blood pressures in pediatric intensive care patients. *Journal of Pediatric Nursing, 26,* 3–12.

Singh, M., Hynie, M., Rivera, T., et al. (2015). An evaluation study of the implementation of stroke best practice guidelines using a knowledge transfer team approach . *Canadian Journal of Neuroscience Nurses, 37*(1), 24–33.

Stewart, M., King, M., Blood, R., et al. (2013). Health inequities experienced by Aboriginal children with respiratory conditions and their parents. *Canadian Journal of Nursing Research, 45*(3), 6–27.

Tilden, V. P. (2000). Preventing scientific misconduct—Times have changed. *Nursing Research, 49,* 243.

Wheeler, D. L. (1997, December 12). Three medical organizations embroiled in controversy over use of placebos in AIDS studies abroad. *Chronicle of Higher Education,* A15–A16.

PART TWO

Qualitative Research

RESEARCH **VIGNETTE**

Creating Qualitatively Derived Knowledge for a Practice Discipline

Sally Thorne, RN, PhD, FAAN, FCAHS
Professor
School of Nursing
University of British Columbia
Vancouver, British Columbia

To build knowledge for a practice discipline with the complexity and dynamism of nursing, ideas must be drawn from a wide variety of perspectives, disciplines, and inquiry approaches. In the practice arena, nurses universally recognize the patient's perspective as among the fundamentally important aspects that must be considered when decisions are made. Beyond what can be gleaned from individual patient-centred approaches, we need general knowledge about how patient perspectives are constituted and expressed, to guide individualized assessments, to help nurses understand what they are looking for, and then to interpret and make sense of what they find. The primacy of this patient-perspective knowledge as a foundational core of disciplinary practice creates the intellectual climate within which nurse researchers have led the way among the applied health disciplines to develop groundbreaking qualitative methodological innovations for understanding health phenomena.

Many techniques used in qualitative research actually originated in the social sciences, in which the study of human complexity has been active for generations. Ever since nurse scholars began to adopt these methods, in the 1980s, they recognized that the knowledge needs of this applied health discipline are quite distinct from those of the more theoretical social sciences; consequently, qualitative research approaches in nursing have evolved from being primarily theoretical and toward being more practically relevant. Practitioners in our discipline tend not to be satisfied with simply building theories; they want to translate what is known into what nurses and other health care providers can potentially use.

To illustrate, nurses have become increasingly unenthusiastic about straightforward description. Instead, they are seeking knowledge that both describes and interprets, telling us not only what seems to be happening but also why that is important. Because they understand that their knowledge products are most valuable when they contribute to the evidentiary basis on which health practice and policy are constructed, nurses increasingly orient their questions and the methods by which they seek to answer them toward the most pressing and hard-to-solve clinical challenges. Nurses who engage in a qualitative study are doing so not merely out of curiosity or theoretical inclination, but rather with a desire to add to the knowledge base that guides practising nurses and their patients in a meaningful way.

I happened to enter graduate studies at the precise time when the worldview of qualitative approaches was emerging as an alternative to the more conventional quantitative science with which nurse scholars had been struggling. The prevailing view at that time was that qualitative researchers were entirely different thinkers than their quantitative colleagues, and the two kinds of research products were completely incommensurate. Thus, my entry into a nursing research career coincided with a time of tension and transition in nursing's methodological universe. Over time, I had the good fortune to be part of the emerging methodological explorations in such areas as the systematic integration of the unique insights derived from both measurement and interpretation into robust knowledge "platforms." Instead of arguing the merits of the various ways of studying phenomena, nurse researchers have increasingly joined together in solving the complex problems faced by clinicians, health care planners, and policymakers. By applying the best parts of those different perspectives in a thoughtful and rational manner, we are trying to build and implement systems of care that provide the best possible conditions for our patients. It is an exciting time to be involved in nursing scholarship!

The kinds of studies that most attract my interest these days are those addressing aspects of health care in which usual nursing practice is not yet as effective as it ought to be and meaningful improvements can be envisioned. For me, clinician–patient communication is one such complex challenge. Although all nurses experientially know how powerful human communication can be in shaping the thoughts, feelings, and behavioural responses that people have to critical events in life, it is extraordinarily difficult to articulate and enforce evidence-informed best practices in this regard.

In cancer care, for instance, communication ought to be a priority, in view of what nurses know of its power to nurture or deflate, inform or misinform, discourage or encourage hope. Because communication is so nuanced, complex, and various, it is not particularly amenable to conventional inquiry methods. Although a few aspects of communication are theoretically quantifiable, much of what can be measured is rather irrelevant to the overall subjective experience of being in a communicative encounter, and this form of evidence provides very little guidance for improving patient experience. Therefore, communication is an ideal phenomenon to be studying from multiple angles, including—of most importance—the perspective of those involved in the encounter. Arguably, interpersonal communication about such difficult issues as a cancer diagnosis is so highly complex that it ought not to be possible; however, nurses know that patients truly benefit from skilled and competent communication, just as they experience harm from miscommunications. Patients should not have to launch their cancer journeys with undue

levels of confusion, fear, anxiety, or emotional distress related to how nurses and others interact with them, and we can gain much from studying a wide range of such experiences to keep refining our understanding of how to communicate well.

In a topic such as cancer communication, although I orient my research questions from the perspective of how a nurse sees the problem, I also recognize the inherent interdisciplinarity of the challenge. I therefore thrive working in strong interprofessional research teams. In the cancer communication studies, about half of the team are nurses, with the rest representing epidemiology, physical therapy, social work, and radiation oncology. In our research program, we have chosen to focus attention on the patient perspective, acknowledging that what we can glean is not in and of itself a "truth" but rather a detectable pattern of subjective material that—together with what we can obtain from other angles of vision—creates an evolving body of rich understanding. Although we recognize the possibility that patient reports could be skewed in particular directions, we have found over many years in this field that they are remarkably authentic to the perceptions that clinicians tell us about what goes on in the practice context. Furthermore, their accounts provide an in-depth and varied contextual understanding to the trends that can be detected quantitatively—why certain kinds of information exchange satisfy some patients and not others, why particular forms of communication

trigger frustration and despair, and so on.

Interpretive description, which we developed as an applied qualitative research approach for the practice disciplines, capitalizes on nursing epistemology to determine what kinds of knowledge are likely to be most useful. While nurse scholars are well informed by various social theories, they rarely assume that any singular theoretical perspective ought to ground or frame their studies. Rather, they often find that a clinical logic model creates the most appropriate intellectual scaffolding upon which to base study design decisions, including all aspects of research orientation and data collection, analysis, and interpretation. In so doing, they design studies that will not only illuminate common patterns but also provide guidance in detecting and making sense of both predictable and infrequent variations, since nursing never deals with standardization in the absence of individualization.

Nurse researchers aspire to the kind of research report that will illuminate relationships between practice elements that may not have been well aligned previously, such that thoughtful clinicians can "see" a practice direction more clearly and be more confident in their practice improvements. In our work, we also aim to help teachers of communication competencies look beyond generalities toward more finely tuned expert practices, understanding how to nurture and support them and to challenge poor practices where they exist.

I genuinely believe that nurses have a pivotal role in shaping the communicative environment in which patients with cancer are informed, guided, supported, and connected throughout their cancer services. I am also convinced that qualitative research provides nurses with some insight that would otherwise be missing in the evidentiary base that allows them to advocate on behalf of patients.

As you read this book and familiarize yourself with the wonderful world of research, I hope that your imagination will be inspired with directions that you might take in your own inquiries on behalf of our profession. Great research really can be a powerful tool for nursing practice! ■

CHAPTER 7

Introduction to Qualitative Research

Julie Barroso | Cherylyn Cameron

LEARNING OUTCOMES

After reading this chapter, you will be able to do the following:

- Describe the quantitative research paradigm.
- Describe the beliefs generally held by qualitative researchers.
- Describe the components of a qualitative research report.
- Identify the links between qualitative research and evidence-informed practice.
- Identify four ways in which qualitative findings can be used in evidence-informed practice.
- Discuss significant issues that arise in conducting qualitative research.

KEY TERMS

bracketing	"grand tour" question	qualitative research
context dependent	inclusion criteria	reflexivity
data saturation	inductive	text
deductive	metasynthesis	triangulation
exclusion criteria	naturalistic setting	
focus group	purposive sample	

STUDY RESOURCES

ⓔ Go to Evolve at http://evolve.elsevier.com/Canada/LoBiondo/Research for the Audio Glossary and Appendix Tables that provide supplemental information for Appendix E.

LET'S SAY THAT YOU ARE READING an article that reports findings that men infected with the human immunodeficiency virus (HIV) are more adherent to their antiretroviral regimens than are HIV-infected women. You wonder why that is so: Why would women be less adherent in taking their medications? Certainly, it is not solely because they are women. Or you are working on a postpartum unit and have just discharged a new mother who has debilitating rheumatoid arthritis. You wonder what the process is by which women with disabilities decide to have children: How do they go about making that decision? These, like so many other questions that nurses have, can be best answered through research conducted with qualitative methods. Qualitative research yields answers to those difficult questions. Although qualitative methods can be used at many different points in a program of research, you can most often use them to answer questions that nurses have when a particular phenomenon in nursing is not well understood.

In this chapter, the basic tenets of qualitative research are reviewed; the components of a qualitative report, qualitative research, and evidence-informed practice are explored; and the issues in qualitative research are examined.

WHAT IS QUALITATIVE RESEARCH?

Qualitative research is a systematic, interactive, and subjective research method used to describe and give meaning to human experiences. This broad term encompasses several methodologies that share many similarities in the conduct of such research. According to Denzin and Lincoln (2011), "qualitative researchers study things in their natural settings, attempting to make sense of, or interpret, phenomena in terms of the meanings people bring to them" (p. 3). A **naturalistic setting** is one that people live in every day. Therefore, the researcher conducting qualitative research goes wherever the participants are: in their homes, schools, communities, and, sometimes, in the hospital or an outpatient setting.

Qualitative studies most often help researchers begin to formulate an understanding of a phenomenon. Although qualitative research has a long history in the social sciences, it is only since 1990 that it has become more accepted in nursing research. For many years, doctoral nursing students were dissuaded from conducting qualitative studies; the push was for the traditional quantitative approach, which was viewed by many authorities in the "hard" sciences as being more credible. Thus, as nursing gained its foothold in academics, doctoral students were urged to conduct research by using the quantitative paradigm, or worldview (beliefs and practices, shared by communities of researchers), to help nursing gain legitimacy in academe. However, as academe and research evolved along two different but parallel channels, qualitative research received greater acceptance; contemporary nurse scholars are trained in qualitative methods. Students are encouraged to use the method that best answers their research questions, instead of using methods that might add a veneer of scientific legitimacy to conducting the research but do not answer the research question at hand.

Qualitative research is discovery oriented; it is explanatory, descriptive in nature. Words, as opposed to numbers, are used to explain a phenomenon. The data gathered in qualitative research come from the text. The term **text** used in this context means that data are in textual form—that is, narrative or words written from interviews that were recorded and then transcribed or notes written from the researcher's observations. Qualitative research lets us see the world through the eyes of another: the woman who struggles to take her antiretroviral medication or the woman with a debilitating illness who has nonetheless carefully thought through what it might be like to have a baby. Qualitative researchers assume that nurses can understand these experiences only if they consider the context in which the experiences take place, and this is why most qualitative research takes place in naturalistic settings.

Another emerging type of data is the use of photovoice. Photovoice, developed by Caroline Wang and Mary Ann Burris (1997), is a participatory health promotion strategy in which people use cameras to document their health and work realities.

WHAT DO QUALITATIVE RESEARCHERS BELIEVE?

Qualitative researchers believe that there are multiple realities; for example, they believe that the experience of having a baby, though some aspects are common to all deliveries, is not the same for any two women and is definitely different for a mother with a disability. Qualitative researchers believe that reality is socially constructed and **context dependent**—that is, the meaning of an observation is defined by its circumstance or the environment. For example, even the experience of reading this book is different for any two students; one may be completely engrossed by the content, while another is reading but is worrying about whether her financial aid application will be approved soon. Figure 7.1 is an illustration of context dependence; what an individual sees depends on who that individual is and what experiences the individual brings to the situation. Qualitative researchers believe that the discovery of meaning is the basis for knowledge. Qualitative researchers know that they must describe the phenomenon under study well. Ideally,

the reader, if even slightly acquainted with the phenomenon, would have an "Aha!" moment in reading a well-written qualitative report.

You may now be saying, "Wow! This sounds great! Qualitative research is for me!" Many nurses feel very comfortable with this approach because they are educated in how to talk to people about the health issues concerning them; they are used to listening and listening well. The most important consideration for any research study, however, is whether the methodology fits the question. It must fit, or else the study will contribute little to the scientific knowledge base for practice. This is also the first question you should ask yourself when you read studies and are considering them as evidence on which to base your practice: Does the methodology fit with the research question under study?

 Research Hint _____
All research is based on a paradigm, but the paradigm is seldom specifically identified in a research report.

DOES THE METHODOLOGY FIT WITH THE RESEARCH QUESTION BEING ASKED?

As stated before, qualitative methods are often best for helping researchers determine the nature of a phenomenon. Sometimes, authors state that they are using qualitative methods because little is known about a phenomenon. That alone is not a good

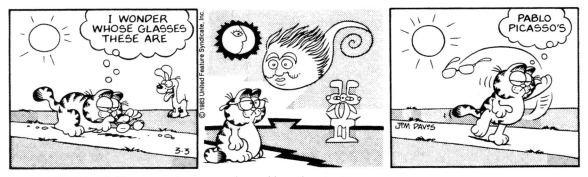

FIG. 7.1   Shifting perspectives: seeing the world as others see it.

STEPS IN THE QUALITATIVE RESEARCH PROCESS

- Review of the literature
- Study design
- Sample
- Setting: recruitment and data collection
- Data collection
- Data analysis
- Findings
- Conclusions

reason for conducting a study, however. Little may be known about a phenomenon because it does not matter! Before researchers ask people to participate in a study, to reveal themselves and their lives to the researchers, the researchers should be asking about things that will help make a difference in people's lives, in how professionals provide nursing care. You should be able to articulate a valid reason for conducting a study, beyond "little is known about . . ."

In the examples at the start of this chapter, we want to know why HIV-infected women are less adherent to their medication regimens, so we can work to change these barriers and anticipate them when our patients are ready to start taking these pills. Similarly, we need to understand the decision-making processes women use to decide whether or not to have a child when they are disabled, so we can guide or advise the next woman who is going through this process. To summarize, we say that a qualitative approach "fits" a research question when the researchers seek to understand the nature or experience of phenomena by attending to personal accounts of persons with direct experiences related to the phenomena. The parts of a qualitative research study are discussed next. Box 7.1 outlines the steps for conducting a qualitative study.

COMPONENTS OF A QUALITATIVE RESEARCH REPORT

Review of the Literature

The first step has already been discussed: being clear that a qualitative approach is the best way to answer the research question. Next, the author presents a quick review of the relevant literature. This may require creativity on the author's part because published research on the phenomenon in question may not exist. However, there are likely to be studies on similar participants, with the same patient population, or on a closely related concept. For example, the author may want to research how women who have a disabling illness make decisions about becoming pregnant. Although no other studies in this particular area may have been conducted, there may be some on decision making in pregnancy when a woman does not have a disabling illness. These would be important inclusions in the review of the literature to show readers that the author is familiar with the research on this process in a nondisabled woman. Or there may be literature on decision making in pregnancy when a woman has a different but not disabling illness, such as cancer or HIV infection.

Assume that the author wanted to examine HIV-infected women's adherence to regimens of antiretroviral therapy. If there is no research available directly on this topic, the author might examine research on adherence to therapy for other chronic illnesses, such as diabetes or hypertension. The author might want to include studies of gender differences in medication adherence; or the author might want to examine the literature on adherence in a stigmatizing illness or to examine appointment adherence for women, to see what facilitates or acts as a barrier to attending health care appointments. The major point is that even though no literature on the author's exact subject may exist, the author should review the literature. In fact, it usually is more challenging to write the review of the literature for a qualitative study because the author must be creative and think of all of the other comparisons he or she needs to make, whether it is on the study subject, relevant study concepts, or similar/dissimilar patient groups.

At the conclusion of reading the review, the most important points you have learned should be clear, and you should be able to articulate the problem to be studied and the purpose for studying it. As discussed in previous chapters, some qualitative researchers conduct a very limited review because they want to be amenable to discovering and learning about the phenomenon under study and not be swayed or otherwise influenced by previous findings in the field.

Study Design

In the next part of the report, the authors should explain the study design—that is, how they will go about answering the research question. In qualitative research, there may simply be a descriptive or naturalistic design, in which the researchers adhere to the general tenets of qualitative research but do not commit to a particular method. However, there are different types of qualitative methods, which are discussed in Chapter 8. What is important, as you read from this point forward, is that the study design is congruent with the philosophical beliefs that qualitative researchers hold. In other words, you would not expect to read about a random sample, a battery of questionnaires administered in a hospital outpatient clinic, or a complicated statistical analysis. Usually, the researchers also indicate that they have received ethical approval from the appropriate research ethics board.

You may read about a pilot study in the opening of the design section; this is work that the researchers performed before undertaking the main study to make sure that the logistics of the proposed study were reasonable: Were they able to recruit participants? Did the questions they asked of participants yield the information they needed? Lack of a pilot study is not a deficit, however.

Sample

The next part of the report is the description of the sample and setting. This section contains critical information that enables you to understand how qualitative research differs from quantitative research. In qualitative studies, the researchers are usually looking for a **purposive sample:** a group consisting of particular people who can elucidate the phenomenon they want to study. Therefore, their recruitment materials must be very specific, so that when people read their recruitment flyers, they know whether they satisfy the criteria. Thus, if the researchers want to talk to HIV-infected women about adherence, they may distribute flyers recruiting for women who are adherent and those who are not. Or they may want to talk to women who qualify for only one of those categories. The researchers who are examining decision making in pregnancy among women with disabling conditions would clearly list the conditions they want to study. For example, they may describe wanting to talk to women with multiple sclerosis or women with rheumatoid arthritis.

Researchers may impose other parameters as well, such as requiring that participants be older than 18 years, or not using illicit drugs, or deciding about a first pregnancy (as opposed to subsequent pregnancies). These parameters are known as **inclusion criteria** (criteria that people must satisfy to participate in a study) and **exclusion criteria** (criteria used to exclude people from participating in a study). It is critical that the authors make these criteria transparent to the reader, so the reader can judge the abilities of the participants to shed light on the phenomenon in question.

Often the researchers make decisions about parameters, such as how to define a "long-term survivor" of a certain illness. In this case, they need to tell you, the reader, why and how they decided who would qualify for this category. Is a long-term survivor someone who has had an illness for 5 years? For 10 years? What is the median survival time for people with this diagnosis? The researchers' decisions should be based on sound scientific rationale.

When the researchers have identified the type of person to include in the research sample, the next step is to develop a strategy for recruiting participants, which means locating and engaging them in the research.

In a research report, the researcher may include a description of the study sample in the findings (it can also be reported in the description of the sample). In any event, besides a demographic description of the study participants, a qualitative researcher should also report on key areas of difference in the sample. For example, in a sample of HIV-infected women, there should be information about stage of illness, what kind and how many pills they must take, how many children they have, and so on. This information helps the reader place the findings into some context.

In qualitative research, there is no set sample size. Qualitative researchers gather participants until data saturation occurs. **Data saturation** is the point in a qualitative study when the information being shared with the researcher from participants becomes repetitive; in other words, the ideas shared by the participants have been shared by previous participants and no new ideas emerge.

Setting: Recruitment and Data Collection

The setting section may actually describe two settings: the setting in which participants were recruited and the setting in which data were collected. Data are usually collected in a naturalistic setting; the participants are not usually brought into a clinic interview room. The setting for data collection is often the participant's home, which can be an incredible window into other aspects of the participant's life. To be in someone else's home is a great privilege and helps the researcher understand what that participant values. For example, persons who are ill may have everything they could need to get through a day clustered around a favourite chair: The researcher might see an oxygen tank, a glass of water, medications, telephone, television, a box of tissues, and so on. This may be an indicator that the participant is someone for whom getting around is tremendously difficult. The researcher will also witness

family dynamics and get a sense of the support structures in place. In any event, a good qualitative researcher considers this setting as additional data to help complete the complex, rich scenario that is being rendered in the study.

Data Collection

In a qualitative study, the data to be collected are usually words: The researcher may interview an individual, interview a group of people in what is called a **focus group,** or observe an individual as she or he goes about a task, such as sorting medications into a pill minder. In each of these cases, however, the data collected are expressed in words. The researcher asks the participant about the phenomenon of interest and then listens. However, the researcher does not have to do this without some technical assistance. Most qualitative researchers use audio recorders to ensure that they have captured the participant's exact words. This also takes some of the pressure off of researchers to write down every single word, and it frees them up to listen fully. The recordings are usually transcribed verbatim, and then the researcher who conducted the interviews listens to the recordings for accuracy. In many studies the researcher will also be taking extensive field notes, jotting down observations of the nonverbal interactions, the setting, and so forth.

The data-collection section should also describe details such as whether informed consent was obtained and the steps from when a participant contacted the researcher to the end of the study visit. It is important to also know how long each interview or focus group lasted and how much time overall the researcher spent "in the field" collecting data.

Another important component in this section is the description of when the researcher decided that the sample was sufficient. In qualitative studies, researchers generally continue to recruit participants until they have reached data saturation. As stated earlier, the number of participants to be selected is usually not predetermined as in quantitative studies; rather, the researchers keep recruiting until they have the data they need. One important exception to this is a study in which a researcher is very interested in getting different types of people in the study. For example, in the study on HIV-infected women and medication adherence, the researchers may want to interview some women who were very adherent in the beginning but then became less so over time, women who were not adherent in the beginning but then became adherent, or women with children and those without children to determine the influence of being a mother on adherence. However, sample sizes tend to be fairly small (fewer than 30 participants) because of the enormous amounts of written text that need to be analyzed by the researcher.

Finally, this section should describe the kinds of questions the researchers asked the participants. These are different from the research question or questions, which should be broad and perhaps written in fairly esoteric language. The interview questions should be clear, be plain, and elicit exactly what the researcher wants to know.

In qualitative studies, there may be a broad overview or **"grand tour" question,** such as "Tell me about taking your medications: the things that make it easier and the things that make it harder," or "Tell me what you were thinking about when you decided to get pregnant." Along with this overview question, there are usually a series of prompts (additional questions) that were derived from the literature; these are areas that the researcher believes are important to cover and that the participant will probably cover, but they are available to remind the researcher in case the material is not mentioned. For example, with regard to medication adherence, the researcher may have read in other studies that motherhood can influence adherence in two very different ways: children can become a reason to live,

which would facilitate taking antiretroviral medication, and children can be all-demanding, leaving the mother with little to no time to take care of herself. Therefore, a neutrally worded question about the influence of children would be a prompt if the participants do not mention it spontaneously.

The sample may be described in the data-collection section or in the "Findings" section.

Data Analysis

Next in the report is the description of data analysis, in which the researcher describes how he or she handled the raw data, which are usually verbatim transcripts of the recorded interviews in a qualitative study. Many qualitative researchers use computer-assisted data analysis programs to help with this task, which can seem overwhelming because of the sheer quantity of data to be dealt with. However, other researchers analyze the data themselves. In either situation, the goal is to find commonalities and differences in the interviews, and then to group these into broader, more abstract, overarching categories of meaning that capture much of the data. For example, in the case regarding pregnancy for women with disabilities, one woman might talk about having discussed the need for assistance with her friends and found that they were willing and able to help her with the baby. Another woman might talk about how she discussed the decision with her mother and sisters and found them to be a ready source of aid. A third woman may say that she talked about this with her church study group, and they told her that they could arrange to bring meals and help with housework during the pregnancy and afterward. On a more abstract level, these women are all talking about social support. Thus, it is possible to find a term that is all-encompassing for these descriptions. In an ideal situation, the authors might even describe an example such as the one you just read, but the page limitations of most journals do not permit this level of detail. Chapter 15 includes a more in-depth exploration on qualitative data analysis methods.

Findings

At last, we come to the results! First, the authors should discuss whether they are describing a process (as in the decision-making example) or a list of circumstances that are functioning in some way (such as a list of barriers to and facilitators for taking medications), a set of conditions that must be present for something to occur (what parents state they need in order to care for a ventilator-dependent child at home), or a description of what it is like to go through some health-related transition (what it is like to become the caretaker of a parent with dementia). This is by no means an all-inclusive list but rather examples to help you know what you should be looking for.

After the description, the authors present the results, usually by breaking them down into units of meaning that help the data come together and solidify to tell a story. It is very useful if the authors describe the logic for breaking down the units as they are presented: Are they discussing the themes from most prevalent to least prevalent? Are they describing a process in temporal terms? Are they starting with topics that were most important to the participant and then moving to less important topics?

After describing how the story will be told, the authors should proceed with a thorough description of the phenomenon, defining each of the themes and fleshing out each theme with a thorough explanation of the role that it plays in the question under study. The authors should also provide quotations that support each of the themes. Ideally, the quotation will be staged, which gives you, the reader, some information about the participant from whom it came: Was it a recent immigrant woman with newly diagnosed HIV infection who did not have children? Was it a woman with disabilities who has chosen to become pregnant but has suffered two miscarriages? Staging of quotes allows you to put the information into some social context.

In a really good report of qualitative research, some of the quotations will give you an "Aha!" feeling: you will have a sense that the researcher has done an excellent job of getting to the core of the problem. Quotations are as critical to qualitative reports as numbers are to a quantitative study.

At the end of the report is the conclusion. The researchers should summarize the results and should compare the findings with those in the existing literature. How are these findings similar to and different from those in the existing literature? The authors can also describe new findings or new conceptual conclusions in this section because the findings may have revealed areas that were not anticipated at the beginning of the study. This is one of the great contributions of qualitative research: opening up new venues of discovery that were not heretofore anticipated. The researchers make suggestions regarding how to use the findings in practice and will discuss whether the findings and the subsequent recommendation are transferable to other patients and settings. After discussing the limitations of the study, researchers often offer further direction for future research.

 Research Hint _____

Values are involved in all research. It is important, however, that they not influence the results of the research.

EVIDENCE-INFORMED PRACTICE

Because nursing is a practice discipline, the most important purpose of nursing research is to use research findings to improve the care of patients. The best way to start to answer questions that have not been addressed or when a new perspective is needed in practice is through the use of qualitative methods. The answers to questions provided by qualitative data reflect important evidence that may offer the first systematic insights about a phenomenon and the setting in which it occurs. Therefore, broadening evidence models beyond a narrow hierarchical perspective is imperative.

QUALITATIVE APPROACH AND NURSING SCIENCE

Qualitative research is particularly well suited to studying the human experience of health, a central concern of nursing science. Because qualitative methods focus on the whole of human experience and the meaning ascribed by individuals living the experience, these methods extend understanding of health beyond traditionally measured units to include the complexity of the human health experience as it occurs in everyday life. This closeness to what is "real" and "everyday" holds the promise of guidance for nursing practice; it is also important for instrument and theory development. In Figure 7.2, three examples are cited to emphasize the capacity of qualitative research methods to (1) guide nursing practice, (2) contribute to instrument development, and (3) develop nursing theory.

ISSUES IN QUALITATIVE RESEARCH

Ethics

Inherent in all research is the protection of human participants. This requirement exists for both quantitative and qualitative research approaches and is discussed in Chapter 6. The basic tenets of ethical practice hold true for the qualitative approach. However, several characteristics of qualitative methods, outlined in Table 7.1 generate unique concerns and necessitate expanding the protection of human participants.

Naturalistic Setting

The central concern that arises when research is conducted in naturalistic settings focuses on the need to obtain consent. Obtaining informed consent is a basic responsibility of the researcher, but it is not always easy in naturalistic settings. For example, when research methods include observing groups of people interacting over time, the complexity of obtaining consent is apparent. These complexities generate controversy and debate among qualitative researchers. The balance between respect for human participants and efforts to collect meaningful data must be continuously negotiated.

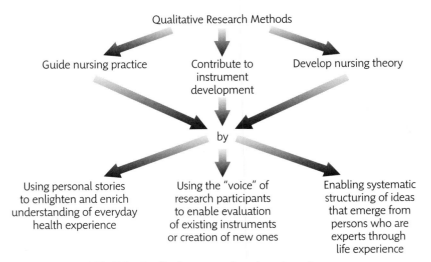

FIG. 7.2 Qualitative approach and nursing science.

TABLE 7.1	
CHARACTERISTICS OF QUALITATIVE RESEARCH THAT GENERATE ETHICAL CONCERNS	
CHARACTERISTICS	**ETHICAL CONCERNS**
Naturalistic setting	Some researchers using methods that rely on participant observation may believe that consent is not always possible or necessary.
Emergent nature of the design	Planning for questioning and observation emerges over the duration of the study. Thus, it is difficult to inform participants precisely of all potential threats before they agree to participate.
Researcher–participant interaction	Relationships developed between the researcher and the participant may blur the focus of the interaction.
Researcher as instrument	In collecting data, the researcher may misinterpret the participant's reality.

The reader should look for evidence that the researcher has addressed this issue of balance by recording attention to the protection of human participants.

Emergent Nature of the Design

The emergent nature of the research design emphasizes the necessity for ongoing negotiation of consent with the participant. During the course of a study, situations change, and what was agreeable at the beginning may become intrusive. Sometimes, as data collection proceeds and new information emerges, the study shifts direction in a way that is not acceptable to the participant.

For example, if the researcher is present in a family's home during a time in which marital discord arises, the family may choose to renegotiate the consent. From another perspective, Morse (1998) discussed the increasing involvement of participants in the research process, which sometimes resulted in participants' request to have their names published in the findings or be included as coauthors. Morse suggested that if the participant originally signed a consent form and then chose

an active identified role, the participant should then sign a "release for publication" form.

The underlying point of this discussion is that the emergent qualitative research process mandates ongoing negotiating of researcher–participant relationships, including the consent relationship. The opportunity to renegotiate consent establishes a relationship of trust and respect, characteristic of the ethical conduct of research.

Researcher–Participant Interaction

The nature of the researcher–participant interaction over time introduces the possibility that the research experience may become therapeutic: a case of research becoming practice. Basic differences exist between the intention of the nurse when conducting research and when engaging in practice (Smith & Liehr, 2003). In practice, the nurse has caring–healing intentions. In research, the nurse intends to understand the perspective of the participant. Such understanding may be a therapeutic experience for the participant. Sometimes talking to a caring listener about things that matter energizes healing, even though this result was incidental. From an ethical perspective, the qualitative researcher is promising only to listen and to encourage the participant's story. If this experience is therapeutic for the participant, it becomes an unplanned benefit of the research.

Several ethical dilemmas may emerge from the qualitative researcher's interaction with participants. Glesne (2011) has described several roles that the qualitative researcher may assume, such as exploiter, intervener or reformer, advocate, and friend. All researchers "use" participants to some extent to meet their own needs, such as status and recognition from ensuing publications, with no recognition of the participants. Furthermore, the researcher is in a position of power (researchers who conduct studies in collaboration with others share the power). Often, the "exploitation" is rationalized by the good that may come of sharing the knowledge obtained from the research. Issues of reciprocity are particularly troublesome for ethnographic researchers, who are immersed in fieldwork for long periods of time (Lipson, 1994).

Other dilemmas are faced when the researcher attempts to intervene in a situation. For example, if the researcher becomes aware of potentially dangerous drug abuse among a group of young adults, should the researcher intervene, with the possible consequence of breaching the confidentiality and, ultimately, the trust of the participants? Finally, as trust and respect are established, researchers may find themselves in the role of confidant, which may, in some cases, lead to friendship. Although some qualitative researchers find the role of friend acceptable if it is based on trust, caring, and collaboration, an inherent danger exists that the data are given in the context of friendship and not for the purposes of research (Glesne, 2011). Investigators may also find it difficult to end the relationship and say goodbye to participants. Fournier, Mill, Kipp, and colleagues (2006) indicated that more attention needs to be given to psychological preparation, focused on exiting the relationship. In participatory action research, the researcher also needs to consider whether there are any long-term obligations to sustain the project (Fournier et al., 2006).

Research Hint

Researchers are privileged to enter the lives of other people and must treat the ensuing relationship with the utmost respect.

Researcher as Instrument

Qualitative research mandates that the researcher become immersed in the field. Understanding how other people think, act, and feel is paramount (Patton, 2002, 2015). Because researchers are interpreting what they observe and experience, their own personal history, experiences, knowledge, and bias may distort the data. The responsibility to remain true to the data requires that the researchers acknowledge any personal bias and interpret findings in a way that accurately reflects the participant's reality. Researchers need to become aware of and monitor their own subjectivity to decrease any distortion of the data. This responsibility is a serious ethical obligation. To accomplish this, researchers should prepare for differences in other cultures and groups by reading, interacting, and seeking out experiences outside of their own norms (Roper & Shapira, 2000). Qualitative researchers frequently write in personal journals during their research activity to monitor and become aware of their personal biases and feelings (Glesne, 2011). Through this process of **reflexivity** in qualitative research, researchers constantly challenge themselves to understand how their perspective may be shaping the method, interviews, analysis, and interpretations. After all, "the interviewer affects the interviewer, and the interviewee affects the interviewer" (Patton, 2015, p. 70). Patton (2015) reminds us that, as a researcher, one needs "to be attentive to and conscious of the cultural, political, social, linguistic, and economic origins of one's own perspective and voice as well as the perspective and voices of those one interviews and those to whom one reports" (p. 70). Louise Racine (2011) noted in her fieldwork with Haitian families in Quebec that her "perceived political affiliation, race, and class (as researcher) had an impact on the research process" (p. 20). Although she initially did not share details about her personal life, she realized that she needed to build trust and equalize power by disclosing who she was. She noted that her political views, which differed from those of her research participants, impacted their willingness to share their lived experiences.

Streubert and Carpenter (2011) recommend that researchers identify their own thoughts, feelings, and perceptions by compartmentalizing them in the process referred to as **bracketing,** in which personal biases about the phenomenon of interest are identified in order to clarify how personal experience and beliefs may influence what is heard and reported. Bracketing is important in both the descriptive phenomenological and the ethnographic traditions and is necessary for the researcher to be "open" and receptive to the phenomenon under study. Bracketing is based on the assumption that people can separate their personal knowledge about a specific phenomenon from their experiences and background. For this reason, bracketing may not always be possible, but, at a minimum, researchers should be aware as much as possible of their own assumptions and how those assumptions may affect their observations and interpretations and thus influence the results of the study.

Triangulation

Triangulation has grown in popularity over the past several years and refers to the combination of several methods. **Triangulation** can be defined as using two pieces of information to locate a third, unique finding. Marshall and Rossman (2011) define it as the act of bringing more than one source of data to bear on a single point. Data from different sources can be used to corroborate, elaborate, or illuminate the phenomenon in question. For example, we might interview a patient and his nurse to triangulate and learn a broader conception of the patient's recovery. Silverman and Marvasti (2008) advocate for beginning from a theoretical perspective or model when using triangulation, and for choosing methods and data that will give an account of structure and meaning from within that perspective. As you read nursing research, you will quickly discover that approaches and methods, such as triangulation, are being combined to contribute to theory building, guide practice, and facilitate instrument development.

Although certain kinds of questions may be answered effectively by combining qualitative and quantitative methods in a single study (see "Mixed Methods" section), this does not necessarily make the findings and related evidence stronger. In fact, if a researcher inappropriately combines methods in a single study, the findings could be weaker and less credible. As a nurse, you need to determine why researchers chose a particular approach for their study and whether this

was an appropriate choice. You are encouraged to follow the ongoing debate about combining methods as nurse researchers strive to determine which research combinations foster understanding and contributions to nursing science.

 Evidence-Informed Practice Tip _____

- Triangulation offers an opportunity for researchers to increase the strength and consistency of evidence provided by the use of both qualitative and quantitative research methods.
- The combination of stories with numbers (qualitative and quantitative research approaches) through use of triangulation may provide the most complete picture of the phenomenon being studied and, therefore, the best evidence for guiding practice.

Five basic types of triangulation have been described (Denzin, 1978; Janesick, 1994):

1. Data triangulation: the use of a variety of data sources in a study. For example, the researcher collects data at different times, in different settings, and from different groups of people.
2. Investigator triangulation: the collaboration of several different researchers or evaluators from divergent backgrounds
3. Theory triangulation: the use of multiple perspectives to interpret a single set of data
4. Methodological triangulation: the use of multiple methods to study a single problem (mixed methods)
5. Interdisciplinary triangulation: the use of other disciplines to increase understanding of the phenomenon (e.g., nursing and sociology)

MIXED METHODS

Use of mixed methods, as defined by Creswell (2014), "involves combining or integration of qualitative and quantitative research and data in a research study" (p. 14). Mixed methods research can take two approaches: the mixing of different research methodologies (defined as the theoretical assumptions underlying the research approach) or the mixing of different research methods (defined as the tools for collecting and analyzing data;

Giddings & Grant, 2007). Mixing methodologies can be more difficult if the assumptions and values underlying the research approaches (i.e., the methodologies being mixed) are from different paradigms.

In spite of the complexity of mixing methodologies and methods, serious readers of nursing research do not take long to determine that approaches and methods are being combined to contribute to theory building, to guide practice, and to facilitate instrument development. Several mixed-methodology research designs have been developed, many from the seminal work of nurse researchers such as Morgan (1998) and Morse (1991). Note that researchers need to determine the primary method (qualitative or quantitative). For example, if the purpose of the study is to describe, discover, or explore, then the theoretical drive is **inductive** (generalizing from specific data), with principal methods that are qualitative. Observations lead to the development of generalizations and, in some cases, theory to explain the

phenomenon. However, if the purpose of the research is to confirm a theory or hypothesis, the underpinning of the research is **deductive** (concluded from data) and, subsequently, a quantitative drive will be used. Theory is tested by the development of a hypothesis and the gathering of data to accept or reject it. This recognition is imperative because it drives the design of the study, from the size of the sample to the analysis of the data.

Morgan (1998) identified several models: for example, (1) small, preliminary, qualitative data providing information useful in the development of a larger quantitative study; (2) limited use of quantitative methods to guide the researcher in decisions pertaining to the larger qualitative project; (3) qualitative methods used to interpret results from a quantitative study; and (4) quantitative methods used to confirm results from the qualitative study. Morse (2003) identified eight different types of multimethod designs with simultaneous or sequential use of qualitative and quantitative methods (Table 7.2).

TABLE **7.2**

TYPES OF MULTIMETHOD DESIGNS

DESIGN	ORDER	COMMENTS
INDUCTIVE PARADIGM		
Qualitative + qualitative	Simultaneous	One method is dominant and forms the basis for the study; paradigm is used when more than one perspective is required
Qualitative → qualitative	Sequential	One method is dominant and forms the basis for the study; the second supplements the first
Qualitative + quantitative	Simultaneous	Inductive drive; paradigm is used when some portion of the phenomenon can be measured
Qualitative → quantitative	Sequential	Inductive drive; paradigm can confirm earlier qualitative findings
DEDUCTIVE PARADIGM		
Quantitative + quantitative	Simultaneous	One method is dominant and forms the basis for the study; paradigm validates the finding of each instrument used
Quantitative → quantitative	Sequential	One method is dominant and forms the basis for the study; paradigm is used to elicit further details
Quantitative + qualitative	Simultaneous	Deductive theoretical drive; paradigm is used when some aspect of the phenomenon is not measurable
Quantitative → qualitative	Sequential	Deductive theoretical drive; paradigm is often used when the findings are unexpected, and the qualitative method is used to find explanations

Mixed-methods research provides researchers with a wider range of tools and options to study phenomena. The variety of methods provides different views and different levels of data.

Table 7.3 synthesizes four studies reporting multimethod analyses. The table notes the conceptual focus of the work, the study purposes, and whether the study suggests implications for theory, practice, and instrument development.

Swanson's (1999) work is a good example of a research program. Utilizing a variety of methodologies and analysis (see Table 7.3), she addressed implications for practice, instrument development, and theory building focused on the issue of caring for women who have had a miscarriage. Her research program included an initial theory-building phase (studies 1 and 2), an instrument development phase (studies 3, 4, and 5), and a phase of testing a practice intervention (study 6). Swanson used the phenomenological method for studies 1 and 2 and quantitative methods for each of her other studies. She did not use more than one method in any of her studies, but her use of multiple methods during the course of her 15-year research program can be likened to examining different facets of one crystal: in this case, the experience of miscarrying. The crystallization process has contributed to theory building, nursing practice, and instrument development. Her practice contribution is highlighted by a case exemplar (Swanson, 1999), which synthesized her years of work with women living through the experience of miscarriage.

To explore the lived experience of transfer students in a collaborative baccalaureate nursing program in Ontario, Cameron (2003) used mixed methodology: the quantitative portion elicited data about a sample, and the qualitative portion consisted of interview questions (see Table 7.3). Data from the quantitative survey supported the findings that emerged from the qualitative methods. The qualitative methods provided depth and substance to the findings from the questionnaire—again, like differing facets of a crystal.

St-Amant, Ward-Griffin, Brown, et al. (2014; see Table 7.3) used a sequential-methods design to study how professional caregivers (RNs) provided care to an elderly relative. They initially used a quantitative survey design to examine the domain of professional and familial caregiving. In the second phase, the researchers used a qualitative grounded theory approach to examine the negotiating strategies utilized by the caregivers.

Stewart, Makwarimba, Letourneau, et al. (2015) used a mixed-method study design to develop and evaluate a social support intervention for Zimbabwean and Sudanese refugee new parents. The social support intervention focused on the use of face-to-face support groups co-led by a peer mentor. Qualitative methods such as group and in-depth individual interviews were conducted to explore the impact of the social support intervention. Several quantitative instruments were used to measure the impact of the intervention on support needs, loneliness and isolation, coping, and parenting stress index.

The studies of Swanson (1999), Cameron (2003), St-Amant et al. (2014), and Stewart et al. (2015) constitute a range of approaches for combining methods in research studies (see Table 7.3). The mixed-methods field continues to evolve as nurse researchers strive to determine which research combinations can deliver an enhanced understanding of human complexity and a substantial contribution to nursing science. Consumers of nursing research are encouraged to follow this ongoing discussion.

Synthesizing Qualitative Evidence: Metasynthesis

The depth and breadth of qualitative research have grown over the years. It has become important to qualitative researchers to synthesize critical amounts of qualitative findings. Qualitative **metasynthesis** is a type of systematic review applied to qualitative research. Unlike quantitative research, in which statistical approaches are used to aggregate or average data by means of meta-analysis, metasynthesis

TABLE 7.3

RESEARCH USING MULTIMETHOD APPROACHES

AUTHOR, YEAR	CONCEPTUAL FOCUS	MULTIMETHOD APPROACH	STUDY PURPOSE	THEORY-BUILDING IMPLICATIONS	PRACTICE IMPLICATIONS	INSTRUMENT DEVELOPMENT IMPLICATIONS
Swanson (1999)	Miscarriage and caring	Six studies, each involving the use of one method	Study 1: To define common themes for women who had recently miscarried	Yes	Yes	—
			Study 2: To describe the human experience of miscarriage and the meaning of caring	Yes	Yes	—
			Study 3: To use descriptive data to create a survey instrument that is based on women's experience of miscarriage	—	—	Yes
			Study 4: To evaluate the relevance of the survey items to create a miscarriage scale	—	—	Yes
			Study 5: To assess the reliability and validity of the miscarriage scale	—	—	Yes
			Study 6: To test the effects of caring, measurement, and time on women's well-being in the first year after miscarriage	Yes	Yes	Yes
Cameron (2003)	Transition resilience	One study involving the use of multiple methods	To explore the lived experience of students transferring from college to university in a collaborative nursing program	Yes	Yes	Yes
St-Amant et al. (2014)	Professionalizing familial care	Phase 1 correlational survey design Phase 2 emergent grounded theory approach	Examine the processed by which registered nurses enact professional care work within the familial care domain	Yes	Yes	—
Stewart et al. (2015)	To design and evaluate a social support intervention for refugee new parents	Conducted group and in-depth individual interviews to explore impacts of the social support intervention. Secondly, several quantitative instruments were used to measure the impact of the intervention on support needs, loneliness and isolation, coping, and parenting stress index	To design and evaluate a social support intervention for refugee new parents	Yes	Yes	Yes

involves integrating qualitative research findings on a topic and is based on comparative analysis and interpretative synthesis of qualitative research findings, whereby the researcher seeks to retain the essence and unique contribution of each study (Sandelowski & Barroso, 2007).

As an example, Sandelowski and Barroso (2005) reported the results of a qualitative metasynthesis and metasummary that integrated the findings of qualitative studies of expectant parents who received a prenatal diagnosis of a fetal abnormality. Using the methods of qualitative research synthesis (meta-analysis and metasummary (see Sandelowski & Barroso, 2007), they analytically reviewed 17 qualitative studies retrieved from multiple databases. On the basis of the synthesis process detailed in the article, clinical implications and the need for further research in the area were identified.

Lombardo, Angus, Lowndes, et al. (2014) wished to explore the contextual conditions under which women access health care, through qualitative metasynthesis. After synthesizing findings from 35 articles reviewed by the six authors of the study, they discovered that in spite of the women's resourcefulness and the utilization of spectrum of resources, systemic problems still needed to be addressed. The authors recommended that "women need to be involved in designing and implementing interventions to improve access to health care" (Lombardo et al., 2014, p. 575).

Essentially, metasynthesis provides a way for researchers to build up a critical amount of qualitative research evidence that is relevant to clinical practice. Sandelowski (2004) cautioned that the use of qualitative metasynthesis is laudable and necessary but that researchers who use metasynthesis methods must clearly understand qualitative methodologies and the nuances of the various qualitative methods. It will be interesting for research consumers to follow the progress of researchers who seek to develop criteria for appraising a set of qualitative studies and to use those criteria to guide the incorporation of these studies into systematic literature reviews.

 Evidence-Informed Practice Tip ___

Qualitative research findings can be used in many ways, including improving ways clinicians communicate with patients and with each other.

CRITICAL THINKING CHALLENGES

- Discuss how a researcher's values could influence the results of a study. Include an example in your answer.
- Can the metaphor "We do not always get closer to the truth as we slice and homogenize and isolate [it]" be applied to both qualitative and quantitative methods? Justify your answer.
- What is the value of qualitative research in evidence-informed practice? Give an example.
- Using the model in Figure 7.2, discuss how you could apply the findings of a qualitative research study about coping with a miscarriage.

KEY POINTS

- All research is based on philosophical beliefs, a worldview, or a paradigm.
- Qualitative research encompasses different methodologies.
- Qualitative researchers believe that reality is socially constructed and is context dependent.
- Researchers' values should be kept as separate as possible from the conduct of research.
- Qualitative research, like quantitative research, follows a process, but the components of the process vary.
- Qualitative research contributes to evidence-informed practice.
- Ethical issues in qualitative research involve issues related to the naturalistic setting, the emergent nature of the design, researcher–participant interaction, and the researcher as instrument.

FOR FURTHER STUDY

ⓔ Go to Evolve at http://evolve.elsevier.com/Canada/LoBiondo/Research for the Audio Glossary and Appendix Tables that provide supplemental information for Appendix E.

REFERENCES

Cameron, C. (2003). The lived experience of transfer students in a collaborative baccalaureate nursing program. (Unpublished doctoral dissertation). University of Toronto.

Creswell, J. W. (2014). *Research design: Qualitative, quantitative and mixed methods approaches* (4th ed.). Thousand Oaks, CA: Sage.

Denzin, N. K. (1978). *The research act: A theoretical introduction to sociological methods.* New York: McGraw-Hill.

Denzin, N. K., & Lincoln, Y. (Eds.), (2011). *The Sage Handbook of qualitative research* (4th ed.). Thousand Oaks, CA: Sage.

Fournier, B., Mill, J., Kipp, W., et al. (2006). Discovering voice: A participatory action research study with nurses in Uganda. *International Journal of Qualitative Methods, 6*(2). Retrieved from http://www.ualberta.ca/~iiqm/backissues/6_2/fournier.pdf.

Giddings, L. S., & Grant, B. M. (2007). A Trojan horse of positivism? A critique of mixed methods research. *Advances in Nursing Science, 30,* 52–60.

Glesne, C. (2011). *Becoming qualitative researchers: An introduction* (4th ed.). Toronto: Pearson.

Janesick, V. J. (1994). The dance of qualitative research design. In N. K. Denzin & Y. S. Lincoln (Eds.), *Handbook of qualitative research* (pp. 209–219). Thousand Oaks, CA: Sage.

Lipson, G. L. (1994). Ethical issues in ethnography. In J. Morse (Ed.), *Critical issues in qualitative research methods* (pp. 333–355). Thousand Oaks, CA: Sage.

Lombardo, A. P., Angus, J. E., Lowndes, R., et al. (2014). Women's strategies to achieve access to healthcare in Ontario, Canada: A meta-synthesis. *Health and Social Care in the Community, 22*(6), 575–587.

Marshall, C., & Rossman, G. B. (2011). *Designing qualitative research* (5th ed.). Los Angeles, CA: Sage.

Morgan, D. (1998). Practical strategies for combining qualitative and quantitative methods: Applications to health research. *Qualitative Health Research, 8,* 362–377.

Morse, J. M. (1991). Approaches to qualitative-quantitative research methodological triangulation. *Nursing Research, 40,* 120–123.

Morse, J. M. (1998). The contracted relationship: Ensuring protection of anonymity and confidentiality. *Qualitative Health Research, 8*(3), 301–303.

Morse, J. M. (2003). Principles of mixed methods and multimethod research design. In A. Tashakkori & C. Teddlie (Eds.), *Handbook of mixed methods in social & behavioural research* (pp. 189–208). Thousand Oaks, CA: Sage.

Patton, M. (2002). *Qualitative research & evaluation methods* (3rd ed.). Thousand Oaks, CA: Sage.

Patton, M. (2015). *Qualitative research & evaluation methods* (4th ed.). Thousand Oaks, CA: Sage.

Racine, L. (2011). The impact of race, gender, and class in a postcolonial feminist fieldwork: A retrospective critique of methodological dilemmas. *Apopria, 3*(1), 15–27.

Roper, J., & Shapira, J. (2000). *Ethnography in nursing research.* Thousand Oaks, CA: Sage.

Sandelowski, M. (2004). Using qualitative research. *Qualitative Health Research, 14*(10), 1366–1386.

Sandelowski, M., & Barroso, J. (2005). The travesty of choosing after positive prenatal diagnosis. *Journal of Obstetrical, Gynecologic & Neonatal Nursing, 34*(4), 307–318.

Sandelowski, M., & Barroso, J. (2007). *Handbook for synthesizing qualitative research.* Philadelphia: Springer.

Silverman, D., & Marvasti, A. (2008). *Doing qualitative research.* Los Angeles: Sage.

Smith, M. J., & Liehr, P. (2003). The theory of attentively embracing story. In M. J. Smith & P. Liehr (Eds.), *Middle range theory for nursing* (pp. 167–187). New York: Springer.

St-Amant, O., Ward-Griffin, C., Brown, J. B., et al. (2014). Professionalizing familiar care: Examining nurses' unpaid family care work. *Advances in Nursing Science, 37*(2), 117–131.

Stewart, M., Makwarimba, E., Letourneau, N. L., et al. (2015). Impacts of support intervention for Zimbabwean and Sudanese refuges parents: "I am not alone." *Canadian Journal of Nursing Research, 47*(4), 113–140.

Streubert, H. J., & Carpenter, D. (2011). *Qualitative research in nursing: Advancing the humanistic imperative* (5th ed.). New York: Wolters Kluwer.

Swanson, K. M. (1999). Research-based practice with women who have had miscarriages. *Image Journal of Nursing Scholarship, 31*(4), 339–345.

Wang, C., & Burris, M. A. (1997). Photovoice: Concept, methodology, and use for participatory assessment. *Human Education and Behavior, 24*(3), 369–387.

CHAPTER 8

Qualitative Approaches to Research

Julie Barroso | Cherylyn Cameron

LEARNING OUTCOMES

After reading this chapter, you will be able to do the following:

- Identify the processes of qualitative research such as phenomenological, grounded theory, ethnographic, and case study methods.
- Recognize the appropriate use of historical methods.
- Recognize the appropriate use of community-based participatory research methods.
- Apply critiquing criteria to evaluate a report of qualitative research.

KEY TERMS

behavioural/materialist
    perspective
case study method
cognitive perspective
community-based
    participatory research (CBPR)
constant comparative method
context
culture
data saturation
domains
emic perspective

ethnographic method
ethnography
etic perspective
external criticism
grounded theory method
hermeneutics
historical research method
instrumental case study
internal criticism
intersubjectivity
intrinsic case study
key informants

lived experience
narrative inquiry
orientational qualitative
    inquiry
participatory action
    research (PAR)
phenomenological method
phenomenology
propositions
qualitative descriptive
snowball sampling
theoretical sampling

STUDY RESOURCES

ⓔ Go to Evolve at http://evolve.elsevier.com/Canada/LoBiondo/Research
    for the Audio Glossary and Appendix Tables that provide supplemental
    information for Appendix E.

QUALITATIVE STUDIES CAN ANSWER THE CRITICAL "why?" questions that result from many evidence-informed practice summaries; a research question may have been answered, but how the answer operates in the caring for people is not explained. As a research consumer you should know that qualitative methods are the best way to start to answer clinical and research questions about what little is known or when a new perspective is needed in practice. The very fact that the number of qualitative research studies has increased exponentially in nursing and other social sciences reflects the urgent need of clinicians to better understand the experience of illness.

This chapter describes a variety of qualitative research methods: phenomenological, grounded theory, ethnographic, qualitative descriptive, case study, historical, and participatory action research. You are encouraged to use the researcher's standpoint as each method is introduced—to imagine how it would be to study an issue of interest from the perspective of each of these methods. No matter which method a researcher uses, there is a demand to embrace the wholeness of humans, focusing on the human experience in natural settings.

The researcher using these methods believes that each unique human being attributes meaning to his or her experience, and experience evolves from his or her social and historical context. Thus, one person's experience of pain is distinct from another's and can be known by the individual's subjective description of it. For example, for the adolescent with rheumatoid arthritis, the researcher interested in studying the adolescent's lived experience of pain spends time in the adolescent's natural settings, such as the home and school. Efforts are directed at uncovering the meaning of pain as it extends beyond the number of medications taken or a rating on a pain scale. Qualitative methods are grounded in the belief that objective data do not capture the whole of the human experience; rather, the meaning of the adolescent's pain emerges within the context of personal history, current relationships, and future plans as the adolescent lives daily life in dynamic interaction with the environment.

The researcher using qualitative methods begins collecting bits of information and piecing them together, building a mosaic or a picture of the human experience being studied. As with a mosaic, when one steps away from the work, the whole picture emerges. This whole picture transcends the bits and pieces and cannot be known from any one bit or piece. In presenting study findings, the researcher strives to capture the human experience and present it so that other people can understand it.

QUALITATIVE RESEARCH METHODS

Thus far, the overview of the qualitative research approach (see Chapter 7) has focused on the importance of evidence offered by qualitative research for nursing science. This overview highlighted how choice of a qualitative approach is reflective of a researcher's worldview and the research question. The topics addressed in the overview provide a foundation for examining the qualitative methods discussed in this chapter. The Critical Thinking Decision Path introduces you to a process for recognizing various qualitative methods by distinguishing areas of interest for each method and noting how the research question might be introduced for each distinct method. In this chapter each of these research traditions is discussed on the basis of views along a continuum from post-positivist to constructivist to social critical theory, as shown in Figure 8.1. The constructivist paradigm (multiple realities) is the basis of most qualitative research, and the positivist or contemporary empiricist paradigm (single reality) is the basis of most empirical analytical or quantitative research. The philosophical foundation and assumptions of qualitative research are discussed in Chapter 2. You may wish to quickly review pp. 26 to 31 to refresh your memory. Make sure that you can differentiate between post-positivism and constructivism. In

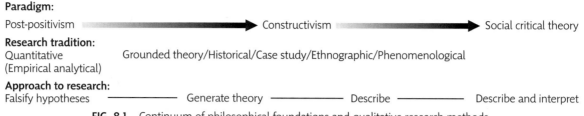

Paradigm:

Post-positivism ━━━━━━━━━━▶ Constructivism ━━━━━━━━━━▶ Social critical theory

Research tradition:
Quantitative   Grounded theory/Historical/Case study/Ethnographic/Phenomenological
(Empirical analytical)

Approach to research:
Falsify hypotheses ───────── Generate theory ───────── Describe ───────── Describe and interpret

FIG. 8.1   Continuum of philosophical foundations and qualitative research methods.

addition to the methods listed in the Critical Thinking Decision Path, several other qualitative research methods are briefly described here.

Phenomenological Method

According to Streubert and Carpenter (2011), "**phenomenology** is a science whose purpose is to describe particular phenomena, or the appearance of things, as lived experience" (p. 73). Phenomenological research is used to answer questions of personal meaning. This method is most useful when the task is to understand an experience in the way that people having the experience understand it and is well suited to the study of phenomena important to nursing. For example, what is the experience of men facing prostate surgery? What is the meaning of pain for people with chronic arthritis? Phenomenological research is an important method with which to begin studying a new topic or a topic that has been studied but needs a fresh perspective.

Phenomenological research is based on phenomenological philosophy, which has changed over time and with different philosophers. Various phenomenological methods exist, including the following:

1. Descriptive phenomenology, which focuses on rich detailed descriptions of the lived world and is based on Edmund Husserl's philosophy
2. Heideggerian phenomenology, which expands description to understanding achieved through searching for the relationships and meanings of phenomena
3. Hermeneutic philosophy, which focuses on interpretation of phenomena

Derived from the Greek word *hermeneuein,* the term **hermeneutics** refers to a theoretical framework in which to understand or interpret human phenomena. Hermeneutic researchers believe that interpretation cannot be absolutely correct or true but must be viewed from the perspective of the historical or cultural context and the original purpose of the text. Researchers "use qualitative methods to establish context and meaning for what people do," and hermeneutists are much clearer about the fact that they are "constructing the reality on the basis of their interpretations of data with the help of the participants who provided data in the study" (Patton, 2002, p. 115). Hermeneutic researchers outline their own perspectives and how they may influence the interpretation and analysis of the data. In many nursing studies, the hermeneutic approach is used to understand a particular phenomenon and scientifically interpret phenomena from text or the written word (Streubert & Carpenter, 2011).

Patton (2015) described many of the different phenomenological approaches in his text *Qualitative Research & Evaluation Methods.* Although he acknowledges the complexity and differing traditions of these approaches, he also states their similarities:

> What these various phenomenological approaches share in common is a focus on exploring how human beings make sense of experience and transform experience into consciousness, both individually and as shared meaning. This requires methodologically, carefully, and thoroughly capturing and describing how people experience some phenomenon—how they perceive it, describe it, feel about it, judge it, remember it, make sense of it, and talk about it with

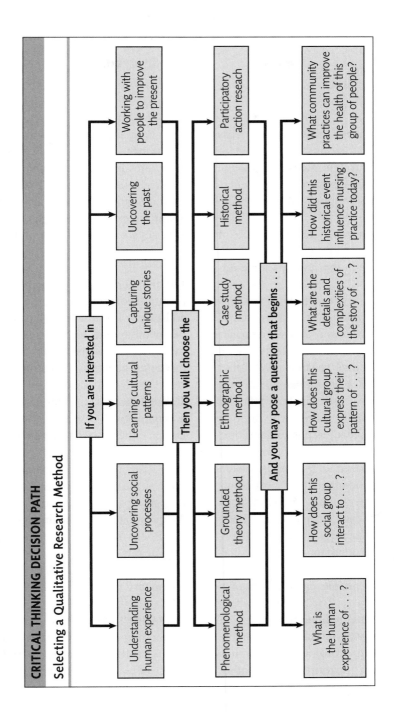

CRITICAL THINKING DECISION PATH

Selecting a Qualitative Research Method

If you are interested in

| Understanding human experience | Uncovering social processes | Learning cultural patterns | Capturing unique stories | Uncovering the past | Working with people to improve the present |

Then you will choose the

| Phenomenological method | Grounded theory method | Ethnographic method | Case study method | Historical method | Participatory action reseach |

And you may pose a question that begins . . . .

| What is the human experience of . . . ? | How does this social group interact to . . . ? | How does this cultural group express their pattern of . . . ? | What are the details and complexities of the story of . . . ? | How did this historical event influence nursing practice today? | What community practices can improve the health of this group of people? |

others. To gather such data, one must take undertake in-depth interviews with people who have directly experienced the phenomenon of interest; that is, they have "lived experience" as opposed to second-hand experience. (p. 115)

The five important concepts or values in phenomenological research (Cohen, 1987) are as follows:

1. The **phenomenological method** is a process of learning and constructing the meaning of human experience through intensive dialogue with persons who are living the experience. This method was developed to understand meanings.

2. Phenomenology was based on a critique of positivism, or the positivist view, which was seen as inappropriate in the study of some human concerns.

3. The object of study is the "life world" *(Lebenswelt),* or lived experience, not contrived situations. In other words, as the philosopher Husserl said, researchers are concerned with the appearance of things *(phenomena)* rather than the things themselves *(noumena).*

4. **Intersubjectivity**—a person's belief that other people share a common world with him or her—is an important tenet in phenomenology. Although phenomena differ, they also share similarities that are based on the similarities in people. The most fundamental of those similarities is that every person has a body in space and time. In other words, the physical body and historical sense lead to similarities in how people experience phenomena. The basic elements, or an essence, of the shared experience are common among people or members of a specific society.

5. The phenomenological reduction, also called *bracketing,* is controversial and more important in some phenomenological approaches than in others (e.g., descriptive methods). Phenomenological reduction means that researchers must be aware of and examine their prejudices or values.

Whatever the form of phenomenological research, you will find the researcher asking a question about the lived experience.

Identifying the Phenomenon

Because the focus of the phenomenological method is the **lived experience**—the undergoing of events and circumstances, as opposed to thinking about these events and circumstances—the researcher is likely to choose this method when studying some dimension of day-to-day existence for a particular group of people. The example used in this chapter is an article by Pooler (2014) about the experiences of living with moderate to very severe chronic lower pulmonary disease.

Structuring the Study

For the purpose of describing structuring in a phenomenological study, the following topics are addressed: The research question, the researcher's perspective, and sample selection. The issue of human participants' protection in research was discussed generally with ethics in Chapter 7.

RESEARCH QUESTION. The question that guides phenomenological research always concerns some human experience. It guides the researcher to ask the participant about some past or present experience. The research question is not exactly the same as the question used to initiate dialogue with the participant, but often the research question and the question used to begin dialogue are very similar. Pooler's (2014) research question to study participants was "What is it like to experience moderate to severe COPD [chronic obstructive pulmonary disease] or asthma?" (p. 3).

RESERACHER'S PERSPECTIVE. When using the phenomenological method, the researcher's perspective is bracketed; that is, the researcher identifies personal biases about the phenomenon of interest in order to clarify how personal experience and beliefs may influence what is heard and reported. The researcher is expected to set aside personal biases—to bracket them—when engaging with the participants. By becoming aware of personal biases, the researcher is more likely to be able to pursue issues of importance introduced by the participant, rather than leading the participant to issues the researcher deems important.

Research Hint

Managing personal bias is an expectation of researchers who use all the methods discussed in this chapter.

The use of phenomenological methods always entails some strategy to identify personal biases and hold them in abeyance while the participant is interviewed. The reader may find it difficult to identify bracketing strategies because they are seldom explicitly identified in a research manuscript. Sometimes the researcher's worldview or assumptions provide insight into biases that have been considered and bracketed. Bracketing is not mentioned in Pooler's (2014) study; again, this is not unusual and does not detract from the quality of the report. Usually, you will find some mention about bracketing if such an issue exists, but not if there are no bracketing issues.

Research Hint

Although the research question may not always be explicitly reported, you may identify it by evaluating the study's purpose or the question/statement posed to the participants.

SAMPLE SELECTION. As you read a report of a phenomenological study, you will find that the selected participant is either living the experience the researcher is querying about or has lived the experience in the past. Because phenomenologists believe that each individual's history is a dimension of the present, a past experience exists in the present moment. Even when a participant is describing an experience occurring in the present, remembered information is being gathered. The 16 participants in the study by Pooler (2014) were 6 females and 10 males, aged 35–77 years old. All of the participants were recruited through purposive sampling from three pulmonary outpatient clinics in Western Canada and were determined by pulmonary function tests to have moderate to very severe COPD or asthma. All of the participants were on disability, unemployed, and/or had taken early retirement due to the severity of the disease. One participant was on a lung transplant list, and five were on long-term home oxygen therapy.

Research Hint

Qualitative studies often involve the use of purposive sampling (see Chapter 7).

Data Gathering

Written or oral data may be collected when the phenomenological method is used. The researcher may pose the query in writing and ask for a written response or may schedule a time to interview the participant and record the interaction. In either case, the researcher may return to ask for clarification of written or recorded transcripts. To some extent, the particular data-collection procedure is guided by the choice of a specific analysis technique. Various analysis techniques require different numbers of interviews. In general, open-ended questions—such as "What comes to mind when you think of . . . ?"—guide the participants to describe their lived experience. During the interview, the researcher attempts to gather more information by asking clarifying questions. **Data saturation** usually guides decisions regarding how many interviews are enough.

Pooler (2014) conducted two open-ended interviews with each participant that were conversational in nature. The object was to collect in-depth stories about their experience. However, several of the participants had shortness of breath, making it challenging to describe their experiences in detail. As a nurse researcher with clinical expertise, Pooler also closely observed the participants' nonverbal behaviour, including their breathing patterns. The questions asked constantly evolved as the researcher analyzed the interviews. She continued to interview participants until no further data or emergent themes were forthcoming and there were enough data to fully describe their experiences.

Data Analysis

As data are collected, data analysis begins. Several techniques are available for data analysis when the phenomenological method is used. Detailed information about specific techniques can be found in the original sources (Colaizzi, 1978; Giorgi, Fischer, & Murray, 1975; Spiegelberg, 1976; van Kaam, 1969). Although the techniques are slightly different from each other, there is a general pattern of moving from the participant's description to the researcher's synthesis of all participants' descriptions. The steps generally include the following:

1. Thorough and sensitive reading of presence with the entire transcription of the participant's description
2. Identification of shifts in participant thought, resulting in division of the transcription into thought segments
3. Specification of significant phrases in each thought segment, in the participant's own words
4. Distillation of each significant phrase to express the central meaning of the segment in the researcher's words
5. Grouping together of segments that contain similar central meanings for each participant
6. Preliminary synthesis of grouped segments for each participant with a focus on the essence of the phenomenon being studied
7. Final synthesis of the essences that have surfaced in all participants' descriptions, resulting in an exhaustive description of the lived experience

As described previously, Pooler (2014) conducted ongoing analysis and used van Manen's approach for analysis. Although not fully described in Pooler's study, there are typically three techniques developed by van Manen (1997) to isolate themes during data analysis: (1) the "wholistic approach" of reading each transcript in its entirety to understand the overall meaning, (2) the "selective approach" to identify meaningful portions of transcript text, and (3) the "line-by-line approach" to discover what each line reveals about the participant's experience.

Describing the Findings

When using the phenomenological method, the nurse researcher constructs a path of information leading from the research question through samples of participants' words and the researcher's interpretation to the final synthesis that elaborates the lived experience. When reading the report of a phenomenological study, you should find that detailed descriptive language is used to convey the complex meaning of the lived experience. Pooler (2014) provided numerous quotations from participants to support her findings. She identified three central themes of slowing down, doing less, and having to stop. For example, a quotation exemplifying the theme of slowing down is as follows:

> "I'll start walking at the same speed as the people I am with are walking. And I can't sustain it. They don't notice that I'm in trouble. And I have to say to them, 'I'm sorry, but you're going to have to slow down because I can't walk at that speed.'" (p. 4)

These direct quotations from participants enable the reader to evaluate the connection between what the participant said and how the researcher labelled it.

Evidence-Informed Practice Tip

Phenomenological research is an important approach for accumulating evidence when researchers study a new topic about which little is known.

Narrative Analysis

When **narrative inquiry** is used as a form of qualitative research, stories of people are collected and examined as the primary source of data (Duffy, 2011; Patton, 2015). The hermeneutic tradition is extended to include in-depth interview transcripts, memoirs, stories, and creative nonfiction. This discipline also draws from the phenomenological tradition in its interest in the lived experience and perceptions of experience. On the basis of the "stories" of people, at times including those of the researcher, researchers using narrative analysis in an attempt to interpret and understand experiences in terms of cultural and social meanings (Patton, 2002; see Practical Application box). As Patton (2015) notes, storytelling and narrative inquiry are not the same thing: The story is data, whereas the narrative analysis "involves interpreting the story, placing it in context, and comparing it with other stories" (p. 128).

Orientational Qualitative Inquiry

In **orientational qualitative inquiry,** an ideology or orientation is used to direct the investigation, including the research question, methodology, fieldwork, and analysis of the findings. Ideologies include feminist, queer, and critical theories (Patton, 2002). For example, a feminist researcher presumes that gender influences all relationships and societal processes. The researcher will attend to "women's ways of knowing" and include the participants throughout the research. Queer theory, which emerged from feminist theory, focuses on lived experience and practice through the lens of gender identity and sexual orientation. For example, Hammond, Holmes, and Mercier (2016) and Holmes, O'Byrne, and Gastaldo (2006, 2007) explored why some gay men continue to have unprotected sex despite the associated health risks. Critical theory focuses on issues of power and justice and how injustice and subjugation shape people's experiences and their view of the world. Rather than studying to merely understand instances of injustice, the critical theorist attempts to critique society, name injustices, and change society. Nurses are particularly interested in addressing and changing oppressive practices that influence health and health care (Browne, 2000). Smith and colleagues (2006) took a critical postcolonial stance in their study on pregnancy and parenting experiences among Indigenous peoples. In the postcolonial stance, issues of power are viewed in terms of the legacy of colonization of Indigenous peoples and the neocolonial present. Racine (2011) combined postcolonial and feminist epistemology in her study of Haitian Canadian caregivers, stating that "postcolonial feminist epistemology not only focuses on patriarchy as a source of oppression, but also examines how social inequities are inscribed within a historical, political, social, cultural, and economic context . . . ." (p. 18).

Grounded Theory Method

In the **grounded theory method,** a systematic set of procedures is used to explore the social processes that guide human interaction and to inductively develop a theory on the basis of those observations. The philosophical spectrum

---

 Practical Application

Lapum, Angus, Peter, and colleagues (2010) used narrative inquiry to examine patients' experiential accounts of technology in open-heart surgery and recovery. Data were collected from two interviews in which the participants were encouraged to tell their story through prompts and questions, such as "Tell me about waking up from surgery." The participants also documented their experiences in journals for several weeks after surgery. The researchers listened, heard, and felt through the stories what was happening to the participants. Although focus was placed on the content of the stories, emphasis was also placed on how the stories were put together: "We attended to facets of temporality, contextuality, plot, scene, and characters in order to understand processes and activities involved in narrative emplotment" (Lapum et al., 2010, p. 756).

of grounded theory ranges from the post-positivist view to the constructivist view (see Figure 8.1). The grounded theory method is based on the sociological tradition of the Chicago School of Symbolic Interactionism, a tradition that reflects on issues related to human behaviour. Glaser and Strauss (1967) developed the method of grounded theory and published the classic first text describing the methodology: *The Discovery of Grounded Theory*. According to Strauss and Corbin (1990), grounded theory

> is one that is inductively derived from the study of the phenomenon it represents. That is, it is discovered, developed, and provisionally verified through systematic data collection and analysis of data pertaining to that phenomenon. Therefore, data collection, analysis, and theory stand in reciprocal relationship with each other. One does not begin with a theory, then prove it. Rather one begins with an area of study and what is relevant to that area is allowed to emerge. (p. 23)

In many qualitative research traditions, explanatory models and theories are described and developed in relation to a human phenomenon under study; grounded theory is distinctive from the other traditional qualitative research methods because its primary focus is on generating theory about dominant social processes. The three major premises that continue to underlie grounded theory research are outlined in Box 8.1.

The purpose of grounded theory, as the name implies, is to generate a theory from data. Grounded

---

BOX **8.1**

MAJOR PREMISES OF GROUNDED THEORY

1. Humans act toward objects on the basis of the meaning that those objects have for them. Meaning is embedded in context and, therefore, it cannot be separated from the context or from the consequences of the meanings in a particular setting.
2. Social meanings arise from social interactions with other people over time and are embedded socially, historically, culturally, and contextually. Therefore, the focus of grounded theory is on social interactions.
3. People use interpretive processes to handle and change meanings in dealing with their situations.

---

theory has contributed substantively to the body of knowledge in the field of nursing. Often, the theories generated from grounded research are then tested empirically. Qualitative data are gathered through interviews and observation. Through analysis of the data, substantive codes are generated and then are clustered into categories. **Propositions** link the concepts to create a foundation that guides further data collection. Additional data that are thought likely to answer generated hypotheses are collected until all categories are "saturated"—that is, no new information is generated. The goal of generating a theory implies that laws drive at least some portion of reality. The truth is sought from relevant groups, for example, patients who are dying.

The context is very important, as was shown in a classic work by Glaser and Strauss (1965). They noted that, at the time of their work, patients were unwilling to talk openly about the process of their own dying, physicians were unwilling to disclose the imminence of death to patients, and nurses were expected not to make these disclosures. This lack of communication led Glaser and Strauss (1965) to their study of the problem of awareness of dying. They described various types of awareness contexts, problems of awareness, and practical uses of awareness theory. Their early fieldwork led to hypotheses and the gathering of additional data, and the framework was refined with further analysis until they formed a systematic substantive theory.

As stated earlier, constructive grounded theory emerged from the seminal work by Glaser and Straus (1967). Charmaz (2014) notes that Glaser and Strauss focused on discovering theory as emerging from data that were separate from the researcher. She argues that

> neither data nor theories are discovered. Rather, we are part of the world we study and the data we collect. And the analyses we produce. We construct our grounded theories through our past and present involvements and interactions with people, perspectives, and research practices. (p. 30)

Identifying the Phenomenon

Researchers typically use the grounded theory method when they are interested in either social processes from the perspective of human interactions or patterns of action and interaction between and among various types of social units (Denzin & Lincoln, 1998). The basic social process is sometimes expressed as a gerund, indicating that change across time as social reality is negotiated. Dahlke, Phinney, Hall, and colleagues (2014) explored nursing practice with hospitalized older adults from a nursing perspective and developed a theory of orchestrating care.

Structuring the Study

RESEARCH QUESTION. Research questions appropriate for the grounded theory method are those that address basic social processes that shape human behaviour. In a grounded theory study, the research question can be a statement or a broad question that permits in-depth explanation of the phenomenon. The researcher does not always need to identify a problem or research question but chooses an area of interest.

RESEARCHER'S PERSPECTIVE. In a grounded theory study, the researcher brings some knowledge of the literature to the study, but an exhaustive literature review is not performed (Streubert & Carpenter, 2011). Therefore, theory emerges directly from data and reflects the contextual values that are integral to the social processes being studied. Thus, the theory product that emerges is "grounded in" the data. This type of study was exemplified in Dahlke et al.'s (2014) article; in the introduction the authors noted that there was little research examining how nurses perceive their practice with hospitalized older adults.

SAMPLE SELECTION. Sample selection involves (1) choosing participants for a purposive sample who are experiencing the circumstance and "are judged to have good knowledge of the study domain" (Wuest, 2011, p. 235) and (2) selecting events and incidents that are related to the social process under investigation. As problems begin to emerge, the researchers may conduct **theoretical sampling,** a sampling method used to select experiences that helps the researchers test ideas and gather complete information about developing concepts. In this method, researchers seek participants who can further clarify the emerging concepts. Dahlke et al. (2014) recruited participants through purposeful, snowball, and theoretical sampling from two units in two separate hospitals in Western Canada. **Snowball sampling** occurs when a participant recommends other participants from his or her contacts. As more and more participants bring on new recruits, the sample appears to grow like a snowball.

Through theoretical sampling, the researchers can target certain groups to test and refine the emerging findings. Researchers may also include key informants to provide clarification on issues such as regulatory and legal issues. **Key informants** are individuals who have special knowledge, status, or communication skills and who are willing to teach the researcher about the phenomenon.

Data Gathering

In the grounded theory method, data are collected through interviews and through skilled observations of individuals interacting in a social setting. Interviews are audio-recorded and then transcribed, and observations are recorded as field notes. Open-ended questions are used initially to identify concepts for further focus. Dahlke et al. (2014) gathered data from 24 participants who were interviewed and from participant observation and examination of documents related to nursing practice. The interviews were semi-structured; eight repeat interviews were conducted to obtain feedback on the emerging theory. The researchers conducted 375 hours of participant observation, at various times of the day and on weekends and holidays. Finally, the documentation gathered was considered to be meaningful in guiding the nursing practice, including care planning and Kardex information.

Data Analysis

A major feature of the grounded theory method is that data collection and analysis occur simultaneously. The process requires systematic, detailed record keeping through the use of field notes and transcribed interview recordings. Hunches about emerging patterns in the data are noted in memos, and the researcher directs activities in the field by pursuing these hunches. This technique of theoretical sampling is used to select participants whose experiences will help the researcher test ideas and gather complete information about developing concepts. The researcher begins by noting indicators or actual events, actions, or words in the data. Concepts, or abstractions, are developed from the indicators (Charmaz, 2000; Strauss, 1987).

The initial analytical process is called *open coding* (Strauss, 1987). Data are examined carefully line by line, categorized into discrete parts, and compared for similarities and differences (Corbin & Strauss, 2008). Data are compared with other data continuously as they are acquired during research. This process is called the **constant comparative method.** Codes in the data are clustered to form categories. The categories are expanded and developed, or they are collapsed into one another. Theory is constructed through this systematic process. As a result, data collection, analysis, and theory generation have a direct reciprocal relationship (Charmaz, 2000; Strauss & Corbin, 1990). Dahlke et al. (2014) analyzed the data concurrently with data collection, as is typical of grounded theory. They further used the constant comparative method described earlier, along with memo writing and the three sets of coding.

Describing the Findings

Grounded theory studies are reported in sufficient detail to provide the reader with the steps in the process, the logic of the method, and the theory that has emerged. In reports of grounded theory studies, descriptive language and diagrams of the process are used as evidence to ensure that the theory reported in the findings remains connected to the data. Instead of providing a description of people's experiences, the focus is to provide theoretical statements about the relationships between the concepts (Wuest, 2011). Dahlke et al. (2014) developed a theory of orchestrating care to explain how nurses continuously manage the work environment to provide care for their hospitalized older adult patients. The nurses accomplished this by understanding the status of their patients and of their medical unit, seeking the aid of other caregivers, and stretching the available resources. The subprocess of building synergy explained how nurses gathered and shared information and worked collaboratively to provide good care. Minimizing strain, a second subprocess, described how the nurses minimized strain through efficient use of the limited resources, supporting and guiding their peers, and reframing practices to provide good care.

 Evidence-Informed Practice Tip _____

When you think about the evidence generated by the grounded theory method, consider whether the theory is useful in explaining, interpreting, or predicting the study phenomenon of interest.

 Research Hint _____

In a report of research in which the grounded theory method was used, you can expect to find a diagrammed model of a theory in which the researcher's findings are synthesized in a systematic way.

Ethnographic Method

Ethnographic research has a long history in the qualitative research tradition and is considered by some authorities to be the oldest of the traditions (Patton, 2015). Anthropologists developed the **ethnographic method,** defined as a method of scientifically describing cultural groups. The Greek root *ethnos* means "people" or "a cultural group." Nurses conduct medical ethnographic studies that focus on health and illness within a cultural system (Roper & Shapira, 2000). Although early ethnographic work addressed the cultural patterns of village life, often in distant locations, nurses now often conduct focused ethnographic research, such as the study of distinct problems within a specific context among a small group of people, or the study of a group's social construction and understanding of a health or illness experience (Roper & Shapira, 2000). Leininger (1985) developed an ethnographic research method called *ethnonursing,* which has since been redefined as "a rigourous, systematic, and in-depth method for studying multiple cultures and care factors within familiar environments of people and to focus on the interrelationships of care and culture to arrive at the goal of culturally congruent care services" (Leininger, 2006, p. 20).

Ethnography (ethnographic research) is the study of cognitive models or patterns of behaviour of people within a culture. Ethnographers seek to understand another way of life from the perspective of the people experiencing it. The following values underlie ethnography:

- Culture is fundamental to ethnographic studies. Culture includes behavioural/materialist and cognitive perspectives. Through the **behavioural/materialist perspective,** culture is observed through a group's patterns of behaviour and customs, its way of life, and what it produces. The **cognitive perspective** is the view that culture consists of the beliefs, knowledge, and ideas that people use as they live. **Culture** refers to the structures of meaning through which people shape experiences.
- Understanding culture requires a holistic perspective that captures the breadth of the beliefs, knowledge, and activities of the group being studied.
- **Context**—the personal, social, and political environment in which a phenomenon of interest (time, place, cultural beliefs, values, and

practices) occurs—is important for an understanding of a culture. Understanding this context requires intensive face-to-face contact over an extended period of time. People are studied where they live, in their natural settings, or where an experience occurs, such as in a hospital or community setting.

- The aim of ethnographic research is to combine the **emic perspective** (the insider's view of the world) with the **etic perspective** (the view of the researcher [outsider]) to develop a scientific generalization about different societies. In other words, generalizations are drawn from special examples or details from participant observation.

An example of ethnographic work that has been useful to nurses is the notion of explanatory models. This idea was developed most by cognitive anthropologists, especially Kleinman (1980). Explanatory models use an interactive approach, emphasizing variations between patients' and practitioners' models of illness. They offer explanations of sickness and treatment, guide choices among available therapies and therapists, and give social meaning to the experience of sickness. These cognitive models vary over time and in response to a particular episode of illness.

Several ethnographic schools of thought exist, three of which are of particular interest to nurse researchers: critical, feminist, and ethnogeriatric. Critical ethnography does not entail the use of different methods; instead, it focuses on beliefs and practices that limit human freedom, justice, and democracy (Usher, 1996). Critical ethnographic researchers make their values explicit; in other words, they document tacit rules that govern human interaction and behaviour. They also explore how dominant social groups oppress those in the minority or those without power. For example, Pauly, McCall, Browne, and colleagues (2015) explored how persons who use illicit drugs encounter stigma and discrimination, resulting in barriers when accessing health care services (see Appendix C). Finally, many critical ethnographers consider study participants to be co-investigators and explore problems and possible solutions with them.

Feminist researchers, like critical ethnographers, focus on oppression and power but apply their work to women. They also consider and analyze the effects of race, class, culture, ethnicity, sexual preference, and other identities as forces that cause and sustain oppression (Macquire, 1996). For example, McDonald (2006) recruited 15 gay women from a university in Western Canada and interviewed them to understand the experience of lesbians who disclose their sexual orientation.

Ethnogeriatrics, as the name implies, focuses on examining the "health and aging issues in the context of cultural beliefs, values, and practices among racial and ethnic minority elders" (Fitzpatrick & Wallace, 2006, p. 179). Ethnogeriatric researchers are interested in the disparities facing older adults from racial and ethnic minorities. The hope is to develop nursing knowledge and culturally appropriate interventions to guide health care systems to be more inclusive of this patient population.

Identifying the Phenomenon

The phenomenon under investigation in an ethnographic study varies in scope from a long-term study of a very complex culture, such as that of the Aborigines (Mead, 1949), to a shorter-term study of a phenomenon within subunits of cultures. Kleinman (1992) notes the clinical utility of ethnography in describing the "local world" of groups of patients who are experiencing a particular phenomenon, such as suffering. The local worlds of patients have cultural, political, economical, institutional, and social-relational dimensions in much the same way that larger, complex societies do. Pauly et al.'s (2015) study of nurse and patient perceptions, in a hospital setting, of illicit substance use provides an introduction to ethnography (see Appendix C).

Structuring the Study

RESEARCH QUESTION. When you review a report of ethnographic research, note that questions are asked about lifeways, or particular patterns of behaviour within the social context of a culture or subculture. Culture is viewed as the system of knowledge and linguistic expressions used by social groups that allows the researcher to interpret or make sense of the world of those groups (Aamodt, 1991). Ethnographic nursing studies address questions that concern how cultural knowledge, norms, values, and other contextual variables influence a person's health care experience. Ethnographers have a broader definition of culture, whereby a particular social context is conceptualized as a culture. In Pauly et al.'s (2015) hospital-based study of nurse and patient perceptions of illicit substance use, the medical unit in a large urban inner-city hospital is seen as a culture appropriate for ethnographic study (see Appendix C).

RESEARCHER'S PERSPECTIVE. When a researcher uses the ethnographic method, the researcher's perspective is that of an interpreter entering an alien world and attempting to make sense of that world from the insider's point of view (Agar, 1986). Like phenomenologists and grounded theory researchers, ethnographers make their own beliefs explicit and bracket, or set aside, their personal biases as they interpret the findings and seek to understand the worldview of other people.

SAMPLE SELECTION. The ethnographer selects a cultural group that is experiencing the phenomenon under investigation. The researcher gathers information from general informants and from key informants. Pauly et al.'s (2015) research took place on two medical units in one large inner-city hospital that served a large population of patients who live in poverty and use illicit drugs (see Appendix C).

Data Gathering

Ethnographic data gathering involves participant observation or immersion in the setting, interviews of informants, and interpretation by the researcher of cultural patterns (Crabtree & Miller, 1992). According to Boyle (1991), ethnographic research in nursing, as in other disciplines, involves interviewing in the natural setting as the major data-collection method. Spradley (1979) identified three categories of questions for ethnographic inquiry: descriptive, or broad, open-ended questions; structural, or in-depth, questions that expand and verify the unit of analysis; and contrast questions, which further clarify and provide criteria for exclusion. Fieldwork is also a major focus of the method. The researchers become immersed in the field by spending extensive time with the group under study. They document their observations, keep a diary of the day's events, and record their impressions and any insights in field notes (Merriam & Tisdell, 2016). Other techniques may include obtaining life histories and collecting material items reflective of the culture. Photographs and films of the informants in their world can be used as data sources.

In Pauly et al.'s (2015) study, data were collected from participant observations, from interviews with 34 people (patients and nurses), and from reviewing hospital documents. The fieldwork was completed after approximately 275 hours of participant observation by two of the researchers, whose field notes documented their observations. The policy documents reviewed included the hospital's mission and value statements and the organizational policies about substance use and harm reduction (see Appendix C).

Data Analysis

As with other qualitative methods, data are collected and analyzed simultaneously. Data analysis proceeds through several levels as the researcher looks for the meaning of cultural symbols in the informant's language. Analysis begins with a search for **domains,** or symbolic categories that include smaller categories. Language is analyzed for semantic relationships, and structural questions are formulated to expand and verify data. Analysis proceeds through increasing levels of complexity until the data, grounded in the informant's reality and synthesized by the researcher, lead to hypothetical propositions about the cultural phenomenon under investigation. Pauly et al. (2015) coded the interviews, field notes, and documents. The data were reviewed to identify patterns of interaction, key concepts, and emerging themes. The emerging themes and data were further conceptualized to higher levels. Each researcher read the data independently and then, with the involvement of advisory groups with expertise in the field, the emergent themes were confirmed (see Appendix C).

Describing the Findings

In ethnographic studies, field notes of observations, interview transcriptions, and sometimes other artifacts such as photographs yield large quantities of data. Rich descriptions are the hallmark of ethnographic research. Wolcott (1994) describes the process of description as sharing "What is going on here?" (p. 12). Charmaz (2000) recommends five techniques in her guidelines for ethnographic writing: pulling the reader in, re-creating experiential mood, adding surprising observations, reconstructing ethnographic experience, and creating closure for the study. Evidence provided by complete ethnographies may be published as monographs. When you critique an ethnographic study, be aware that the report of findings usually provides examples from data, thorough descriptions of the analytical process, and statements of the hypothetical propositions and their relationship to the ethnographer's frame of reference.

Pauly et al. (2015) described three different constructs of illicit drug use that highly stigmatized the use of illicit substances, as viewed in the health care setting. These were described as (1) illicit drug use as an individual failing, (2) illicit drug use after a criminal activity, and (3) illicit drug use as a disease of addiction (see Appendix C).

 Evidence-Informed Practice Tip ___

Evidence generated by ethnographic studies answers questions about how cultural knowledge, norms, values, and other contextual variables influence the health experience of a particular patient population in a specific setting.

Qualitative Descriptive Method

Many qualitative researchers use the **qualitative descriptive** method, related to phenomenological, grounded theory, and ethnography, when researchers want to provide a comprehensive summary of the experiences of their participants. As Sandelowski (2000) describes, "Researchers conducting qualitative descriptive studies stay close to their data and to the surface of words and events. . . . Qualitative descriptive study is the method of choice when straight descriptions of phenomena are desired" (p. 334). Qualitative descriptive researchers do not highly abstract the data; the data are presented as they are. However, descriptive research requires validity, with multiple observers accurately documenting the same event. Researchers use a variety of methods when sampling, collecting data, doing analysis, and displaying data. Similar to other types of qualitative research, purposeful sampling is used where the goal is to gather rich data until such time data saturation occurs. Data in qualitative descriptive research are similar to data in other types of qualitative research where the researchers use interviewing (both individual and group), observation, and examination of documents (Lambert & Lambert, 2012). The data analysis is not as prescriptive as in other types of qualitative research; it focuses on content analysis derived from the data themselves and is constantly analyzed as data are collected. The data are presented in a straightforward summary. Qualitative descriptive research is used when researchers desire a straightforward description of a phenomenon (Lambert & Lambert, 2012).

Case Study Method

Case study as a research method involves an in-depth description of the essential dimensions and processes of the phenomenon being studied. Merriam and Tisdell (2016) defined it as "an in-depth description and analysis of a bounded system" (p. 37). This is what differentiates a case study from other qualitative inquiries: The unit of analysis is intrinsically bounded. A limited number of participants can be included. Case study research, rooted in sociology, is described slightly differently by major thinkers who write about this method, such as Yin, Stake, Merriam, and Creswell. For the purpose of introducing this research method, Stake's view is emphasized here. The **case study method** is about studying the peculiarities and commonalities of a specific case over time to provide an in-depth description of the essential dimensions and processes of the phenomenon—familiar ground for practising nurses. Stake (2003) has noted that case study is not a methodological choice but rather a choice of what to study. Case study can include quantitative data, qualitative data, or both, but it is defined by its focus on uncovering an individual case. Stake (2003) distinguishes intrinsic from instrumental case study. **Intrinsic case study** is research undertaken to have a better understanding of the case—nothing more, nothing less. "The researcher at least temporarily subordinates other curiosities so that the stories of those 'living the case' will be teased out" (Stake, 2003, p. 122). In **instrumental case study** the researcher is pursuing insight into an issue or wants to challenge some generalization.

Case studies can be used for a variety of purposes, such as to present data gathered with another method, as a teaching device, or as a research method (Yin, 1994, 2014). Case studies have been used in various disciplines, including nursing, political science, sociology, business, social work, economics, and psychology. Nurses have a long and continuing tradition of using case studies for teaching and learning about patients (e.g., Parsons, 1911). Nightingale (1858/1969) stressed the importance of coming to know patients and of basing practice on experience. She noted that knowing how to provide care requires the nurse to learn about the patient's life. In case studies, these details are described, and the lessons that can be learned from the particular patient are made clear. Persons who have had a particular experience can provide insights that are both valuable and unavailable to those who have not had this experience. Obtaining these descriptions through the use of case studies can serve a variety of functions: It can make practitioners and researchers aware of patients' experiences, clarify the concepts included in an experience or general label, be used in policy decision making, and support theory building by identifying hypotheses for testing with further research (Cohen & Saunders, 1996).

An example of a case study is that by Maddalena, Bernard, Etowa, and colleagues (2010), who examined the experiences and recollections of primary caregivers of African Canadians dying from cancer. The researchers were also interested in the use of complementary and alternative medicine and home remedies at the end of life.

Identifying the Phenomenon

Although some definitions of case study demand that the focus of research be contemporary, Stake's (1995, 2003) defining criterion of attention to the single case broadens the scope of the phenomenon for study. By using a single case, Stake designated a focus on an individual, a family, a community, or an organization—some complex phenomenon that mandates close scrutiny for understanding. In the case study by Maddalena and colleagues (2010), the focus was on the experiences of caregivers of

patients of African Canadian descent who died of cancer. The authors chose three case studies of families of African Canadian descent in Nova Scotia.

Structuring the Study

RESEARCH QUESTION. The research question for a case study is one that provokes the curiosity of the researcher. Stake (2003) has suggested that research questions be developed around issues that serve as a foundation to uncover complexity and pursue understanding. Although researchers pose questions to begin discussion, the initial questions are never all-inclusive. Rather, the researcher uses an iterative process of "growing questions" in the field; that is, as data are collected to address these questions, other questions emerge to guide the researcher in the process of untangling the complex story. Therefore, research questions evolve over time and are re-created in case study research. As an example, initially Maddalena and colleagues (2010) were interested in the experiences and recollections of the caregivers of African Canadian cancer patients at the end of life. Later, they also became interested in the use of complementary and alternative therapies and home remedies used at the end of life.

RESEARCHER'S PERSPECTIVE. When the researcher begins with questions developed around suspected issues of importance, the perspective of the researcher is reflected in the questions; this is sometimes referred to as an *etic perspective*. As the researcher begins engaging the phenomenon of interest, the story unfolds and leads the way, shifting from an etic (researcher-based) to an emic (story-based) perspective (Stake, 2003). The reader may recognize a shift from etic to emic perspective when stories spin off of the original questions posed by the researcher. Maddalena and colleagues (2010), with the exception of the first author, self-identified as African Canadian, which provided, at least initially, a strong etic perspective.

SAMPLE SELECTION. Sample selection is one of the areas of which scholars in the field present differing views, ranging from choosing only the most common cases to choosing only the most unusual cases (Aita & McIlvain, 1999). Stake (2003) advocates selecting cases that may offer the best opportunities for learning. For example, if several heart transplant recipients are available for the researcher to study, practical factors will influence the opinion of which patient offers the best opportunity for learning. It is more practical to study patients who live in the area and can be easily visited at home or in the medical centre than to study someone living in another country. The researcher may want to choose someone who has an actively participating family, because most transplant recipients reside in a family setting. No choice is perfect when a case is selected. There is much to learn about any one individual, situation, or organization during case study research, regardless of the contextual factors influencing the unit of analysis.

Using purposive sampling, Maddalena and colleagues (2010) followed specific inclusion criteria: (1) that the caregivers were African Canadian and (2) that they provided care for someone who had died in the previous 3 years. Three case studies were examined: one rural family, one urban family, and one recently arrived immigrant family. From these families, a total of seven participants—three primary and four secondary caregivers—were identified. The different experiences of the primary and secondary caregivers provided a richer understanding of the experience and validated the findings.

Data Gathering

Data are gathered through the use of interview, observation, document review, and any other methods by which researchers accumulate evidence that enables understanding of the complexity of the case. The researcher will do what is needed to get a sense of the environment and the relationships that provide the context for the case.

Stake (1995) advocates development of a data-gathering plan to guide the progress of the study from definition of the case through decisions regarding reporting. Little explicit information may be provided about data gathering in the report of research.

The primary source of data in Maddalena and colleagues' (2010) study was individual in-depth interviews with the primary caregivers. Secondary caregivers were also interviewed to provide more depth and thus facilitated triangulation. Follow-up interviews were also conducted to seek clarification of issues raised in the first interview.

Data Analysis and Describing Findings

Data analysis is closely tied to data gathering and description of findings as the case study story is generated: "Qualitative case study is characterized by researchers spending extended time, on site, personally in contact with activities and operations of the case, reflecting, revising descriptions and meanings of what is going on" (Stake, 2003, p. 450). Reflecting and revising meanings are the work of the case study researcher, who has recorded data, searched for patterns, linked data from multiple sources, and devised preliminary thoughts regarding the meaning of collected data. This reflective dynamic evolution is the iterative process of creating the case study story that can be thought of as the evidence. As the reader of a case study, you may have difficulty determining how data analysis was conducted because the research report generally does not list research activities. Findings are embedded in (1) a chronological development of the case, (2) the researcher's story of coming to know the case, (3) the descriptions of individual case dimensions, and (4) vignettes that highlight case qualities (Stake, 1995).

In Maddalena and colleagues' (2010) study, the verbatim-transcribed interviews were coded manually individually by four members of the research team. The team met to compare coding and engage in the analysis of the data. Once the team reached consensus, a thematic and discourse analysis was used to further analyze the data. As prevalent themes emerged, each was explored in the context of how culture influenced their experiences during the time from initial diagnosis through interactions with the health system to death and bereavement. With the researchers' etic view of the Black community and culture, the team made sense of the data through the shared historical and cultural experiences of the Black community. Using a discourse analysis approach, the researchers examined each of the themes in terms of their social, political, and historical contexts. The researchers found that the end of life for African Canadians was characterized by end-of-life care provided by family in the home setting, community involvement, a focus on spirituality, and a preference for home care over institutionalized care. In the home setting, the caregivers were faced with a myriad of challenges. Common among the three case studies was the use of complementary and alternative methods and home remedies. In each of the three case studies, the use of prayer was considered a complementary method.

 Evidence-Informed Practice Tip _____

Case studies are a way of providing in-depth, evidence-informed discussion of clinical topics that can be used to guide practice.

Historical Research Method

The **historical research method** is a systematic approach for understanding the past through collection, organization, and critical appraisal of facts. One of the goals in historical methodology is to shed light on the past so that it can guide the present and the future: "Through historical research, we can better understand how nurses in the present can assume control of their practice, education, and roles in the contemporary healthcare system" (Lundy, 2011, p. 383). The attention in nursing to historical methodology was initiated by Teresa E. Christy, who elaborated the method

(Christy, 1975) and the need (Christy, 1981) for historical research long before most nurse scholars accepted it as a legitimate research method. More recently, Lusk (1997) has summarized important information for the nurse interested in understanding historical research. She has provided guidance for choosing a topic, acquiring data, addressing ethical issues, analyzing data, and reporting findings.

When you appraise a study in which the historical method was used, expect to find the research question embedded in the phenomenon to be studied. The question is stated implicitly rather than explicitly.

The three theoretical frameworks that guide historical research are as follows (Streubert & Carpenter, 2011):

1. Biographical history: an exploration of the life of an individual to understand the effects of the time and culture on the person's life
2. Social history: an exploration of the prevailing values and beliefs in a particular period by examining everyday events
3. Intellectual history: an exploration of the ideas of a particular individual or a group of people

An example of biographical history is the book about Gertrude Richard Ladner (i.e., her family and nursing life), in which the authors present new ideas about nursing and family life in the late nineteenth and early twentieth centuries in Western Canada (Zerr, Zilm, & Grant, 2006). Although the authors believed that Ladner represented the ordinary life of women and nurses in that time, they discovered that she was more than a handmaiden for the physicians with whom she worked. Many of the details included in the book were gathered from her personal journal, providing a record of the work of nurses, their day-to-day experiences, and nursing knowledge that informed their practice.

Reeves, Macmillan, and van Soeren (2010) applied a sociohistorical analysis of historical documents to understand how modern health care professions emerged from sixteenth-century craft guilds. Their analysis provides an understanding of how the historical practice of protecting and promoting one's own members of the guild is one of the roots of today's barriers to effective collaboration and interprofessional teamwork.

Data sources provide the sample for historical research. The more clearly a researcher delineates the historical event being studied, the more specifically data sources can be identified. Data may include written or video documents, interviews with persons who witnessed the event, photographs, and other materials that shed light on the subject. Sometimes pivotal information cannot be retrieved and must be eliminated from the list of possible sources. To determine which data sources were used when you review a published study, look at the reference list. Sources of data may be primary or secondary. Primary sources are eyewitness accounts provided by varying sorts of communication appropriate to the time. Secondary sources provide a view of the phenomenon from another person's perspective rather than a first-hand account.

Validity of documents is established by external criticism; reliability is established by internal criticism. In **external criticism,** the authenticity of the data source is judged. The researcher seeks to ensure that the data source is indeed what it seems to be. For instance, if the researcher is reviewing a handwritten letter of Florence Nightingale, some of the validity issues are the following:

- Are the ink, paper, and wax seal on the envelope representative of Nightingale's time?
- Is the wax seal one that Nightingale used in other authentic data sources?
- Is the writing truly Nightingale's?

Only if the data source passes the test of external criticism does the researcher begin internal criticism. **Internal criticism** is the process of judging the reliability or consistency of information within the historical document (Christy, 1975). To judge reliability, the researcher must become familiar with the time in which the data

emerged. A sense of the context and language of the time is essential to understanding a document. The meaning of a word in one era may not be equivalent to the meaning in another era. Knowing the language, customs, and habits of the historical period is critical for judging reliability. The researcher assumes that a primary source provides a more reliable account than does a secondary source (Christy, 1975). The further a source is from an eyewitness account, the more questionable is its reliability. The researcher using historical methods attempts to establish fact, probability, or possibility (Box 8.2).

During the analytical stage, the researcher begins the process of interpretation of meaning. Often working with incomplete records, the historian researcher is reaching beyond the evidence to make inferences. The report usually contains extensive samples of the data, along with evidence of reliability and validity: "A critical description of historical evidence, an evaluation of

---

| BOX **8.2** |

ESTABLISHING FACT, PROBABILITY, AND POSSIBILITY WITH THE HISTORICAL METHOD

FACT

Two independent primary sources that agree with each other
or
One independent primary source that receives critical evaluation and one independent secondary source that is in agreement and receives critical evaluation and no substantive conflicting data

PROBABILITY

One primary source that receives critical evaluation and no substantive conflicting data
or
Two primary sources that disagree about particular points

POSSIBILITY

One primary source that provides information but is not adequate to receive critical evaluation
or
Only secondary or tertiary sources

Adapted from Christy, T. E. (1975). The methodology of historical research: A brief introduction. *Image*, *24*(3), 189–192.

its historical significance to contemporary society, and creative narratives are provided in the written research report, including the derived interferences" (Lundy, 2011, p. 391).

Research Hint

When you critique a study based on the historical method, expect not to find a report of data analysis but simply a description of findings synthesized into a continuous narrative.

Evidence-Informed Practice Tip

The presentation of a historical study should be logical, consistent, and easy to follow.

Participatory Action Research

Based on orientational qualitative inquiry, **participatory action research (PAR)** is a method in which a goal is to change society. According to the tenets of PAR, all forms of knowledge, including indigenous knowledge, are of value and can be applied to practical problems. The researcher studies a particular setting to identify areas in which improvements in practice are needed (Glesne, 2011). After possible solutions are identified, action is taken to implement changes in partnership with the "stakeholders." Careful attention is given to evaluating the process to ensure that the changes have the desired effect. PAR requires careful collaboration with the research participants and focuses on practical problems that are particular to a practice setting or community (Streubert & Carpenter, 2011). Stringer and Genat (2004) define action research as

a systematic, participatory approach to inquiry that enables people to extend their understanding of problems or issues and to formulate actions directed towards the resolution of those problems or issues . . . action research seeks local understandings that are specifically relevant to the particular context of a study. (p. 4)

Community-based participatory research (CBPR) is a method by which the voice of a community is systematically accessed in order to

plan context-appropriate action. According to Holkup, Tripp-Reimer, Salois, et al. (2004), CBPR

provides an alternative to traditional research approaches that assume a phenomenon may be separated from its context for purposes of study. . . . CBPR recognizes the importance of involving members of a study population as active and equal participants, in all phases of the research project, if the research process is to be a means of facilitating change. (p. 162)

Change or action is the intended outcome of CBPR, and *action research* is a term related to CBPR. Some scholars would consider CBPR a sort of action research and would group both action research and CBPR within the tradition of critical science (Fontana, 2004).

Evidence-Informed Practice Tip

Although qualitative in its approach to research, CBPR leads to an action component in which a nursing intervention is implemented and evaluated for its effectiveness in a specific patient population.

In his book *Action Research,* Stringer (1999) distills the research process into three phases: "look," "think," and "act." Stringer defines the "look" as "building the picture" by getting to know stakeholders so that the problem is defined on their terms and the problem definition is reflective of the community context. The "think" phase addresses interpretation and analysis of what was learned in the "look" phase; the researcher is charged with connecting the ideas of the stakeholders so that they provide evidence that is understandable to the community group (Stringer, 1999). Finally, in the "act" phase, Stringer advocates for planning, implementing, and evaluating, on the basis of information collected and interpreted in the other phases of research.

Identifying the Phenomenon

PAR evolved from the work of Lewin (1948), who viewed action research as a means for solving practical social problems and for enacting change for the improvement of communities. PAR is heavily used as a research methodology in education, and in the health professions, PAR methods are used to improve health care services in communities. PAR has been applied to health and wellness programs, program evaluation, care plans, community nursing, and health care delivery and policy. Studies have ranged from issues and conditions stemming from chronic illness, pregnancy and childbirth, pain management, and incontinence to rehabilitation (Stringer & Genat, 2004). For example, MacDonald, Martin-Misener, Steenbeek, et al. (2015) were interested in Mi'kmaq women's experiences with Pap screening (see Appendix A). Their study is used in the following section to illustrate PAR.

Structuring the Study

RESEARCH QUESTION. The first step in structuring the PAR study, as in other qualitative methods, is to frame the research question and to identify who is affected by or has an effect on the problem. Because of the emergent nature of PAR, researchers can begin with a tentative problem and questions and then refine or reframe them as they enter the field. Recall the look–think–act cycle of Stringer (1999) described earlier. In the "look" phase, the researcher explores the problem by "asking who is involved, what is happening, and how, where and when events and activities occur" (p. 36). Reflecting on their observations, researchers, in collaboration with the stakeholders, can fine-tune the final research question, which serves as a guide to the study. As mentioned earlier, MacDonald et al. (2015) explored the experiences of Mi'kmaq women with Pap screening. Utilizing talking circles and individual in-depth interviews with Mi'kmaq women and interviews with health care providers, the researchers explored the historical and social contexts that impacted the women's experiences. The women were considered active participants who provided input into the research process,

including the development of the research questions, participant recruitment, data collection, and analysis.

RESEARCHER'S PERSPECTIVE. When using PAR methods, the researcher is no longer the expert but acts more as a consultant. In their case study of Mi'kmaq women's experiences with Pap screening, MacDonald et al. (2015) used participatory methodology, involving pregnant Indigenous women and parenting Indigenous families. MacDonald et al. upheld the principles of PAR and principles of respectful research with Indigenous people by enabling the community to participate, valuing all participants' viewpoints and experiences, and using collaborative decision making throughout all aspects of the research process, from recruitment to dissemination of findings. In PAR, the participants are co-researchers and are engaged in the research process as it emerges. This involvement requires processes that are democratic, participatory, empowering, and life-enhancing (Stringer & Genat, 2004). PAR investigators, like ethnographers, immerse themselves in the field for deep understanding and to build trust and credibility. For example, MacDonald et al. (2015) frequented the health centre and attended community events.

SAMPLE SELECTION. Because it is not possible to include everyone who may have a "stake" or interest in the research question, researchers purposively select a sample of participants who represent varied perspectives, experiences, and backgrounds. Participants may be people who have the widest range of differences in their experiences, particularly interesting backgrounds or experiences; those who are typical; and those with particular knowledge of the phenomenon under study. For example, MacDonald et al. (2015) worked with community facilitators who assisted in recruitment of the participants, utilizing purposive and snowball sampling. The initial talking-circle participants recruited by the community facilitators were purposefully selected Indigenous women of diverse ages, socioeconomic backgrounds, education, and Pap screening experiences. The purpose of the talking circle was to facilitate collaboration with the community and to co-design the study. This group recruited a few other women to the study. The 16 women who were eventually recruited for the more in-depth interviews had to fit certain criteria, such as identify as Indigenous Mi'kmaq, be between 21 and 75 years of age, and have had a least one Pap screening (see Appendix A).

Data Gathering

In the "look" phase, data are gathered from a variety of sources; interviews are the principal means for understanding the experiences of the participants. PAR also includes observation in the field, gathering and reviewing of relevant documents, and the examination of relevant materials and equipment. A literature review may add information to enhance the understanding of the data emerging from the interviews and other sources. MacDonald et al. (2015) interviewed the 16 women to hear their stories about their beliefs, attitudes, and experiences related to Pap screening. All but one woman participated in a second interview in which they reviewed the initial analysis of the first interviews to provide feedback on the data interpretation, preliminary findings, and emerging themes. This is a hallmark of CPBR: the participants are involved in all steps of the research process (see Appendix A).

Data Analysis

In the "think" phase, the researchers think about and reflect on all of the data gathered. The purpose of data analysis is to distill and reduce the volume of information into a manageable and organized set of concepts or ideas. The process in PAR must directly capture the experiences of the participants and be distilled in such a way "that it makes sense to them all" (Stringer & Genat, 2004).

Stringer and Genat (2004) have identified two approaches to analysis. The first, based on

"epiphanic moments" (Denzin, 1998), focuses on the significant experiences as the primary units of analysis, giving voice to the participants' experiences. A second process involves the categorization and coding of data to reveal patterns and themes. Regardless of the process used, PAR allows the participants to make sense of their experience and then to use the new understanding to make a positive change.

In MacDonald et al.'s (2015) study, the participants read and validated the initial interview and provided input on the analysis. The researchers then changed some of their initial coding and themes based on the participant and community facilitator feedback. Critical to this process was the opportunity for the participants to ensure that the names of the themes and subthemes were appropriately titled from an Indigenous perspective and accurately reflected their experiences (see Appendix A).

Describing the Findings

In accordance with Stringer's (1999) look–think–act framework, the next step is to present the outcomes to the participants and other nonparticipant stakeholders so that they understand what is happening. Several dissemination mechanisms may be used because formal academic writing is not accessible for most lay participants. The results may be shared in written reports, oral presentations, or performances. Written narrative accounts and storytelling are often used to describe the findings. The next, and most important, step is to apply the findings to solve the research problem or issue that instigated the study. This action portion of PAR parallels the nursing process of identification of goals and objectives, intervention, and, finally, evaluation. The action plans should include the following (Stringer & Genat, 2004):

Why: A statement of the overall purpose
What: A set of objectives to be obtained
How: A sequence of tasks and steps for each objective

Who: The people responsible for each task and activity

Where: The place where the tasks will be done

When: The time for initiation and completion

The researcher should also arrange for ongoing evaluation of the process. As with the exploratory phase, stakeholders are intimately involved in each step of the action plan, from identifying the plan to implementing it. The participants in MacDonald et al.'s (2015) study identified five themes and subthemes and presented them in a diagram (see Appendix A) and in excerpts from the data. They found that, despite challenging circumstances, many women still accessed Pap screening. They stated that providers of health care for Indigenous people need to appreciate the impact of historical trauma and interpersonal violence and to individualize Pap screening policies, as the best practice guideline does not always apply to Indigenous people (see Appendix A).

QUALITATIVE APPROACH: NURSING METHODOLOGY

The qualitative methodologies elaborated throughout this chapter are derived from other disciplines, such as sociology, anthropology, and philosophy. In the discipline of nursing, these methodologies are used to conduct research. However, as the discipline matures, methodology based on nursing ontology (belief system) has emerged. Madeleine Leininger (1996), Rosemarie Rizzo Parse (1997), and Margaret Newman (1997) are nurse theorists who have created research methods specific to their theories. In Table 8.1, the methodologies of these theorists are compared. Each method was developed over years and tested by other researchers. Each researcher has attempted to advance nursing knowledge through inquiry that is congruent with the specific nursing theory.

In this section of the chapter, we have explored several different traditions and methods of qualitative research; however, many researchers are now combining a number of related or different methods to frame their naturalistic study. Remember that qualitative inquiry is evolving and changing. As Glesne (2011) has noted, "The open, emergent nature of qualitative inquiry means a lack of standardization; there are no clear criteria to package into neat research steps" (p. 25). As you read more qualitative research studies, you will note many interesting designs, all amenable

TABLE **8.1**

NURSING RESEARCH METHODOLOGIES

ASPECT	LEININGER (1996)	PARSE (1997)	NEWMAN (1997)
Theory	Culture care	Human becoming	Health as expanding consciousness
Research methodology	Ethnonursing is centred on learning from people about their beliefs, experiences, and culture care information.	Parse's research methodology is the study of universal health experiences through true presence both with participants sharing life stories and with transcribed data to uncover meaning.	Newman's method focuses on pattern recognition and uses multiple interviews, involving collaboration, to arrive at recognized life patterns.
Research example	Use of culture care theory with Anglo-American and African American older adults in a long-term care setting (McFarland, 1997)	The lived experience of serenity: using Parse's research method (Kruse, 1999)	Pattern of expanding consciousness in women in creative movement and narrative as modes of expression (Picard, 2000)

to exploring the complexity of the human experience. MacDonald et al. (2015), in their study on Mi'kmaq women's experiences with Pap screening, combined a CBPR study using postcolonial feminist perspectives and Indigenous principles. Ford-Gilboe, Wuest, and Merritt-Gray (2005) applied a feminist perspective to their grounded theory on the basic social processes of health promotion among lone-parent families recovering from intimate family violence.

In summary, the term *qualitative research* is an overriding description of multiple methods with distinct origins and procedures. In spite of distinctions, each method shares a common nature that guides data collection from the perspective of the participants to create a story that synthesizes disparate pieces of data into a comprehensible whole that provides evidence and promises direction for building nursing knowledge.

APPRAISING THE EVIDENCE

Qualitative Research

Although general criteria for critiquing qualitative research are proposed in the following Critiquing Criteria box, each qualitative method has unique characteristics that influence what you may expect in the published research report, and journals often have page restrictions that penalize qualitative researchers because it can be difficult to fully explain all of the steps discussed in Chapter 4 in a few pages. The criteria for critiquing are formatted to evaluate the selection of the phenomenon, the structure of the study, data gathering, data analysis, and description of the findings. Each question of the criteria focuses on factors discussed throughout the chapter. Appraising qualitative research is a useful activity for learning the nuances of this research approach. You are encouraged to identify a qualitative study of interest and apply the criteria for critiquing. Keep in mind that qualitative methods are the best way to start answering clinical and research questions that previously have not been addressed in research studies or that do not lend themselves to a quantitative approach. The answers provided by qualitative data reflect important evidence that may provide the first insights into a patient population or clinical phenomenon.

CRITIQUING CRITERIA

Qualitative Approaches

IDENTIFYING THE PHENOMENON

1. Is the phenomenon focused on human experience within a natural setting?
2. Is the phenomenon relevant to nursing, health, or both?

STRUCTURING THE STUDY
Research Question

3. Does the question specify a distinct process to be studied?
4. Does the question identify the context (participant group/place) of the process that will be studied?
5. Does the choice of a specific qualitative method fit with the research question?

Researcher's Perspective

6. Are the biases of the researchers reported?
7. Do the researchers provide a structure of ideas that reflect their beliefs?

Sample Selection

8. Is it clear that the selected sample is experiencing the phenomenon of interest?

DATA GATHERING

9. Are data sources and methods for gathering data specified?
10. Is there evidence that participant consent is an integral part of the data-gathering process?

DATA ANALYSIS

11. Can the dimensions of data analysis be identified and logically followed?

12. Is the participant's reality clearly described?
13. Is there evidence that the researcher's interpretation captured the participant's meaning?
14. Have other professionals confirmed the researcher's interpretation?

DESCRIBING THE FINDINGS

15. Are examples provided to guide the reader from the raw data to the researcher's synthesis?
16. Does the researcher link the findings to existing theory or literature, or is a new theory generated?

CRITICAL THINKING CHALLENGES

- How does the researcher select a specific type of qualitative research method to answer the research question?
- Do findings from qualitative research studies need to be validated in subsequent studies?
- How can a nurse researcher select a qualitative research method when he or she is attempting to accumulate evidence regarding a new topic about which little is known?
- How can the case study approach to research be applied to evidence-informed practice?

KEY POINTS

- Qualitative research is the investigation of human experiences in naturalistic settings, pursuing meanings that inform theory, practice, instrument development, and further research.
- Qualitative research studies are guided by research questions.
- Data saturation occurs when the information being shared with the researcher becomes repetitive.
- Qualitative research methods include five basic elements: identifying the phenomenon, structuring the study, gathering the data, analyzing the data, and describing the findings.
- The phenomenological method is a process of learning and constructing the meaning of human experience through intensive dialogue with persons who are living the experience.
- The grounded theory method is an inductive approach that implements a systematic set of procedures to arrive at theory about basic social processes.
- The ethnographic method focuses on scientific descriptions of cultural groups.
- The case study method focuses on a selected phenomenon over a short or long time to provide an in-depth description of its essential dimensions and processes.

- The historical research method is the systematic compilation of data and the critical presentation, appraisal, and interpretation of facts regarding people, events, and occurrences of the past.
- CBPR is a method that systematically accesses the voice of a community to plan context-appropriate action.

FOR FURTHER STUDY

e Go to Evolve at http://evolve.elsevier.com/Canada/LoBiondo/Research for the Audio Glossary and Appendix Tables that provide supplemental information for Appendix E.

REFERENCES

Aamodt, A. A. (1991). Ethnography and epistemology: Generating nursing knowledge. In J. M. Morse (Ed.), *Qualitative nursing research: A contemporary dialogue* (pp. 29–40). Newbury Park, CA: Sage.

Agar, M. H. (1986). *Speaking of ethnography*. Beverly Hills, CA: Sage.

Aita, V. A., & McIlvain, H. E. (1999). An armchair adventure in case study research. In B. Crabtree & W. L. Miller (Eds.), *Doing qualitative research* (2nd ed., pp. 253–268). Thousand Oaks, CA: Sage.

Boyle, J. S. (1991). Field research: A collaborative model for practice and research. In J. M. Morse (Ed.), *Qualitative nursing research: A contemporary dialogue*. Newbury Park, CA: Sage.

Browne, A. J. (2000). The potential contribution of critical social theory to nursing science. *Canadian Journal of Nursing Research, 32*(2), 35–55.

Charmaz, K. (2000). Grounded theory: Objectivist and constructivist methods. In N. K. Denzin & Y. S. Lincoln (Eds.), *Handbook of qualitative research* (2nd ed., pp. 509–535). Thousand Oaks, CA: Sage.

Charmaz, K. (2014). *Constructing grounded theory: A practical guide through qualitative analysis* (2nd ed.). Thousand Oaks, CA: Sage.

Christy, T. E. (1975). The methodology of historical research: A brief introduction. *Nursing Research, 24*(3), 189–192.

Christy, T. E. (1981). The need for historical research in nursing. *Research in Nursing & Health, 4*(2), 227–228.

Cohen, M. Z. (1987). A historical overview of the phenomenological movement. *Image, 19*(1), 31–34.

Cohen, M. Z., & Saunders, J. (1996). Using qualitative research in advanced practice. *Advanced Practice Nursing Quarterly, 2*(3), 8–13.

Colaizzi, P. (1978). Psychological research as a phenomenologist views it. In R. S. Valle & M. King (Eds.), *Existential phenomenological alternatives for psychology* (pp. 48–71). New York: Oxford University Press.

Corbin, J., & Strauss, A. (2008). *Basics of qualitative research.* Los Angeles: Sage.

Crabtree, B. F., & Miller, W. L. (1992). *Doing qualitative research.* Newbury Park, CA: Sage.

Dahlke, S. A., Phinney, A., Hall, W. A., et al. (2014). Orchestrating care: Nursing practice with hospitalised older adults. *International Journal of Older People Nursing, 10,* 252–262.

Denzin, N. K. (1998). The practices and politics of interpretation. In N. K. Denzin & Y. S. Lincoln (Eds.), *Collecting and interpreting qualitative materials* (pp. 458–498). Thousand Oaks, CA: Sage.

Denzin, N. K., & Lincoln, Y. S. (1998). *The landscape of qualitative research.* Thousand Oaks, CA: Sage.

Duffy, M. (2011). Narrative inquiry: The method. In P. Munhall (Ed.), *Nursing research: A qualitative perspective* (5th ed., pp. 421–440). Mississauga, ON: Jones & Bartlett Learning.

Fitzpatrick, J. J., & Wallace, M. (Eds.), (2006). *Encyclopedia of nursing research* (2nd ed.). New York: Springer.

Fontana, J. S. (2004). A methodology for critical science in nursing. *Advances in Nursing Science, 27,* 93–101.

Ford-Gilboe, M., Wuest, J., & Merritt-Gray, M. (2005). Strengthening capacity to limit intrusion: Theorizing family health promotion in the aftermath of woman abuse. *Qualitative Health Research, 15,* 477–601.

Giorgi, A., Fischer, C. L., & Murray, E. L. (Eds.), (1975). *Duquesne studies in phenomenological psychology.* Pittsburgh: Duquesne University Press.

Glaser, B., & Strauss, A. (1965). *Awareness of dying.* Chicago: Aldine de Gruyter.

Glaser, B. G., & Strauss, A. L. (1967). *The discovery of grounded theory: Strategies for qualitative research.* Chicago: Aldine.

Glesne, C. (2011). *Becoming qualitative researchers: An introduction* (4th ed.). Toronto: Pearson.

Hammond, C., Holmes, D. & Mercier, M. (2016). Breeding new forms of life: A critical reflection on extreme variances of bareback sex. *Nursing Inquiry, 23*(3), 267–277.

Holkup, P. A., Tripp-Reimer, T., Salois, et al. (2004). Community-based participatory research: An approach to intervention research with a Native American community. *Advances in Nursing Science, 27,* 162–175.

Holmes, D., O'Byrne, P., & Gastaldo, D. (2006). Raw pleasure as limit experience: A Foucauldian analysis of unsafe anal sex between men. *Social Theory and Health, 4,* 319–333.

Holmes, D., O'Byrne, P., & Gastaldo, D. (2007). Setting the space for sex: Architecture, desire and health issues in gay bathhouses. *International Journal of Nursing Studies, 44*(2), 273–284.

Kleinman, A. (1980). *Patients and healers in the context of culture.* Berkeley, CA: University of California Press.

Kleinman, A. (1992). Local worlds of suffering: An interpersonal focus for ethnographies of illness experience. *Qualitative Health Research, 2,* 127–134.

Kruse, B. G. (1999). The lived experience of serenity: Using Parse's research method. *Nursing Science Quarterly, 12,* 143–150.

Lambert, V. A., & Lambert, C. E. (2012). Qualitative descriptive research: An acceptable design. *Pacific Rim International Journal of Nursing Research, 16*(4), 255–256.

Lapum, J., Angus, J. E., Peter, E., et al. (2010). Patients' narrative accounts of open-heart surgery and recovery: Authorial voice of technology. *Social Science & Medicine, 70,* 754–762.

Leininger, M. (1985). Life-health-care history: Purposes, methods and techniques. In M. M. Leininger (Ed.), *Qualitative research methods in nursing* (pp. 119–132). New York: Grune & Stratton.

Leininger, M. M. (1996). Culture care theory. *Nursing Science Quarterly, 9,* 71–78.

Leininger, M. M. (2006). *Culture care, diversity and universality: A worldwide nursing theory* (2nd ed.). Mississauga, ON: Jones & Bartlett.

Lewin, K. (1948). *Resolving social conflicts.* New York: Harper.

Lundy, K. S. (2011). Historical research. In P. Munhall (Ed.), *Nursing research: A qualitative perspective* (5th ed., pp. 381–397). Mississauga, ON: Jones & Bartlett Learning.

Lusk, B. (1997). Historical methodology for nursing research. *Image, 29,* 355–359.

MacDonald, C., Martin-Misener, R., Steenbeek, A., et al. (2015). Honouring stories: Mi'kmaq women's experiences with Pap screening in Eastern Canada. *Canadian Journal of Nursing Research, 47*(1), 72–96.

Macquire, P. (1996). Considering more feminine participatory research: What's congruency got to do with it? *Qualitative Inquiry, 2,* 106–118.

Maddalena, V. J., Bernard, W. T., Etowa, J., et al. (2010). Cancer care experiences and the use of complementary and alternative medicine at the end of life in Nova Scotia's Black communities. *Journal of Transcultural Nursing, 21*(2), 114–122.

McDonald, C. (2006). Lesbian disclosure: Disrupting the taken for granted. *Canadian Journal of Nursing Research, 38,* 42–57.

McFarland, M. R. (1997). Use of culture care theory with Anglo and African American elders in long-term care settings. *Nursing Science Quarterly, 10,* 186–192.

Mead, M. (1949). *Coming of age in Samoa.* New York: New American Library/Mentor Books. (Original work published 1928)

Merriam, S. B., & Tisdell, E. J. (2016). *Qualitative research: A guide to design and implementation.* San Francisco: Jossey-Bass.

Newman, M. A. (1997). Evolution of the theory of health as expanding consciousness. *Nursing Science Quarterly, 10,* 22–25.

Nightingale, F. (1969). *Notes on nursing: What it is and what it is not.* New York: Dover. (Original work published 1858)

Parse, R. R. (1997). Transforming research and practice with the human becoming theory. *Nursing Science Quarterly, 10,* 171–174.

Parsons, S. (1911). The case method of teaching nursing. *American Journal of Nursing, 11,* 1009–1011.

Patton, M. (2002). *Qualitative research & evaluation methods* (3rd ed.). Thousand Oaks, CA: Sage.

Patton, M. (2015). *Qualitative research & evaluation methods* (4th ed.). Thousand Oaks, CA: Sage.

Pauly, B., McCall, J., Browne, A. J., et al. (2015). Toward cultural safety: Nurse and patient perceptions of illicit substance use in a hospitalized setting. *Advances in Nursing Science, 38*(2), 121–135.

Picard, C. (2000). Patterns of expanding consciousness in midlife women: Creative movement and narrative as modes of expression. *Nursing Science Quarterly, 13,* 150–157.

Pooler, C. (2014). Living with chronic lower pulmonary disease: Disruptions of the embodied phenomenological self. *Global Qualitative Nursing Research,* 1–11.

Racine, L. (2011). The impact of race, gender, and class in a postcolonial feminist fieldwork: A retrospective critique of methodological dilemmas. *Apopria, 3*(1), 15–27.

Reeves, S., Macmillan, K., & van Soeren, M. (2010). Leadership of interprofessional health and social care teams: A socio-historical analysis. *Journal of Nursing Management, 18,* 258–264.

Roper, J., & Shapira, J. (2000). *Ethnography in nursing research.* Thousand Oaks, CA: Sage.

Sandelowski, M. (2000). What ever happened to qualitative description? *Research in Nursing and Health, 23,* 334–340.

Smith, D., Edwards, N., Varcoe, C., et al. (2006). Bringing safety and responsiveness into the forefront of care for pregnant and parenting Aboriginal people. *Advances in Nursing Science, 29*(2), E27–E44.

Spiegelberg, H. (1976). *The phenomenological movement* (Vols. I–II). The Hague: Martinus Nijhoff.

Spradley, J. P. (1979). *The ethnographic interview.* New York: Holt, Rinehart, & Winston.

Stake, R. E. (1995). *The art of case study research.* Thousand Oaks, CA: Sage.

Stake, R. E. (2003). Case studies. In N. K. Denzin & Y. S. Lincoln (Eds.), *Strategies of qualitative inquiry* (2nd ed., pp. 134–164). Thousand Oaks, CA: Sage.

Strauss, A. L. (1987). *Qualitative analysis for social scientists.* New York: Cambridge University Press.

Strauss, A., & Corbin, J. (1990). *Basics of qualitative research: Grounded theory procedures and techniques.* Newbury Park, CA: Sage.

Streubert, H. J., & Carpenter, D. R. (2011). *Qualitative research in nursing: Advancing the humanistic imperative* (5th ed.). Philadelphia: Wolters Kluwer.

Stringer, E. T. (1999). *Action research* (2nd ed.). Thousand Oaks, CA: Sage.

Stringer, E. T., & Genat, W. J. (2004). *Action research in health.* Thousand Oaks, CA: Sage.

Usher, P. (1996). Feminist approaches to research. In D. Scott & R. Usher (Eds.), *Understanding educational research* (pp. 120–143). New York: Routledge.

van Kaam, A. (1969). *Existential foundations in psychology.* New York: Doubleday.

van Manen, M. (1997). *Researching lived experience: Human science for an action sensitive pedagogy* (2nd ed.). London, ON: Althouse Press.

Wolcott, H. F. (1994). *Transforming qualitative data: description, analysis and interpretation.* Thousand Oaks, CA: Sage.

Wuest, J. (2011). Grounded theory: The method. In P. Munhall (Ed.), *Nursing research: A qualitative perspective* (5th ed., pp. 225–256). Mississauga, ON: Jones & Bartlett Learning.

Yin, R. (1994). *Case study research: Design and methods* (2nd ed.). Thousand Oaks, CA: Sage.

Yin, R. (2014). *Case study research: Design and methods* (5th ed.). Thousand Oaks, CA: Sage.

Zerr, S. J., Zilm, G., & Grant, V. (2006). *Labor of love. A memoir of Gertrude Richards Ladner, 1879 to 1976.* Delta, BC: ZGZ.

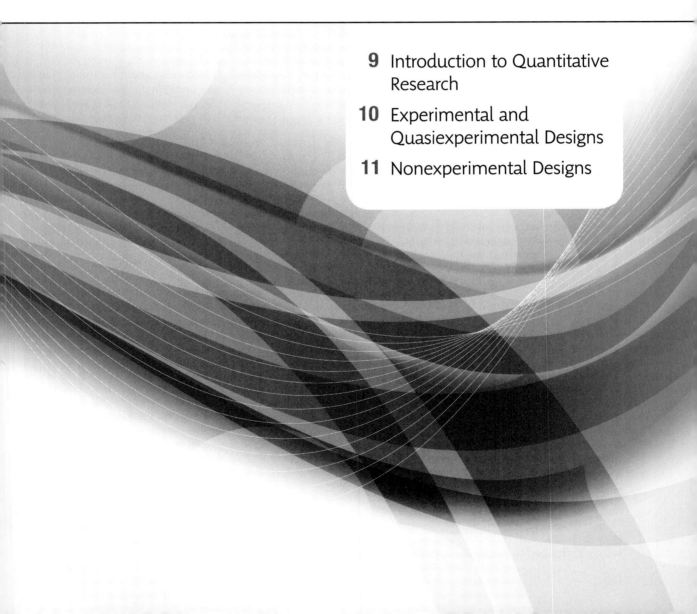

PART THREE

Quantitative Research

RESEARCH **VIGNETTE**

Tackling the Prevention of Falls among Older Adults

Nancy C. Edwards, RN, BScN, MSc, PhD
Full Professor
School of Nursing
University of Ottawa
Ottawa, Ontario

In the late 1980s, while working as a clinical nurse consultant at the Ottawa Public Health Department, I was asked to assist with a needs assessment of older adults living in low-income apartment buildings in Ottawa. The survey covered a wide range of topics, and at the last minute, the public health nurses decided to add a few questions about older adults' experiences with falls. The findings were startling: they revealed a high incidence of falls and injuries. Published epidemiological studies indicated that our findings were not spurious. Indeed, one-third of all older adults fall annually, and approximately 25% of falls result in some sort of injury.

Soon after this survey was conducted, our then medical officer of health, Dr. Steve Corber, spoke to me about the possibility of setting up and evaluating a fall prevention initiative. Dr. Corber suggested that preventing falls should become a program focus within the health department. I was working with a senior nursing manager, Maureen Murphy, at the time, and we were interested in a more theoretical question: the relative contribution of self-care versus collective action initiatives to promote health. However, we decided to meld these two interests, and a randomized controlled trial was born!

With funding from the Ontario Ministry of Health and Long-Term Care, we compared the effect of fall prevention clinics and a community action strategy on the incidence of falls among older adults living in 48 apartment buildings. I worked closely with the fall prevention team as we piloted and implemented the two interventions. Although we did not detect a change in the rate of falls, we did note improvements in some behavioural outcomes for fall prevention among older adults in the community action buildings in comparison with the control buildings.

Many important issues surfaced during this trial and became the basis for a program of research. We became interested in the role of the built environment in falls. In some of our study buildings, older adults who had difficulties getting into and out of the bathtub described their failed efforts to persuade landlords to have grab bars installed. Landlords were refusing them permission because the installation of grab bars was thought to "lower property values." In essence, aesthetics trumped safety.

Several qualitative and quantitative studies ensued. Older adults described the embarrassment of using grab bars and other assistive devices. A survey of older adults in apartment buildings with and without universally installed grab bars identified barriers to accessing grab bars. A comparison of low-income and public apartment buildings with private apartment buildings indicated that older adults living in low-income buildings were much more likely to have access to grab bars than were older adults living in private buildings.

Concerns about bathroom grab bars and safe stairs became a focus for our regional fall prevention coalition. We began to consider what research was necessary to inform changes to building code recommendations in Canada. It became apparent that, to complement our community-based studies, we needed the expertise of researchers who were able to design and conduct laboratory studies to determine what grab bar configurations are optimal to assist transfers into and out of a bathtub.

From both the laboratory and the community studies, we were able to identify the configuration of grab bars that older adults find easiest to use. We determined that older adults are 2.8 times more likely to use universally installed grab bars consistently, in comparison with grab bars they had installed themselves, after other factors were adjusted. We also documented both the high proportion of falls in bathrooms and on stairs and the high rates of injury that result from these falls, in comparison with falls occurring in other locations.

In a subsequent community study funded by the Canadian Institutes of Health Research, we identified stair hazards prevalent in private homes and in public buildings. Older adults were asked to identify the most common locations of hazardous stairs. Churches and community centres were among the locations most frequently identified. Independent raters also assessed indoor and outdoor stairs, both those identified by older adults as hazardous in the community and the stairs that the raters used in their own homes or apartment buildings. The most common hazards were the lack of contrast marking on the edge of the stairs, inadequate tread length, risers that were too high, and nonuniform risers. Although older adults were able to identify hazardous stairs they had difficulty navigating, fewer than 25% of them had specific suggestions for ways to improve stair safety.

Our research findings on bathroom and stair falls are now being used to inform policy change. For example, I submitted a request to the National Research Council for an additional requirement to the building codes for the universal installation of grab bars in showers and bathtubs in all residential homes. Included with the submission was an estimate of the costs of such a requirement and the cost savings that would be incurred. These estimates are an important consideration for committee members who review code change requests. I have also been a member of several National Research Council task groups and subgroups reviewing potential code changes for stairs, handrails, ramps, and guards. This has provided me with important insights about how research evidence and other inputs influence the code change process. Our research on stair falls is being reviewed as part of the evidence for changes to the building codes in the current cycle of building code changes.

Bridging the interface between research and policy is a critical knowledge translation strategy. Informing and influencing policy change requires the engagement of an informed public. We've used various outreach strategies, including "fireside chats" on fall prevention via CHNET-Works (http://www.chnet-works.ca), a series of resolutions presented to nongovernmental organizations (e.g., Canadian Public Health Association) calling for evidence-informed changes to building codes that pertain to bathtub grab bars and safe stairs, the production of videos and other resources on fall prevention for health care providers and the lay public, and letters to the editor in response to newspaper articles about housing renovations. Our work on preventing falls has reinforced the importance of interdisciplinary research in the design of community health interventions. Substantial health care changes in populations such as older adults will come about only through long-term research and policy change efforts. "Quick fixes" are rare. As a researcher, I need to be prepared to work actively with colleagues at the local, provincial, and national levels and to use a wide repertoire of knowledge translation strategies. ∎

CHAPTER 9

Introduction to Quantitative Research

Geri LoBiondo-Wood | Mina D. Singh

LEARNING OUTCOMES

After reading this chapter, you will be able to do the following:

- Define research design.
- Identify the purpose of the research design.
- Define control as it affects the research design.
- Compare and contrast the elements that affect control.
- Begin to evaluate the degree of control that should be exercised in the design.
- Define internal validity.
- Identify the threats to internal validity.
- Define external validity.
- Identify the conditions that affect external validity.
- Identify the links between study design and evidence-informed practice.
- Evaluate the design by using the critiquing questions.

KEY TERMS

accuracy	feasibility	objectivity
attrition	Hawthorne effect	pilot study
bias	history threat	randomization
constancy	homogeneity	reactivity
control	instrumentation threats	selection bias
control group	internal validity	selection effects
experimental group	maturation	testing effect
external validity	measurement effects	
extraneous variable	mortality	

STUDY RESOURCES

ⓔ Go to Evolve at http://evolve.elsevier.com/Canada/LoBiondo/Research for the Audio Glossary and Appendix Tables that provide supplemental information for Appendix E.

THE WORD *DESIGN* IMPLIES THE ORGANIZATION of elements into a masterful work of art. In the world of art and fashion, the word conjures up images of processes and techniques that are used to express a total concept. When an individual creates something, process and form are employed. The form, process, and degree of adherence to structure depend on the aims of the creator.

The same can be said of the research process. The research process does not need to be a sterile procedure, but it should be one in which the researcher develops a masterful work within the limits of a problem and the related theoretical basis. The framework that the researcher creates is the design. When reading a study, the research consumer should be able to recognize that the research problem, purpose, literature review, theoretical framework, and hypothesis all interrelate with, complement, and assist in the operationalization of the design (Figure 9.1). The degree to which a fit exists between these design elements determines the strength of the study and of the consumer's confidence in the evidence provided

by the findings and their potential applicability to practice.

Nursing practice is concerned with a variety of activities that require varying degrees of process and form, such as the provision of quality care, cost-effective patient care, responses of patients to disease, and factors that affect caregivers. When nurses administer patient care, they draw on the nursing process. Previous chapters stressed the importance of theory and knowledge of subject matter to research. How a researcher structures, implements, or designs a study affects the results of a research project.

To grasp the implications and the use of research, you need to understand the central issues in the design of a research project. This chapter provides an overview of the meaning, purpose, and issues related to quantitative research design. Chapters 10 and 11 discuss specific types of quantitative designs.

PURPOSE OF THE RESEARCH DESIGN

The purpose of the research design is to provide the plan for answering research questions. These questions can result in research driven by a researcher's curiosity or interest in a theoretical question. This process is called *basic research,* and its motivation is to expand nursing knowledge. In contrast, *applied research* is designed to solve clinical problems rather than to acquire knowledge for knowledge's sake; thus, the goal is to improve the patient's health care condition.

The design in quantitative research then becomes the vehicle for hypothesis testing or answering research questions, whether they are basic or applied. The design involves a *plan,* a *structure,* and a *strategy.* These three design concepts guide a researcher in writing the hypothesis or research questions, conducting the project, and analyzing and evaluating the data. The overall purpose of the research design is twofold: to aid in the solution of research problems and to maintain control (see Practical

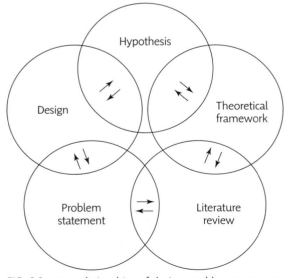

FIG. 9.1 Interrelationships of design, problem statement, literature review, theoretical framework, and hypothesis.

Practical Application

A research example that demonstrates how the design can aid in answering a research question and maintain control is the study by Maheu, Meschino, Hu, and colleagues (2015). The main purpose of their study was to test the feasibility and preliminary effects of a psycho-educational telephone (PET) intervention to reduce distress in women who receive uninformative BRCA 1/2 results. To maintain control, the researchers had strict sample characteristics. Inclusion criteria were as follows: (1) a breast cancer (BC) diagnosis; (2) a significant family history of BC; (3) a scheduled appointment to receive their test result; and (4) ability to understand and read English. Exclusion criteria were as follows: women who had an identified BRCA 1/2 mutation in the family at the study's beginning or received notice of one during the course of the study. By establishing the specific sample criteria and participant eligibility, the researchers were able to maintain control over the study's conditions and suggest an extension of the study's outcome with further research.

Application box). All research is an attempt to answer questions. The design, coupled with the methods and analysis, is the mechanism for finding solutions to research questions. **Control** is defined as the measures that the researcher uses to hold the conditions of the study uniform and avoid possible impingement of **bias** (distortion of the results) on the dependent variable or outcome.

Various considerations, including the type of design, affect the accomplishment of the study. These considerations include **objectivity**—the use of facts without distortion by personal feelings or bias—in the conceptualization of the problem; accuracy; feasibility; control of the experiment; internal validity; and external validity. Statistical principles underlie the many forms of control, but it is more important that the research consumer have a clear conceptual understanding of statistics and how they inform the research questions.

The type of design used in a study also affects its application to practice. Chapters 10 and 11 present a number of experimental, quasiexperimental, and nonexperimental designs. The type of design used in a study is linked to the level of evidence, and, in turn, the contribution of a study's findings is linked to evidence-informed practice. As discussed in Chapter 1, the term *evidence-informed practice* is currently being used instead of *evidence-based practice* because it is more inclusive in that it encompasses many forms of evidence, such as clinical experience and judgement with research utilization. As you critically appraise the design, take into account other aspects of a study's design, which are reviewed in this chapter.

OBJECTIVITY IN THE CONCEPTUALIZATION OF THE PROBLEM

In the conceptualization of the problem, objectivity is derived from a review of the literature and development of a theoretical framework (see Figure 9.1). Using the literature, the researcher assesses the depth and breadth of available knowledge about the problem. The literature review and theoretical framework should show that the researcher reviewed the literature critically and objectively (see Chapters 2 and 5), because this conceptualization of the problem affects the type of design chosen. For example, for a question about the relationship of the length of a breastfeeding education program, either an experimental or a correlational design may be recommended (see Chapters 10 and 11), whereas for a question regarding the physical changes in a woman's body during pregnancy and the maternal perception of the unborn child, a survey or correlation study may be advised (see Chapter 11). The literature review should reflect the following:

- When the problem was studied
- The aspects of the problem that were studied
- Where the problem was investigated
- By whom the problem was investigated
- The gaps or inconsistencies in the literature

Research Hint_____

A review that incorporates the aspects presented here allows the research consumer to judge the objectivity of the problem area and therefore whether the design chosen is suitable for investigating the problem.

ACCURACY

Accuracy in determining the appropriate design is also accomplished through the theoretical framework and review of the literature (see Chapters 2 and 5). **Accuracy** means that all aspects of a study systematically and logically follow from the research problem. The beginning researcher is wise to answer a question involving few variables that does not require the use of sophisticated designs. The simplicity of a research project does not render it useless or of a lesser value for practice. Although the project is simple, the researcher should not forgo accuracy. The research consumer should believe that the researcher chose a design that was consistent with the research problem and offered the maximum amount of control.

Many clinical problems have not yet been researched, so a preliminary, or pilot, study is a wise approach to testing the accuracy of a study design before a larger study is undertaken. A **pilot study** is a small, simple study conducted as a prelude to a larger study. The key is the accuracy, validity, and objectivity used by the researcher in attempting to answer the question. Accordingly, you should read various types of research reports and assess whether and how the criteria for each step of the research process were followed. Many nursing journals publish not only sophisticated clinical research projects but also smaller clinical studies whose results can be applied to practice.

FEASIBILITY

When you, as a consumer of research, critique the study design, you must also be aware of the pragmatic consideration of feasibility. **Feasibility** is the capability of the study to be successfully carried out. Sometimes, the reality of feasibility does not truly sink in until the researcher begins the study. When you review a study, you should consider feasibility, including availability of the participants, timing of the research, time required for the participants to take part in the study, costs, and analysis of the data (Table 9.1). Studies in which researchers are testing feasibility are also called *pilot studies* (see Practical Application box).

An example of a feasibility study is one conducted by Vahabi and Damba (2015). They examined the feasibility of a culturally and gender-specific dance program to promote physical activity for South Asian immigrant women in the Greater Toronto Area. Specifically, the researchers implemented a 6-week Bollywood dance fitness program for South Asian women. The results indicated that it was "feasible and acceptable" to implement the program, given the study's high participation rate and participants' overall satisfaction with the program.

Before a large experimental study (such as a randomized clinical trial) is conducted, it is helpful to first conduct a pilot study with a small number of participants to determine the feasibility of participant recruitment, the intervention, the data-collection protocol, the likelihood that

---

Practical Application ▬▬▬

Baumbusch, Dahlke, and Phinney (2014) conducted a pilot study to compare the knowledge and perceptions of nurse educators and clinical instructors in nursing care of older adults, as a first step toward developing strategies to support clinical instructors' professional development in this area of practice. The results showed that, although clinical instructors had foundational knowledge about older adults, they had significantly less specialized knowledge about nursing care of older adults than nurse educators, thus development in this area was supported.

TABLE **9.1**

PRAGMATIC CONSIDERATIONS IN DETERMINING THE FEASIBILITY OF A RESEARCH PROBLEM

FACTOR	PRAGMATIC CONSIDERATION
Time	The research problem must be able to be studied within a realistic period of time. All researchers have deadlines for completion of a project. The scope of the problem must be circumscribed enough to provide ample time for the completion of the entire project. Research studies generally take longer than anticipated to complete.
Participant availability	The researcher must determine whether a sufficient number of eligible participants will be available and willing to take part in the study. If a researcher has a "captive" audience (e.g., students in a class-room), it may be relatively easy to enlist their cooperation. When a study involves the participants' independent time and effort, they may be unwilling to participate when they will receive no apparent reward for doing so. Other potential participants may have fears about harm or confidentiality and be suspicious of the research process in general. Participants with unusual characteristics, such as rare diseases, are often difficult to locate. People are generally cooperative about taking part in a study, but a researcher must consider needing a larger participant pool than will actually participate. At times, when reading a research report, the researcher may note how the procedures were liberalized or the number of participants was altered—probably as a result of some unforeseen pragmatic consideration.
Facility and equipment availability	All research projects require some kind of equipment, such as questionnaires, telephones, stationery, stamps, technical equipment, or another apparatus. Most research projects also require the availability of a facility for the work, such as a hospital site for data collection, a laboratory space, or a computer centre for data analysis.
Money	Many research projects require some expenditure of money. Before embarking on a study, the researcher probably itemized the expenses and estimated the total cost of the project. This estimation of cost provides a clear picture of the budgetary needs for items such as books, stationery, postage, printing, technical equipment, telephone and computer charges, and salaries. These expenses can range from about $200 for a small-scale student project to hundreds of thousands of dollars for a large-scale federally funded project.
Researcher experience	The selection of the research problem should be based on the nurse's experience and interest. It is much easier to develop a research study related to a topic that is either theoretically or experientially familiar. Selecting a problem that is of interest to the researcher is essential for maintaining enthusiasm when the inevitable successes and failures occur.
Ethics	Research problems that place unethical demands on participants are not feasible for study. Researchers must take ethical considerations seriously. The consideration of ethics may affect the choice of the design and the methodology.

participants will complete the study, the reliability and validity of new measurement tools, and the costs of the study. These pragmatic considerations are not presented as a step in the research process, as are the theoretical framework and methods, but they do affect every step of the process and therefore should be considered when you assess a study. For example, the student researcher may or may not have funding or accessible services. When you critique a study,

note the credentials of the author or authors and whether the investigation was part of either a student project or a fully funded grant project. If the project was a student project, the standards of critiquing are applied more liberally than for projects conducted by an experienced researcher or clinician with a doctoral degree. Finally, the pragmatic issues raised affect the scope and breadth of an investigation and, therefore, its generalizability.

CONTROL

When developing a study, a researcher attempts to use a design to maximize the degree of control over the tested variables. Control involves holding the conditions of the study constant and establishing specific sampling criteria, as described by McQueen, Montelpare, and Dennis (2013) in their study of validating a Breastfeeding Self-Efficacy Scale among Indigenous women, in which the inclusion criteria were breastfeeding Indigenous women, the ability to read and speak English, and telephone accessibility for follow-up. Women were excluded from the study if breastfeeding could be precluded by infant prematurity or illness or if there were multiple births or maternal complications.

An efficient design can maximize results, decrease errors, and control pre-existing conditions that may affect outcome. To accomplish these tasks, the research design and methods should demonstrate the researcher's efforts at control. For example, to validate the Breastfeeding Self-Efficacy Scale–Short Form and to test their hypotheses and apply control, McQueen and colleagues (2013) determined that a sample size of 102 at 8-week follow-up was adequate for analysis, as the minimum required for psychometric testing of an instrument is 70 (5 participants for each of the 14 items).

When research designs are critiqued, the issue of control is always raised but with varying levels of flexibility. The issues discussed here will become clearer as you review the various types of designs.

Control is accomplished by ruling out extraneous variables that compete with the independent variables as an explanation for a study's outcome. An **extraneous variable** (also called a *mediating variable*) interferes with the operations of the phenomena being studied (e.g., age and gender). Means of controlling extraneous variables include the following:

- Use of a homogeneous sample
- Use of consistent data-collection procedures

- Manipulation of the independent variable
- Randomization

An investigator might be interested in how a new smoking cessation program (independent variable) affects smoking behaviour (dependent variable). The independent variable is assumed to affect the outcome, or dependent variable. An investigator needs to be relatively sure that the decrease in smoking is truly related to the smoking cessation program rather than to another variable, such as motivation.

The following example illustrates and defines these concepts further. El-Masri, Fox-Wasylyshyn, Springer, and associates (2014) compared the effects of three types of radiation treatment on prostate cancer. To rule out the effects of extraneous variables on function, bother, and well-being (dependent variable) among men with prostate cancer, demographic information was collected, including age, marital status, living arrangements, history of cancer, stage of cancer, and mode of cancer detection. Although the design of the research study alone does not inherently provide control, an appropriately designed study with the necessary controls can increase an investigator's ability to answer a research question.

 Evidence-Informed Practice Tip _____

As you read a report, assess whether the study includes a tested intervention and whether the report contains a clear description of the intervention and how it was controlled. If the details are not clear, the intervention may have been administered differently among the participants, which would affect the interpretation of the results.

Homogeneous Sampling

In the example of smoking cessation, extraneous variables may affect the dependent variable. The characteristics of a study's participants are common extraneous variables. Age, gender, length of time smoked, amount smoked, and even smoking rules may affect the outcome in the smoking cessation example, even though they are extraneous or outside the study's design. As a control for these and other similar problems, the researcher's participants should demonstrate **homogeneity,** or similarity with regard to the extraneous variables relevant to the particular study (see Chapter 12). Extraneous variables are not fixed but must be reviewed, and their inclusion in the analyses is based on the study's purpose and theoretical base. By using a sample of homogeneous participants, the researcher has used a straightforward step of control.

For example, McInnis-Perry, Weeks, and Stryhn (2013) explored the emotional and informational social support needs of community-dwelling Canadians aged 65 and older in Atlantic provinces. They ensured the homogeneity of the sample by using the following sampling criteria: Participants were aged 65 years or older, and they lived in Prince Edward Island, New Brunswick, Newfoundland, Labrador, or Nova Scotia. The sample was therefore homogeneous with regard to age, language, and location of home. This control step limits the generalizability or application of the outcomes to other populations when the outcomes are analyzed and discussed (see Chapter 17). The results can then be generalized only to a similar population of individuals. Homogeneity could be considered limiting, but not necessarily, because no treatment or program is applicable to all populations, and educated consumers of research must take into consideration the differences in populations.

 Research Hint

When reviewing studies, remember that it is better to have a "clean" study, whose results can be used to make generalizations about a specific population, than a "messy" study, whose results may be poorly or not at all generalizable.

If the researcher believes that one of the extraneous variables is important, it may be included in the design. In the smoking cessation example, if individuals are working in an area where smoking is not allowed and this condition is considered to be important to the study, the researcher could account for it in the design and set up a control condition for it. This condition can be established by comparing two different work areas: one where smoking is allowed and one where it is not. Of importance is that before the data are collected, the researcher should have identified, planned for, and controlled the important extraneous variables.

Constancy in Data Collection

Another basic but critical component of control is constancy in data-collection procedures. **Constancy** refers to the ability of the data-collection design to hold the conditions of the study to a cookbook-like recipe. In other words, for the purpose of collecting data for the study, each participant is exposed to the same environmental conditions, timing of data collection, data-collection instruments, and data-collection procedures (see Chapter 13).

An example of constancy in data collection is illustrated in the study by Carriere, Carriere, Ayas, and associates (2014). The objective of this study was to determine barriers to achieving a time-to-target temperature goal in post–cardiac arrest patients treated with mild therapeutic hypothermia. Two researchers systematically and comprehensively reviewed all study charts, once a month for 6 months, with guidance from recommendations from a literature review. At the end of the 6 months, a random chart audit was completed by an investigator to check for interrater reliability. This type of control aided the investigators' ability to draw conclusions, discuss the findings, and cite the need for further research in this area. For the consumer, constancy demonstrates a clear, consistent, and specific means of data collection.

Thomas, Elliott, Rao, and colleagues (2012) explored the effects of motivational interviewing–based coaching on cancer pain management. Data were collected from each subject in the same manner and under the same conditions by trained data collectors. This type of control helped the investigators' ability to draw conclusions, discuss limitations, and cite the need for further research. It also demonstrates a clear, consistent, and specific means of data collection. When interventions are implemented, researchers will often describe the training and supervision of interventionists and/or data collectors that took place to ensure constancy. All study designs should demonstrate constancy (fidelity) of data collection, but studies that test an intervention require the highest level of intervention fidelity.

Manipulation of the Independent Variable

A third means of control is manipulation of the independent variable. *Manipulation* refers to the administration of a program, treatment, or intervention to only one group within the study but not to the other participants in the study. The first group is known as the **experimental group,** and the other group is known as the **control group,** or comparison group. In a control group, the variables under study are held at a constant or comparison level. For example, Weinert, Cudney, Comstock, and colleagues (2014) examined whether a computer intervention would increase self-efficacy in chronic illness self-management skills and improve quality of life. The experimental group received the computer intervention, the control group did not.

Experimental and quasiexperimental designs involve manipulation, whereas in nonexperimental designs, the independent variable is not manipulated. This lack of manipulation does not decrease the usefulness of a nonexperimental design. The use of a control group in an experimental or quasiexperimental design is related to the research question and, again, its theoretical framework.

Blinding is a technique used in experimental and quasiexperimental research in which the participants are not aware of whether they are receiving the intervention. *Double blinding* is a technique in which both the researchers and the participants are not aware of who is receiving the intervention and who is in the control group. For example, Kundu, Lin, Oron, and colleagues (2014) conducted a single-site, double-blind, randomized controlled study investigating the effects of Reiki therapy on postoperative pain management in children. Postoperatively, the participants' pain scores were recorded both by a blinded observer and by their assigned nurse, who was also blinded to group assignment in the control or experimental group.

 Research Hint _____

Be aware that the lack of manipulation of the independent variable does not mean that the study is weaker. The level of the problem, the amount of theoretical work, and the research that has preceded the project affect the researcher's choice of the design. If the problem is amenable to a design in which the independent variable can be manipulated, the power of a researcher to draw conclusions will increase, provided that all of the considerations of control are equally addressed.

Randomization

Researchers may also choose other forms of control, such as randomization. **Randomization** is a sampling selection procedure in which each participant in a population has an equal chance of being assigned to either the experimental group or the control group. Randomization eliminates bias, aids in the attainment of a representative sample, and can be used in various designs. Weinert and colleagues (2014) had 309 participants in their study. Each of these participants were randomly assigned to either the control or experimental group. Randomization can also be accomplished with paper-and-pencil-type instruments. By randomly ordering items on the instruments, the investigator can assess whether a difference in responses is correlated with the order of the items. Randomization may be especially important in longitudinal studies, in which bias from giving the same instrument to the same participants on a number of occasions can be a problem (see Chapter 12).

QUANTITATIVE CONTROL AND FLEXIBILITY

The same level of control cannot be exercised in all types of designs. At times, when a researcher wants to explore an area in which little or no literature on the concept exists, the researcher will probably use an exploratory design. In this type of study, the researcher is interested in describing or categorizing a phenomenon in a group of individuals. Koopman, LeBlanc, Fowler, and colleagues (2016) used an exploratory design to investigate the relationship between hope, coping, and quality of life in adults with myasthenia gravis, as this had not been studied before. They concluded that nurses should use interventions to continue to support hope, quality of life, and coping in this group of individuals. In critiquing this type of study, the issue of control should be applied in a highly flexible manner because of the preliminary nature of the work.

If from a review of a study you determine that the researcher intended to conduct a correlational study (an examination of the relationship between or among the variables), then the issue of control takes on more importance. Control must be exercised as strictly as possible. At this intermediate level of design, it should be clear to the reviewer that the researcher considered the extraneous variables that may affect the outcomes.

All aspects of control are strictly applied to studies that use an experimental design. The reader should be able to locate in the research report how the researcher met these criteria: whether the conditions of the research were constant throughout the study, the assignment of participants was random, and experimental and control groups were used. Because of the control exercised in the study, the reader can determine

that all issues related to control were considered and the extraneous variables were addressed.

 Evidence-Informed Practice Tip _____

Remember that establishing evidence for practice is determined by assessing the validity of each step of the study, assessing whether the evidence assists in planning patient care, and assessing whether patients respond to the evidence-informed care.

INTERNAL AND EXTERNAL VALIDITY

Consumers of research must believe that the results of a study are valid, based on precision, and faithful to what the researcher wanted to measure. To form the basis of further research, practice, and theory development, a study must be credible and dependable. The two important criteria for evaluating the credibility and dependability of the results are internal validity and external validity. Threats to validity are listed in Box 9.1, and a discussion of each threat follows.

Internal Validity

Internal validity is the degree to which the experimental treatment, not an uncontrolled condition, resulted in the observed effects. To establish

---

BOX **9.1**

THREATS TO VALIDITY

INTERNAL VALIDITY
History threats
Maturation effects
Testing effects
Instrumentation threats
Mortality (attrition)
Selection bias

EXTERNAL VALIDITY
Selection effects
Reactive effects
Measurement effects

internal validity, the researcher rules out other factors or threats as rival explanations of the relationship between the variables. Threats to internal validity may be numerous and are considered by researchers in planning a study and by consumers before implementing the results in practice (Campbell & Stanley, 1996). Research consumers should note that the threats to internal validity are most clearly applicable to experimental designs, but attention to factors that can compromise outcomes should be considered to some degree in all quantitative designs. If these threats are not considered, they could negate the results of the research by affecting the design. Threats to internal validity include history threats, maturation effects, testing effects, instrumentation threats,

mortality **(attrition),** and selection bias. Table 9.2 provides examples of these threats.

History Threats

Not only the independent variable but also another specific event may affect the dependent variable, either inside or outside the experimental setting. This threat to internal validity is referred to as the **history threat.** For example, in a study on the effects of a breastfeeding education program on the length of time of breastfeeding, government-sponsored breastfeeding promotions on television and in newspapers could affect the length of time of breastfeeding and would be considered a threat of history (see Table 9.2).

TABLE **9.2**

EXAMPLES OF INTERNAL VALIDITY THREATS	
THREAT	**EXAMPLE**
History threat	A study tested a teaching intervention in one hospital and compared outcomes to those of another hospital in which usual care was given. During the final months of data collection, the control hospital implemented a heart failure critical pathway; as a result, data from the control hospital (cohort) was not included in the analysis.
Maturation effect	Breitenstein, Gross, Fogg, et al. (2012) evaluated the 1-year efficacy outcomes of a parenting program to promote parenting competency. Although the program had significant positive outcomes in parental self-efficacy, the authors noted that the children's maturation may have accounted for observed behaviour problems in the children.
Testing effect	A researcher wishes to measure acute pain with a repeated-measures design during a lengthy procedure. The researcher must consider the results in view of the possible bias of repeating the pain measurements over a short period of time. The measurements may prime the patients' responses, and the practice of reporting pain repeatedly on the same instrument during a procedure may influence the results. El-Masri et al. (2014) explored the impact of prostrate cancer radiation treatment on functions, bother, and well-being. They obtained patient responses through self-report, which the researchers noted to be a possible limitation.
Instrumentation threat	Li, Powers, Melnyk, et al. (2012) discussed issues that possibly affected instrumentation, such as the reliance on chart reviews, family caregiver self-reports, perceptions of patient status as data-collection strategies, and spacing of data-collection time points.
Mortality (attrition)	Thomas and colleagues (2012) noted that they had participant losses in all three of their groups and that the lack of statistical significance in their findings may have been related to an inadequate sample size, even though the intervention had a positive outcome.
Selection bias	Newman, Doran, and Nagle (2014) controlled for selection bias by establishing selection criteria in their study on critical care nurses' information-seeking behaviour, in Ontario. They indicated that there may be sample bias, as the sample consisted of nurses who consented during the annual renewal process and may not reflect all Ontario critical care nurses.

Maturation Effects

Maturation refers to the developmental, biological, or psychological processes that operate within an individual as a function of time; these processes are external to the events of the investigation. For example, suppose that a researcher wished to evaluate the effect of a specific teaching method on the achievements of baccalaureate students on a skills test. The investigator would record the students' abilities before and after the teaching method. Between the pretest and the posttest, the students would have grown older and wiser. The growth or change is unrelated to the investigation, and the differences between the two testing periods may be explained by such maturation rather than by the experimental treatment.

Maturation effects could also occur in a study of the relationship between two methods of teaching about children's knowledge of self-care measures. Posttests of student learning must be conducted relatively soon after the teaching sessions are completed. Such a short interval allows the investigator to conclude that the results were the outcome of the design of the study and not maturation in a population of children who are learning new skills rapidly. Maturation is more than change that results from an age-related developmental process; maturation can also be related to physical changes (see Table 9.2).

Testing Effects

Taking the same test repeatedly could influence participants' responses the next time the test is completed. For example, the effect on the participant's posttest score as the result of having taken a pretest is known as a **testing effect.** The effect of taking a pretest may sensitize an individual and improve the score on the posttest. Individuals generally score higher when they take a test a second time, regardless of the treatment. The differences between posttest and pretest scores may be a result not of the independent variable but rather of the experience gained through the testing. For example, in one study the same case study was used as pretest and posttest to explore an educational tool for registered nurses learning to provide nursing care for acutely ill patients (Gillespie & Shackell, 2014). Whether the significant increase in knowledge of oxygen supply and demand, cellular oxygen, and priority interventions resulted from the teaching and learning strategies or was the effect of taking the test more than once was difficult to determine. Table 9.2 provides another example of a testing effect.

Instrumentation Threats

Instrumentation threats are changes in the variables or observational techniques that may account for changes in the obtained measurement. For example, a researcher may wish to study various types of thermometers (e.g., tympanic, digital, electronic, chemical indicator, plastic strip, and mercury) to compare the accuracy of the mercury thermometer with the other temperature-taking methods. To prevent instrumentation threats, the researcher must check the calibration of the thermometers according to the manufacturer's specifications before and after data collection.

Another example concerns techniques of observation or data collection. If a researcher has several raters collecting observational data, they all must be trained in a similar manner. If they are not similarly trained, or even if they are similarly trained but unable to conduct the study as planned, a lack of consistency may occur in their ratings; therefore, a threat to internal validity will occur.

To avoid instrumentation threats in an evaluation of the effectiveness of evidence-informed strategies to limit interruptions during medication administration times in three cardiac care units, observation was carried out by the study's staff members (Flynn, Evanish, Fernald, et al., 2016). In an effort to further minimize instrumentation threat, a prior study (interrater reliability) was conducted to establish agreement among trained data collectors. This study resulted in 96% agreement among the collectors. (For another example, see Table 9.2.) Although the researcher can take steps to prevent problems of instrumentation, the threat of instrumentation may still occur. When a research critiquer finds such a threat, it must be evaluated within the total context of the study.

Mortality/Attrition

Mortality or attrition is the loss of study participants from the first data-collection point (pretest) to the second data-collection point (posttest). If the participants who remain in the study are not similar to those who dropped out, the results could be affected. The loss of participants may be from the sample as a whole, or, in a study that has both an experimental group and a control group, more of the participants may drop out from one group than from the other group; this effect is known as *differential loss of participants*. For example, in a study of the ways in which a media campaign affects the incidence of breastfeeding, if most dropouts were non-breastfeeding women, the perception given could be that exposure to the media campaign increased the number of breastfeeding women, whereas the effect of experimental attrition led to the observed results. See Table 9.2 for an example of a study in which mortality (attrition) may have influenced the results.

Selection Bias

If precautions are not used to gain a representative sample, **selection bias**—the threat to internal validity that arises when pretreatment differences exist between the experimental group and the control group—could result from the way the participants were chosen. Selection effects are a problem in studies in which the individuals themselves decide whether to participate in a study. Suppose an investigator wishes to assess whether a new smoking cessation program contributes to smoking cessation. If the new program is offered to all smokers, chances are that only individuals who are more motivated to stop smoking will take part in the program. Assessment of the

effectiveness of the program is problematic because the investigator cannot know for certain whether the new program encouraged smoking cessation behaviours or whether only highly motivated individuals joined the program. To avoid selection bias, the researcher could randomly assign participants to either the new teaching method group or a control group that receives a different type of instruction. Table 9.2 provides another example of selection bias.

 Research Hint

The list of threats to internal validity is not exhaustive. More than one threat can be found in a study, depending on the type of study design. Finding a threat to internal validity in a study does not invalidate the results and is usually acknowledged by the investigator in the "Results" or "Discussion" section of the study.

 Evidence-Informed Practice Tip

Avoiding threats to internal validity in clinical research can be difficult. However, this reality does not render studies that have threats useless. It is important to take the threats into consideration and weigh the total evidence of a study for not only its statistical meaningfulness but also its clinical meaningfulness.

External Validity

External validity concerns the generalizability of an investigation's findings to additional populations and to other environmental conditions. To achieve external validity, variation in the conditions and the types of participants should lead to the same results. The goal of the researcher is to select a design that maximizes both internal and external validity, although attaining this goal is not always possible. If it is not possible, the researcher must attain the minimum criterion of external validity.

The factors that may affect external validity are related to the selection of participants, study conditions, and type of observations. These factors are termed *selection effects, reactive effects,*

CRITICAL THINKING DECISION PATH

Potential Threats to a Study's Validity

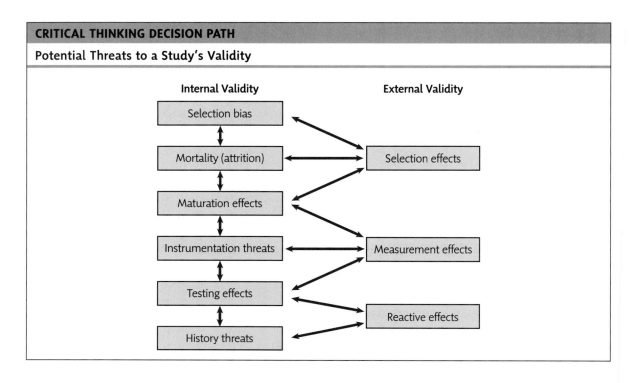

and *testing effects*. You may notice the similarity in the names of the factors of selection and testing and those of the threats to internal validity. When considering factors as internal threats, the reader assesses them as they relate to the *independent* and *dependent* variables within the study; when assessing them as external threats, the reader considers them in terms of the generalizability, or use outside the study with other populations and settings.

The Critical Thinking Decision Path displays the ways in which threats to internal and external validity can interact. This path is not, however, exhaustive with regard to the type of threats and their interaction. In comparison with problems of internal validity, generalizability issues are typically more difficult to deal with because they mean that the researcher is assuming that other populations are similar to the one being tested.

Selection Effects

Selection concerns the generalizability of the results to other populations. An example of **selection effects** is when the researcher cannot attain the ideal sample population. At times, the number of available participants may be low, or they may not be accessible to the researcher. The researcher may then need to choose a nonprobability method of sampling, not a probability method. Therefore, the type of sampling method used and how participants are assigned to research conditions will affect the generalizability of findings to other groups, or the external validity. In the following quotations, the authors have noted selection effects:

- "The study was limited from a sample size perspective ($n = 31$), even though all NPs [nurse practitioners] in the jurisdiction were invited to participate." (Borycki, Sangster-Gormley, Schreiber, et al., 2014, p. 62)

- "The small numbers of participants working with specific age groups did not allow for meaningful between-group analysis." (Creamer, Mill, Austin, et al., 2014, p. 28)
- "Although our sample size was drawn from a broad geographic pool, the 47 managers who participated may not reflect the views of all managers in more than 400 intensive care units in Canada)." (Edwards, McMillan, & Fallis, 2013, p. 34)
- "The findings in this study must be considered with the limitations of sample size . . . obtaining a larger sample from other sites that perform TAVI [transcatheter aortic valve implantation] would have provided a more representative sample of the population." (Forman, Currie, Lauck, et al., 2015, p. 566)

These remarks are cautionary, but they also point out the usefulness of the findings for practice and for future research aimed at building the data in these areas.

Reactive Effects

Reactivity is defined as the participants' responses to being studied. Participants may behave in a certain way with the investigator not because of the study procedures but merely as an independent response to being studied. This response is also known as the **Hawthorne effect,** named after Western Electric Corporation's Hawthorne plant, where a study of working conditions was conducted in the 1930s. The researchers developed several different working conditions, such as turning up the lights, piping in music loudly or softly, and changing work hours. They found that no matter what was done, the workers' productivity increased. They concluded that production increased as a result of the workers' knowing that they were being studied rather than because of the experimental conditions.

For example, in a randomized controlled study, Bennett, Lyons, Winters-Stone, and colleagues (2007) tested the effect of telephone-based motivational interviewing on increasing physical activity and improving physical fitness, thus improving health self-efficacy in adults living in rural areas. The researchers noted that the physical activity counsellors knew to which group (control or experimental) the participants were assigned, which may have allowed the control group to become aware of components of the experimental treatment. The researchers also noted that each participant also participated in a 6-minute walk test in which a strict protocol was used, but it was also possible that conversation before the test might have influenced performance rate. The researchers made recommendations about how to avoid such threats in future studies.

Measurement Effects

Administration of a pretest in a study affects the generalizability of the findings to other populations; the resulting changes are known as **measurement effects.** Just as pretesting affects the posttest results within a study, pretesting affects the posttest results and generalizability outside the study. For example, suppose a researcher wants to conduct a study with the aim of changing attitudes toward acquired immune deficiency syndrome (AIDS). To accomplish this task, an education program on the risk factors for AIDS is incorporated. To test whether the education program changes attitudes toward AIDS, tests are given before and after the teaching intervention. The pretest on attitudes allows the participants to examine their attitudes regarding AIDS. The participants' responses on follow-up testing may differ from those of individuals who were given the education program and did not see the pretest. Therefore, when a study is conducted and a pretest is given, it may prime the participants and affect their subsequent answers, which in turn can affect the generalizability of the findings.

Research Hint_____

When you review a study, be aware of the internal and external threats to validity. These threats do not render a study useless; instead, they make it more useful to you. Recognition of the threats allows researchers to build on data and allows consumers to think through what part of the study can be applied to practice. Specific threats to validity depend on the type of design and generalizations that the researcher hopes to make.

Other threats to external validity depend on the type of design and methods of sampling used by the researcher but are beyond the scope of this text. Campbell and Stanley (1996) offered detailed coverage of the issues related to internal and external validity.

APPRAISING THE EVIDENCE

Quantitative Research

Critiquing the design of a study requires knowledge of the overall implications of a particular design for the study as a whole (see Critiquing Criteria box). Researchers want to consider the level of evidence provided by the design and how the study can be used to improve or change practice. Minimizing threats to internal and external validity enhances the strength of evidence for any quantitative design. The concept of the research design is all-inclusive and parallels the concept of the theoretical framework. The research design is similar to the theoretical framework in that it deals with a piece of the research study that affects the whole. This chapter has introduced the meaning, purpose, and important factors of design choice, as well as the vocabulary that accompanies these factors. Several criteria for evaluating the design can be drawn from this chapter. Remember that the criteria are applied differently with various designs. Differences in application do not mean that the research consumer will find a haphazard approach to design but rather that each design has particular criteria that allow the consumer to classify the design by type (e.g., experimental or nonexperimental). These criteria must be met and addressed in conducting an experiment. The particulars of specific designs are addressed in Chapters 10 and 11. The following discussion primarily pertains to the overall evaluation of a quantitative research design.

The research outcome should demonstrate that an objective review of the literature and the establishment of a theoretical framework guided the choice of the design. No explicit statement regarding these areas is made in a research article. A consumer can evaluate the design by critiquing the theoretical framework (see Chapter 2)

and literature review (see Chapter 5). Is the question new and not extensively researched? Has a great deal of research been conducted on the question, or is the question a new or different way of looking at an old question? Depending on the level of the question, the investigators make certain choices. These choices enable researchers to look for differences in a controlled, comparative manner.

The research consumer should be alert for the methods that investigators use to maintain control (e.g., homogeneity in the sample, consistent data-collection procedures, manipulation of the independent variable, and randomization). As discussed in Chapter 10, all of these criteria must be met for an experimental design. As you begin to understand the types of designs (i.e., experimental, quasiexperimental, and nonexperimental designs, such as survey and relationship designs), you will find that control is applied in varying degrees or—as in the case of a survey study—the independent variable is not manipulated (see Chapter 11). The level of control and its applications presented in Chapters 10 and 11 provide the remaining knowledge for fully critiquing the aspects of a study's design.

Once you have established whether the necessary control or uniformity of conditions has been maintained, you must determine whether the study is believable or valid. You should ask whether the findings are the result of the variables tested—and thus internally valid—or whether another explanation is possible. To assess this aspect, you should review the threats to internal validity. If the investigator's study was systematic, was well grounded in theory, and followed the criteria for each of

APPRAISING THE EVIDENCE—cont'd

Quantitative Research

the processes, you will probably conclude that the study is internally valid.

In addition, you must know whether a study has external validity or generalizability to other populations or environmental conditions. External validity can be claimed only after internal validity has been established. If the credibility of a study (internal validity) has not been established, a study has no generalizability to other populations (external validity). Determination of external validity is related directly to the sampling method (see Chapter 12). If the study is not representative of any one group or phenomenon of interest, external validity may

be limited or not present. The establishment of internal and external validity requires not only knowledge of the threats to internal and external validity but also knowledge of the phenomena being studied, which allows critical judgements to be made about the linkage of theories and variables for testing. You should find that the design follows from the theoretical framework, literature review, research question, and hypotheses. You should believe, on the basis of clinical knowledge and knowledge of the research process, that the investigators are not, as the expression goes, comparing apples with oranges.

CRITIQUING CRITERIA

1. Is the type of study design employed appropriate?
2. Does the researcher use the various concepts of control that are consistent with the type of design chosen?
3. Does the design seem to reflect feasibility?
4. Does the design flow from the proposed research question, theoretical framework, literature review, and hypothesis?
5. What are the threats to internal validity?
6. What are the controls for the threats to internal validity?
7. What are the threats to external validity?
8. What are the controls for the threats to external validity?
9. Is the design appropriately linked to the levels of evidence hierarchy?

CRITICAL THINKING CHALLENGES

- Consider the following statement: "All research attempts to solve problems." How would you support or refute this statement?
- As a consumer of research, you recognize that control is an important concept in the issue of research design. You are critiquing an assigned experimental study as part of your "open-book" midterm examination. From what is written, you cannot determine how the researchers kept the conditions of the study constant. How does this characteristic affect the study's use in an evidence-informed practice model?
- Box 9.1 lists six major threats to the internal validity of an experimental study. Prioritize them, and defend the one that you deem the essential, or number one, threat to address in a study.
- You are critiquing the research design of an assigned study as a consumer of research. How

does the research design influence the findings of evidence in the study?
- How do threats to external validity contribute to the strength and quality of evidence provided by the findings of a research study?

KEY POINTS

- The purpose of the design is to provide the format of masterful and accurate research.
- Many types of designs exist. No matter which type of design the researcher uses, the purpose remains the same.
- The research consumer should be able to locate within the study a sense of the question that the researcher wished to answer. The question should be proposed with a plan or scheme for the accomplishment of the investigation.

Depending on the question, the consumer should be able to recognize the steps taken by the investigator to ensure control.

- The choice of the specific design depends on the nature of the question. To specify the nature of the research question, the design must reflect the investigator's attempts to maintain objectivity, accuracy, pragmatic considerations, and, most important, control.
- Control affects not only the outcome of a study but also its future use. The design should also reflect how the investigator attempted to control threats to both internal and external validity.
- Internal validity must be established before external validity can be established. Both are considered within the sampling structure.
- No matter which design the researcher chooses, it should be evident to the reader that the choice was based on a thorough examination of the research question within a theoretical framework.
- The design, research question, literature review, theoretical framework, and hypothesis should all be interrelated.
- The choice of the design is affected by pragmatic issues. At times, two different designs may be equally valid for the same question.
- The choice of design affects the study's level of evidence.

FOR FURTHER STUDY

ⓔ Go to Evolve at http://evolve.elsevier.com/Canada/LoBiondo/Research for the Audio Glossary and Appendix Tables that provide supplemental information for Appendix E.

REFERENCES

Baumbusch, J., Dahlke, S., & Phinney, A. (2014). Clinical instructors' knowledge and perceptions about nursing care of older people. *Nursing Education in Practice*, *14*, 434–440.

Bennett, J. A., Lyons, K. S., Winters-Stone, K., et al. (2007). Motivational interviewing to increase physical activity in long-term cancer survivors: A randomized controlled trial. *Nursing Research*, *56*(1), 18–27.

Borycki, E., Sangster-Gormley, E., Schreiber, R., et al. (2014). Electronic record adoption and use among nurse practitioners in British Columbia. *Canadian Journal of Nursing Research*, *46*(1), 44–65.

Breitenstein, S. M., Gross, D., Fogg, L., et al. (2012). The Chicago Parent Program: Comparing 1-year outcomes for African American and Latino parents of young children. *Research in Nursing & Health*, *5*, 475–489.

Campbell, D., & Stanley, J. (1996). *Experimental and quasi-experimental designs for research*. Chicago: Rand-McNally.

Carriere, S. A., Carriere, K., Ayas, N., et al. (2014). Barriers to achieving a time-to-target temperature goal in post-cardiac arrest patients treated with mild therapeutic hypothermia. *Dynamics*, *25*(4), 27–32.

Creamer, A. M., Mill, J., Austin, W., et al. (2014). Canadian nurse practitioners' therapeutic commitment to persons with mental illness. *Canadian Journal of Nursing Research*, *46*(4), 13–32.

Edwards, M. P., McMillan, D. E., & Fallis, W. M. (2013). Napping during breaks on night shift: Critical care managers' perceptions. *Dynamics*, *24*(4), 30–35.

El-Masri, M., Fox-Wasylyshyn, S. M., Springer, C. D., et al. (2014). Exploring the impact of prostrate cancer radiation treatment on functions, bother, and well-being. *Canadian Journal of Nursing Research*, *46*(2), 42–56.

Flynn, F., Evanish, J. Q., Fernald, J. M., et al. (2016). Progressive care nurses improving patient safety by limiting interruptions during medication administration. *Critical Care Nurse*, *36*(4), 19–35.

Forman, J., Currie, L., Lauck, S., et al. (2015). Exploring changes in functional status while waiting for transcatheter aortic valve implantation. *European Journal of Cardiovascular Nursing*, *14*(6), 560–569.

Gillespie, M., & Shackell, E. (2014). Exploring the effectiveness of the oxygen supply and demand framework in nursing education. *Dynamics*, *25*(4), 22–36.

Koopman, W. J., LeBlanc, N., Fowler, S., et al. (2016). Hope, coping, and quality of life in adults with myasthenia gravis. *Canadian Journal of Neuroscience Nursing*, *38*(1), 56–64.

Kundu, A., Lin, Y., Oron., et al. (2014). Reiki therapy for postoperative oral pain in pediatric patients: Pilot data from a double-blind, randomized clinical trial. *Complementary Therapies in Clinical Practice*, *20*, 21–25.

Li, H., Powers, B. A., Melnyk, B. M., et al. (2012). Randomized controlled trial of CARE: An intervention to improve outcomes of hospitalized elders and family caregivers. *Research in Nursing & Health*, *35*(5), 533–549.

Maheu, C., Meschino, W. S., Hu, W., et al. (2015). Pilot testing of a psycho-educational telephone intervention for women receiving uninformative BRCA ½ genetic test results. *Canadian Journal of Nursing Research*, *47*(1), 53–71.

McInnis-Perry, G., Weeks, L. E., & Stryhn, H. (2013). Age and gender differences in emotional support and informational social support insufficiency for older adults in Atlantic Canada. *Canadian Journal of Nursing Research*, *45*(4), 50–68.

McQueen, K. A., Montelpare, W. J., & Dennis, C.-L. (2013). Breastfeeding and Aboriginal women: Validation of the breastfeeding self-efficacy scale-short form. *Canadian Journal of Nursing Research*, *45*(2), 58–75.

Newman, K., Doran, D., & Nagle, L. M. (2014). The relation of critical care nurses' information-seeking behavior with perception of personal control, training, and non-routineness of the task. *Dynamics*, *25*(1), 13–18.

Thomas, M. L., Elliott, J. E., Rao, S. M., et al. (2012). A randomized clinical trial of education or motivational-interviewing–based coaching compared to usual care to improve cancer pain management. *Oncology Nursing Forum*, *39*(1), 39–49.

Vahabi, M., & Damba, C. (2015). A feasibility study of a culturally and gender-specific dance to promote physical activity for South Asian immigrant women in the greater Toronto area. *Women's Health Issues*, *25*(1), 79–87.

Weinert, C., Cudney, S., Comstock, B., et al. (2014). Computer intervention: Illness self-management/quality of life of rural women. *Canadian Journal of Nursing Research*, *46*(1), 26–43.

CHAPTER 10

Experimental and Quasiexperimental Designs

Susan Sullivan-Bolyai | Carol Bova | Mina D. Singh

LEARNING OUTCOMES

After reading this chapter, you will be able to do the following:

- List the criteria necessary for inferring cause-and-effect relationships.
- Distinguish the differences between experimental and quasiexperimental designs.
- Define problems with internal validity that are associated with experimental and quasiexperimental designs.
- Describe the use of experimental and quasiexperimental designs for evaluation research.
- Critically evaluate the findings of selected studies in which cause-and-effect relationships were tested.
- Apply levels of evidence to experimental and quasiexperimental designs.

KEY TERMS

a priori
after-only design
after-only nonequivalent
    control group design
antecedent variable
attrition
control
dependent variable
evaluation research
experiment
experimental design

formative evaluation
independent variable
intervening variable
manipulation
mortality
nonequivalent control
    group design
one-group pretest–posttest
    design
posttest–only control group
    design

pre-experimental design
quasiexperiment
quasiexperimental design
randomization
Solomon four-group design
summative evaluation
testing effects
time series design
true experiment

STUDY RESOURCES

ⓔ Go to Evolve at http://evolve.elsevier.com/Canada/LoBiondo/Research
   for the Audio Glossary and Appendix Tables that provide supplemental
   information for Appendix E.

CHAPTER 9 PROVIDED AN OVERVIEW OF the meaning, purpose, and issues related to quantitative research design. This chapter provides a discussion of specific types of quantitative designs, inasmuch as choosing the correct design is crucial for hypothesis testing or answering research questions. The design involves a *plan,* a *structure,* and a *strategy,* which guide a researcher in writing the hypothesis or research questions, conducting the project, and analyzing and evaluating the data. Each design has specific characteristics to maintain control: for example, homogeneity in the sample, consistent data-collection procedures, manipulation of the independent variable, and randomization.

One of the fundamental purposes of scientific research in any profession is to determine cause-and-effect relationships. Nurses, for example, are concerned with developing effective approaches to maintaining and restoring wellness. Testing such nursing interventions to determine how well they actually work—that is, evaluating the outcomes in terms of efficacy and cost-effectiveness—is accomplished with the use of experimental and quasiexperimental designs. These designs differ from nonexperimental designs in one important way: The researcher actively seeks to bring about the desired effect and does not passively observe behaviours or actions. In other words, the researcher is interested not merely in observing customary patient care but in making something beneficial happen. Experimental and quasiexperimental studies are also important to consider in relation to evidence-informed practice because they provide level II and level III evidence. The findings of such studies provide the validation of clinical practice and the rationale for changing specific aspects of practice (see Chapter 20).

Experimental designs are particularly suitable for testing cause-and-effect relationships because they help eliminate potential alternative explanations (threats to validity) for the findings. Inferring causality requires that the following three criteria be met:

1. The causal variable and effect variable must be associated with each other.
2. The cause must precede the effect.
3. The relationship must not be explainable by another variable.

When you critique studies in which experimental and quasiexperimental designs were used, the primary focus is on the validity of the conclusion that the experimental treatment, or the **independent variable,** caused the desired effect on the outcome, or **dependent variable.** The validity of the conclusion depends on how well the researcher controlled the other variables that may explain the relationship studied. Thus, the focus of this chapter is to explain how various types of experimental and quasiexperimental designs control extraneous variables.

The purpose of this chapter is to acquaint you with the issues involved in interpreting studies that have an **experimental design** (characterized by three properties: randomization, control, and manipulation) or a **quasiexperimental design** (in which random assignment is not used, but the independent variable is manipulated, and certain mechanisms of control are used). Examples of these designs are listed in Box 10.1. The Critical Thinking Decision Path shows an algorithm that influences a researcher's choice of experimental or quasiexperimental design.

BOX **10.1**

SUMMARY OF EXPERIMENTAL AND QUASIEXPERIMENTAL RESEARCH DESIGNS

EXPERIMENTAL DESIGNS
1. True experimental (pretest–posttest control group) design
2. Solomon four-group design
3. After-only design

QUASIEXPERIMENTAL DESIGNS
1. Nonequivalent control group design
2. After-only nonequivalent control group design
3. One-group pretest–posttest design
4. Time series design

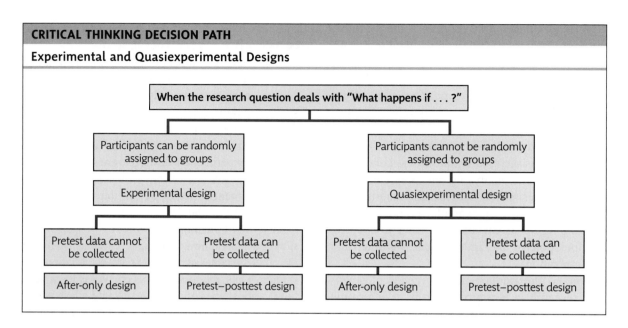

CRITICAL THINKING DECISION PATH

Experimental and Quasiexperimental Designs

When the research question deals with "What happens if . . . ?"

Participants can be randomly assigned to groups

Participants cannot be randomly assigned to groups

Experimental design

Quasiexperimental design

Pretest data cannot be collected

Pretest data can be collected

Pretest data cannot be collected

Pretest data can be collected

After-only design

Pretest–posttest design

After-only design

Pretest–posttest design

TRUE EXPERIMENTAL DESIGN

An **experiment** is a scientific investigation that makes observations and collects data according to explicit criteria. A **true experiment**—also known as a *pretest–posttest control group design* or *classic experiment*—has three identifying properties: randomization, control, and manipulation. These properties allow for other explanations of the phenomenon to be ruled out and thereby provide the strength of the design for testing cause-and-effect relationships.

A research study in which an experimental design is used is commonly called a *randomized control trial* (RCT). An RCT or experimental design is considered to be the best research design, "the gold standard," for providing information about cause-and-effect relationships. An individual RCT generates level II evidence because only minimal bias is introduced by this design. The higher level of evidence that a design produces, the more likely the results are to offer an unbiased estimate of the effect of an intervention and the more confident you can be that the intervention will be effective and produce the same results over and over again.

An example of an RCT is a study conducted by Dehcheshmeh and Rafiei (2015) to compare music therapy and Hoku point ice massage to relieve labour pains during delivery, which were the two experimental groups. The control group was usual labour care. The women were randomly assigned to one of the three groups.

Randomization

Randomization, or random assignment to a group, is required for a study to be considered a true experimental design. It involves the assignment of participants to either the experimental or the control group on a purely random basis. In other words, each participant has an equal and known probability of being assigned to any group. Random assignment may be performed individually or by groups (for examples, see Newman, Doran, & Nagle, 2014; Weinert, Cudney, Comstock, et al., 2014). Random assignment to experimental or control groups allows for the elimination of any systematic bias that may affect the dependent variable being studied. In randomization, it is assumed that any important intervening variable (a condition that occurs during the study that affects the dependent variable) will occur in an equal distribution between the groups. Randomization minimizes variance and decreases selection bias. Participants are randomly assigned to groups through several procedures, such as a table of random numbers or computer-generated number sequences. Whatever method is used, it is important that the process be truly random, that it be tamper-proof, and that the group assignment is concealed. Note that random assignment to groups is different from the random sampling discussed in Chapter 12.

Control

Control refers to the introduction of one or more constants into the experimental situation. Control is acquired by manipulating the causal or independent variable, randomly assigning participants to a group, carefully preparing experimental protocols, and using comparison groups. In experimental research, the comparison group is the control group, or the group that receives the usual treatment rather than the innovative, experimental treatment.

Manipulation

As discussed previously, experimental designs are characterized by the researcher "doing something" to at least some of the participants. The experimental treatment is administered to some participants in the study but not to others, or different amounts of it are administered to different groups. This difference in how the treatment is provided is the **manipulation** of the independent variable. The independent variable might be a treatment, a teaching plan, or a medication. The effect of this manipulation is measured to determine the result of the experimental treatment.

The concepts of control, randomization, and manipulation and their application to experimental design are sometimes confusing for students. These concepts allow researchers to have confidence

in the causal inferences they make by allowing them to rule out other potential explanations.

Consider the use of control, randomization, and manipulation in the following example. Sherrard, Duchesne, Wells, and colleagues (2015) used an RCT to examine whether the use of an interactive voice response follow-up system would improve adherence to best practice guidelines for acute coronary syndrome (ACS). Randomization was achieved by using a single list of random numbers with a permuted block-design, which was generated by an independent statistician. The use of random assignment meant that all patients who met the study criteria had an equal and known chance of being assigned to the control group or the experimental group. The use of random assignment to groups helps ensure that the two study groups are comparable with regard to pre-existing factors that might affect the outcome of interest, such as gender, age, and length of stay in the hospital. Also, the researchers in this example checked statistically whether the procedure of random assignment did, in fact, produce groups that were similar at baseline.

Evidence-Informed Practice Tip _____

In health care research, the term *randomized control trial* (RCT) often refers to a true experimental design. These designs are being used more frequently in nursing research, which is critical to evidence-informed practice initiatives.

The degree of control exerted over the experimental conditions in Sherrard and colleagues' (2015) study is illustrated by its detailed description of the implementation of the interactive voice response (telephone calls). This included the scheduled timing and duration of each phone call. This control helped ensure that all members of the experimental group received similar treatment, and it assists the reader in understanding the process of the experiments. The control group provided a comparison against which the experimental group could be judged.

In Sherrard and colleagues' (2015) study, receiving the interactive voice response was the manipulated treatment. Patient outcomes were measured for all participants, including increased medication adherence, emergency department (ED) visits, hospitalization, and unplanned visits. The primary outcome variable was a composite outcome of increased adherence to medication and decreased adverse events. By comparing the experimental intervention with the use of usual care, Sherrard and colleagues could claim that the evidence was sufficient to state that patients with ACS were more likely to receive care as recommended by best practice guidelines using interactive voice technology, compared with those who received the usual care.

The use of the experimental design allows researchers to rule out many of the potential threats to internal validity of the findings, such as selection bias, history, and maturation effects (see Chapter 9). The strength of the true experimental design lies in its ability to help the researcher control the effects of any extraneous variables—alternative events that could explain the findings—that might constitute threats to internal validity. Such extraneous variables can be either *antecedent* or *intervening*.

The **antecedent variable** occurs before the study but may affect the dependent variable and confound the results. Factors such as age, gender, socioeconomic status, and health status might be important antecedent variables in nursing research because they may affect dependent variables, such as recovery time and ability to integrate health care behaviours. Antecedent variables that might have affected the dependent variables in the study by Sherrard and colleagues (2015) include age, gender, income, level of education, and severity of ACS diagnosis. Random assignment to groups helps ensure that the groups are similar with regard to these variables so that differences in the dependent variable may be attributed to the experimental treatment. However, the researcher should check, and report, how the groups actually compared with regard to such variables.

An **intervening variable** is a condition that occurs during the course of the study and is not part of the study; however, the intervening variable affects the dependent variable and can affect the study outcomes. An example of an intervening variable that might have affected the outcomes of Sherrard and colleagues' (2015) study is the new onset of an illness that is unrelated to that of ACS in the participants of the study. This can lead to changes in the primary outcome measured in the study (ED visits, hospitalization).

Types of Experimental Designs

Several different experimental designs exist (Campbell & Stanley, 1966). Each is based on the classic design called the *true experiment*, diagrammed in Figure 10.1. Above the description diagram, symbolic notations are routinely used:

- R represents random assignment (for both the experimental group and the control group).
- O signifies observation through data collection on the dependent variable.
- O_1 signifies pretest data collection.
- O_2 represents posttest data collection.
- X represents exposure to the intervention.

Therefore, in Figure 10.1, note that the participants were assigned randomly *(R)* to the experimental or the control group. The experimental treatment *(X)* was given only to participants in the experimental group, and the pretests *(O_1)* and posttests *(O_2)* are the measurements of the dependent variables that were made before and after the experimental treatment was performed. In all true experimental designs, participants are randomly assigned to groups, an experimental treatment is introduced to some of the participants, and the effects of the treatment are observed. The variation in designs primarily concerns the number of observations that are made.

As shown in Figure 10.1, participants are randomly assigned to the two groups, experimental and control, so that antecedent variables

A. True or classic experiment

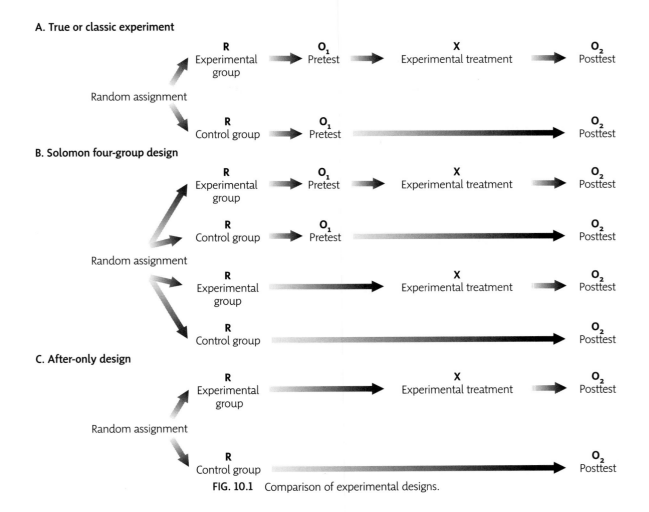

FIG. 10.1 Comparison of experimental designs.

are controlled. Next, pretest measurements or observations are made so that the researcher has a baseline for determining the effect of the independent variable. The researcher then introduces the experimental variable to one of the groups and measures the dependent variable again to see whether it has changed. The control group receives no experimental treatment, but the dependent variable in that group is also measured later for comparison with the experimental group. The degree of difference between the two groups at the end of the study indicates the confidence the researcher has that a causal link exists between the independent and dependent variables.

Because random assignment and the control inherent in this design minimize the effects of many threats to internal validity, the true experimental design is a strong design for testing cause-and-effect relationships.

However, the design is not perfect. Some threats cannot be controlled in true experimental studies (see Chapter 9). People tend to drop out of studies that require their participation over an extended period. The influence over the outcome of an experiment of people dropping out or dying is commonly known as **attrition** or **mortality.** If the number or type of people who drop out of the experimental group differs from that of the control group, a mortality/attrition effect might explain the findings. When you read such a work, examine the sample and the results carefully to see whether dropouts or deaths occurred.

Testing effects—the effects on the scores of a posttest as the result of having taken a pretest—also can be a problem in these studies because the researcher is usually administering the same test twice, and participants tend to score better the second time just by learning the test. Researchers can circumvent this problem in one of two ways: They might use different forms of the same test for the two measurements, or they might use a more complex experimental design called the Solomon four-group design.

The **Solomon four-group design,** shown in Figure 10.1, consists of two groups that are identical to those used in the classic experimental design plus two additional groups: an experimental after-group and a control after-group. As the diagram shows, all four groups have randomly assigned *(R)* participants, as in all experimental studies. However, the addition of these latter two groups helps rule out testing threats to internal validity that the before- and after-groups may experience. For example, suppose a researcher is interested in the effects of counselling on the self-esteem of patients with chronic illness. Just taking a test of self-esteem *(O₁)* may influence how the participants report themselves. The items might make the participants think more about how they view themselves so that the next time they fill out the questionnaire *(O₂)*, their self-esteem might appear to have improved. In reality, however, their self-esteem may be the same as it was before; the scores are different only because the participants had previously taken the test. The use of this design with the two groups that do not receive the pretest allows for evaluating the effect of the pretest on the posttest in the first two groups. (See Practical Application box for another example of use of the Solomon four-group design.)

Although this design helps evaluate the effects of testing, the threat of mortality/attrition remains a problem, as in the classic experimental design.

A less frequently used experimental design is the **after-only design,** shown in Figure 10.1. This design, which is sometimes called the **posttest–only control group design,** is composed of two randomly assigned groups *(R),* but in contrast to the true experimental design, neither group is given a pretest or other measures. Again, the independent variable is introduced to the experimental group *(X)* and not to the control group. The process of randomly assigning the participants to groups is assumed to be sufficient to ensure a lack of bias so that the researcher can still determine whether the treatment *(X)* created significant differences between the two groups *(O₁* and *O₂).* This design is particularly useful when testing effects are expected to be a major problem and the number of available participants is too limited for a Solomon four-group design.

An example of this design would be a study of an intervention on postoperative pain management, inasmuch as pain cannot be measured before surgery and only an after-only design is required.

Research Hint

Remember that mortality/attrition is a problem in most experimental studies because data are usually collected more than once. The researcher should demonstrate that the groups are equivalent both when they enter the study and at the final analysis.

Field and Laboratory Experiments

Experiments also can be classified by setting. Field experiments and laboratory experiments share the properties of control, randomization, and manipulation and involve the same design characteristics but are conducted in different environments. Laboratory experiments take place in an artificial setting created specifically for the purpose of research. In the laboratory, the researcher has almost total control over the features of the environment, such as temperature, humidity, noise level, and participant conditions. Conversely, field experiments are exactly what the name implies: experiments that take place in a real, pre-existing social setting, such as a hospital or clinic, where the phenomenon of interest usually occurs.

Because most experiments in the nursing literature are field experiments and control is such an important element in the conduct of experiments, studies conducted in the field are subject to treatment contamination by factors specific to the setting that the researcher cannot control. However, studies conducted in the laboratory are by nature "artificial" because the setting is created for the purpose of research. Thus, laboratory experiments, although stronger with regard to internal validity questions than field studies, have more problems with external validity. For example, a participant's behaviour in the laboratory may be quite different from the person's behaviour in the real world; this dichotomy presents problems in generalizing findings from the laboratory to the real world. Therefore, when you read research reports, you need to consider the possible effect of the experiment's setting on the findings of the study.

Consider a hypothetical study on different types of wound treatment gels and creams for the management of pressure ulcers. This study could be performed in a laboratory with animals, which would have allowed complete control over the external environment of the study—a variable that might be important in studying wound healing. However, researchers cannot guarantee that the results found in a study in a laboratory would be applicable to human patients in hospital settings; thus, some external validity would be lost.

Advantages and Disadvantages of the Experimental Design

As previously discussed, experimental designs are the most appropriate design for testing cause-and-effect relationships because the design enables the researcher to control the experimental situation. Therefore, experimental designs offer better corroboration than if the independent variable is manipulated in such a way that certain consequences can be expected. Such studies are important because one of nursing's major research priorities is documenting outcomes to provide a basis for changing or supporting current nursing practice.

Experimental designs are not commonly used in nursing research, for several reasons. First, experimentation is conducted under the assumption that all the relevant variables involved in a phenomenon have been identified. For many areas of nursing research, this is simply not the case, and descriptive studies need to be completed before experimental interventions can be applied. Second, these designs have some significant disadvantages. One problem with an experimental design is that many variables important in predicting outcomes of nursing care are not amenable to experimental manipulation. It is well known that health status varies with age and socioeconomic status. No matter how careful a researcher is, no one can assign participants randomly by age or a certain level of income. In addition, it may be technically possible to manipulate some variables, but their nature may preclude their actually manipulation.

For example, if a researcher tried to randomly assign groups to study the effects of cigarette smoking and asked the experimental group to smoke two packs of cigarettes a day, that researcher's ethics would be seriously questioned. It is also potentially true that such a study would not work because nonsmokers randomly assigned to the smoking group would be unlikely to comply with the research task. Thus, sometimes even when a researcher plans to conduct a true experiment, participants dropping out of the study or other factors may, in effect, make the study a quasiexperiment.

Quasiexperimental designs are considered when it is not possible to randomly assign participants or when a control group is lacking. For example, Robertson and Carter (2013) found a decrease in pneumonia rates in neurologically impaired patients in the hospital. Randomly assigning participants to a control and experimental group was not feasible, therefore a retrospective study group was used for the control condition, while a prospective group received the intervention. Another problem with experimental designs is that they may be difficult or impractical to perform in field settings. It may be quite difficult to randomly assign patients on a hospital floor to different groups when they might talk to each other about the different treatments. Experimental procedures also may be disruptive to the usual routine of the setting. If several nurses are involved in administering the experimental program, it may be impossible to ensure that the program is administered in the same way to each participant.

Because of these problems in carrying out true experiments, researchers frequently turn to another type of research design to evaluate cause-and-effect relationships. Such designs, because they seem experimental but lack some of the control of the true experimental design, are called *quasiexperiments.*

QUASIEXPERIMENTAL DESIGNS

Quasiexperimental designs are intended to test cause-and-effect relationships; however, in a quasiexperimental design, full experimental control is not possible. A **quasiexperiment** is a research design in which the researcher initiates an experimental treatment, but some characteristic of a true experiment is lacking. Control may not be possible because of the nature of the independent variable or the nature of the available participants. Quasiexperimental designs usually lack the element of randomization, as described earlier with the Robertson and Carter (2013) study. In other cases, the control group may be missing. However, like experiments, quasiexperiments involve the introduction of an experimental treatment.

In comparison with the true experimental design, quasiexperimental designs are used similarly. Both types of designs are used when the researcher is interested in testing cause-and-effect relationships. However, the basic problem with the quasiexperimental approach is a weakened confidence in making causal assertions. Because of the lack of some controls in the research situation, quasiexperimental designs are subject to contamination by many, if not all, of the threats to internal validity discussed in Chapter 9.

Types of Quasiexperimental Designs

Many different quasiexperimental designs exist. Only the ones most commonly used in nursing research are discussed in this book. To illustrate, the symbols and notations introduced earlier in the chapter are used. Refer to the true experimental design shown in Figure 10.1 and compare it with the **nonequivalent control group design** shown in Figure 10.2. Note that the latter design looks exactly like that of the true experiment except that participants are not randomly assigned to groups.

For example, suppose a researcher is interested in the effects of a new diabetes education

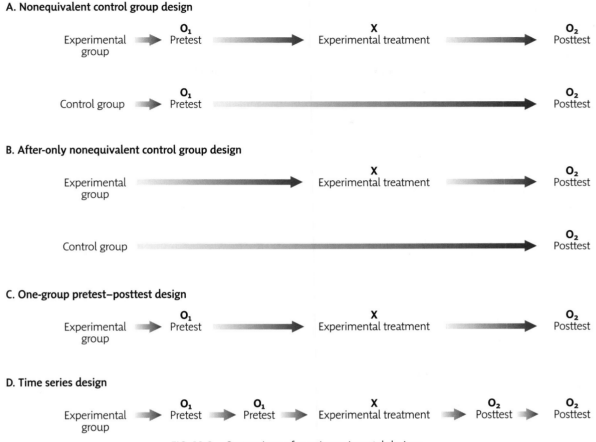

A. Nonequivalent control group design

Experimental group → O_1 Pretest →→→→ X Experimental treatment →→→→ O_2 Posttest

Control group → O_1 Pretest →→→→→→→→→→→→ O_2 Posttest

B. After-only nonequivalent control group design

Experimental group →→→→ X Experimental treatment →→→→ O_2 Posttest

Control group →→→→→→→→→→→→ O_2 Posttest

C. One-group pretest–posttest design

Experimental group → O_1 Pretest →→→→ X Experimental treatment →→→→ O_2 Posttest

D. Time series design

Experimental group → O_1 Pretest → O_1 Pretest → X Experimental treatment → O_2 Posttest → O_2 Posttest

FIG. 10.2   Comparison of quasiexperimental designs.

program on the physical and psychosocial outcomes of patients with newly diagnosed diabetes. If the conditions were right, the researcher might be able to randomly assign participants to either the group receiving the new program or the group receiving the usual program, but for any number of reasons, that design might not be possible (e.g., nurses on the unit where patients are admitted might be so excited about the new program that they cannot help but include the new information for all patients). Thus, the researcher has two choices: to abandon the experiment or to conduct a quasiexperiment. To conduct a quasiexperiment, the researcher might find a similar unit where the new program has not been introduced

and study the patients with newly diagnosed diabetes who are admitted to that unit as a comparison group. The study would then involve the quasiexperimental type of design.

Studies in which both quantitative and qualitative methods are used are called *mixed-methods studies.*

 Research Hint_____

Remember that researchers often make trade-offs and sometimes use a quasiexperimental design instead of an experimental design because it may be pragmatically impossible to randomly assign participants to groups. The fact that the design is not "pure" does not decrease the value of the study, although the utility of the findings may be decreased.

The nonequivalent control group design is commonly used in nursing research studies conducted in field settings. The basic problem with the design is the weakening of the researcher's confidence in assuming that the experimental and comparison groups are similar at the beginning of the study. Threats to internal validity, such as selection bias, maturation effects, testing effects, and mortality (attrition), are possible with this design. However, the design is relatively strong because the gathering of the data at the time of the pretest allows the researcher to compare the equivalence of the two groups on important antecedent variables before the independent variable is introduced.

An example of the nonequivalent control group design is that of Lauzière, Chevarie, Poirier, and colleagues (2013). The purpose of this project was to evaluate the effect of participating in an interdisciplinary-led education program on systolic and diastolic blood pressure. The intervention was implemented through four weekly education sessions of 1 to 2 hours' duration. A total of 40 participants were recruited for the study. As a nonequivalent control group design, the pretest done in the study was a baseline measurement of the participants' blood pressure, height, weight, waist circumference, and body mass index. These measurements were then compared with the posttest measurements in order to determine the effectiveness of the intervention.

Suppose that the researcher did not measure the participants' responses before the introduction of the new treatment (or the researcher was hired after the new program began) but later decided that data demonstrating the effect of the program would be useful. Perhaps, for example, a third party asks for such data to determine whether it should pay the extra cost of the new teaching program. Sometimes the outcomes simply cannot be measured before the intervention, as with prenatal interventions that are expected to affect birth outcomes. The study that could be conducted would have an **after-only nonequivalent control group design,** illustrated in Figure 10.2. This design is similar to the after-only experimental design, but randomization is not used to assign participants to groups. In this design, the two groups are assumed to be equivalent and comparable before the introduction of the independent variable *(X)*. Thus, the soundness of the design and the confidence that the researchers can have in the findings depend on the soundness of this assumption of preintervention comparability. Often, the assumption that the two nonrandomly assigned groups are comparable at the outset of the study is difficult to assert because the validity of the statement cannot be assessed.

In the example of the teaching program for patients with newly diagnosed diabetes, measuring the participants' motivation after the teaching program would not reveal whether their motivations differed before they received the program, and it is possible that the teaching program would motivate individuals to learn more about their health problem. Therefore, the researcher's conclusion that the teaching program improved physical status and psychosocial outcome would be subject to the alternative conclusion that the results were an effect of pre-existing motivations (selection effect) in combination with greater learning by participants so motivated (selection–maturation interaction). Nonetheless, this design is frequently used in nursing research because opportunities for data collection are often limited and because this design is particularly useful when testing effects may be problematic.

An approach used by researchers when only one group is available is to study that group over a longer period—that is, to test participants before an intervention and again afterward. This quasiexperimental design is called a **time series design** and is illustrated in Figure 10.2. Time series designs are useful for determining trends, as in a study on the underutilization of evidence-informed best practice in symptom management among cancer patients in an oncology unit (Allard & Jalbert, 2011). The nurses completed the same questionnaire at three points (before intervention, 1 month after intervention, and 6 months after intervention). The questionnaire measured overall utilization of research results through three questions. Sometimes data are collected many times before the introduction of the treatment to establish a baseline point of reference on outcomes. The experimental treatment is then introduced, and data are collected multiple times afterward to determine a change from baseline. The broad range and number of data-collection points help rule out alternative explanations, such as history effects. However, a testing threat to internal validity is ever present because of multiple data-collection points, and without a control group, the threats of selection bias and maturation effects cannot be ruled out (see Chapter 9).

To rule out some alternative explanations for the findings of a **one-group pretest–posttest design,** researchers typically measure the phenomenon of interest over a longer period and introduce the experimental treatment sometime during the course of the data-collection period (see Figure 10.2). Even with the absence of a control group, the broader range of data-collection points helps rule out threats to validity such as history threats. Obviously, the earlier example of teaching patients with diabetes does not lend itself to this design because researchers do not have access to the patients before the diagnosis.

 Research Hint_____

One of the reasons replication is so important in nursing research is that many problems cannot be subjected to experimental methods. Therefore, the consistency of findings across many patient populations helps support a cause-and-effect relationship even when an experiment cannot be conducted.

Advantages and Disadvantages of Quasiexperimental Designs

Because of the problems inherent in interpreting the results of studies with quasiexperimental

designs, you may wonder why anyone would use them. Quasiexperimental designs are used frequently because they are practical and feasible, and the results are generalizable. These designs are more adaptable to the real-world practice setting than controlled experimental designs. In addition, for some hypotheses, these designs may be the only way to evaluate the effect of the independent variable of interest.

The weaknesses of the quasiexperimental approach involve mainly the inability to establish clear cause-and-effect relationships. However, if the researcher can rule out any plausible alternative explanations for the findings, such studies can lead to increased knowledge about causal relationships. Researchers have several options for ruling out these alternative explanations. They may control extraneous variables **a priori** (before initiating the intervention) by design.

Researchers can also use methods to control extraneous variables statistically. In some cases, common-sense knowledge of the problem and the population can suggest that a particular explanation is not plausible. Nonetheless, replicating such studies is important to support the causal assertions developed through the use of quasiexperimental designs.

The literature on cigarette smoking is an excellent example of how findings from many studies, experimental and quasiexperimental, can be linked to establish a causal relationship. A large number of well-controlled experiments with laboratory animals randomly assigned to smoking and nonsmoking conditions have documented that lung disease does develop in "smoking" animals. Although such evidence is suggestive of a link between smoking and lung disease in humans, it is not directly transferable because animals and humans are different. Because humans cannot be randomly assigned to smoking and nonsmoking groups, for ethical and other reasons, researchers interested in this problem must use quasiexperimental data to test their hypotheses about smoking and lung disease.

Several different quasiexperimental designs have been used to study this problem, and all have yielded similar results: A causal relationship does exist between cigarette smoking and lung disease. Note that the combination of results from both experimental and quasiexperimental studies led to the conclusion that smoking causes lung disease, because the studies together meet the causal criteria of relationship, timing, and lack of an alternative explanation.

The tobacco industry has argued that because the studies on humans are not true experiments, another explanation is possible for the relationships that have been found. For example, these relationships suggest that the tendency to smoke is linked to the tendency for lung disease to develop, and smoking is merely an unimportant intervening variable. The reader needs to review the evidence from studies to determine whether the cause-and-effect relationship postulated is believable.

Evidence-Informed Practice Tip

Findings from studies with experimental designs are considered level II evidence, and those from studies with quasiexperimental designs are considered level III evidence. Quasiexperimental designs are lower on the hierarchy of evidence because of a lack of a research control, which limits the ability to establish confident cause-and-effect statements that influence clinical decision making.

PRE-EXPERIMENTAL DESIGNS

Pre-experimental designs follow similar experimental steps but do not include a control or comparison group. There is only a single group, with no comparison with an equivalent or nonequivalent nontreatment group. Examples are the one-group pretest–posttest ($O_1 \rightarrow X \rightarrow O_2$) and the one-group posttest-only ($X \rightarrow O_1$) designs, where X is the treatment or intervention, and O is the data-collection points.

In the one-group pretest–posttest design, data are collected before and after an experimental

Practical Application

Davison, Szafron, Gutwin, and colleagues (2014) conducted a one-group pretest–posttest design study to measure the preferences and values of men newly diagnosed with prostate cancer, using a Web-based decision support technology. The intervention in the study was the Web-based Decision Support Intervention-Prostate Cancer (DSI-PC) program. Each participant acted as his own control by being tested twice: before having a treatment consultation and after making a treatment decision. Findings revealed that the DSI-PC intervention led to an increase in the men's level of satisfaction with their treatment decisions and with their level of involvement in decision making.

treatment on this one group of participants. In this type of design, the participants act as their own controls, and no randomization occurs. Because controls and randomization are important characteristics that enhance the internal validity of the study, the evidence generated by the findings of this type of pre-experimental design needs to be interpreted with careful consideration of the design limitations.

The advantage of these designs is that they can be used to evaluate treatments, ruling out ineffective treatments before large-scale experimental or quasiexperimental studies are initiated. The disadvantage of this design is that without a control or comparison group, it is difficult to make any conclusions as to whether the treatment, (X) really caused the outcomes or changes.

EVALUATION RESEARCH AND EXPERIMENTATION

As the science of nursing expands and the cost of health care rises, nurses and other health care providers have become increasingly concerned with the ability to document the costs and the benefits of nursing care (see Chapter 1). This task is a complex process, but at its heart is the ability to evaluate or measure the outcomes of nursing care to inform health care decision making. Such studies usually are associated with quality assurance, quality improvement, and evaluation. Studies of evaluation or quality assurance do exactly what the name implies: They are concerned with the determination of the quality of nursing and health care and with the assurance that the public is receiving high-quality care.

Quality assurance and quality improvement in nursing are current and important topics for nursing care. Many early studies of quality assurance documented whether nursing care met predetermined standards. The goal of quality improvement studies is to evaluate the effectiveness of nursing interventions and to provide direction for further improvement in the achievement of quality clinical outcomes and cost-effectiveness.

Evaluation research is the use of scientific research methods and procedures to evaluate a program, treatment, practice, or policy. In evaluation research, analytical means are used to document the worth of an activity such as an intervention, but such research is not a different design. Both experimental and quasiexperimental designs (as well as nonexperimental designs) are used to determine the effect or outcomes of a program. When these designs are used in evaluating a program, the term *evaluation research* is used. Bigman (1961) listed the following purposes and uses of evaluation research:

1. To discover whether and how well the objectives are being fulfilled
2. To determine the reasons for specific successes and failures
3. To direct the course of the experiment with techniques for its effectiveness
4. To reveal principles that underlie a successful program
5. To base further research on the reasons for the relative success of alternative techniques
6. To redefine the means to be used for attaining objectives and to redefine subgoals in view of research findings

According to Clarke (2001), the following four levels of evaluation research are being highlighted in health care, especially nursing research: evaluation of the effectiveness of clinical interventions; evaluation of the effect of new ways of delivering health care; evaluation of structured programs aimed at specific patient groups; and evaluation of the quality of service. In many evaluation research studies, investigators use mixed methods, with both quantitative and qualitative information.

Evaluation studies may be either formative or summative. In **formative evaluation,** a program is assessed as it is being implemented; usually, the focus is on evaluation of the process of a program rather than the outcomes. In **summative evaluation,** the outcomes of a program are assessed after completion of the initial program.

Kuehn, Chircop, Downe-Wamboldt, and colleagues (2011) used a summative evaluation to assess the effect of a North American nursing exchange program on student cultural awareness. In contrast, Doran, Reid-Haughian, Chilcote, and colleagues (2013) used a formative evaluation to evaluate the implementation of a clinical information system in a community setting. Knowledge related to summative (outcomes) and formative (process) evaluation of programs is important in translating research into clinical practice.

The use of experimental and quasiexperimental designs in studies of quality improvement and evaluation enables researchers to determine not only whether care is adequate but also which method of care is best under certain conditions. Furthermore, such studies can be used to determine whether a particular type of nursing care or intervention is cost-effective—that is, that the care or intervention does what it is intended to do but at lower or equivalent cost. Cost studies are usually incorporated into the evaluation of an intervention. For example, Keeler, Haas, Nieswiadomy, and colleagues (2015) wanted to estimate the cost of central catheter–related bloodstream infection (CRBSI) in Canadian blood and marrow cell transplant recipients with a central catheter. The authors compared the costs associated with care of patients who had CRBSI to those for patients who did not have CRBSI. Keeler and colleagues found that care for patients with CRBSI cost the system an extra $44,816.48 per incident.

In an era of health care reform and cost containment for health expenditures, evaluating the relative costs and benefits of new programs of care has become increasingly important. Relatively few studies in nursing and medicine have been dedicated to such evaluation, but in terms of outcomes, nursing costs and cost savings will be important in future studies.

Research Hint

According to Gaudine and Lamb (2015), the term *quality assurance* in health care has been replaced with the term *quality improvement (QI)*, as quality can be improved, not assured. The purpose of QI is thus to bring about immediate improvement to processes and outcomes by using a systematic, evidence-informed approach and compare organizations' quality to standards or benchmarks. QI projects in health care focus on improving patient, staff, and institutional outcomes. The steps are to identify which outcomes need to be improved, discern how they will be improved, and develop a strategy to implement and evaluate QI outcomes. Thus, QI projects include an evaluation. These projects are site specific, and the results may not be generalizable knowledge to other groups or sites.

APPRAISING THE EVIDENCE

Experimental and Quasiexperimental Designs

As discussed earlier in the chapter, various designs for research studies differ in the amount of control the researcher has over the antecedent and intervening variables that may affect the results of the study. True experimental designs, which yield level II evidence, offer the most possibility for control, whereas nonexperimental designs, which yield level IV, V, or VI evidence, offer the least. Quasiexperimental designs, which yield level III evidence, offer evidence that lies somewhere in between. Research designs must balance the needs for internal validity and external validity in order to produce useful results. In addition, judicious use of design requires that the chosen design be appropriate to the problem, free of bias, and capable of answering the research question.

Questions that you should pose when reading studies that test cause-and-effect relationships are listed in the Critiquing Criteria box. All of these questions should help you judge, with confidence, whether a causal relationship exists.

For studies in which either experimental or quasiexperimental designs are used, first try to determine the type of design that was used. Often, a statement describing the design of the study appears in the abstract and in the "Methods" section of the article. If such a statement is not present, you should examine the study for evidence of the following three characteristics: control, randomization, and manipulation. If all are discussed, the design is probably experimental. Conversely, if the study

involves the administration of an experimental treatment but does not involve the random assignment of participants to groups, the design is quasiexperimental. Next, try to identify which of the variations within these two types of designs was used. Determining the answer to these questions gives you a head start because inherent in each design are particular threats to validity, and this step makes it easier to critically evaluate the study. The next question to ask is whether the researcher required a solution to a cause-and-effect problem. If so, the study is suited to these designs. Finally, think about the conducting of the study in the setting. Is it realistic to think that the study could be conducted in a clinical setting without some contamination?

The most important question to ask as you read experimental studies is "What else could have happened to explain the findings?" Thus, the author must provide adequate accounts of how the procedures for randomization, control, and manipulation were carried out. The study should include a description of the procedures for random assignment to such a degree that the reader can determine the likelihood for any one participant to be assigned to a particular group. The description of the independent variable also should be detailed. The inclusion of this information helps the reader decide whether the treatment given to some participants in the experimental group might differ from what was given to others in the

APPRAISING THE EVIDENCE—cont'd

Experimental and Quasiexperimental Designs

same group. In addition, threats to validity, such as testing effects and mortality (attrition), should be addressed. Otherwise, the conclusions of the study could potentially be erroneous and less believable to the reader.

This question of potential alternative explanations or threats to internal validity for the findings is even more important when you critically evaluate a quasiexperimental study because these study designs cannot possibly control for many plausible alternative explanations. A well-written report of a quasiexperimental study systematically reviews potential threats to the validity of the findings. Then your work as the reader is to decide whether the author's explanations make sense. When critiquing evaluation research, you should look for a

careful description of the program, policy, procedure, or treatment being evaluated. In addition, you may need to determine the design used to evaluate the program and assess the appropriateness of the design for the evaluation. Once you have discerned the design, you can assess threats to validity for the appropriate design in determining the appropriateness of the author's conclusions in relation to the outcomes. As with all research, the results of studies with these designs need to be generalizable to a larger population of people than was actually studied. Thus, researchers need to decide whether the experimental protocol eliminated some potential participants and whether this weakness affected not only internal validity but also external validity.

CRITIQUING CRITERIA

1. What design is used in the study?
2. Is the design experimental or quasiexperimental?
3. Is the problem one of a cause-and-effect relationship?
4. Is the method used appropriate to the problem?
5. Is the design suited to the setting of the study?

EXPERIMENTAL DESIGNS

1. What experimental design is used in the study, and is it appropriate?
2. How are randomization, control, and manipulation applied?
3. Are there reasons to believe that alternative explanations exist for the findings?
4. Are all threats to validity, including mortality (attrition), addressed in the report?

5. Whether the experiment was conducted in the laboratory or a clinical setting, are the findings generalizable to the larger population of interest?

QUASIEXPERIMENTAL DESIGNS

1. What quasiexperimental design is used in the study, and is it appropriate?
2. What are the most common threats to the validity of the findings of this design?
3. What are the plausible alternative explanations, and have they been addressed?
4. Are the author's explanations of threats to validity acceptable?
5. What does the author say about the limitations of the study?
6. Do other limitations related to the design exist that are not mentioned?

EVALUATION RESEARCH

1. Do the authors identify a specific problem, practice, policy, or treatment that they will evaluate?
2. Do the authors identify the outcomes to be evaluated?
3. Is the problem analyzed and described?
4. Is the program to be analyzed described and standardized?
5. Do the authors identify the measurement of the degree of change (outcome) that occurs?
6. Do the authors determine whether the observed outcome is related to the activity or to one or more other causes?

CRITICAL THINKING CHALLENGES

- Discuss the barriers to nurse researchers in meeting the three criteria of a true experimental design.
- How is it possible to have a research design that includes an experimental treatment intervention

and a control group and yet is not considered a true experimental study? How does this affect the usefulness of the findings in an evidence-informed practice?

- Argue your case for supporting or not supporting the following claim: "The fact that true experimental design is not used does not decrease the value of the study, even though it may decrease the utility of the findings in practice." Include examples with your rationale.

▪ Respond to the following question: Why are experimental studies considered the best evidence for an evidence-informed practice model? Justify your answer.

depends on the ability of the researcher to rule out plausible threats to the validity of the findings, such as history threats, selection bias, and maturation and testing effects.
- The level of evidence (level III) provided by quasiexperimental designs weakens confidence that the findings were the result of the intervention rather than extraneous variables.
- The overall purpose of critiquing such studies is to assess the validity of the findings and to determine whether these findings are worth incorporating into the nurse's personal practice.

KEY POINTS

- Experimental designs or randomized clinical trials provide the strongest evidence (level II) in terms of whether an intervention or treatment affects patient outcomes.
- Two types of design commonly used in nursing research to test hypotheses about cause-and-effect relationships are experimental and quasiexperimental designs. Both are useful for the development of nursing knowledge because they test the effects of nursing actions and lead to the development of prescriptive theory.
- True experiments are characterized by the ability of the researcher to control extraneous variation, manipulate the independent variable, and randomly assign participants to research groups.
- Experiments conducted in clinical settings or in the laboratory provide the best evidence in support of a causal relationship because the following three criteria can be met: (1) the independent and dependent variables are related to each other; (2) the independent variable chronologically precedes the dependent variable; and (3) the relationship cannot be explained by the presence of a third variable.
- Researchers frequently use quasiexperimental designs to test cause-and-effect relationships because experimental designs are often impractical or unethical.
- Quasiexperiments may lack either randomization or the comparison group, or both, which are characteristics of true experiments. Their usefulness in studying causal relationships

FOR FURTHER STUDY

ⓔ Go to Evolve at http://evolve.elsevier.com/Canada/LoBiondo/Research for the Audio Glossary and Appendix Tables that provide supplemental information for Appendix E.

REFERENCES

Allard, N., & Jalbert, C. (2011). Towards using evidence in oncology: Identified issues and suggested solutions. *Canadian Oncology Nursing Journal, 21*(3), 163–168, 169–173.

Bigman, S. K. (1961). Evaluating the effectiveness of religious programs. *Review of Religious Research, 2,* 99–110.

Campbell, D., & Stanley, J. (1966). *Experimental and quasiexperimental designs for research.* Chicago: Rand-McNally.

Clarke, A. (2001). Evaluation research in nursing and health care. *Nurse Researcher, 8*(3), 4–14.

Davison, B. J., Szafron, M., Gutwin, C., et al. (2014). Using a web-based decision support intervention to facilitate patient–physician communication at prostate cancer treatment discussions. *Canadian Oncology Nursing Journal, 24*(4), 241–247.

Dehcheshmeh, F. S., & Rafiei, H. (2015). Complementary and alternative therapies to relieve labor pain: A comparative study between music therapy and Hoku point ice massage. *Complementary Therapies in Clinical Practice, 21,* 229–232.

Doran, D. M., Reid-Haughian, C., Chilcote, A., et al. (2013). A formative evaluation of nurses' use of electronic devices in a home care setting. *Canadian Journal of Nursing Research, 45*(1), 54–73.

Gaudine, A., & Lamb, M. (2015). *Nursing leadership and management: Working in Canadian healthcare organizations*. North York, ON: Pearson Canada.

Keeler, M., Haas, B. K., Nieswiadomy, M., et al. (2015). Tunnelled central venous catheter-related bloodstream infection in Canadian blood stem cell transplant recipients. *Canadian Oncology Nursing Journal*, *25*(3), 311–318.

Kuehn, A. F., Chircop, A., Downe-Wamboldt, B., et al. (2011). Evaluating the impact of a North American nursing exchange program on student cultural awareness. *International Journal of Nursing Education Scholarship*, *8*(1), Article 1.

Lauzière, T. A., Chevarie, N., Poirier, M., et al. (2013). Effects of an interdisciplinary education program on hypertension: A pilot study. *Canadian Journal of Cardiovascular Nursing*, *23*(2), 12–19.

Newman, K., Doran, D., & Nagle, L. M. (2014). The relation of critical care nurses' information-seeking behaviour with perception of personal control, training, and non-routineness of the task. *Dynamics (Pembroke, Ont.)*, *25*(1), 13–18.

Robertson, T., & Carter, D. (2013). Oral intensity: Reducing non-ventilator-associated hospital-acquired pneumonia in care-dependent, neurologically impaired patients. *Canadian Journal of Neuroscience Nursing*, *35*(2), 10–17.

Rubel, S. K., Miller, J. W., Stephens, R. L., et al. (2010). Testing decision aid for prostate cancer screening. *Journal of Health Communications*, *15*, 307–321.

Sherrard, H., Duchesne, L., Wells, G., et al. (2015). Using interactive voice response to improve disease management and compliance with acute coronary syndrome best practice guidelines: A randomized controlled trial. *Canadian Journal of Cardiovascular Nursing*, *25*(1), 10–15.

Weinert, C., Cudney, S., Comstock, B., et al. (2014). Computer intervention: Illness self-management/quality of life of rural women. *Canadian Journal of Nursing Research*, *46*(1), 26–43.

CHAPTER 11

Nonexperimental Designs

Geri LoBiondo-Wood | Judith Haber | Mina D. Singh

LEARNING OUTCOMES

After reading this chapter, you will be able to do the following:

- Describe the overall purpose of nonexperimental designs.
- Describe the characteristics of survey and relationship/difference designs.
- Define the differences between survey and relationship/difference designs.
- List the advantages and disadvantages of surveys and each type of relationship/difference design.
- Identify methodological, secondary analysis, and meta-analysis research.
- Identify the purposes of methodological, secondary analysis, and meta-analysis research.
- Discuss relational inferences versus causal inferences as they relate to nonexperimental designs.
- Identify the criteria used to critique nonexperimental research designs.
- Apply the critiquing criteria to the evaluation of nonexperimental research designs as they appear in research reports.
- Apply levels of evidence to nonexperimental designs.

KEY TERMS

cohort
correlational study
cross-sectional study
descriptive/exploratory survey
developmental study
epidemiological study
ex post facto study
hierarchical linear
    modelling (HLM)

incidence
longitudinal study
meta-analysis
methodological research
nonexperimental research
    design
prediction study
prevalence
prospective study

psychometrics
relationship/difference
    study
retrospective data
retrospective study
secondary analysis
survey study

STUDY RESOURCES

ⓔ Go to Evolve at http://evolve.elsevier.com/Canada/LoBiondo/Research
for the Audio Glossary and Appendix Tables that provide supplemental
information for Appendix E.

MANY PHENOMENA OF INTEREST AND RELEVANCE to nursing do not lend themselves to an experimental design. For example, nurses studying pain may be interested in knowing the amount of pain, variations in the amount of pain, and patients' responses to postoperative pain. The investigator would not design an experimental study that would potentially intensify a patient's pain just to study the pain experience; that would be unethical. Instead, the researcher would use a nonexperimental design to examine the factors that contribute to the variability in a patient's postoperative pain experience. Nonexperimental research designs are used in studies when the researcher wishes to construct a picture of a phenomenon; examine events, people, or situations as they naturally occur; or test relationships and differences among variables. Nonexperimental designs may enable the researcher to understand how a phenomenon occurs at one point or over a period of time.

In experimental research, the independent variable is manipulated; in a **nonexperimental research design,** the independent variable is not manipulated. In nonexperimental research, the independent variables have occurred naturally, and the investigator cannot directly control them by manipulation. In contrast, in an experimental design, the researcher actively manipulates one or more variables. The researcher in a nonexperimental design explores relationships or differences among the variables. Nonexperimental research requires a clear, concise research problem or hypothesis that is based on a theoretical framework. Even though the researcher does not actively manipulate the variables, the concepts of control (see Chapter 9) should be considered as much as possible.

Researchers do not agree on how to classify nonexperimental studies. A continuum of quantitative research designs is shown in Figure 11.1. This chapter divides nonexperimental designs into *survey studies* and *relationship/difference studies,* as illustrated in Box 11.1. These categories are flexible; nonexperimental studies may be classified in a different way in other sources. Some studies belong exclusively to one of these categories, whereas other studies have the characteristics of more than one category or more than one design label. As you read the research literature, you will often find that researchers who are conducting a nonexperimental study use several design classifications. This chapter introduces the various types of nonexperimental designs, their advantages and disadvantages, the use of nonexperimental research, the issues of causality, and the critiquing process as it relates to nonexperimental research. The Critical Thinking Decision Path outlines the path to the choice of a nonexperimental design.

 Evidence-Informed Practice Tip _____

When you critically appraise nonexperimental studies, be aware of possible sources of bias that can be introduced at any point in the study.

BOX **11.1**

SUMMARY OF NONEXPERIMENTAL RESEARCH DESIGNS

SURVEY STUDIES
- Descriptive
- Exploratory
- Comparative

RELATIONSHIP/DIFFERENCE STUDIES
- Correlational
- Developmental
  - Cross-sectional
  - Longitudinal or prospective
  - Retrospective or ex post facto

Nonexperimental ⟹ Quasiexperimental ⟹ Experimental

FIG. 11.1 Continuum of quantitative research designs.

CRITICAL THINKING DECISION PATH

Nonexperimental Design Choices

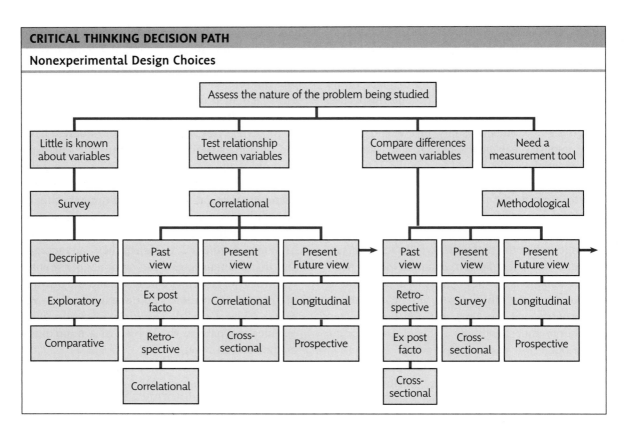

SURVEY STUDIES

The broadest category of nonexperimental designs is the survey study. In a **survey study**—further classified as *descriptive, exploratory,* or *comparative*—detailed descriptions of existing variables are collected, and the data are used to justify and assess current conditions and practices or to make more plans for improving health care practices. When you read research, you will find that the terms *exploratory, descriptive, comparative,* and *survey* may be used either alone, interchangeably, or together to describe the design of a study (Table 11.1). For example, investigators may use a **descriptive/exploratory survey** to search for accurate information about the characteristics of particular participants, groups, institutions, or situations or about the frequency of a phenomenon's occurrence, particularly when little

is known about the phenomenon. The data are used to justify or assess current conditions or to make plans for improvement of conditions. Qualitative researchers also use the term *descriptive* in their reports, as in the study by Small, Kushner, and Neufeld (2013), who used a qualitative descriptive design to examine the perspective of professionals on youth smoking prevention. You will be able to determine the difference in study type by checking in the analysis and findings sections, inasmuch as the qualitative descriptive study entails the use of the analyses outlined in Chapter 15, whereas the descriptive correlational or survey studies entail the use of descriptive and inferential statistical analyses.

In survey studies, the types of variables of interest can be classified as opinions, attitudes, or facts. For example, Edwards, McMillan, and

TABLE 11.1	
EXAMPLES OF STUDIES WITH MORE THAN ONE DESIGN LABEL	
DESIGN TYPE	**STUDY'S PURPOSE**
Descriptive with repeated measures	This study examines how nurses working in campus health clinics identify smokers and provide cessation support (Lawrence, Travis, & Lawler, 2012).
Descriptive, correlational	This descriptive correlational study examines relationships between mild stroke functional and psychosocial outcomes over the early post-discharge period among dyads of mild stroke patients and their spousal caregivers (Green, & King, 2011).
Cross-sectional, descriptive, correlational	This study describes family members' perception of informational support, anxiety, satisfaction with care, and their relationships in order to guide further refinement of a local informational support initiative and its eventual evaluation (Bailey, Sabbagh, Loiselle, et al., 2010).
Explanatory, correlational	This study's aim was to determine the stressors, academic performance, and learned resourcefulness in baccalaureate nursing students (Goff, 2011).
Retrospective, cross-sectional	The purpose of this investigation was to explore the barriers and facilitators to exercise in individuals with cancer in Ontario (Fernandez, Franklin, Amlani, et al., 2015).
Prospective, cohort	The authors describe the Geriatric Emergency Management–Falls Intervention Team (GEM-FIT) project, a nurse-led research initiative to improve fall prevention in older adults through interdisciplinary collaboration (Merrett, Thomas, Stephens, et al., 2011).

Fallis (2013) conducted an online survey to explore critical care nurse managers' perception of experiences with their nursing staff's napping practices on night shift. In another example, Newman, Doran, and Nagle (2014) did a cross-sectional survey collected from 177 critical care nurses who were randomly selected. The aim of the study was to examine the relationship between critical care nurses' information-seeking behaviour and perception of personal control, training, and non-routineness of the task. Fact variables in survey studies include attributes of individuals, such as gender, income level, political and religious affiliations, ethnicity, occupation, and educational level. For example, McInnis-Perry, Weeks, and Stryhn (2013) surveyed Canadians aged 65 years and older in the Atlantic provinces and found that their social needs are not being met and that these needs increase with age. The researchers also found that more men than women report having no support.

Data in survey research can be collected through a questionnaire or an interview (see Chapter 13). For example, Borycki, Sangster-Gormley, Schreiber, and colleagues (2014) administered a Web-based questionnaire to understand the adoption and use of electronic medical records by nurse practitioners in British Columbia. Another example is the study by Schofield, Forchuk, Montgomery, and associates (2016), who used a face-to-face structured interview to compare personal health practices between individuals with mental illness and the general Canadian population.

Survey researchers study either small or large samples of participants recruited from defined populations. The sample can be either broad or narrow and can be made up of people or institutions. For example, if a primary care rehabilitation unit based on a case-management model is to be established in a hospital, researchers might survey prospective applicants' attitudes with regard to case management before the unit staff members are selected. In a broader example, if a hospital is contemplating converting all patient care units to a case-management model, a survey might be conducted to determine the attitudes of a representative sample of nurses in the hospital toward case management. The data might provide the basis for projecting the in-service needs of nursing with regard to case management. The scope and depth of a survey are a function of the nature of the problem.

In surveys, investigators attempt only to relate one variable to another or to assess differences between variables; they do not attempt to determine causation. The two major advantages of surveys are the great deal of information that can be obtained from a large population in a more economical manner than face-to-face interviews and the surprising accuracy of survey research information. If a sample is representative of the population (see Chapter 12), a relatively small number of participants can accurately represent the views of the population.

However, survey studies have several disadvantages. First, the information obtained in a survey tends to be superficial. The breadth rather than the depth of the information is emphasized. Second, conducting a survey requires a great deal of expertise in various research areas. The survey investigator must have skills in sampling techniques, questionnaire construction, interviewing, and data analysis to elicit reliable and valid data. Third, large-scale surveys can be time consuming and costly, although the use of on-site personnel can reduce costs.

Research Hint

Research consumers should recognize that a well-constructed survey can provide a wealth of data about a particular phenomenon of interest, even though causation is not being examined.

Evidence-Informed Practice Tip

Evidence obtained from a survey population may be coupled with clinical expertise and applied to a similar population to develop an educational program to enhance knowledge and skills in a particular clinical area. For example, a survey designed to measure nursing staff's knowledge and attitudes about evidence-informed practice may yield data that are used to develop a staff development course in evidence-informed practice.

RELATIONSHIP/DIFFERENCE STUDIES

Investigators endeavour to trace the relationships or differences between variables that can provide a deeper insight into a phenomenon. This type of study can be classified as a **relationship/difference study.** The following types of relationship/difference studies are discussed here: *correlational studies* and *developmental studies.*

Correlational Studies

In a **correlational study,** an investigator examines the relationship between two or more variables. The researcher is not testing whether one variable causes another variable or how different one variable is from another variable. Instead, the researcher is testing whether the variables covary; in other words, as one variable changes, does a related change occur in the other variable? The researcher using this design is interested in quantifying the strength of the relationship between the variables or in testing a hypothesis about a specific relationship. The positive or negative direction of the relationship is also a central concern (see Chapter 16 for an explanation of the correlation between variables).

In their correlational study, Laschinger and Nosko (2015) explored the relationship between nurses' exposure to workplace bullying and post-traumatic stress disorder. These researchers were not testing a cause-and-effect relationship.

Another example of correlational research is the study by Creamer, Mill, Austin, and colleagues (2014), who wanted to determine how Canadian nurse practitioners rate their levels of therapeutic commitment, role competency, and role support when working with persons with mental health problems. They found that these three subscales were correlated, especially role competency and therapeutic commitment.

Correlational studies offer researchers and research consumers the following advantages:
- An increased flexibility when investigating complex relationships among variables

- An efficient and effective method of collecting a large amount of data about a problem
- A potential for practical application in clinical settings
- A potential foundation for future experimental research studies
- A framework for exploring the relationship between variables that cannot be inherently manipulated

The correlational design has a quality of realism and is particularly appealing because it suggests the potential for practical solutions to clinical problems. However, there are disadvantages of correlational studies:

- Inability to manipulate the variables of interest
- No randomization in the sampling procedures because the study deals with pre-existing groups; therefore, generalizability is decreased
- Inability to determine a causal relationship between the variables because of the lack of manipulation, control, and randomization

One of the most common misuses of a correlational design is the researcher's conclusion that a causal relationship exists between the variables. In their correlational study, Meyer, O'Brien-Pallas, Doran, and colleagues (2014) examined the influence of front-line managers' characteristics and scope of responsibilities on teamwork. They appropriately concluded that leadership practices, clinical support roles, and compressed operational hours had positive effects on teamwork, whereas the number of nondirect report staff and areas assigned had negative effects. The report concluded with some very thoughtful recommendations: that additional research across sectors is needed to explicate the influence of managerial scope of responsibility on the quality and efficiency of team services and on team health, safety, satisfaction, retention, and clinical outcomes (p. 53).

Correlational studies may be further labelled *descriptive correlational* or *predictive correlational*. A study by Wong, Elliott-Miller, Laschinger, and colleagues (2015) is an example of predictive

correlational study. The goal of study was to examine the relationships between span of control (SOC) and managers' job and unit performance outcomes. The researchers concluded that a combination of SOC and core self-evaluation significantly predicted role overload, work control, and job satisfaction, but only SOC significantly predicted unit adverse outcomes.

The inability to draw causal statements should not lead you to conclude that a nonexperimental correlational study has a weak design. In terms of evidence for practice, researchers—on the basis of the literature review and their findings—frame the utility of the results in view of previous research and therefore help establish supportive evidence of the applicability of the results to a specific patient population. A correlational design is very useful for clinical research studies because many of the phenomena of clinical interest are beyond the researcher's ability to manipulate, control, and randomize.

Developmental Studies

Nonexperimental designs in which a time perspective is used can be further subclassified. A **developmental study** is concerned not only with the existing status and the relationship and differences among phenomena at one point in time but also with changes that occur as a function of time. The following three types of developmental study designs are discussed here: *cross-sectional*, *longitudinal* or *prospective*, and *retrospective* or *ex post facto*. Remember that in the literature, studies may be designated by more than one design name. This practice is accepted because many studies have elements of several nonexperimental designs. Table 11.1 provides examples of studies classified with more than one design label.

Cross-Sectional Studies

In a **cross-sectional study,** researchers examine data at one time; in other words, the data are collected on only one occasion with the same participants rather than with the same participants at several times.

An example of a cross-sectional study is provided by Rajacich, Freeman, Armstrong-Stassen, and colleagues (2014), who investigated the environmental work factors in the acute care setting and their influence on male registered nurses' job satisfaction and intention to stay in the profession. Another cross-sectional study approach is to simultaneously collect data on the study's variables from different **cohort** (participants) groups. An example of a cross-sectional study with different cohort groups was conducted by Fox, Sidani, and Brooks (2010), who used a naturalistic cohort design to determine the relationship between bed rest and orthostatic intolerance of sitting in adults residing in chronic care facilities. Cohorts represented different amounts of bed rest that were occurring naturally: "no bed rest," "two to four days" of bed rest, and "five to seven days" of bed rest. In cross-sectional studies, researchers can investigate relationships and correlations, differences and comparisons, or both. For instance, Fox and colleagues (2010) posed research questions that allowed the researchers to investigate both differences and relationships among and between variables.

 ### Evidence-Informed Practice Tip ____

Replication of significant findings in nonexperimental studies, with similar or different populations or both, increases your confidence in the conclusions offered by the researcher and the strength of evidence generated by consistent findings from more than one study.

Longitudinal or Prospective Studies

In contrast to the cross-sectional design, the **longitudinal study** or **prospective study** (also referred to as *repeated-measures* studies) involves collecting data from the same group at different times. Researchers also use longitudinal studies to explore differences and relationships.

For example, the investigator conducting a study with children with diabetes could use a longitudinal design. In that case, the investigator could collect yearly data or monitor the same children over a number of years to compare changes in the variables at different ages. By collecting data from each participant at yearly intervals, the investigator obtains a longitudinal perspective of the diabetic process.

In one longitudinal study, Goldie, Prodan-Bhalla, and Mackay (2012) collected data from a sample of 103 postoperative cardiac surgery patients over a year. The purpose of the study was to compare the effectiveness of acute care nurse practitioner–led care to that of hospitalist-led care in a postoperative cardiac unit. In another longitudinal study, Benzies, Mychasiuk, and Tough (2015) investigated how patterns of postpartum psychological distress at 8 weeks postpartum are associated with maternal concerns about their children's emotional and behavioural problems at the age of 3 years.

Cross-sectional and longitudinal designs have many advantages and disadvantages. When assessing the appropriateness of a cross-sectional study versus a longitudinal study, the research consumer should first assess the researcher's goal in view of the theoretical framework. For example, in a hypothetical study of infant colic, the researchers are investigating a developmental process; therefore, a longitudinal design seems more appropriate. However, the disadvantages inherent in a longitudinal design also must be considered. The period of data collection may be long because of the time the participants take to progress to each data-collection point. In the infant colic study, it might take the researchers between 12 and 18 months to collect the data from the total sample. Threats to internal validity, such as testing and attrition, also are ever-present and unavoidable in a longitudinal study (see Chapter 16). As a result, longitudinal designs are costly in terms of time, effort, and money. Moreover, confounding variables could affect interpretation of the results. Participants in these studies may respond in a socially desirable way that they believe is congruent with the investigators' expectations (see discussion of the Hawthorne effect, in Chapter 9).

Despite the pragmatic constraints imposed by a longitudinal study, the researcher should proceed with this design if the theoretical framework supports a longitudinal developmental perspective. The advantages of a longitudinal study are that participants are monitored separately and thereby serve as their own controls; an increased depth of responses can be obtained; and early trends in the data can be analyzed. The researcher can assess changes in the variables of interest over time and explore both relationships and differences between variables.

Cross-sectional studies, in comparison with longitudinal studies, are less time consuming and less expensive and are thus more manageable for the researcher. Because large amounts of data can be collected at one time, the results are more readily available. In addition, the confounding variable of maturation, which results from the passage of time, is not present. However, the investigator's ability to establish an in-depth developmental assessment of the interrelationships of the phenomena being studied is reduced. Thus, the researcher is unable to determine whether the change that occurred is related to the change that was predicted because the same participants were not monitored over a period of time. In other words, the participants are unable to serve as their own controls (see Chapter 10).

In summary, longitudinal studies begin in the present and end in the future, and cross-sectional studies encompass a broader perspective of a cross-section of the population at one specific time.

 Evidence-Informed Practice Tip ____

The quality of evidence provided by a longitudinal cohort study is stronger than that from other nonexperimental designs because the researcher can determine the incidence of a problem and its possible causes.

Retrospective or Ex Post Facto Studies

A **retrospective study** is essentially the same as an **ex post facto study.** Epidemiologists primarily use the term *retrospective,* whereas social scientists prefer the term *ex post facto.* In either case, the dependent variable has already been affected by the independent variable, and the investigator attempts to link current events to past events.

When scientists wish to explain causality or the factors that determine the occurrence of events or conditions, they prefer to use an experimental design. However, they cannot always manipulate the independent variable or use random assignments. In cases in which experimental designs cannot be employed, ex post facto studies may be used. *Ex post facto* literally means "from after the fact." These studies also are known as *causal-comparative* studies or *comparative* studies. As this design is discussed further, you will see that ex post facto research is similar to quasiexperimental research because in both, differences between variables are examined.

In retrospective studies, a researcher hypothesizes, for example, that variable X (cigarette smoking) is related to and a determinant of variable Y (lung cancer), but X, the presumed cause, is not manipulated, and participants are not randomly assigned to groups. Instead, the researcher chooses a group of participants who have experienced X (cigarette smoking) in a normal situation and a control group of participants who have not experienced X. The behaviours, performances, or conditions (lung tissue) of the two groups are compared in order to determine whether the exposure to X had the effect predicted by the hypothesis. Table 11.2 illustrates this example and reveals that although cigarette smoking appears to be a determinant of lung cancer, the researcher is still not able to conclude that a causal relationship exists between the variables because the independent variable has not been

TABLE 11.2		
PARADIGM FOR THE EX POST FACTO DESIGN		
GROUPS (NOT RANDOMLY ASSIGNED)	**INDEPENDENT VARIABLE (NOT MANIPULATED BY INVESTIGATOR)**	**DEPENDENT VARIABLE**
Exposed group: cigarette smokers	X: cigarette smoking	Y_e: lung cancer
Control group: nonsmokers		Y_c: no lung cancer

manipulated and the participants were not randomly assigned to groups.

Another example of a retrospective study is that of Laforme, Jubinville, Gravel, and colleagues (2014), who were interested in user profiles and reasons for calls to an epilepsy hotline. They collected **retrospective data** (data that have already been recorded) on 5,189 telephone queries to a specific epileptologist between January 2004 and 2011, and to two epileptologists from 2010 onward. The study revealed that the majority of calls (72%) were made by patients themselves, followed by family members (16%) and health care providers (11%). Most were related to medication (25%), notification of seizures (23%), appointments or tests (12%), and adverse effects (9%).

The advantages of the retrospective design are similar to those of the correlational design. The additional benefit of the retrospective design is that it offers a higher level of control than a correlational study. For example, in a cigarette smoking study, the lung tissue samples from nonsmokers and smokers could be compared. This comparison would enable the researcher to establish the existence of a differential effect of cigarette smoking on lung tissue. However, the researcher would remain unable to draw a causal link between the two variables. This inability is the major disadvantage of the retrospective design.

Another disadvantage of retrospective research is that an alternative hypothesis may be the reason for the documented relationship. If the researcher obtains data from two existing groups of participants, such as one that has been exposed to X and one that has not, and the data support the hypothesis that X is related to Y, the researcher cannot be sure whether X or an extraneous variable is the cause of the occurrence of Y. Finding naturally occurring groups of participants who are similar in all ways except for their exposure to the variable of interest is very difficult. The possibility always exists that the groups differ in another way (e.g., in exposure to another lung irritant, such as asbestos), which can affect the findings of the study and produce spurious results. Consequently, when you read about such a study, you need to cautiously evaluate the conclusions drawn by the investigator.

 Research Hint

When you read research reports, you will find that, at times, researchers classify a study's design with more than one design label. This classification is correct because research studies often reflect aspects of more than one design.

Longitudinal or prospective (cohort) studies are less common than retrospective studies because it can take a long time for the phenomenon of interest to become evident in a prospective study. For example, if researchers were studying pregnant women who regularly consume alcohol, it would take 9 months for the effect of low birth weight in the participants' infants to become evident. The problems inherent in a prospective study are therefore similar to those of a longitudinal study. However, longitudinal or prospective studies are considered stronger than retrospective studies because of the degree of control that can be imposed on extraneous variables that might confound the data.

Research Hint

Remember that nonexperimental designs can test relationships, differences, comparisons, or predictions, depending on the purpose of the study.

PREDICTION AND CAUSALITY IN NONEXPERIMENTAL RESEARCH

Researchers and research consumers are concerned with the issues of prediction and causality in explaining cause-and-effect relationships. Historically, researchers have said that only experimental research can support the concept of causality. For example, nurses are interested in discovering what causes anxiety in many settings. If nurses can uncover the causes, they can perhaps develop interventions that would prevent or decrease the anxiety. Causality makes it necessary to order events chronologically; therefore, if nurses find in a randomized experiment that event 1 (stress) occurs before event 2 (anxiety) and that participants who experienced stress were anxious, whereas those in the unstressed group were not, then the hypothesis that stress causes anxiety is supported. If these results occurred in a nonexperimental study in which some participants underwent the stress of surgery and were anxious, whereas others did not have surgery and were not anxious, an association or relationship would be said to exist between stress (surgery) and anxiety. The results of a nonexperimental study, however, do not imply that the stress of surgery caused the anxiety.

Many variables (e.g., anxiety) that nurse researchers wish to study to explore causation cannot be manipulated, nor would it be wise to try to manipulate the variables. However, studies that can assert a predictive or causal sequence are needed. In view of this need, many nurse researchers use several analytical techniques that can explain the relationships among variables to establish predictive or causal links. These techniques are called *causal modelling* (see the following Practical Application box), *model testing,* and *associated causal analysis* (Kaplan, 2008; Schumacker & Lomax, 2004).

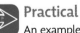

Practical Application

Samuels-Dennis, Ford-Gilboe, Wilk, and colleagues (2010) used causal modelling to validate a theoretical model that highlights the process through which posttraumatic stress disorder (PTSD) develops among women. The results revealed that mothers' strains and personal resources played a significant mediating role in the relationship between cumulative trauma and PTSD.

You will also find the terms *path analysis, LISREL, analysis of covariance structures, structural equation modelling* (SEM), and **hierarchical linear modelling (HLM)** (Raudenbush & Bryk, 2002) used to describe the statistical techniques (see Chapter 16) used in these studies. An HLM is a type of regression analysis that allows for analysis of hierarchically structured data simultaneously at all levels (see the following Practical Application box for an example of the use of HLM).

In a **prediction study,** a model may be tested to assess which independent variables can best explain one or more dependent variables in order to make a forecast or prediction derived from particular phenomena. For example, Stephenson, DeLongis, Steele, and colleagues (2017) examined the role of maternal posttraumatic growth in changes in behavioural problems among siblings of children with complex chronic health

Practical Application

An example of HLM appeared in a study by Laschinger, Nosko, Wilk, et al. (2014), who tested a multilevel model examining the effects of unit empowerment and perceived support for professional nursing practices on unit effectiveness and individual nurse well-being. The findings indicated that nurses' shared perception of structural empowerment on their units indirectly influenced their shared perception of unit effectiveness through perceived unit support for professional nursing practice, which, in turn, had a significant positive direct effect on unit effectiveness. Higher core-self-evaluation had a direct and indirect effect on job satisfaction through increased psychological empowerment.

conditions. Results from a time-lagged multi-level regression revealed that higher levels of maternal posttraumatic growth predicted subsequent declines in parent-reported internalizing, externalizing, and total behavioural problems among healthy siblings. In another example, Goff (2011) conducted an explanatory correlational study to explore learned resourcefulness, stressors, and academic performance in baccalaureate nursing students. Goff found that levels of personal and academic stressors were evident but were not significant predictors of academic performance. Age was a significant predictor of academic performance.

In another example, Wing, Regan, and Laschinger (2013) tested a model based on Kanter's theory of structural empowerment to examine the relationship between new graduate nurses' perceptions of structural empowerment, workplace incivility, and mental health symptoms. Wing and associates explained the development of the model and the premise of the study. The explanation enables readers of the study to clearly understand the purpose and aim of the research and the test of the model with regression analyses. Although Wing and associates did not test a cause-and-effect relationship between the chosen independent predictor variables and the dependent criterion variable, the study did demonstrate a theoretically meaningful model of how variables work together in a group in a particular situation.

Research Hint

Nonexperimental clinical research studies have progressed to the point at which prediction models are used to explore or test relationships between independent variables and dependent variables.

As nurse researchers develop their programs of research in a specific area, more tests of models will be available. The statistics used in model-testing studies are advanced, but the beginning

research consumer should be able to read the article, understand the purpose of the study, and determine whether the model generated was logical and developed with a solid basis from the literature and past research.

A full description of the techniques and principles of causal modelling is beyond the scope of this text.

Evidence-Informed Practice Tip

Research studies that entail the use of nonexperimental designs and provide level IV evidence can build the foundation for a program of research that leads to experimental designs in which the effectiveness of nursing interventions can be tested.

ADDITIONAL TYPES OF QUANTITATIVE STUDIES

Other types of quantitative studies complement the science of research. These additional designs provide a means of viewing and interpreting phenomena to provide further breadth and knowledge to nursing science and practice. These types of quantitative studies are methodological research, systematic review, meta-analysis, integrative review, secondary analysis, and epidemiological studies.

Methodological Research

Methodological research is the development and evaluation of data-collection instruments, scales, and techniques. As noted in Chapters 13 and 14, methodology has a strong influence on research. The most significant and important aspect of methodological research addressed in measurement development is **psychometrics**—the theory and development of measurement instruments (such as questionnaires) and measurement techniques (such as observational techniques) through the research process. Thus, psychometrics is concerned with the measurement of a concept, such as anxiety or interpersonal conflict, with reliable and valid tools. (See Chapter 14 for a discussion of reliability and validity.)

Nurse researchers have used the principles of psychometrics to develop and test measurement instruments that focus on nursing phenomena. Nurse researchers also use instruments developed in other disciplines, such as psychology and sociology, in which tools have been psychometrically tested. Sound measurement tools are critical for the reliability and validity of a study. A study's purpose, problems, and procedures may be clear, and the data analysis may be correct and consistent, but if the measurement tool has inherent psychometric problems, the findings will be rendered questionable or of limited utility.

The main problem for nurse researchers is locating appropriate measurement tools. Many of the phenomena of interest in nursing practice and research are intangible, such as interpersonal conflict, caring, coping, and maternal–fetal attachment. The intangible nature of various phenomena, and yet the need to measure them, places methodological research in an important position in research. Methodological research differs from other designs of research. First, it does not include all of the research process steps discussed in Chapter 3. Second, to implement methodical research techniques, the researcher must have a sound knowledge of psychometrics or must consult with a researcher knowledgeable in psychometric techniques. The methodological researcher is not interested in the relationship of the independent variable to a dependent variable or in the effect of an independent variable on a dependent variable. Instead, the methodological researcher is interested in identifying an intangible construct (concept) and making it tangible with a paper-and-pencil instrument or observation protocol.

A methodological study includes the following steps:

- Defining the construct, or concept, or behaviour to be measured
- Formulating the tool's items
- Developing instructions for users and respondents
- Testing the tool's reliability and validity

A sound, specific, and exhaustive literature review is necessary to identify the theories underlying the steps in this construct. The literature review provides the basis of item formulation. Once the items have been developed, the researcher assesses the tool's reliability and validity (see Chapter 14). Various aspects of these procedures may differ according to the tool's use, purpose, and stage of development.

In an example of methodological research, Kennedy, Tomblin-Murphy, Martin-Misener, and associates (2015) documented the psychometric properties of the Nursing Competence Self-Efficacy Scale.

Common considerations that researchers incorporate into methodological research are outlined in Table 11.3. Many more examples of methodological research can be found in the nursing research literature (Akhtar-Danesh, Valaitis, Schofield, et al., 2010; Pagano, O'Shea, Campbell, et al., 2015; Roberts & Ward-Smith, 2010). Psychometric or methodological studies are found primarily in journals that report research. The *Journal of Nursing Measurement* is devoted to the publication of information on instruments, tools, and approaches for measurement of variables.

The specific procedures of methodological research are beyond the scope of this book, but you are urged to look closely at the tools used in studies.

Systematic Review

A *systematic review* is a summation and assessment of research studies found in the literature based on a clearly focused question that uses systematic and explicit methods to identify, select, critically appraise, and analyze relevant data from the selected studies to summarize the findings in a focused area (Liberati, Altman, Tetzlaff, et al., 2009; Moher, Liberati, Tetzlaff, et al., 2009). The strength of evidence provided by systematic reviews is a key component for developing a practice based on evidence. The qualitative counterpart to a systematic review is meta-synthesis, which uses qualitative principles to assess qualitative research and is

TABLE 11.3

COMMON CONSIDERATIONS IN THE DEVELOPMENT OF MEASUREMENT TOOLS

CONSIDERATION	COMMENT
The well-constructed scale, test, interview schedule, or other form of index should consist of an objective, standardized measure of samples of a behaviour that has been clearly defined. Observations should be made on a small but carefully chosen sampling of the behaviour of interest, thus creating confidence that the samples are representative.	A new tool should be based on a thorough review of previous theoretical and research literature to ensure validity.
The tool should be standardized; that is, a set of uniform items and response possibilities are uniformly administered and scored.	Without specific criteria and rating procedures, the evaluations of the items would be based on the subjective impressions, which may have varied significantly between observers and conditions.
The items of a measurement tool should be unambiguous; they should be clear-cut, concise, exact statements with only one idea per item. Negative stems or items with negatively phrased response possibilities result in ambiguity in meaning and scoring.	For example, in constructing a tool to measure job satisfaction, a nurse scientist writes the following item: "I never feel that I don't have time to provide good nursing care." The response format consists of "Agree," "Undecided," and "Disagree." A response of "Disagree" will likely not reflect the respondent's true intention because of the confusion that is created by the double-negative phrasing "never . . . don't."
The type of items used in any one test or scale should be restricted to a limited number of variations. Participants who are expected to shift from one kind of item to another may fail to provide a true response as a result of the distraction of making such a change.	Mixing true-or-false items with questions that require a yes-or-no response and items that provide a response format of five possible answers can lead to a high level of measurement error.
Items should not provide irrelevant clues. Unless carefully constructed, an item may furnish an indication of the expected response or answer. Furthermore, the correct answer or expected response to one item should not be given by another item.	An item that provides a clue to the expected answer may contain value words that convey cultural expectations, such as "A good wife enjoys caring for her home and family."
The items of a measurement tool should not be made difficult by requiring unnecessarily complex or exact operations. Furthermore, the difficulty of an item should be appropriate to the level of the participants being assessed. Limiting each item to one concept or idea helps accomplish this objective.	A test constructed to evaluate learning in an introductory course in research methods may contain an item that is inappropriate for the designated group, such as "A non-linear transformation of data to linear data is a useful procedure before a hypothesis of curvilinearity is tested."
The diagnostic, predictive, or measurement value of a tool depends on the degree to which it serves as an indicator of a relatively broad and significant area of behaviour, known as the *universe of content* for the behaviour. As already emphasized, a behaviour must be clearly defined before it can be measured. The definition is developed from the universe of content: that is, the information and research findings that are available for the behaviour of interest. The items should reflect that definition. The extent to which the test items appear to accomplish this objective is an indication of the validity of the instrument.	Two nurse researchers are studying the construct of quality of life. Each nurse has defined this construct in a different way. Consequently, the measurement tool that each nurse devises will include different questions. The questions on each tool will reflect the universe of content for quality of life as defined by each researcher.
The instrument also should adequately cover the defined behaviour. The primary consideration is whether the number and nature of items in the sample are adequate. If the sample has too few items, the accuracy or reliability of the measure must be questioned. In general, the sample should have a minimum of 10 items for each independent aspect of the behaviour of interest.	For example, few people would be satisfied with an assessment of intelligence if the scale were limited to three items.
The measure must prove its worth empirically through tests of reliability and validity.	The researcher should demonstrate to the reader that the scale is accurate and measures what it purports to measure (see Chapter 14).

described in Chapter 5. In a systematic review, statistical methods such as a meta-analysis may or may not be used to analyze the studies reviewed. A systematic review provides the most powerful and useful evidence available to guide practice: level I evidence (see Chapter 3). Systematic reviews that use multiple randomized clinical trials (RCTs) to combine study results offer stronger evidence (level I) in estimating the magnitude of an effect for an intervention.

You will also find reviews of an area of research or theory synthesis termed *integrative reviews*, discussed later in the chapter. Systematic and integrative reviews are not designs per se, but methods for searching and integrating the literature related to a specific clinical issue. These methods take the results of many studies in a specific area, assesses the studies critically for reliability and validity (quality, quantity, and consistency), and synthesize findings to inform practice. Meta-analysis provides level I evidence— the highest level of evidence, as it involves statistically analyzing and integrating the results of many studies. Systematic reviews and meta-analyses also grade the level of design or evidence of the studies reviewed. Of all the review types, a meta-analysis provides the strongest summary support because it summarizes studies using data analysis. Box 11.2 outlines the path for completing a systematic review.

The components of a systematic review are the same as in a meta-analysis (Box 11.3) except for the analysis of the studies. An example of a systematic review is that by Fowles, Cheng, and Mills (2012), on the effectiveness of maternal health–promoting interventions. In this review, the authors
- Synthesized the literature from studies on the effectiveness of interventions promoting maternal health in the first year after childbirth.
- Included a clear clinical question; all of the sections of a systematic review were presented, except there was no statistical meta-analysis (combination of studies data) of the studies as a whole because the interventions

---

> **BOX 11.2**
>
> **COMPLETING A SYSTEMATIC REVIEW**
>
> A systematic review is a summary of the quantitative research literature that used similar designs based on a focused clinical question. The goal is to bring together all of the studies concerning a focused clinical question and, using rigorous inclusion and exclusion criteria, assess the strength and quality of the evidence provided by the chosen studies in relation to:
> - Sampling issues
> - Internal validity (bias) threats
> - External validity
> - Data analysis
>
> The purpose is to report, in a consolidated fashion, the most current and valid research on intervention effectiveness and clinical knowledge, which will ultimately be the basis for evidence-informed decision making about the applicability of findings to clinical practice.
>
> Once the studies in a systematic review are gathered from a comprehensive literature search (see Chapter 5), they are assessed for quality and synthesized according to quality or focus; then practice recommendations are made and presented in an article. More than one person independently evaluates the studies to be included or excluded in the review. Generally, the articles critically appraised are discussed in the article and presented in a table format within the article, which helps you to easily identify the specific studies gathered for the review and their quality. The most important principle to assess when reading a systematic review is how the author(s) of the review identified the studies to evaluate and how they systematically reviewed and appraised the literature that leads to the reviewers' conclusions.

and outcomes varied across the studies reviewed.

Each study in this review was considered individually, not collectively, for its sample size, effect size, and its contribution to knowledge in the area, based on a set of criteria.

Although systematic reviews are highly useful, they also have to be reviewed for potential bias. Thus the studies in a review need to be carefully critiqued for scientific rigour in each step of the research process.

Meta-Analysis

A **meta-analysis** is a systematic summary using statistical techniques to assess and combine studies

BOX 11.3

SYSTEMATIC REVIEW COMPONENTS WITH OR WITHOUT META-ANALYSIS

- Introduction
- Review rationale and a clear clinical question (PICOT)
- Methods
- Information sources, databases used, and search strategy identified: how studies were selected and data extracted as well as the variables extracted and defined
- Description of methods used to assess risk of bias, summary measures identified (e.g., risk, ratio); identification of how data is combined, if studies are graded what quality appraisal system was used (see Chapters 1, 17, and 18)
- Results
- Number of studies screened and characteristics, risk of bias within studies, if a meta-analysis there will be a synthesis of results including confidence intervals, risk of bias for each study, and all outcomes considered
- Discussion
- Summary of findings including the strength, quality, quantity, and consistency of the evidence for each outcome
- Any limitations of the studies, conclusions, and recommendations of findings for practice
- Funding
- Sources of funding for the systematic review

of the same design to obtain a precise estimate of effect (impact of an intervention on the dependent variable/outcomes or association between variables) (Borenstein, Hedges, Higgins, et al., 2009). The terms *meta-analysis* and *systematic review* are often used interchangeably. The main difference is that, as noted earlier, a meta-analysis includes a statistical assessment of the studies reviewed. Meta-analysis involves statistically analyzing the data from each of the studies, treating all the studies reviewed as one large data set in order to obtain a precise estimate of the effect (impact) of the results (outcomes) of the studies in the review. Johnston (2005) has noted that the meta-analysis of a number of RCTs gives due weight to the sample size of the studies included and provides an estimate of treatment effect; in other words, a meta-analysis helps determine whether the intervention makes a difference.

Meta-analysis involves a rigorous process of summary and determining the impact of a number of studies rather than the impact derived from a single study alone (see Chapter 10). After the clinical question is identified and the search of the review of published and unpublished literature is completed, a meta-analysis is conducted in two phases:

Phase I: The data are extracted (i.e., outcome data, sample sizes, and measures of variability from the identified studies).

Phase II: The decision is made as to whether it is appropriate to calculate what is known as a pooled average result (effect) of the studies reviewed.

Effect sizes are calculated using the difference in the average scores between the intervention and control groups from each study (Higgins & Green, 2011). Each study is considered a unit of analysis. A meta-analysis takes the effect size (see Chapter 12) from each of the studies reviewed to obtain an estimate of the population (or the whole) to create a single effect size of all the studies. Thus the effect size is an estimate of how large a difference there is between intervention and control groups in the summarized studies. For example, in the meta-analysis by Murphy, Lipp, and Powles (2012), the researchers studied the question "Does counselling follow-up of women who had a miscarriage improve psychological well-being?" (see Appendix E). The studies that assessed this question were reviewed, and each was weighted for its impact or effect on improving psychological well-being. This estimate helps health care providers decide which intervention, if any, is more useful for improving well-being after a miscarriage.

In addition to calculating effect sizes, authors of meta-analyses use multiple statistical methods to present and depict the data from studies reviewed (see Chapters 19 and 20). One of these methods is a forest plot, sometimes called a *blob-bogram*. A forest plot graphically depicts the results of analyzing a number of studies. Figure 11.2

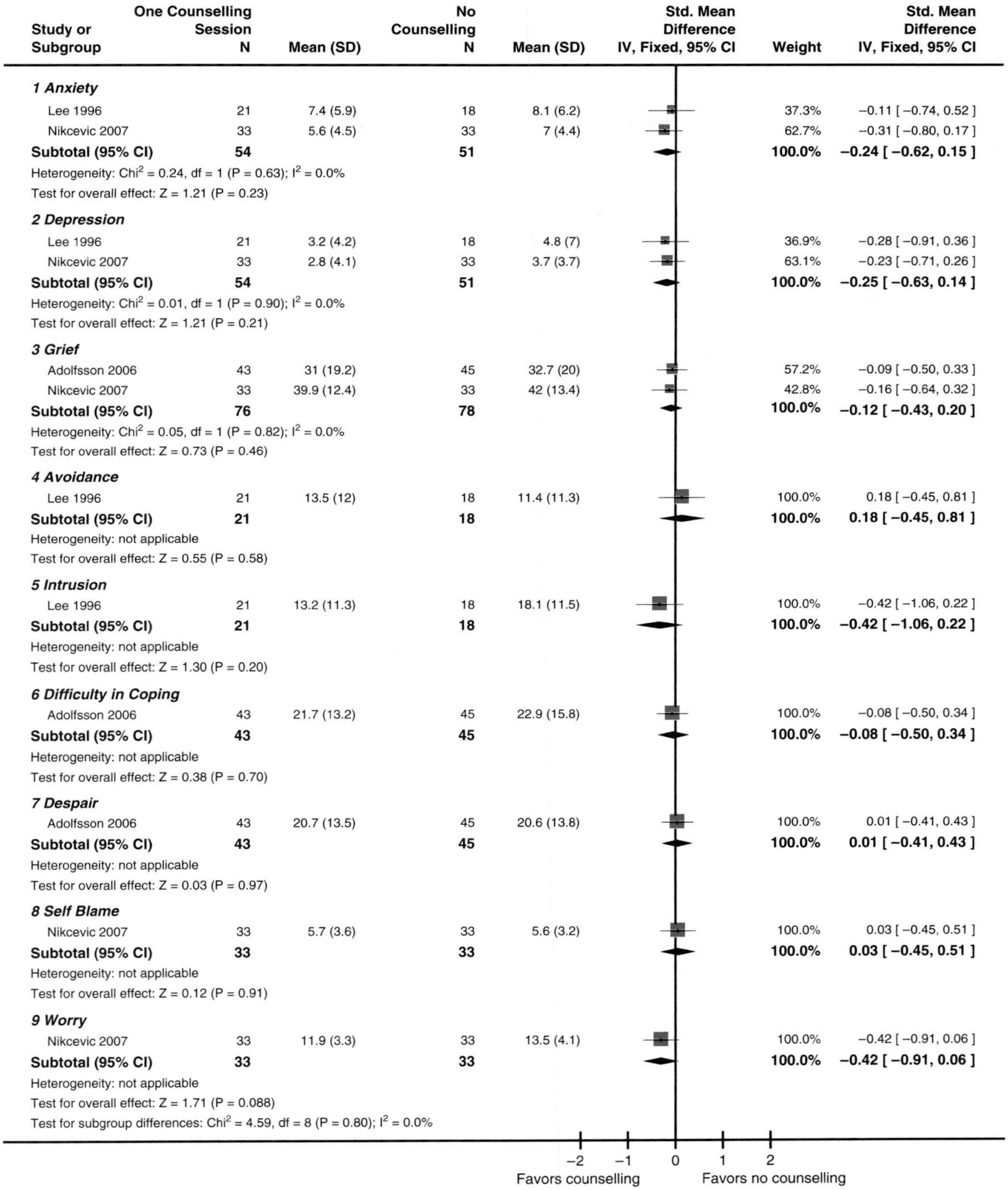

Study or Subgroup	One Counselling Session N	Mean (SD)	No Counselling N	Mean (SD)	Std. Mean Difference IV, Fixed, 95% CI	Weight	Std. Mean Difference IV, Fixed, 95% CI
1 Anxiety							
Lee 1996	21	7.4 (5.9)	18	8.1 (6.2)		37.3%	−0.11 [−0.74, 0.52]
Nikcevic 2007	33	5.6 (4.5)	33	7 (4.4)		62.7%	−0.31 [−0.80, 0.17]
Subtotal (95% CI)	**54**		**51**			**100.0%**	**−0.24 [−0.62, 0.15]**
Heterogeneity: Chi^2 = 0.24, df = 1 (P = 0.63); I^2 = 0.0%							
Test for overall effect: Z = 1.21 (P = 0.23)							
2 Depression							
Lee 1996	21	3.2 (4.2)	18	4.8 (7)		36.9%	−0.28 [−0.91, 0.36]
Nikcevic 2007	33	2.8 (4.1)	33	3.7 (3.7)		63.1%	−0.23 [−0.71, 0.26]
Subtotal (95% CI)	**54**		**51**			**100.0%**	**−0.25 [−0.63, 0.14]**
Heterogeneity: Chi^2 = 0.01, df = 1 (P = 0.90); I^2 = 0.0%							
Test for overall effect: Z = 1.21 (P = 0.21)							
3 Grief							
Adolfsson 2006	43	31 (19.2)	45	32.7 (20)		57.2%	−0.09 [−0.50, 0.33]
Nikcevic 2007	33	39.9 (12.4)	33	42 (13.4)		42.8%	−0.16 [−0.64, 0.32]
Subtotal (95% CI)	**76**		**78**			**100.0%**	**−0.12 [−0.43, 0.20]**
Heterogeneity: Chi^2 = 0.05, df = 1 (P = 0.82); I^2 = 0.0%							
Test for overall effect: Z = 0.73 (P = 0.46)							
4 Avoidance							
Lee 1996	21	13.5 (12)	18	11.4 (11.3)		100.0%	0.18 [−0.45, 0.81]
Subtotal (95% CI)	**21**		**18**			**100.0%**	**0.18 [−0.45, 0.81]**
Heterogeneity: not applicable							
Test for overall effect: Z = 0.55 (P = 0.58)							
5 Intrusion							
Lee 1996	21	13.2 (11.3)	18	18.1 (11.5)		100.0%	−0.42 [−1.06, 0.22]
Subtotal (95% CI)	**21**		**18**			**100.0%**	**−0.42 [−1.06, 0.22]**
Heterogeneity: not applicable							
Test for overall effect: Z = 1.30 (P = 0.20)							
6 Difficulty in Coping							
Adolfsson 2006	43	21.7 (13.2)	45	22.9 (15.8)		100.0%	−0.08 [−0.50, 0.34]
Subtotal (95% CI)	**43**		**45**			**100.0%**	**−0.08 [−0.50, 0.34]**
Heterogeneity: not applicable							
Test for overall effect: Z = 0.38 (P = 0.70)							
7 Despair							
Adolfsson 2006	43	20.7 (13.5)	45	20.6 (13.8)		100.0%	0.01 [−0.41, 0.43]
Subtotal (95% CI)	**43**		**45**			**100.0%**	**0.01 [−0.41, 0.43]**
Heterogeneity: not applicable							
Test for overall effect: Z = 0.03 (P = 0.97)							
8 Self Blame							
Nikcevic 2007	33	5.7 (3.6)	33	5.6 (3.2)		100.0%	0.03 [−0.45, 0.51]
Subtotal (95% CI)	**33**		**33**			**100.0%**	**0.03 [−0.45, 0.51]**
Heterogeneity: not applicable							
Test for overall effect: Z = 0.12 (P = 0.91)							
9 Worry							
Nikcevic 2007	33	11.9 (3.3)	33	13.5 (4.1)		100.0%	−0.42 [−0.91, 0.06]
Subtotal (95% CI)	**33**		**33**			**100.0%**	**−0.42 [−0.91, 0.06]**
Heterogeneity: not applicable							
Test for overall effect: Z = 1.71 (P = 0.088)							
Test for subgroup differences: Chi^2 = 4.59, df = 8 (P = 0.80); I^2 = 0.0%							

−2 −1 0 1 2
Favors counselling   Favors no counselling

FIG. 11.2 An example of a forest plot. *CI,* confidence interval; *df,* degrees of freedom; *IV,* independent variable; *SD,* standard deviation.

is an example of a forest plot from the study by Murphy and colleagues (2012).

Evidence-Informed Practice Tip ____

Evidence-informed practice methods such as meta-analysis increase your ability to manage the ever-increasing volume of information produced to develop the best evidence-informed practices.

Figure 11.2 displays three studies that compared use of one counselling session versus no counselling sessions at 4 months after miscarriage, using different psychological measures of well-being. Each study analyzed is listed. To the right of the listed study is a horizontal line that identifies the effect size estimate for each study. The box on the vertical line represents the effect size of each study and the diamond is the effect or significance of the combined studies. The boxes to the left of the 0 line mean that counselling was favoured or produced a significant effect. The box to the right of the line indicates studies in which counselling was not favoured or significant. The diamond is a more precise estimate of the interventions as it combines the data from the studies. The exemplar provided is basic, as meta-analysis is a sophisticated methodology.

A well-done meta-analysis assesses for bias in studies and provides clinicians a means of deciding the merit of a body of clinical research. Besides the repository of meta-analyses found in The Cochrane Library, published by The Cochrane Collaboration (see Appendix E), meta-analyses can be found published in journals. For example, Cullen, Augenstine, Kaper, and colleagues (2011) conducted a meta-analysis with studies that assessed the feasibility and safety of prehospital hypothermia via data extraction from randomized controlled studies. The article presents an introduction, details of the methods used to search the literature (databases, search terms, and years), data extraction, and analysis. The article also includes an evidence table of the studies reviewed, description of how the data were summarized, results of the meta-analysis, forest plot of the reviewed studies (see Chapter 19), conclusions, and implications for practice and research.

The Cochrane Collaboration

The largest repository of meta-analyses is the Cochrane Collaboration/Review. The Cochrane Collaboration is an international organization that prepares and maintains a body of systematic reviews that focus on health care interventions (Box 11.4). The reviews are found in the Cochrane Database of Systematic Reviews. The Cochrane Collaboration collaborates with a wide range of health care individuals with different skills and backgrounds for developing reviews. These partnerships assist with developing reviews that minimize bias while keeping current with assessment of health care interventions, promoting access to the database, and ensuring the quality of the reviews (Higgins & Green, 2011). Murphy and colleagues' (2012) meta-analysis can be found in the Cochrane Collaboration Database (see Appendix E). The steps of a Cochrane

---

BOX 11.4

COCHRANE REVIEW SECTIONS

- Review information: Authors and contact person
- Abstract
- Plain language summary
- The review
- Background of the question
- Objectives of the search
- Methods for selecting studies for review
- Type of studies reviewed
- Types of participants, types of intervention, types of outcomes in the studies
- Search methods for finding studies
- Data collection
- Analysis of the located studies, including effect sizes
- Results including description of studies, risk of bias, intervention effects
- Discussion
- Implications for research and practice
- References and tables to display the data
- Supplementary information (e.g., appendices, data analysis)

BOX **11.5**

COCHRANE LIBRARY DATABASES

- Cochrane Database of Systematic Reviews: Full-text Cochrane reviews
- Database of Abstracts of Review of Effects (DARE): Critical assessments and abstracts of other systematic reviews that conform to quality criteria
- Cochrane Central Register of Controlled Trials (CENTRAL): Information of studies published in conference proceedings and other sources not available in other databases
- Cochrane Methodology Register (CMR): Bibliographic information on articles and books on reviewing research and methodological studies

BOX **11.6**

INTEGRATIVE REVIEW EXAMPLES

- Cahill, LoBiondo-Wood, Bergstrom, and colleagues (2012) published an integrative review of brain tumour symptoms as an antecedent to uncertainty. This review included a purpose, description of the methods used (databases searched, years included), key terms used, and parameters of the search. These components allow others to evaluate and replicate the search. Twenty-one nonexperimental design studies that assessed brain tumour symptoms and uncertainty were found and reviewed in the text and via a table format.
- Kestler and LoBiondo-Wood (2012) published an integrative review of symptom experience in children and adolescents with cancer. The review was a follow-up of a 2003 review published by Docherty and was completed to assess the progress that has been made since the 2003 research publication on the symptoms of pediatric oncology patients. The review included a description of the search strategy used, including databases, years searched, terms used, and the results of the search. Literature on each symptom was described, and a table of the 52 studies reviewed was included.

Report mirror those of a standard meta-analysis except for the plain language summary. This useful feature is a straightforward summary of the meta-analysis. The Cochrane Library also publishes several other useful databases (Box 11.5).

Integrative Review

Critical reviews of an area of research without a statistical analysis or a theory synthesis are termed *integrative reviews*. An integrative review is the broadest category of review (Whittemore, 2005; Whittemore & Knafl, 2005). It can include theoretical literature, research literature, or both. An integrative review may include methodology studies, a theory review, or the results of differing research studies with wide-ranging clinical implications (Whittemore, 2005). An integrative review can include quantitative or qualitative research, or both. Statistics are not used to summarize and generate conclusions about the studies. Several examples of an integrative review are found in Box 11.6. Recommendations for future research are suggested in each review.

Secondary Analysis

Secondary analysis also is not a design but a form of research in which the previously collected and analyzed data from one study are reanalyzed for a secondary purpose. The original study may be either an experimental or a nonexperimental

design. For example, Dunlop and Fox-Wasylyshyn (2011) conducted a secondary analysis to examine the factors associated with whether or not individuals with acute myocardial infarction (AMI) attribute their symptoms to the heart. The original study was a descriptive study that examined the factors associated with a delay in seeking care in patients with AMI. In another study, Beuthin, Holroyd, Stephenson, and colleagues (2012) conducted a secondary analysis of data from a larger hermeneutic study, designed to help health providers better understand the day-to-day experience of medication use and decision making by older adults living in the community. Data were available from 21 participants selected from Vancouver Island.

Epidemiological Studies

In an **epidemiological study,** factors affecting the health and illness of populations are examined in relation to the environment. The purview of public health for many years, epidemiological studies are investigations of the distribution, determinants, and dynamics of health and disease. In these studies, investigators attempt to link effects with cause; however, a clear understanding of the causes is often not possible, especially when the illness or problem has already occurred and the method is to look retrospectively at the evidence.

Some of the questions that epidemiological researchers attempt to answer are "Did exposure to a certain environment affect health?" and "Does staff shortage or do organizational issues affect burnout?" Research cannot answer such questions directly but can establish a statistically significant association between exposure to causative factors and disease or the effects of ill health.

Two frequently conducted types of epidemiological studies are studies of **prevalence** (the number of people affected by a disease or health problem) and studies of **incidence** (the number of cases occurring in a particular period).

TOOLS FOR EVALUATING INDIVIDUAL STUDIES

As the importance of practising from a base of evidence has grown, so has the need to have tools or instruments available that can assist practitioners in evaluating studies of various types. When evaluating studies for clinical evidence, it is first important to assess whether the study is valid. At the end of each chapter of this text are critiquing questions that will aid you in assessing whether studies are valid and whether the results are applicable to your practice. In addition to these questions, there are standardized appraisal tools that can assist with appraising the evidence. The international collaboration Critical Appraisal Skills Programme (CASP), whose focus is on teaching critical appraisal, developed tools known as Critical Appraisal Skills Programme Checklists that provide an evidence-informed approach for assessing the quality, quantity, and consistency of

specific study designs (CASP, 2017). These instruments are part of an international network that provides consumers with specific questions to help assess study quality. Each checklist has a number of general questions as well as design-specific questions. The tools centre on assessing a study's methodology, validity, and reliability. The questions focus on the following:

1. Are the study's results valid? Understanding the steps of research methodology, especially threats to internal validity as described in the previous and subsequent chapters, will assist in this process (see Chapters 9 through 16).
2. What are the results? This means can you rely on the results (analysis) or the study's findings (see Chapters 16 and 17).
3. Are the findings applicable to your practice? Chapters 19 and 20 are aimed at helping you with this decision.

Each CASP guideline is divided into one of the above three areas in a study. There are eight critical appraisal checklists. The checklist with instructions can be found at http://www.casp-uk.net. The design-specific CASP tools with checklists are available online and include the following:

- Systematic reviews
- Randomized controlled studies
- Cohort studies
- Diagnostic studies
- Case-control studies
- Economic evaluations
- Qualitative studies
- Clinical prediction rule

CLINICAL PRACTICE GUIDELINES

Clinical practice guidelines are systematically developed statements or recommendations that link research and practice and serve as a guide for practitioners. Guidelines have been created to assist in bridging practice and research and are developed by professional organizations, government agencies, institutions, or convened expert panels. Guidelines provide clinicians with an algorithm for clinical management, to assist in decision making for specific diseases (e.g., colon cancer) or for treatments (e.g., pain management). Not all guidelines are well developed and, like research, must be assessed before implementation (see Chapter 9). Guidelines should present scope and purpose of the practice, detail who the development group included, demonstrate scientific rigour, be clear in their presentation, demonstrate clinical applicability, and demonstrate editorial independence. An example is the National Comprehensive Cancer Network, which is an interdisciplinary consortium of 21 cancer centres across the world. Interdisciplinary groups develop practice guidelines for practitioners and education guidelines for patients. These guidelines are accessible at http://www.nccn.org.

The research findings in a clinical practice guideline need to be evaluated for quality, quantity, and consistency. Practice guidelines can be either expert-based or evidence-informed. Evidence-informed practice guidelines are those developed using a scientific process. This process includes first assembling a multidisciplinary group of experts in a specific field. This group is charged with completing a rigorous search of the literature and completing an evidence table that summarizes the quality and strength of the evidence on which the practice guideline is derived (see Chapters 19 and 20). For various reasons, not all areas of clinical practice have a sufficient research base; therefore, expert-based practice guidelines are developed. Expert-based guidelines depend on having a group of nationally known experts in the field who meet and solely use opinions of experts along with whatever research evidence is developed to date. If limited research is available for such a guideline, a rationale should be presented for the practice recommendations.

Many national organizations develop clinical practice guidelines. It is important to know which one to apply to your patient population. For example, there are numerous evidence-informed practice guidelines developed for the management of pain. These guidelines are available from organizations such as the Oncology Nurses Society, American Academy of Pediatrics, National Comprehensive Cancer Network, National Cancer Institute, American College of Physicians, and American Academy of Pain Medicine. As a consumer of evidence, you need to be able to evaluate each of the guidelines and decide which is the most appropriate one for your patient population.

The Agency for Healthcare Research and Quality (AHRQ) supports the National Guideline Clearinghouse (NGC). The NGC's mission is to provide health care providers from all disciplines with objective, detailed information on clinical practice guidelines that are disseminated, implemented, and issued. The NGC encourages groups to develop guidelines for implementation via their site; it is a very useful site to find well-developed clinical practice guidelines on a wide range of health- and illness-related topics. Specific guidelines can be found on the AHRQ Effective Health Care Program website.

Evaluating Clinical Practice Guidelines

As the number of evidence-informed practice guidelines increases, it becomes more important that you critique these guidelines with regard to the methods used for guideline formulation and consider how they might be used in practice. Critical areas that should be assessed when critiquing evidence-informed practice guidelines include the following:

- Date of publication or release and authors
- Endorsement of the guideline
- Clear purpose of what the guideline covers and patient groups for which it was designed
- Types of evidence (research, nonresearch) used in guideline formulation
- Types of research included in formulating the guideline (e.g., "We considered only randomized

and other prospective controlled trials in determining efficacy of therapeutic interventions.")

- Description of the methods used in grading the evidence
- Search terms and retrieval methods used to acquire evidence used in the guideline
- Well-referenced statements regarding practice
- Comprehensive reference list
- Review of the guideline by experts
- Whether the guideline has been used or tested in practice and, if so, with what types of patients and what types of settings

Evidence-informed practice guidelines that are formulated using rigorous methods provide a useful starting point for nurses to understand the evidence base of practice. However, more research may be available since the publication of the guideline, and refinements may be needed. Although information in well-developed, national, evidence-informed practice guidelines are a helpful reference, it is usually necessary to localize the guideline using institution-specific evidence-informed policies, procedures, or standards before application within a specific setting.

There are several tools for appraising the quality of clinical practice guidelines. The Appraisal of Guidelines Research and Evaluation II (AGREE II) instrument is one of the most widely used tools to evaluate the applicability of a guideline to practice (Brouwers, Kho, Browman, et al., 2010). The AGREE II was developed to assist in evaluating guideline quality, provide a methodological strategy for guideline development, and inform practitioners about what information should be reported in guidelines and how it should be reported. The AGREE II is available online and replaces the original AGREE tool. The instrument focuses on six domains with a total of 23 questions rated on a 7-point scale and two final assessment items that require the appraiser to make overall judgments of the guideline based on how the 23 items were rated. Along with the instrument itself, the AGREE Enterprise website offers guidance on tool usage and development. The AGREE II has been tested for reliability and validity. The guideline assesses the following components of a practice guideline:

1. Scope and purpose of the guideline
2. Stakeholder involvement
3. Rigour of guideline development
4. Clarity of presentation of the guideline
5. Applicability of the guideline to practice
6. Demonstrated editorial independence of the developers

APPRAISING THE EVIDENCE

Systematic Reviews and Clinical Practice Guidelines

For each of the review methods described—systematic review, meta-analysis, integrative review, and clinical practice guidelines—think about each method as one that progressively sifts and sorts research studies and the data until the highest quality of evidence is used to arrive at the conclusions. First the researcher combines the results of all the studies that focus on a specific question. The studies considered of lowest quality are then excluded and the data are reanalyzed. This process is repeated sequentially, excluding studies until only the studies of highest quality available are included in the analysis. An alteration in the overall results as an outcome of this sorting and separating process suggests how sensitive the conclusions are to the quality of studies included (Whittemore, 2005). No matter which type of review is completed, it is important to understand that the research studies reviewed still must be examined through your evidence-informed practice lens. This means that evidence that you have derived through your critical appraisal and synthesis or through other researchers' review must be integrated with an individual clinician's expertise and patients' wishes. The criteria for critiquing systematic reviews and clinical practice guidelines are presented in the Critiquing Criteria boxes.

CRITIQUING CRITERIA

Systematic Reviews

1. Does the PICOT (Population, Intervention, Comparison, Outcome, Time) question used as the basis of the review match the studies included in the review?
2. Are the review methods clearly stated and comprehensive?
3. Are the dates of the review's inclusion clear and relevant to the area reviewed?
4. Are the inclusion and exclusion criteria for studies in the review clear and comprehensive?

5. What criteria were used to assess each of the studies in the review for quality and scientific merit?
6. If studies were analyzed individually, were the data clear?
7. Were the methods of study combination clear and appropriate?
8. If the studies were reviewed collectively, how large was the effect?
9. Are the clinical conclusions drawn from the studies relevant and supported by the review?

Clinical practice guidelines, though they are systematically developed and

make explicit recommendations for practice, may be formatted differently. Practice guidelines should reflect the components listed. Guidelines can be located on an organization's website, on the Registered Nurses' Association of Ontario website (http://rnao.ca/bpg), on the AHRQ website (http://www.AHRQ.gov), or on MEDLINE (see Chapters 3 and 20). Well-developed guidelines are constructed using the principles of a systematic review.

CRITIQUING CRITERIA

Clinical Practice Guidelines

1. Is the date of publication or release current?
2. Are the authors of the guideline clear and appropriate to the guideline?
3. Is the clinical problem and purpose clear in terms of what the guideline covers and patient groups for which it was designed?

4. What types of evidence (research, nonresearch) were used in formulating the guideline, and are they appropriate to the topic?
5. Is there a description of the methods used to grade the evidence?
6. Were the search terms and retrieval methods used to acquire research and nonresearch evidence used in the guideline clear and relevant?

7. Is the guideline well referenced and comprehensive?
8. Are the recommendations in the guideline sourced according to the level of evidence for its basis?
9. Has the guideline been reviewed by experts in the appropriate field of discipline?
10. Who funded the guideline development?

Evidence-informed practice requires that you determine—based on the strength and quality of the evidence provided by the systematic review, coupled with your clinical expertise and patient values—whether or not you would consider a change in practice. For example, the meta-analysis by Murphy and colleagues (2012) in Appendix E details the important findings from the literature, some that could be used in nursing practice and some that need further research.

Evidence-Informed Practice Tip _____

Evidence-informed practice methods, such as systematic reviews, increase a nurse's ability to manage the

ever-increasing volume of information produced to develop the best practices that are evidence informed.

Research Hint _____

As you read the literature, you will find studies with labels such as *outcomes research, needs assessments, evaluation research,* and *quality assurance.* These studies are not designs per se; instead, these studies are conducted with either experimental or nonexperimental designs. Studies with these labels are designed to test the effectiveness of health care techniques, programs, or interventions. When reading such a research study, you should assess which design was used and whether the principles of the design, sampling strategy, and analysis are consistent with the study's purpose.

APPRAISING THE EVIDENCE

Nonexperimental Designs

The criteria for critiquing nonexperimental designs are presented in the Critiquing Criteria box. When you critique nonexperimental research designs, keep in mind that such designs offer the researcher the least amount of control. The first step in critiquing nonexperimental research is to determine which type of design was used in the study. Often, a statement describing the design of the study appears in the abstract and in the "Methods" section of the report. If such a statement is not present, you should closely examine the report for evidence of which type of design was employed. You should be able to discern that either a survey or a relationship design was used, as well as the specific subtype. For example, you would expect an investigation of self-concept development in children from birth to 5 years of age to be a relationship study with a longitudinal design.

Next, you should evaluate the theoretical framework and underpinnings of the study to determine whether a nonexperimental design was the most appropriate approach to the problem. For example, in many of the studies on pain discussed throughout this text, the relationship between pain and any of the independent variables under consideration cannot be manipulated. For such studies, a nonexperimental correlational, longitudinal, or cross-sectional design is appropriate. Investigators use one of these designs to examine the relationship between the variables in naturally occurring groups. Sometimes, you may think that it would have been more appropriate for the investigators to use an experimental or a quasiexperimental design. However, you must recognize that pragmatic or ethical considerations also may have guided the researchers in their choice of design (see Chapters 6 and 10).

You should assess whether the problem is at a level of experimental manipulation. Often, researchers merely wish to examine whether relationships exist between variables. Therefore, when you critique such studies, you should be able to determine the purpose of the study. If the purpose of the study does not include the expectation of a cause-and-effect relationship, you need not look for one. However, be wary when the researcher in a nonexperimental study suggests a cause-and-effect relationship in the findings.

Finally, the factor or factors that influence changes in the dependent variable are often ambiguous in nonexperimental designs. As with all complex phenomena, multiple factors can contribute to variability in the participants' responses. When an experimental design is not used for controlling some of these extraneous variables that can influence results, the researcher must strive to provide as much control of these variables as possible within the context of a nonexperimental design.

When it has not been possible to randomly assign participants to treatment groups as an approach to controlling an independent variable, the researcher may use a strategy of matching participants for identified variables. For example, in a study of birth weight, pregnant women could be matched with regard to variables such as weight, height, smoking habits, drug use, and other factors that might influence the birth weights of their infants. The independent variable of interest, such as the type of prenatal care, would then be the major difference in the groups. You would then feel more confident that the only difference between the two groups was the differential effect of the independent variable because the other factors in the two groups were theoretically the same. However, you should also remember that other influential variables—such as income, education, and diet—might have been present but were not considered in matching. Threats to internal and external validity represent a major influence on the interpretation of a nonexperimental study because they impose limitations on the generalizability of the results.

If you are critiquing one of the additional types of research discussed, you must first identify the type of research used; then you must understand its specific purpose and format. The format and methods of secondary analysis, methodological research, and meta-analysis vary; knowing how they vary allows you to assess whether the process was applied appropriately. Some of the basic principles of these methods were presented in this chapter. The specific criteria for evaluating these designs are beyond the scope of this text; the references provided can assist you in this process. Even though the format and methods vary, all research has a central goal: to answer questions scientifically.

CRITIQUING CRITERIA

1. Which nonexperimental design is used in the study?
2. In accordance with the theoretical framework, is the rationale for the type of design evident?
3. How is the design congruent with the purpose of the study?
4. Is the design appropriate for the research problem?
5. Is the design suited to the data-collection methods?
6. Does the researcher present the findings in a manner congruent with the design used?
7. Does the researcher theorize beyond the relational parameters of the findings and erroneously infer cause-and-effect relationships between the variables?
8. Are alternative explanations for the findings possible?
9. How does the researcher discuss the threats to internal and external validity?
10. How does the researcher deal with the limitations of the study?

CRITICAL THINKING CHALLENGES

■ Discuss which type of nonexperimental design might help validate the defining characteristics of a particular nursing diagnosis you use in practice. Do you think it is possible for nurses and patients to serve as the participants in this type of study?
■ The midterm group (five-student) assignment for your research class is to critique an assigned quantitative study. To proceed, you must first decide the study's overall type. You think it is an ex post facto nonexperimental design, whereas the other students think it is an experimental design because the study has several explicit hypotheses. How would you convince the other students that you are correct?
■ You are completing your senior practicum on a surgical step-down unit. The nurses completed an evidence-informed practice protocol for patient-controlled analgesics. Some of the nurses want to implement it immediately, whereas others want to implement it with only some patients. You think that it should be implemented as a research study. Could either of the ways the nurses want to implement the protocol be considered in a research study?
■ You are part of a journal club at your hospital. Your group has been examining a phenomenon specific to your patient population and noticed that 20 correlational studies on the topic have been published. Your group decides to perform a meta-analysis of the data. What steps need to be considered in performing the meta-analysis?

What level of evidence would you expect to obtain with this method? Explain your answer.
■ In reviewing a clinical practice guideline, think about what types of evidence (research, nonresearch) were used in formulating the guideline and whether they are appropriate to the topic. Is there a description of the methods used to grade the evidence? Were the search terms and retrieval methods that were used to acquire research and nonresearch evidence in the guideline clear and relevant? Is the guideline well referenced and comprehensive? Are the recommendations in the guideline sourced according to the level of evidence for its basis?

KEY POINTS

- Nonexperimental research designs are used in studies that make an account of events as they naturally occur. The major difference between nonexperimental and experimental research is that in nonexperimental designs, the independent variable is not actively manipulated by the investigator.
- Nonexperimental designs can be classified either as survey studies or as relationship/difference studies.
- Survey studies and relationship/difference studies are both descriptive and exploratory in nature.
- In survey research, the investigator collects detailed descriptions of existing phenomena

and uses the data either to justify current conditions and practices or to make more intelligent plans for improving them.

- In relationship/difference studies, researchers endeavour to explore the relationships or differences between variables in order to provide deeper insight into the phenomena of interest.
- In correlational studies, researchers examine relationships.
- Developmental studies are further divided into categories of cross-sectional, longitudinal (prospective), and retrospective (ex post facto) studies.
- Methodological research, secondary analysis, meta-analysis, epidemiological studies, and clinical practice guidelines are examples of other means of adding to the body of nursing research. Both the researcher and the reader must consider the advantages and disadvantages of each design.
- Nonexperimental research designs do not enable the investigator to establish cause-and-effect relationships between the variables. You must be wary of nonexperimental studies in which researchers make causal claims about the findings, unless a causal modelling technique is used.
- Nonexperimental designs offer the researcher the least amount of control. Threats to validity represent a major influence on the interpretation of a nonexperimental study because they impose limitations on the generalizability of the results and, as such, should be fully assessed by the critical reader.
- The critiquing process is directed toward evaluating the appropriateness of the selected nonexperimental design in relation to factors such as the research problem, the theoretical framework, the hypothesis, the methodology, and the data analysis and interpretation.
- Although nonexperimental designs do not provide the highest level of evidence (level I), they do provide a wealth of data that become useful for formulating both level I and level II studies that are aimed at developing and testing nursing interventions.

FOR FURTHER STUDY

(e) Go to Evolve at http://evolve.elsevier.com/ Canada/LoBiondo/Research for the Audio Glossary and Appendix Tables that provide supplemental information for Appendix E.

REFERENCES

Akhtar-Danesh, N., Valaitis, R. K., Schofield, R., et al. (2010). A questionnaire for assessing nurses' learning needs. *Western Journal of Nursing Research, 32*(8), 1055–1072.

Bailey, J. J., Sabbagh, M., Loiselle, C. G., et al. (2010). Supporting families in the ICU: A descriptive correlational study of informational support, anxiety, and satisfaction with care. *Intensive & Critical Care Nursing, 26*(2), 114–122.

Benzies, K., Mychasiuk, R., & Tough, S. (2015). What patterns of postpartum psychological distress are associated with maternal concerns about their children's emotional and behavioral problems at the age of three years? *Early Child Development Care, 185*(1), 1–16.

Beuthin, R. E., Holroyd, A., Stephenson, P. H., et al. (2012). Metaphors and medication: Understanding medication use by seniors in everyday life. *Canadian Journal of Nursing Research, 44*(3), 150–168.

Borenstein, M., Hedges, L. V., Higgins, J. P. T., et al. (2009). *Introduction to meta-analysis*. Chichester, UK: Wiley.

Borycki, E. M., Sangster-Gormley, E., Schreiber, R., et al. (2014). How are electronic medical records used by nurse practitioners? *Studies in Health Technology Information, 205*, 196–200.

Brouwers, M., Kho, M. E., Browman, G. P., et al. (2010). AGREE II: Advancing guideline development, reporting and evaluation in healthcare. *Canadian Medical Association Journal, 182*, E839–E842.

Cahill, J., LoBiondo-Wood, G., Bergstrom, N., et al. (2012). Brain tumor symptoms as antecedents to uncertainty: An integrative review. *Journal of Nursing Scholarship, 44*(2), 145–155.

Creamer, A. M., Mill, J., Austin, W., et al. (2014). Canadian nurse practitioners' therapeutic commitment to persons with mental illness. *Canadian Journal of Nursing Research, 46*, 13–32.

Critical Appraisal Skills Programme. (2017). *Critical appraisal skills programme: Making sense of evidence*. Retrieved from http://www.casp-uk.net.

Cullen, D., Augenstine, D., Kaper, L. L., et al. (2011). Therapeutic hypothermia initiated in the pre-hospital setting. *Advanced Emergency Nursing Journal, 33*(4), 314–321.

Docherty, S. L. (2003). Symptom experiences of children and adolescnets with cancer. *Annual Review of Nursing Research, 21,* 123–149.

Dunlop, T., & Fox-Wasylyshyn, S. (2011). Predictors of cardiac symptom attribution among AMI patients. *Canadian Journal of Cardiovascular Nursing, 21*(3), 14–22.

Edwards, M. P., McMillan, D. E., & Fallis, W. M. (2013). Napping during breaks on night shift: Critical care nurse managers' perceptions. *Dynamics (Pembroke, Ont.), 24*(4), 30–35.

Fernandez, S., Franklin, J., Amlani, N., et al. (2015). Physical activity and cancer: A cross-sectional study on the barriers and facilitators to exercise during cancer treatment. *Canadian Oncology Nursing Journal, 25*(1), 37–48.

Fowles, E. R., Cheng, H. R., & Mills, S. (2012). Postpartum health promotion interventions: A systematic review. *Nursing Research, 61*(4), 269–282.

Fox, M. T., Sidani, S., & Brooks, D. (2010). The relationship between bed rest and sitting orthostatic intolerance in adults residing in chronic care facilities. *Journal of Nursing and Healthcare of Chronic Illness, 2*(3), 187–196.

Goff, A.-M. (2011). Stressors, academic performance, and learned resourcefulness in baccalaureate nursing students. *International Journal of Nursing Education Scholarship, 8*(1), Article 1.

Goldie, C. L., Prodan-Bhalla, N., & Mackay, M. (2012). Nurse practitioners in postoperative cardiac surgery: Are they effective? *Canadian Journal of Cardiovascular Nursing, 22*(4), 8–15.

Green, T. L., & King, K. M. (2011). Relationships between biophysical and psychosocial outcomes following minor stroke. *Canadian Journal of Neuroscience Nursing, 33*(2), 15–23.

Higgins, J. P. T., & Green, S. (2011). *Cochrane handbook for systematic reviews of interventions version 5.1.0.* Retrieved from http://handbook.cochrane.org.

Johnston, L. (2005). Critically appraising quantitative evidence. In B. M. Melnyk & E. Fineout-Overholt (Eds.), *Evidence-based practice in nursing and healthcare* (pp. 79–126). Philadelphia: Lippincott Williams & Wilkins.

Kaplan, D. (2008). *Structure equation modeling: Foundations and extensions.* Thousand Oaks, CA: Sage.

Kennedy, E., Tomblin-Murphy, G., Martin-Misener, R., et al. (2015). Development and psychometric assessment of the Nursing Competence Self-Efficacy Scale. *Journal of Nursing Education, 54*(10), 550–558.

Kestler, S. A., & LoBiondo-Wood, G. (2012). Review of symptom experiences in children and adolescents with cancer. *Cancer Nursing, 35*(2), E31–E49.

Laforme, A., Jubinville, S., Gravel, M., et al. (2014). Retrospective analysis of phone queries to an epilepsy clinic hotline. *Canadian Journal of Neuroscience Nursing, 36*(3), 41–45.

Laschinger, H. K., & Nosko, A. (2015). Exposure to workplace bullying and post-traumatic stress disorder symptomology: The role of protective psychological resources. *Journal of Nursing Management, 23*(2), 252–262.

Laschinger, H. K. S., Nosko, A., Wilk, P., et al. (2014). Effects of unit empowerment and perceived support for professional nursing practice on unit effectiveness and individual nurse well-being: A time-lagged study. *International Journal of Nursing Studies, 51*(12), 1615–1623.

Lawrence, K. G., Travis, E. H., & Lawler, S. A. (2012). Tobacco intervention practices of postsecondary campus nurses in Ontario. *Canadian Journal of Nursing Research, 44*(4), 142–159.

Liberati, A., Altman, D. G., Tetzlaff, J., et al. (2009). The PRISMA statement for reporting sys-tematic reviews and meta-analyses of studies that evaluate health care interventions: Explanation and elaboration. *Annals of Internal Medicine, 151*(4), w65–w94.

McInnis-Perry, G., Weeks, L. E., & Stryhn, H. (2013). Age and gender differences in emotional and informational social support insufficiency for older adults in Atlantic Canada. *Canadian Journal of Nursing Research, 45*(4), 50–68.

Merrett, A., Thomas, P., Stephens, A., et al. (2011). A collaborative approach to fall prevention. *Canadian Nurse, 105*(8), 24–29.

Meyer, R. M., O'Brien-Pallas, L., Doran, D., et al. (2014). Boundary spanning by nurse managers: Effects of managers' characteristics and scope of responsibility on teamwork. *Nursing Leadership (Toronto, Ont.), 27*(2), 42–55.

Moher, D., Liberati, A., Tetzlaff, J., et al. (2009). Preferred reporting items for systematic reviews and meta-analyses: The PRISMA statement. *PLOS Medicine, 62*(10), 1006–1012.

Murphy, F. A., Lipp, A., & Powles, D. L. (2012). Follow-up for improving psychological well-being for women after a miscarriage (review). *Cochrane Database System Review, 3,* 1–39.

Newman, K., Doran, D., & Nagle, L. M. (2014). The relation of critical care nurses' information-seeking behaviour with perception of personal control, training, and non-routineness of the task. *Dynamics (Pembroke, Ont.)*, *25*(1), 13–18.

Pagano, M. P., O'Shea, E. R., Campbell S. H., et al. (2015). Validating the Health Communication Assessment Tool© (HCAT). *Clinical Simulation in Nursing*, *11*(9), 402–410.

Rajacich, D., Freeman, M., Armstrong-Stassen, M., et al. (2014). Commuter migration: Work environment factors influencing nurses' decisions regarding choice of employment. *Nursing Leadership*, *27*(2), 56–67.

Raudenbush, S., & Bryk, A. (2002). *Hierarchical linear models: Applications and data analysis methods* (2nd ed.). Newbury Park, CA: Sage.

Roberts, C. A., & Ward-Smith, P. (2010). Choosing a career in nursing: Development of a career search instrument. *International Journal of Nursing Education Scholarship*, *7*(1), Article 2.

Samuels-Dennis, J., Ford-Gilboe, M., Wilk, P., et al. (2010). Cumulative trauma, personal and social resources, and post-traumatic stress symptoms among income-assisted single mothers. *Journal of Family Violence*, *25*(6), 603–617.

Schofield, R., Forchuk, C., Montgomery, P., et al. (2016). Comparing personal health practices: Individuals with mental illness and the general Canadian population. *Canadian Nurse*, *112*(5), 23–27.

Schumacker, R. E., & Lomax, R. C. (2004). *A beginner's guide to structural equation modeling*. Hillsdale, NJ: Erlbaum.

Small, S. P., Kushner, K. E., & Neufeld, A. (2013). Smoking prevention among youth: A multipronged approach involving parents, schools, and society. *Canadian Journal of Nursing Research*, *45*(3), 116–135.

Stephenson, E., DeLongis, A., Steele, R., et al. (2017). Siblings of children with a complex chronic health condition: Maternal posttraumatic growth as a predictor of changes in child behavior problems. *Journal of Pediatric Psychology*, *42*(1), 104–113.

Whittemore, R. (2005). Combining evidence in nursing research: Methods and implications. *Nursing Research*, *54*(1), 56–62.

Whittemore, R., & Knafl, K. (2005). The integrative review: Updated methodology. *Journal of Advanced Nursing*, *52*(5), 546–553.

Wing, T., Regan, S., & Laschinger, H. K. S. (2013). The influence of empowerment and incivility on the mental health of new graduate nurses. *Journal of Nursing Management*, *23*, 632–643.

Wong, C. A., Elliott-Miller, P., Laschinger, H. K. S., et al. (2015). Examining the relationships between span of control and manager job and unit performance outcomes. *Journal of Nursing Management*, *23*, 156–168.

PART FOUR

Processes Related to Research

RESEARCH **VIGNETTE**

Minimizing the Harmful Outcomes Associated with Newborn Pain

Marsha Campbell-Yeo, PhD, NNP, BC RN
Assistant Professor
School of Nursing
Clinician Scientist
IWK Health Centre
Dalhousie University
Halifax, Nova Scotia

As a neonatal nurse practitioner (NNP) and a mother, I know that no parent wants to see their child in pain. Sadly, the parents of sick and/or preterm infants see their children in pain regularly. Preterm and sick babies often experience an average of 12 painful procedures every single day. To make matters worse, the majority of these procedures are conducted with little or no pain relief. As recently as the 1980s, it was commonly thought that babies could not feel pain and even surgeries were performed without anaesthetic. It was only through research that we now know that not only do babies experience the immediate pain and stress of a painful procedure, but untreated or undertreated pain during a baby's early life leads to immediate and long-term consequences, such as alteration in their brain microstructure associated with learning and motor delays, behaviour problems, and lower academic achievement later in life.

As someone who had provided intensive care to babies and their families for over 25 years, it was clearly evident to me that in addition to seeing the suffering endured by the babies and their families, nurses told me how stressful it was to repeatedly be asked to perform painful procedures on babies without the benefit of really knowing what they could do to provide optimal relief. I was driven to use research to examine how we, as nurses and health care providers, could minimize the harmful outcomes associated with newborn pain. In addition, I wanted to determine the best ways to ensure that this evidence actually reached and benefited patients through practice uptake and change in the clinical setting. One of the first things that my colleagues and I did was try to look beyond all the medical technology used in the neonatal intensive care unit (NICU) and consider interventions that blended high-tech care with a more humanistic approach. Historically, we knew that mothers have always been a critical component of infant survival and well-being, but I noticed that mothers were not always incorporated into their infant's care in the critical care setting. Moreover, we knew that, in addition to frequent exposure to pain and stress, the developmental trajectory of vulnerable preterm infants could be further negatively influenced by the separation of the mother and baby dyad, a too common occurrence in the NICU. I decided to research this topic to explore how mothers and families could be better involved in the care of their newborns, to minimize infant pain and improve the long-term outcomes for preterm and sick newborns and their families. As a clinician, I had seen first-hand the positive impact that human touch (e.g., skin-to-skin contact, facilitated tucking, breastfeeding, and massage) could have on infants and mothers. I became particularly interested in skin-to-skin contact (SSC), commonly referred to as kangaroo care (KC), which is the upright holding of a diaper-clad infant on his or her mother's chest. SSC has been associated with numerous immediate benefits in a nonpain context in both developed and developing countries.

In collaboration with my PhD supervisor, Dr. Celeste Johnston, I began a series of studies to determine the effect of SSC on preterm babies' behavioural response when provided during a routine heel lance procedure. We were able to demonstrate significant reduction in composite pain scores, measured using the Premature Infant Pain Profile, a valid and reliable pain assessment tool. We found pain-relieving benefits for babies born between 32 and 36 weeks gestational age and even babies delivered as early as 28 weeks gestational age (Johnston, Filion, Campbell-Yeo, et al., 2008). We also determined that while SSC provided by mothers appeared to have the greatest benefit, dads or alternate providers, such as aunts, grandmothers, and nurses, could help too (Johnston, Campbell-Yeo, & Filion, 2011)! I was the first to examine the effects of putting preterm twins in the same incubator to see if this would reduce their stress response to the many needle procedures that they undergo. The thought behind this process, called *co-bedding*, was that it may be helpful for the twins (who might be face-to-face, back-to-back, or in the spooning position), as this could provide comfort due to the human contact, the familiar smell, or just the company. In a randomized trial, we found that co-bedded preterm twins recovered more quickly (heart rate and oxygen saturation) and had a more stable stress response (lower cortisol levels) than twins cared for in separate incubators (Campbell-Yeo, Johnston, Joseph, et al., 2012). We also found that co-bedding had no adverse effects on either the twin who had the painful procedure or the other twin (Campbell-Yeo, Johnston, Joseph, et al., 2014).

We then decided to create a synthesis of all the evidence examining the impact that mothers and families can have in minimizing their baby's pain through SSC. I co-led a review, "Skin-to-Skin Care for Procedural Pain in Neonates (Johnston, Campbell-Yeo, Fernandes, et al., 2014). This Cochrane review found that SSC between mothers and babies significantly decreased pain in preterm and full-term infants during a single painful procedure such as heel lance, venipuncture, and intramuscular injection when compared with no treatment and appeared to be equally effective as sweet-tasting solutions, considered standard of care. From this finding, I decided to expand on the idea and explore whether the

beneficial effects of SSC would be sustained over time and could minimize pain when used during all of the common needle-related procedures experienced in the NICU. I ran a clinical trial called "Trial of Repeated Analgesia in Kangaroo Care" (TRAKC), which investigated how preterm babies who received SSC differed developmentally at discharge from the NICU compared with babies who only got a sweet-tasting solution (sucrose) during their painful procedures (Campbell-Yeo, Johnston, Benoit, et al., 2013). Our preliminary findings tell us that it does. We would never have been able to answer these important clinical questions without the dedication and support of all the nurses and neonatal team in our NICU to ensure that the babies' group allocation was maintained during their entire hospital stay. It definitely takes a village to conduct clinical research. We are now following up with these babies at 18 months of age (TRAKC18) to see if the SSC provided during painful procedures in early life influences how these toddlers respond to pain, their relationship with their mothers, and their current behavioural development (Campbell-Yeo & Dol, 2000–2016). We are excited to soon be able to answer these questions.

One thing we also found was that while nurses who were provided education related to the use of SSC reported feeling more comfortable and had less concerns about using SSC in their practice, their actual use of SSC over a 6-month period did not change (Benoit, Campbell-Yeo, Johnston,

et al., 2016). Some of the reasons for this included ergonomic concerns, unit routines, and lack of maternal presence. I felt that I had to find a way to let moms and dads know the positive impact that they can have on reducing the pain newborns experience in their early lives. We asked parents and many told us that they thought the Internet was the best way to find out information about their baby. Thus, I decided to create a parent-friendly video, titled *The Power of a Parent's Touch* (Campbell-Yeo, Chambers, Taddio, et al., 2014). This video is meant to empower parents to help them minimize their baby's pain during their stay in the NICU. The English video launched in December of 2014 and has now been translated using subtitles in seven languages (Portuguese, Spanish, French [Canada], German, Russian, Arabic, and Chinese [traditional]) and has a significant reach. To date, it has been viewed over 160,000 times in over 152 countries.

It is not just the 1 in 10 babies that are born preterm worldwide that experience untreated pain. Untreated pain is an issue for every baby, even those that are born healthy. All babies undergo painful procedures in their first few days, with many experiencing up to 20 injections during their early years. Nurses are one of the primary providers that perform needle-related procedures and have the greatest parental interactions. Not only is it imperative that nurses utilize effective interventions to relieve pain, but they should also support parents to advocate for better pain relief and encourage their active involvement and partnership in their child's pain management. Parents are one of the most under-utilized resources to help manage and relieve procedural pain. We need to change that because parents can make a substantial difference. ■

REFERENCES

Benoit, B., Campbell-Yeo, M., Johnston, C., et al. (2016). Staff nurse utilization of kangaroo care as an intervention for procedural pain in preterm infants. *Advances in Neonatal Care, 16*(3), 229–238.

Campbell-Yeo, M., Chambers, C. C., Taddio, A., et al. (2014, December 2). *The power of a parent's touch* [Video file]. Retrieved from https://www.youtube.com/watch?v=3nqN9c3FWn8.

Campbell-Yeo, M., & Dol, J. (2000–2016). *Trial of Repeated Analgesia with Kangaroo Care—18-month follow-up (TRAKC18)*. Bethesda, MD: National Library of Medicine (US). Retrieved from https://clinicaltrials.gov/ct2/show/NCT02694692.

Campbell-Yeo, M., Johnston, C., Benoit, B., et al. (2013). Trial of repeated analgesia with kangaroo mother care. *BMC Pediatrics, 13*, 182.

Campbell-Yeo, M., Johnston, C. C., Joseph, K. S., et al. (2012). Co-bedding and recovery time after heel lance in preterm twins: Results of a randomized trial [NCT00917631]. *Pediatrics, 130*(3), 500–506.

Campbell-Yeo, M., Johnston, C. C., Joseph, K. S., et al. (2014). Co-bedding between preterm twins attenuates stress response following heel lance: Results of a randomized trial. *Clinical Journal of Pain, 30*(7), 598–604.

Johnston, C. C., Campbell-Yeo, M., Fernandes, A., et al. (2014). Skin-to-skin care for procedural pain in neonates (full review). *Cochrane Database System Reviews, 1*, CD008435.

Johnston, C. C., Campbell-Yeo, M., & Filion, F. (2011). Paternal versus maternal kangaroo care for procedural pain in preterm neonates. *Archives of Pediatrics & Adolescent Medicine, 165*(9), 792–796.

Johnston, C. C., Filion, F., Campbell-Yeo, M., et al. (2008). Kangaroo mother care diminishes pain from heel lance in very preterm neonates: A crossover trial. *BMC Pediatrics, 8*, 13.

CHAPTER 12

Sampling

Judith Haber | Mina D. Singh

LEARNING OUTCOMES

After reading this chapter, you will be able to do the following:

- Identify the purpose of sampling.
- Define population, sample, and sampling.
- Compare a population and a sample.
- Discuss the eligibility criteria for sample selection.
- Define nonprobability sampling and probability sampling.
- Identify the types of strategies for both nonprobability and probability sampling.
- Identify the types of qualitative sampling.
- Compare the advantages and disadvantages of specific nonprobability and probability sampling strategies.
- Discuss the contribution of nonprobability and probability sampling strategies to the strength of evidence provided by study findings.
- Discuss the factors that influence determination of sample size.
- Discuss the procedure for drawing a sample.
- Identify the criteria for critiquing a sampling plan.
- Use the critiquing criteria to evaluate the "Sample" section of a research report.

KEY TERMS

accessible population
cluster sampling
convenience sampling
data saturation
delimitations
effect size
element
eligibility criteria
heterogeneity
homogeneous
matching

multistage sampling
network sampling
nonprobability sampling
pilot study
population
probability sampling
purposive sampling
quota sampling
random selection
representative sample
sample

sampling
sampling frame
sampling interval
sampling unit
simple random sampling
snowball effect sampling
stratified random sampling
systematic sampling
target population
theoretical sampling

STUDY RESOURCES

SAMPLING IS THE PROCESS OF SELECTING representative units of a population for study in a research investigation. Although sampling is a complex process, it is a familiar one. In their daily lives, people gather knowledge, make decisions, and formulate predictions on the basis of sampling procedures. For example, nursing students may make generalizations about the overall quality of nursing professors as a result of their exposure to a sample of nursing professors during their undergraduate programs. Patients may make generalizations about a hospital's food or quality of nursing care during a 1-week hospital stay. Limited exposure to a limited portion of these phenomena forms the basis of people's conclusions, so much of their knowledge and many of their decisions are based on their experience with samples.

Researchers also derive knowledge from samples. Many questions in scientific and naturalistic research cannot be answered without the use of sampling procedures. For example, when the effectiveness of a new education intervention for diabetic patients is tested, the intervention is administered to a sample of the population. The researcher must come to some conclusions without giving the intervention to the entire population of diabetic patients. To obtain the experiences or outcomes of engaging in this education, the researcher needs to select the appropriate sampling strategy in accordance with the research design and question. This is done to avoid erroneous conclusions or making generalizations from a nonrepresentative sample. Thus, research methodologists have expended considerable effort to develop sampling theories and procedures that produce accurate and meaningful information.

Essentially, researchers sample representative segments of the population because sampling the entire population of interest to obtain relevant information is rarely feasible or necessary.

This chapter will familiarize you with the basic concepts of sampling as they pertain to the principles of quantitative and qualitative research designs, nonprobability and probability sampling, sample size, and the related critiquing process.

SAMPLING CONCEPTS

Population

A **population** is a well-defined set that has certain specified properties or characteristics from which data can be gathered and analyzed. A population can be composed of people, animals, objects, or events. For example, if a researcher is studying undergraduate nursing students, the type of educational preparation of the population must be specified. In this example, the population consists of undergraduate students enrolled in a generic baccalaureate nursing program. Examples of other possible populations might be all female patients admitted to a certain hospital for lumpectomies for treatment of breast cancer during 2016, all children with asthma in the province of Alberta, or all men and women with a diagnosis of schizophrenia in North America. These examples illustrate that a population may be broadly defined and potentially involve millions of people, or it may be narrowly specified to include only a few people.

When you read a research report, you should consider whether the researcher has identified the population descriptors that form the basis for the inclusion (eligibility) or exclusion criteria (delimitations) that are used to select the sample from the array of all possible units, whether people, objects, or events. Consider the population previously defined as undergraduate nursing students enrolled in a generic baccalaureate program. Would this population include both part-time and full-time students? Would it include students who had previously attended another nursing program? What about international students? At which level (first year through senior year) would students qualify? As much as possible, the researcher must specifically delineate the exact criteria used to decide whether an individual would be classified as a member of a given population. The population descriptors that provide the basis for inclusion (eligibility) criteria should be evident in the sample; in other words, the characteristics of the population and the sample should be congruent. The degree of congruence is evaluated to assess the representativeness of the sample. For example, if a population is defined as full-time, Canadian-born, senior-level nursing students enrolled in a generic baccalaureate nursing program, the sample would be expected to reflect these characteristics.

Think about the concept of inclusion criteria, or **eligibility criteria** (characteristics of a population that meet requirements for inclusion in a study), applied to a research study in which the participants are patients. For example, in an investigation of the effects of music on dyspnea during exercise in individuals with chronic obstructive pulmonary disease (COPD), the participants had to meet all of the following inclusion (eligibility) criteria:

1. A confirmed medical diagnosis of COPD (i.e., chronic bronchitis, emphysema, or both)
2. Ability to speak and read English
3. Ability to ambulate independently
4. Experiencing dyspnea at least once a week
5. An increase in the level of dyspnea of at least two points on the Borg scale after a 6-minute walk

Examples of exclusion criteria, or **delimitations** (characteristics that restrict the population to a homogeneous group of participants), include gender, age, marital status, socioeconomic status, religion, ethnicity, level of education, age of children, health status, and diagnosis. In a study examining changes in functional status between time of eligibility assessment and transcatheter aortic valve implantation (TAVI), Forman, Currie, Lauck, and colleagues (2015) established the following exclusion criteria: patients undergoing a TAVI in conjunction with another surgical procedure, non-English-speaking individuals, participants who scored less than 25/30 on the Mini–Mental State Examination (MMSE) at the time of eligibility assessment, and those who scored less than 20/30 on the MMSE during the assessment of functional status. These exclusion criteria were selected because of their potential effect to confound functional status with lower mental state.

As another example, in an exploratory mixed-methods study investigating patient quality of life, caregiver burden, and family outcomes after aggressive surgical interventions for severe stroke, Green, Demchuk, and Newcommon (2015) stated clear inclusion and exclusion criteria. The inclusion criteria were age ≥ 16 years at the time of the stroke; initial stroke classified as severe; patients who had undergone surgical intervention for stroke, including decompression craniotomy and/or clot removal for malignant middle cerebral artery infarctions; subarachnoid hemorrhage; able to read and understand English; able to provide informed consent; and able to complete survey questionnaires, either in person or by telephone. Exclusion criteria included patients with severe cognitive impairment or receptive or global aphasia, no identified caregiver, and unable to read and understand English or provide informed consent.

The **heterogeneity,** or dissimilarities, of a sample group inhibits the researchers' ability to interpret the findings meaningfully and to make generalizations. It is much wiser to study only one **homogeneous** group—that is, a group with limited variation in attributes or characteristics, or to include specific groups as distinct subsets of the sample and study the groups comparatively, as was the case in Ostry, Maggi, Hershler, and colleagues' (2010) study. These researchers sought to determine mental health outcomes in sawmill workers in British Columbia. They compared rural workers with urban workers and, after controlling for socioeconomic variables, concluded that rural sawmill workers had better outcomes.

Remember that exclusion criteria or delimitations are not established in a casual or meaningless way but are established to control for extraneous variability or bias. Each exclusion criterion should have a rationale, presumably related to a potential contaminating effect on the dependent variable. Carefully established sample exclusion criteria increase the precision of the study and contribute to accuracy while constraining the generalizability or transferability of the findings (see Chapter 9).

The population criteria establish the **target population**—that is, the entire set of cases about which the researcher would like to make generalizations. A target population might include all undergraduate nursing students enrolled in generic baccalaureate programs in Canada. Because of time, money, and personnel, however, using a target population is often not feasible. An **accessible population**—one that meets the population criteria and is available—is used instead. For example, an accessible population might include all full-time generic baccalaureate students attending school in Manitoba. Pragmatic factors must also be considered in identifying a potential population of interest.

 Research Hint

Often, researchers do not clearly identify the population under study, or the population is not clarified until the "Discussion" section, when an effort is made to discuss the group (population) to which the study findings can be generalized.

A population is not restricted to human participants. The population may consist of hospital records; blood, urine, or other specimens taken from patients at a clinic; historical documents; or laboratory animals. For example, a population might consist of all urine specimens collected from patients in the Mount Sinai Hospital antepartum clinic or all patient charts on file at a day surgery centre. A population can be defined in a variety of ways. Of importance is that the basic unit of the population be clearly defined, because the generalizability of the findings is a function of the population criteria.

 Evidence-Informed Practice Tip

Consider whether the sample selection was biased, thereby influencing the validity of the evidence provided by the outcomes of the study.

Samples and Sampling

Sampling is a process of selecting a portion or subset of the designated population to represent the entire population. A **sample** is a set of elements that make up the population; an **element** is the most basic unit about which information is collected. The most common element in nursing research is individuals, but other elements (e.g., places or objects) can form the basis of a sample or population. For example, a researcher plans a study to compare the effectiveness of different nursing interventions on reducing falls in older adults in long-term care facilities. Four facilities, each of which having a different treatment protocol, are identified as the sampling units—not the nurses themselves or the treatment alone. A sampling unit can be an organization, a group, or an individual person.

The purpose of sampling is to increase the efficiency of a research study. Examining every element or unit in the population would not be feasible. When sampling is done properly, the researcher can draw inferences and make generalizations about the population without examining each unit in the population.

In qualitative research, the results can have good generalizability to the population under study. Sampling procedures that entail the formulation of specific criteria for selection ensure that the characteristics of the phenomena of interest will be, or are likely to be, present in all of the elements being studied. The researcher's efforts to ensure that the sample is representative of the target population provide a stronger position from which to draw conclusions from the sample findings that are generalizable to the population (see Chapter 9).

After reviewing a number of research studies, you will recognize that samples and sampling procedures vary in terms of merit. The foremost criterion in evaluating a sample is its representativeness. A **representative sample** has key characteristics that closely approximate those of the population. For instance, if 70% of the population in a study of child-rearing practices consisted of women and 40% were full-time employees, a representative sample should reflect these characteristics in the same proportions.

The representativeness of a sample cannot be guaranteed without access to a database about the entire population. Because it is difficult and inefficient to assess an entire population, the researcher must employ sampling strategies that minimize or control for sample bias. If an appropriate sampling strategy is used, the sample data will almost always enable a reasonably accurate understanding of the phenomena under investigation.

Evidence-Informed Practice Tip ____

Determining whether the sample is representative of the population being studied in journal articles will influence both your interpretation of the evidence provided by the findings and your decision making about the findings' relevance to the your patient population and practice setting.

SAMPLING STRATEGIES USED IN QUANTITATIVE RESEARCH

Sampling strategies are generally grouped into two categories: *nonprobability sampling* and *probability sampling*. In **nonprobability sampling,** elements are chosen through nonrandom methods. The drawback of this strategy is that each element's probability of being included in the samples cannot be estimated. In other words, ensuring that every element has a chance for inclusion in the nonprobability sample is not possible. In **probability sampling,** some form of random selection is used when the sample units are chosen. This type of sample enables the researcher to estimate the probability that each element of the population will be included in the sample. Probability sampling is the more rigorous sampling strategy used in quantitative research and is more likely to result in a representative sample.

The remainder of this section is devoted to a discussion of different types of nonprobability and probability sampling strategies. A summary of sampling strategies appears in Table 12.1. You may refer to this table as the various nonprobability and probability strategies are discussed in the following sections. Note that if there is bias in sampling, it will distort the analysis and the findings of the study.

Research Hint _____

Research articles are not always explicit about the type of sampling strategy that was used. If the sampling strategy is not specified, assume that in a quantitative study, a convenience sample was used and that in a qualitative study, a purposive sample was used.

Nonprobability Sampling

Because of a lack of random selection, the nonprobability sampling strategy is less generalizable than probability sampling because it tends to produce less representative samples. Such samples are more feasible for the researcher to obtain, however, and most samples—in nursing

TABLE 12.1

SUMMARY OF SAMPLING STRATEGIES

SAMPLING STRATEGY	EASE OF DRAWING A REPRESENTATIVE SAMPLE	RISK OF BIAS	REPRESENTATIVENESS OF THE SAMPLE
NONPROBABILITY			
Convenience	Very easy	Greater than in any other sampling strategy	Because samples tend to be self-selecting, representativeness is questionable
Quota	Relatively easy	Contains an unknown source of bias that affects external validity	Builds in some representativeness by using knowledge about the population of interest
Purposive	Relatively easy	Bias increases with greater heterogeneity of the population; conscious bias is also a danger but is offset with maximal variation	Very limited ability to generalize because the sample is handpicked from a quantitative view, but this approach is necessary for the qualitative researcher to choose participants on the basis of the phenomenon under study
Network	Can be easy if the network is accessible	Minimal if a thorough sampling plan is developed	Represents the event, incident, or experience being studied
Theoretical	Requires a two-stage process; can be prolonged	Minimal if a thorough sampling plan is developed	Typically begins with another type of sampling, such as convenience or criterion sampling aimed at variation in the phenomenon, and thus represents aspects of the theory being constructed
PROBABILITY			
Simple random	Laborious	Low	Maximized; the probability of nonrepresentativeness decreases with increased sample size
Stratified random	Time-consuming	Low	Enhanced
Cluster	Less time consuming than simple or stratified sampling	Subject to more sampling errors than is simple or stratified sampling	Less representative than simple or stratified sampling
Systematic	More convenient and efficient than is simple, stratified, or cluster sampling	Bias in the form of nonrandomness can be inadvertently introduced	Less representative if bias occurs as a result of coincidental nonrandomness

research and the research of other disciplines— are nonprobability samples. When a nonprobability sample reflects the target population through the careful use of inclusion and exclusion criteria, you can have more confidence in the representativeness of the sample and the external validity of the findings. The major types of nonprobability sampling used in quantitative research are *convenience sampling* and *quota sampling*.

Convenience Sampling

Convenience sampling is the use of the most readily accessible persons or objects as participants in a study. The participants may include volunteers, the first 25 patients admitted to a certain hospital with a particular diagnosis, all of the people who enrolled in a certain program during the month of September, or all of the students enrolled in a certain course at a particular university during 2015. The participants are convenient and accessible to the researcher; hence the term *convenience sample.*

As an example, in developing a model to determine factors influencing job satisfaction over time, Cummings, Raymond-Seniuk, Lo, and associates (2013) used convenience sampling to obtain for their study 338 full-time and part-time nurses who provided direct care to cancer patients in a variety of settings. In another study, El-Masri, Omar, and Groh (2015) used a convenience sample of 311 participants to evaluate the effectiveness of a nurse practitioner–led outreach program on the health outcomes, emergency department (ED) transfers, and hospital admissions of long-term care residents. In their study exploring quality of life, caregiver burden, and family outcomes, Green and associates (2015) also obtained a convenience sample from patients who were discharged home from a large tertiary care facility after undergoing aggressive surgical intervention after a severe stroke.

The advantage of a convenience sample is that it can be an easy way for the researcher to obtain participants. The researcher may need to be concerned only with obtaining a sufficient number of participants who meet the same criteria. The major disadvantage of a convenience sample is that the risk of bias is greater than in any other type of sample (see Table 12.1). Because convenience samples entail voluntary participation, the probability that researchers will recruit people who feel strongly about the issue being studied is increased, which may favour certain outcomes of the study. The problem of bias is related to the tendency of convenience samples to be self-selecting; in other words, the researcher obtains information only from the people who volunteer

to participate. In this case, the following questions must be raised:

- What motivated some of the people to participate and others not to participate?
- What kind of data would have been obtained if nonparticipants had also responded?
- How representative of the population are the people who did participate?

For example, a researcher may stop people on a street corner to ask their opinion on an issue; place advertisements in the newspaper; put signs in local churches, community centres, or supermarkets; or search specific agencies websites to recruit volunteers for a particular study. To describe the practices, attitudes, and beliefs of nursing educators in Quebec with regard to teaching smoking cessation strategies to undergraduate students, Lepage, Dumas, and Saint-Pierre (2015) recruited participants by drawing up a list of emails from educational institutions websites. To assess the degree to which a convenience sample approximates a random sample, a researcher can compare the convenience sample data with the known demographic information and examine variability around the mean. In this manner, the researcher checks for the representativeness of the convenience sample and the extent to which bias is or is not evident.

Because recruiting research participants is crucial for nurse researchers, innovative recruitment strategies are sometimes used. For example, a researcher may offer to pay the participants for their time. A relatively new method of accessing and recruiting participants is through online computer networks (e.g., disease-specific chat rooms and bulletin boards).

In evaluating a research report, you should recognize that the convenience sample strategy, although the most common, is the weakest form of sampling strategy in quantitative research in terms of generalizability. When a convenience sample is used, researchers should analyze and interpret the data cautiously. When you critique a research study in which this sampling strategy was used, you should be skeptical about the external validity of the findings (see Chapter 9).

Quota Sampling

Quota sampling refers to a form of nonprobability sampling in which knowledge about the population of interest is used to ensure some representativeness about the sample (see Table 12.1). Through quota sampling, the researcher identifies a particular strata of the population, and the quota sample proportionally represents the strata. For example, the data in Table 12.2 reveal that of the 5,000 nurses in a particular city, 20% are diploma graduates, 40% are post–RN degree graduates, and 40% are baccalaureate graduates. Each of these strata should be proportionately represented in the sample. In this case, the researcher used a proportional quota sampling strategy and decided to include 10% of a population of 5,000 (i.e., 500 nurses). On the basis of the proportion of each stratum in the population, 100 diploma graduates, 200 post-RN graduates, and 200 baccalaureate graduates were the quotas established for the three strata. The researcher recruited participants who met the eligibility criteria of the study until the quota for each stratum was filled. In other words, once the researcher obtained the necessary 100 diploma graduates, 200 post-RN graduates, and 200 baccalaureate graduates, the sample was complete with regard to both the research design and other pragmatic matters, such as economy.

The researcher systematically ensures that proportional segments of the population are included in the sample. For example, in Im, Chang, Ko, and colleagues' (2012) study exploring midlife women's attitudes toward physical activity, the researchers stratified a quota sample of 542 subjects by ethnicity and socioeconomic status. An example of nonproportional quota sampling is in the study by Fox, Sidani, and Brooks (2010), who examined differences in sleep complaints among adults with varying amounts of bed rest who were residing in extended-care facilities for chronic disease management. The three cohorts (comparative, moderate, and high) reflected different amounts of bed rest that were naturally occurring. To ensure equal representation of the different amounts of bed rest, nonproportional quota sampling was used.

The characteristics chosen to form the strata are selected according to a researcher's judgement on the basis of knowledge of the population and the literature review. The criterion for selection should be a variable that reflects important differences in the independent variables under investigation. Age, gender, religion, ethnicity, medical diagnosis, socioeconomic status, level of completed education, and occupation are among the variables that are likely to be important in stratifying samples in nursing research investigations.

In critiquing a research strategy, you need to determine whether the sample strata appropriately reflect the population under consideration and whether the variables used are homogeneous enough to ensure a meaningful comparison. Even when the researcher has addressed these factors, you must remember that a quota strategy is a nonprobability sample and thus includes an

TABLE **12.2**

NUMBERS AND PERCENTAGES OF STUDENTS IN STRATA OF A QUOTA SAMPLE OF 5,000 GRADUATES OF NURSING PROGRAMS IN A PARTICULAR CITY

CATEGORIES	DIPLOMA GRADUATES	ASSOCIATE DEGREE GRADUATES	BACCALAUREATE GRADUATES
Strata	1,000 (20%)	2,000 (40%)	2,000 (40%)
Quota sample	100	200	200

unknown source of bias that affects the external validity. The people who choose to participate may not be typical of the population in terms of the variables being measured, and assessing the possible biases that may be operating is not possible. When the phenomena being investigated are relatively similar within the population, the risk of bias may be minimal; however, in heterogeneous populations, the risk of bias is greater.

 Evidence-Informed Practice Tip _____

> When you think about applying study findings to your clinical practice, consider whether the participants in the sample are similar to your own patients.

Probability Sampling

The primary characteristic of probability sampling is the random selection of elements from the population. In **random selection,** each element of the population has an equal and independent chance of being included in the sample. In the hierarchy of evidence, probability sampling represents the strongest type of sampling strategy. That means there is greater confidence that the sample is representative rather than biased and that it more closely reflects the characteristics of the population of interest. Four commonly used probability sampling strategies are *simple random sampling, stratified random sampling, cluster sampling,* and *systematic sampling.*

Random selection of sample participants should not be confused with random assignment of participants. As discussed in Chapter 10, *randomization* refers to the assignment of participants to either an experimental or a control group on a purely random basis.

Simple Random Sampling

Simple random sampling is a laborious and carefully controlled process. Because the principles of simple random sampling are incorporated in the more complex probability designs, the principles of this strategy are presented.

In **simple random sampling,** the researcher defines the population (a set), lists all units of the population (a **sampling frame**), and selects a sample of units (a subset) from which the sample will be chosen. For example, if Canadian hospitals specializing in the treatment of cancer were the sampling unit, a list of all such hospitals would be the sampling frame. If certified adult nurse practitioners constituted the accessible population, a list of those nurses would be the sampling frame.

Once a list of the population elements has been developed, the best method of selecting a sample is to employ a table of random numbers containing columns of digits, as shown in Figure 12.1. Such tables can be generated by computer programs. For example, Mackenzie, Ireland, Moore, and associates (2013), who evaluated the effectiveness of a nursing intervention on the management of blood pressure in patients who have had a stroke, used a random sampling with the help of a centralized telephone randomization system. The system generated a random blocking table, which ensured even distribution of the control and experimental group in all the four sites of the study. After assigning consecutive numbers to units of the population, the researcher starts at any point on the table of random numbers and reads consecutive numbers in any direction (i.e., horizontally, vertically, or diagonally). When a number is read that corresponds with the written unit on a card, that unit is chosen for the sample. The investigator continues to read until a sample of the desired size is drawn. As an example, Rajacich, Kane, Lafreniére, et al. (2014) used simple random sampling to select 1,300 male nurses working in acute-care settings in Ontario to study environmental work factors on job satisfaction and intention to stay in the profession.

The advantages of simple random sampling are as follows:
- The sample selection is not subject to the conscious biases of the researcher.
- The representativeness of the sample is maximized in relation to the population characteristics.

1,000 random integers between 0 and 99

40	23	0	29	10	94	17	58	12	85	13	25	80	84	72	74	54	63	55	31
32	98	59	23	74	97	51	42	21	87	48	64	54	38	84	68	14	17	35	48
84	34	84	14	53	65	67	37	2	45	84	21	71	34	10	80	72	27	11	13
86	37	24	89	23	4	44	40	72	81	44	69	25	44	34	34	34	75	50	50
50	58	85	8	22	24	73	20	63	35	60	87	91	92	96	80	19	22	87	24
1	87	43	82	9	31	40	88	33	28	82	73	18	6	48	64	59	45	34	3
21	19	42	76	84	67	29	68	8	66	93	89	96	28	12	14	38	47	52	65
32	66	33	21	81	97	39	76	67	27	97	22	76	89	41	11	91	29	6	66
16	82	42	75	35	42	92	90	77	24	21	8	36	16	5	54	89	51	57	85
74	32	63	65	93	96	18	36	82	72	39	69	37	97	51	17	36	71	38	30
50	94	4	66	17	37	10	53	8	29	67	74	88	38	11	59	60	91	56	17
71	47	81	18	53	98	7	87	29	37	22	93	13	6	95	7	95	71	14	6
71	93	48	16	33	19	46	21	60	44	52	91	52	58	10	9	41	31	35	18
20	94	13	99	45	6	53	54	1	25	79	28	1	48	36	26	68	37	59	7
75	22	69	56	62	40	64	45	40	99	94	14	98	84	22	38	24	87	43	71
16	87	41	0	88	83	11	37	71	78	22	39	43	37	75	84	84	11	55	58
92	90	80	2	30	37	84	55	56	50	3	71	24	13	62	74	82	44	90	32
96	89	31	32	37	45	70	67	80	55	58	9	55	60	61	55	86	44	27	77
38	29	36	94	65	39	56	29	29	65	88	13	71	38	71	8	81	66	31	44
20	6	61	66	90	13	70	60	92	53	87	49	34	42	14	47	75	33	26	9
63	44	94	21	14	13	41	80	39	72	29	3	25	89	44	88	13	49	18	58
13	32	93	90	31	75	86	95	18	51	61	59	84	95	67	54	40	30	29	63
26	35	48	81	19	24	36	36	76	16	46	5	93	41	97	46	79	54	95	49
89	74	96	95	94	69	31	60	16	69	76	42	28	71	69	34	46	55	20	42
50	39	28	64	20	68	60	33	92	82	61	70	5	68	95	88	12	85	18	94
55	86	5	96	87	69	75	93	54	79	0	57	45	8	86	59	25	21	9	29
75	35	1	2	86	62	70	83	85	13	97	37	13	73	16	38	36	23	54	11
74	50	1	77	87	92	68	87	57	36	17	47	0	97	78	72	72	45	54	51
34	24	35	13	26	42	22	75	47	2	34	87	15	50	65	27	5	72	28	68
73	33	42	65	91	24	44	84	71	55	70	1	27	30	8	61	65	61	18	92
7	55	12	6	61	17	23	95	91	58	60	30	35	61	34	27	75	44	35	64
10	94	18	4	3	19	21	37	28	55	76	25	10	29	80	64	8	81	20	32
20	48	92	87	95	58	57	73	42	1	12	81	94	85	63	97	24	19	93	51
81	10	92	49	70	15	76	4	36	92	62	99	78	32	86	74	43	22	98	46
66	67	82	94	67	75	16	88	84	98	0	52	37	0	43	9	0	51	2	62
84	92	36	11	3	52	44	65	45	67	97	86	92	2	50	5	93	66	73	40
36	29	98	46	88	23	28	44	8	71	69	43	53	16	87	21	56	23	37	24
15	11	82	30	59	94	23	30	40	25	87	26	24	30	44	53	33	65	72	55
89	57	49	79	83	88	42	45	41	93	38	24	15	80	97	18	61	12	13	42
23	36	65	9	64	26	93	37	26	44	42	17	45	68	27	77	74	56	49	34
9	93	90	61	45	40	75	85	64	66	36	89	72	43	99	90	92	10	10	85
53	94	30	31	62	92	82	30	94	56	40	4	50	53	9	74	87	2	36	36
18	69	77	38	89	78	30	68	71	92	22	93	91	74	52	1	97	69	71	42
50	20	76	36	6	20	75	56	36	5	14	70	9	78	23	33	91	33	25	72
30	46	1	10	16	72	69	26	94	39	80	36	36	68	92	74	22	74	41	42
59	47	7	92	77	55	2	12	5	24	0	30	25	62	83	36	92	96	36	75
93	22	3	20	82	44	16	69	98	72	30	57	77	15	90	29	32	38	3	48
9	55	27	41	40	94	77	14	54	10	25	75	1	74	72	15	69	80	33	58
70	8	3	5	46	89	28	86	40	6	25	40	81	26	63	97	87	48	26	41
19	6	89	31	80	60	13	89	17	69	38	93	58	55	54	69	74	33	8	55

FIG. 12.1 A table of random numbers.

- The differences in the characteristics of the sample and the population are purely a function of chance.
- The probability of choosing a nonrepresentative sample decreases as the size of the sample increases.

You must remember, however, that although a researcher may use a carefully controlled sampling procedure that minimizes error, no guarantee exists that the sample will be representative. Factors such as sample heterogeneity and participant dropout may jeopardize the representativeness of the sample despite the most stringent random sampling procedure. In examining the relationship between critical care nurses' information-seeking behaviour, perception of personal control, training, and the non-routineness of tasks, Newman, Doran, and Nagle (2014) drew the sample from a population of critical care nurses working in hospitals in Ontario, Canada, to reduce heterogeneity. A random sample was drawn from the College of Nurses of Ontario database.

The major disadvantage of simple random sampling is that it is a time-consuming and inefficient method of obtaining a random sample. (Consider the task of listing all baccalaureate nursing students in Canada.) With random sampling, it may also be impossible to obtain an accurate or complete listing of every element in the population. Imagine, for example, trying to obtain a list of all completed suicides in Toronto for 2014. Although suicide may have been the cause of death, another cause (e.g., cardiac failure) often appears on the death certificate. It would be difficult to estimate how many elements of the target population would be eliminated from consideration. Bias would definitely be an issue, despite the researcher's best efforts. Thus, the evaluator of a research article must exercise caution in generalizing from reported findings, even when random sampling is the stated strategy, if the target population has been difficult or impossible to list completely.

Stratified Random Sampling

Stratified random sampling requires that the population be divided into strata or subgroups. The subgroups or subsets that the population is divided into are homogeneous. An appropriate number of elements from each subset is randomly selected on the basis of the proportion in the population. The goal of this strategy is to achieve a greater degree of representativeness. Stratified random sampling is similar to the proportional stratified quota sampling strategy discussed earlier in this chapter. The major difference is that stratified random sampling involves a random selection procedure for obtaining sample participants. Figure 12.2 illustrates the use of stratified random sampling.

The population is stratified according to any number of attributes, such as age, gender, ethnicity, religion, socioeconomic status, or level of education completed. The variables selected to make up the strata lead to subgroups that share one or more of the attributes being studied (see Practical Application box). The following questions can be asked in the selection of a stratified sample:

- Does a critical variable or attribute exist that provides a logical basis for stratifying the sample?
- Does the population list contain sufficient information about the attributes that will be used to divide the sample into subsets?
- Is it appropriate for each subset to be equal in size, or is it more appropriate for each subset to be proportionally stratified on the basis of the proportion of each subset in the population?
- If proportional sampling is being used, is the number of participants in each subset sufficient as a base for meaningful comparisons?
- Once the subset comparison has been determined, are random procedures used for selection of the sample?

Sawatzky, Ratner, Richardson, and colleagues (2012) used stratified random sampling to examine

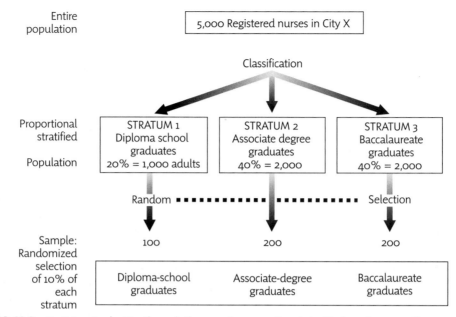

Entire population

5,000 Registered nurses in City X

Classification

Proportional stratified

Population

| STRATUM 1 Diploma school graduates 20% = 1,000 adults | STRATUM 2 Associate degree graduates 40% = 2,000 | STRATUM 3 Baccalaureate graduates 40% = 2,000 |

Random ● Selection

Sample: Randomized selection of 10% of each stratum

100   200   200

| Diploma-school graduates | Associate-degree graduates | Baccalaureate graduates |

FIG. 12.2   Participant selection through the use of a proportional stratified random sampling strategy.

Practical Application

Koopman, LeBlanc, Fowler, and associates (2016) explored the relationship between hope, coping, and quality of life in adults with myasthenia gravis. The researchers stratified a sample of 100 patients to match the proportion of these patients according to the type of myasthenia gravis in the population: 25% ocular myasthenia gravis, and 75% generalized myasthenia gravis.

---

the extent to which the relationship between adverse stress and depression is mediated by university students' perceived ability to manage their stress. The data were obtained via one Canadian university's spring 2006 ($n = 2,147$) and 2008 ($n = 2,292$) National College Health Assessment (NCHA) surveys. Students were randomly selected and then stratified according to whether they were undergraduate, graduate, or international and by campus location.

As illustrated in Table 12.1, a stratified random sampling strategy has the following advantages: (1) the representativeness of the sample is enhanced; and (2) the risk of bias is low (i.e., the researcher has a valid basis for making comparisons among subsets if information about the critical variables has been available). A third advantage is that the researcher is able to oversample a disproportionately small stratum to adjust for the researchers' underrepresentation, statistically weigh the data accordingly, and continue to make legitimate comparisons.

The obstacles encountered by a researcher in using this strategy include (1) the difficulty of obtaining a population list containing complete critical variable information; (2) the time-consuming effort of obtaining multiple enumerated lists; (3) the challenge of enrolling proportional strata; and (4) the time and money involved in carrying out a large-scale study with a stratified sampling strategy. In critiquing the study, you must question the appropriateness of this sampling strategy for the problem under investigation.

Wong, Laschinger, and Cziraki (2014) used a disproportional stratified sample to ensure that nurses from each province were represented in their study examining nurses' perceptions of incentives for pursuing management roles. It is appropriate for the researcher to strive to represent all strata proportionately in the study sample.

Multistage Sampling (Cluster Sampling)

Multistage sampling, or **cluster sampling,** involves a successive random sampling of units (clusters) that meet sample eligibility criteria; this sampling progresses from large to small. A **sampling unit** is an element or set of elements used for selecting the sample. The first-stage sampling unit consists of large units or clusters. The second-stage sampling unit consists of smaller units or clusters. Third-stage sampling units are even smaller.

Consider an example in which a sample of nurse practitioners is desired. The first sampling unit is a random sample of hospitals, obtained from a provincial nurses' association list, that meet the eligibility criteria (e.g., size, type). The second-stage sampling unit consists of a list of acute care nurse practitioners (ACNPs) practising at each hospital selected in the first stage (i.e., the list obtained from the vice president for nursing at each hospital). The criteria for inclusion in the list of ACNPs are as follows: (1) participants must be certified ACNPs with at least 2 years' experience as an ACNP; (2) at least 75% of the ACNPs' time must be spent in providing care directly to patients in acute or critical care practices; and (3) the participants must be in full-time employment at the hospital. The second-stage sampling strategy calls for random selection of two ACNPs from each hospital who meet the eligibility criteria.

When multistage sampling is used in relation to large national surveys, provinces are used as the first-stage sampling unit, followed by successively smaller units (such as counties, cities, districts, and blocks) as the second-stage sampling unit and then households as the third-stage sampling unit.

Sampling units or clusters can be selected by simple random or stratified random sampling methods (see Practical Application box). Suppose that the hospitals described in the preceding example are grouped into four strata according to size (i.e., number of beds) as follows: (1) 200 to 299; (2) 300 to 399; (3) 400 to 499; and (4) 500 or more. Stratum 1 comprises 25% of the population; stratum 2 comprises 30% of the population; stratum 3 comprises 20% of the population; and stratum 4 comprises 25% of the population. Thus, either a simple random or a proportional stratified sampling strategy can be used to randomly select hospitals that would proportionately represent the population of hospitals in the provincial nurses' association list.

The main advantage of cluster sampling, as stated in Table 12.1, is that it is considerably more economical in terms of time and money than other types of probability sampling, particularly when the population is large and geographically dispersed or when a sampling frame of the elements is not available. However, cluster sampling has two major disadvantages: (1) more sampling errors tend to occur than with simple random or stratified random sampling, and (2) the appropriate handling of the statistical data from cluster samples is very complex.

In critiquing a research report, you need to consider whether the use of cluster sampling is

---

> ### Practical Application
>
> Babenko-Mould, Iwasiw, Andrusyszyn, and associates (2012) used a multilevel sampling design in their study examining the effects of clinical practice environments on clinical teacher and nursing student outcomes. The first level was 352 nursing students within 64 clinical teachers.
>
> Laschinger, Read, Wilk, et al. (2014) used a cluster sample of 525 nurses in 49 nursing units in 25 acute care hospitals, across all regions in Ontario, to study the influence of nursing unit empowerment and social capital on unit effectiveness and nurse perceptions of patient care quality.

justified in light of the research design, as well as other pragmatic matters, such as economy.

Systematic Sampling

Systematic sampling is a sampling strategy that involves the selection of every "*k*th" case drawn from a population list at fixed intervals, such as every tenth member listed in the directory of the College and Association of Registered Nurses of Alberta (CARNA). Systematic sampling might be used to recruit every "*k*th" person who enters a hospital lobby or who is hospitalized with a diagnosis of acquired immune deficiency syndrome (AIDS) in 2015. When systematic sampling is used, the population must be narrowly defined (e.g., as consisting of all people entering or leaving the hospital lobby) for the sample to be considered a probability sample. If older adults were sampled systematically on entering a hospital lobby, the resulting sample would not be a probability sample because not every older adult would have a chance of being selected. As such, systematic sampling can sometimes represent a nonprobability sampling strategy.

Systematic sampling strategies can be designed, however, to fulfill the requirements of a probability sample. First, the listing of the population (sampling frame) must be random in relation to the variable of interest. For example, suppose that participants were being selected from every tenth hospital room for a study on patient satisfaction with nursing care. In the hospital where the study was being conducted, every tenth room happened to be a private room. Patients in private rooms might respond differently regarding their satisfaction than patients in semiprivate rooms. Because of the nonrandom arrangement of the rooms, bias may be introduced.

Second, the first element or member of the sample must be selected randomly. In this case, the researcher—who has a population list, or sampling frame—first divides the population *(N)* by the size of the desired sample *(n)* to obtain the sampling interval width *(k)*. The **sampling interval** is the standard distance between the elements chosen for the sample. For example, to select a sample of 50 family nurse practitioners from a population of 500 family nurse practitioners, the sampling interval would be as follows:

$$k = \frac{500}{50} = 10$$

Essentially, every tenth case on the family nurse practitioner list would be sampled. Thus, if the starting point was participant 5, the next person chosen would be 15th, then 25th, etc.

Once the sampling interval has been determined, the researcher uses a table of random numbers (see Figure 12.1) to obtain a starting point for the selection of the 50 participants. If the population size is 500 and a sample size of 50 is desired, a number between 1 and 500 is randomly selected as the starting point. In this instance, if the first number is 51, the family nurse practitioners corresponding to numbers 51, 61, 71, and so forth would be included in the sample of 50.

Another procedure recommended in many texts is to randomly select the first element from within the first sampling interval. If the sampling interval is 5, a number between 1 and 5 is selected as the random starting point. For example, the number 3 is randomly chosen. Keeping in mind the sampling interval of 5, the next elements selected would correspond to the numbers 8, 13, 18, and so on, until the sample was obtained. Although this procedure is technically correct, choosing a random starting point from across the total population of elements is more attractive because every element has a chance to be chosen for the sample during the first selection step.

Systematic sampling and simple random sampling are essentially the same type of procedure. The advantage of systematic sampling is that the results are obtained in a more convenient and efficient manner (see Table 12.1). The disadvantage of systematic sampling is that bias in the form of nonrandomness can be inadvertently introduced into the procedure. This problem may occur if the population list is arranged so that a certain type of element is listed at intervals that coincide with the sampling interval. For example, if every tenth nursing student on a population list of all types of nursing students in Ontario was a baccalaureate student and the sampling interval was 10, baccalaureate students would be over-represented in the sample.

Cyclical fluctuations are also a factor in systematic sampling. For example, if a list is kept of nursing students using the college library each day to do computer literature searches, a biased sample would probably be obtained if every seventh day, such as Sunday, is chosen as the sampling interval because probably fewer and perhaps different nursing students use the library on Sundays than on weekdays. Therefore, caution must be exercised about departures from randomness because they affect the representativeness of the sample and, as a result, the external validity of the study.

You should note whether a satisfactory random selection procedure was performed. If randomization was not used, the systematic sampling may have become a nonprobability quota sample. You need to be cognizant of this issue because the implications related to interpretation and generalizability are drastically altered when a nonprobability sample is involved.

For example, in their study, Ridout, Aucoin, Browning, and associates (2014) explored the incidence of failure to communicate vital information as patients progressed through the six phases of the perioperative process. One thousand eight hundred fifty-eight eligible surgical cases were identified, and 293 charts needed to be reviewed to achieve a power of 0.8 and determine a difference at the 0.05 level. Every sixth record that met the criteria was used for the study. Because randomization was not used at any phase of this multilevel sampling procedure, you would consider this study to be a nonprobability stratified sample with the external validity limitations of that sampling strategy (see Chapter 9).

 Evidence-Informed Practice Tip ____

The sampling strategy, whether probability or nonprobability, must be appropriate for the study design and evaluated in relation to the level of evidence provided by the design.

Special Sampling Strategies

Several special sampling strategies are used in nonprobability sampling. **Matching** is a special strategy used to construct an equivalent comparison sample group by filling it with participants who are similar to each participant in another sample group in terms of pre-established variables, such as age, gender, level of education, medical diagnosis, or socioeconomic status. Theoretically, any variable other than the independent variable that could affect the dependent variable should be matched. In reality, the more variables matched, the more difficult it is to obtain an adequate sample size.

For example, Graziotti, Hammond, Messinger, and colleagues (2012) examined strategies to maximize retention in longitudinal studies involving high-risk families. The researchers conducted a follow-up study of 1,388 children, half of whom were initially identified as cocaine or opiate exposed ($n = 658$), who were then matched to a non-cocaine- or non-opiate-exposed control ($n = 730$), based on gestational age, race, and gender.

SAMPLING STRATEGIES USED IN QUALITATIVE RESEARCH

Because nonprobability sampling is the best method of obtaining individuals who are key informants of a phenomenon, these sampling methods are widely used in qualitative research. As described in Chapter 7, qualitative research methods are conducted to gain both insights into and in-depth meaning about experiences, incidents, or events. In qualitative research, the sampling procedure is governed by the methodology used. Many sampling strategies are used in qualitative sampling, but the most common approaches are *convenience sampling, network sampling, purposive sampling,* and *theoretical sampling.*

Convenience Sampling

Convenience sampling is also used in qualitative research to access participants of a particular phenomenon. Salami, Nelson, McGillis-Hall, and associates (2014) used convenience sampling to explore the experiences of Philippine-educated nurses who migrated through the Live-In Caregiver program in Ontario.

Network Sampling

Network sampling, sometimes referred to as **snowball effect sampling** or *snowballing,* is a strategy used for locating samples that are difficult or impossible to locate in other ways. This sampling strategy takes advantage of social networks and the tendency of friends to share characteristics. When a few participants with the necessary eligibility criteria are found, the researcher asks for their assistance in getting in touch with other people with similar characteristics that meet these criteria.

Network sampling was study by O'Byrne, Bryan, Hendriks, et al. (2014), who studied how gay and bisexual men perceived the criminal prosecution of persons living with HIV and who do not disclose their HIV status. They recruited participants by raising awareness of the project within AIDS service agencies, distributed posters in venues frequented by gay men, and used snowball sampling by giving participants a supply of the research assistant's business cards to pass on to others who might be willing to participate.

In a qualitative participatory study, MacDonald, Martin-Misener, Steenbeek, and colleagues (2015) explored Mi'kmaq women's experiences with Pap screening within the contexts that shaped their experiences (see Appendix A). Sixteen women were recruited using purposive and snowball sampling. Indigenous women were recruited by community facilitators by purposive

sampling. Then, those who participated informed other women in the community about the study.

Today, online computer networks, as described in the following section on purposive sampling, can be used to assist researchers in recruiting participants who are otherwise difficult to locate, thereby taking advantage of the networking or snowball effect. The Critical Thinking Decision Path illustrates the relationship between the type of sampling strategy and the appropriate generalizability.

Purposive Sampling

Purposive sampling is an increasingly common strategy in which the researcher's knowledge of the population and its elements is used to handpick the cases to be included in the sample. The researcher usually selects participants who are considered typical of the population.

For example, Dahlke and Baumbusch (2015) used a subset of purposive sampling, maximum variation purposive sampling, to locate more experienced nurses in their qualitative study. Maximum variation purposive sampling is the "process of deliberately selecting a heterogeneous sample and observing commonalities in their experiences" (Morse, 1994, p. 229).

A purposive sample is also used when a highly unusual group is being studied, such as a population with a rare genetic disease (e.g., Tay-Sachs disease). In this case, the researcher would describe the sample characteristics precisely to ensure that the reader will have an accurate picture of the participants in the sample. This type of sample can also be used to study the differential effect of risk factors in a specific population longitudinally. In another situation, the researcher may wish to interview individuals who reflect a particular characteristic. For example, Hawkins and Rodney (2015) studied the journey of nurses from the Philippines seeking RN licensure and employment in Canada. Purposive sampling was used to identify nurses educated in the Philippines

CRITICAL THINKING DECISION PATH

Assessing the Relationship between the Type of Sampling Strategy and the Appropriate Generalizability

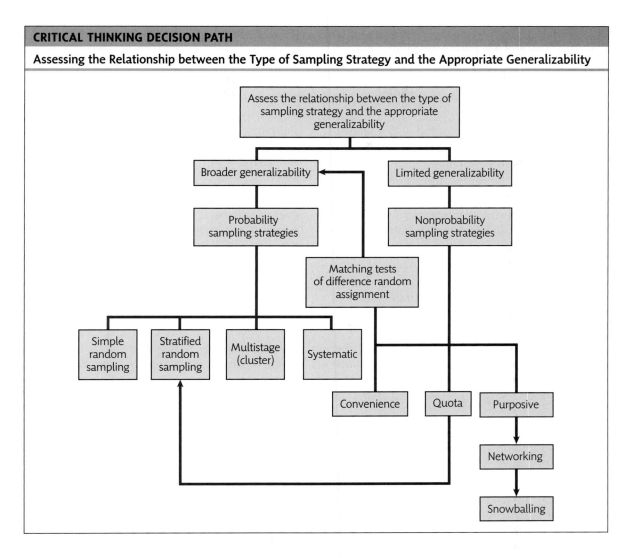

who had sought or had considered seeking Canadian RN licensure.

Today, computer networks (e.g., online services) can be of great value in helping researchers access and recruit participants for purposive samples. For instance, Freeman, Beaulieu, and Crawley (2015) used emails and public notices at schools of nursing to recruit 92 nurse graduates who were considering migrating abroad in order to explore the graduates' job values and expectations.

The researcher who uses a purposive sample assumes that errors of judgement in overrepresenting or underrepresenting elements of the population in the sample will tend to balance each other. The validity of this assumption, however, cannot be determined objectively. You must be aware that the more heterogeneous the population, the greater the chance that bias is introduced in the selection of a purposive sample. As indicated in Table 12.1, conscious bias in the selection of participants remains a constant concern. Therefore, the findings from a study involving a purposive sample should be regarded with caution. As with any nonprobability sample, the ability to generalize is very limited. The following are several instances when a purposive sample may be appropriate:

- The effective pretesting of newly developed instruments with a purposive sample of diverse types of people
- The validation of a scale or test with a known-groups technique
- The collection of exploratory data in relation to an unusual or highly specific population, particularly when the total target population remains unknown to the researcher
- The collection of descriptive data (e.g., as in qualitative studies) with which researchers seek to describe the lived experience of a particular phenomenon (e.g., postpartum depression, caring, hope, or surviving childhood sexual abuse)
- The focus of the study population when it is related to a specific diagnosis (e.g., type 1 diabetes, multiple sclerosis), a specific condition (e.g., legal blindness, terminal illness), or a specific demographic characteristic (e.g., same-sex twin pairs)

Many types of purposive sampling exist (Palys, 2008), but the following three types of cases are the most often used:

1. Typical cases: cases that are "normal" or "average" among those being studied
2. Deviant or extreme cases: cases that represent unusual manifestations of the phenomenon of interest
3. Confirming or disconfirming cases: cases that are exceptions, that represent variation, or for which an initial elaborate analysis is necessary

In any type of purposive sampling, sampling is stopped when **data saturation** occurs—that is, when the information being shared with the researcher becomes repetitive.

Criterion sampling is also a form of purposive sampling. The researcher needs to have a set of criteria for a sample, and all cases that meet these criteria are selected. It is important that the criteria are established so that cases that

are chosen will yield rich data relevant to the research problem being explored—for example, all patients who were in a smoking cessation program and have resumed smoking. This criterion would enable an understanding of what is needed to support individuals who wish to quit smoking.

Theoretical Sampling

Theoretical sampling is associated with grounded theory research. As you learned in Chapter 8, the goal of grounded research is theory generation; thus, a theoretical sampling strategy is used to fully elaborate and validate variations in the data by finding examples of a theoretical construct (Sandelowski, 1995). In **theoretical sampling,** the researcher selects experiences that will help test ideas and gather complete information about developing concepts. Sampling is stopped when theory saturation or redundancy occurs.

Theoretical sampling was used by Jansen, McWilliam, Forbes, and associates (2013), who explored the social-interaction processes of knowledge translation related to urinary incontinence. Jansen and associates used constant comparison to guide the initial coding of concepts and the theoretical sampling process. The views, situations, and experiences of different family members were compared, and data from the same individuals were gathered at different times.

 Research Hint _____

Look for a brief discussion of a study's sampling strategy in the "Methods" section of a research article. Some articles have a separate subsection with the heading "Sample," "Participants," or "Study Participants." A statistical description of the characteristics of the actual sample often does not appear until the "Results" section of a research article.

SAMPLE SIZE: QUANTITATIVE

No single rule can be applied to the determination of a sample's size. When researchers estimate sample size, they must consider many factors, such as the following:

- The type of design used
- The type of sampling procedure used
- The type of formula used for estimating the optimal sample size
- The degree of precision required
- The heterogeneity of the attributes under investigation
- The relative frequency at which the phenomenon of interest occurs in the population (i.e., a common versus a rare health problem)
- The projected cost of using a particular sampling strategy

The sample size should be determined before the study is conducted. A general rule is always to use the largest sample possible. The larger the sample, the more likely it is to be representative of the population; smaller samples produce less accurate results.

An exception to the rule about sample size is the **pilot study,** which is a small sample study conducted as a prelude to a larger-scale (parent) study. The pilot study typically is conducted with similar methods and procedures that both yield preliminary data for determining the feasibility of conducting a larger-scale study and establish that sufficient scientific evidence exists to justify subsequent, more extensive research.

Hertzog (2008) summarized methods for justifying sample sizes on the basis of the aim of the pilot study. This author suggests that a sample size as small as 10 to 15 participants per group may be sufficient for the decisions being made. For pilot studies involving group comparisons, 10 to 20 participants per group may be enough. On the other hand, if a researcher is developing or testing an instrument, it is suggested that each group comprise 35 to 40 participants. For example, Cossette, Frasure-Smith, Robert, et al. (2012) conducted a pilot study on nursing interventions to address smoking cessation in cardiac patients post–hospital discharge and used a sample of 20 patients per group. This pilot was intended to

provide a preliminary assessment of effect size and trend.

The principle of "larger is better" holds true for both probability and nonprobability samples. Results based on small samples (fewer than 10 participants) tend to be unstable; the values fluctuate from one sample to the next. Small samples tend to increase the probability of obtaining a markedly nonrepresentative sample. As the sample size increases, the mean more closely approximates the population values; thus, fewer sampling errors are introduced.

An example of this concept is illustrated by a study in which the average monthly consumption of sleeping pills was investigated for patients on a rehabilitation unit after a cerebrovascular accident. The data in Table 12.3 indicate that the population consisted of 20 patients whose average consumption of sleeping pills was 15.2 per

TABLE 12.3

COMPARISON OF POPULATION AND SAMPLE VALUES AND AVERAGES IN A STUDY OF SLEEPING PILL CONSUMPTION

NUMBER IN GROUP	GROUP	NUMBER OF SLEEPING PILLS CONSUMED (VALUES EXPRESSED MONTHLY)	AVERAGE
20	Population	1, 3, 4, 5, 6, 7, 9, 11, 13, 15, 16, 17, 19, 21, 22, 23, 25, 27, 29, 30	15.2
2	Sample 1A	6, 9	7.5
2	Sample 1B	21, 25	23.0
4	Sample 2A	1, 7, 15, 25	12.0
4	Sample 2B	5, 13, 23, 29	17.5
6	Sample 3A	3, 4, 11, 15, 21, 25	13.3
6	Sample 3B	5, 7, 11, 19, 27, 30	16.5
10	Sample 4A	3, 4, 7, 9, 11, 13, 17, 21, 23, 30	13.8
10	Sample 4B	1, 4, 6, 11, 15, 17, 19, 23, 25, 27	13.8

month. The population of 20 patients was divided into sets of two simple random samples with sizes of 2, 4, 6, and 10. Each sample average in the right column represents an estimate of the population average, which is known to be 15.15. In most cases, the population value was unknown to the researchers, but because the population is so small, it could be calculated. In Table 12.3, note that with a sample size of two, the estimate might have been wrong by as much as eight sleeping pills in sample 1B. As the sample size increases, the averages get closer to the population value, and the differences in the estimates between samples A and B also get smaller. Large samples permit the principles of randomization to work effectively (i.e., to counterbalance atypical values in the long run).

The sample size can be estimated with the use of a statistical procedure known as *power analysis* (see Chapter 16). A simple example illustrates this concept. Suppose that a researcher wants to determine the effect of nurse preoperative teaching on patient postoperative anxiety. Patients are randomly assigned to an experimental group or a control group. How many patients should be used in the study? When using power analysis, the researcher must estimate how large a difference will be observed between the groups (i.e., the difference in the mean amount of postoperative anxiety after the experimental preoperative teaching program). This difference is called the **effect size.** If a small difference is expected, the sample must be large (in this case, 196 patients in each group) to ensure that the differences will be revealed in a statistical analysis. If a medium-size difference is expected, the total sample size would be 128 (64 in each group). When expected differences are large, a small sample size can ensure that differences will be revealed through statistical analysis.

An example is illustrated by the study of El-Masri and colleagues (2015), who evaluated the effectiveness of a nurse practitioner–led outreach program for long-term care homes utilizing observations. Before data collection, they conducted a power analysis, with an alpha value set at .05 and the power set at .80; the power analysis indicated that 848 observations were needed to yield an odds ratio of 1.5 for the primary outcome of emergency department transfer. Alpha is the probability of making a type I error (rejecting the null hypothesis when the null hypothesis is true).

Power analysis is an advanced statistical technique that is commonly used by researchers and is a requirement for external funding. When power analysis is not used, research studies may be based on samples that are too small, which may lead to a lack of support for the researcher's hypotheses and to a type I error (rejecting a null hypothesis when it should have been accepted); in other words, the researcher finds significant results when none exist (see Chapter 16). A researcher may also commit a type II error (accepting a null hypothesis when it should have been rejected) if the sample is too small; in other words, the sample is too small to detect treatment effects (see Chapter 16).

Despite the principles related to determining sample size that have been identified in this chapter, you should be aware that large samples do not ensure representativeness or accuracy. A large sample cannot compensate for faulty research design. The proportion of the population that is sampled does not provide a guarantee of accurate results. Accurate results can be obtained from only a small fraction of a large population. For example, a 10% probability sample of a population containing 1,500 elements will yield more precise results than will a nonprobability 0.01% sample of a population with 100,000 elements.

You should evaluate the sample size in terms of (1) how representative the sample is of the target population and (2) to which population the researcher wishes to generalize the results of the study. The goal of sampling is to gather a sample as representative as possible with as few sampling errors as possible.

SAMPLE SIZE: QUALITATIVE

In qualitative research, no power analyses are conducted a priori to determine sample size requirements. According to Sandelowski (1995), sample size is determined by the purpose and type of the sampling and the research method to be used. Morse (1994) recommended about six participants for phenomenological studies and about 30 to 50 cases for ethnographies and grounded theory studies. These suggestions do not constitute a hard-and-fast rule because a one-person case study may be sufficient for a phenomenological study. When you critique a study, you need to note how the researcher has explained the sampling plan and what limitations have been stated. Participants are added to the sample until data saturation is reached (i.e., new data no longer emerge during the data-collection process). The fittingness of the data is a more important concern than the representativeness of participants (see Chapter 14).

Research Hint

Remember to look for some rationale about the sample size and the strategies that the researcher has used (e.g., matching, test of differences on demographic variables) to ascertain or build in sample representativeness.

Evidence-Informed Practice Tip

Research designs and types of samples are often linked. You would expect to see experimental designs in which probability sampling strategies were used; if a nonprobability purposive sampling strategy is used to recruit participants to such a study, you would expect the participants to then be randomly assigned to intervention and control groups.

SAMPLING PROCEDURES

The criteria for selecting a sample vary according to the sampling strategy. Regardless of which strategy is used, the procedure must be systematically organized. Such organization will eliminate the bias that occurs when sample selection is carried out inconsistently. Bias in sample representativeness and generalizability of findings are important sampling issues that have generated national concern.

For example, many of the landmark adult health studies (e.g., the Framingham Heart Study and the Baltimore Longitudinal Study of Aging) historically excluded women as participants. The findings of these studies were generalized from men to all adults despite the lack of female representation in the samples. Findings based on Euro-American or Euro-Canadian data cannot be generalized to Punjabis, Chinese, West Indians, or any other cultural group. Consequently, careful identification of the target population is a crucial step in the process. For example, O'Keefe-McCarthy, McGillion, Nelson, and associates (2014) cautioned that the limited ethnicity (White) is a limiting factor in using their Prodromal Symptoms-Screening Scale.

In order to establish conclusions about, for example, psychosocial stressors related to all patients with a first-time myocardial infarction, both men and women must be included in the target population. As another example, to establish conclusions about the incidence of extrapyramidal adverse effects of haloperidol (Haldol) in a psychiatric ward among Chinese patients in comparison with Euro-Canadians, the target population must be diverse. Sometimes, however, the target population must be gender specific, as when breast or prostate cancer or aspects of pregnancy or menopause are studied.

Several general steps (Figure 12.3) ensure the identification of a consistent approach by the researcher. Initially, the target population (i.e., the entire group of people or objects about whom the researcher wants to establish conclusions or make generalizations) must be identified. The target population may consist, for example, of all female patients with a first-time diagnosis of breast cancer, all children with asthma, all pregnant teenagers, or all doctoral nursing students in Canada.

Next, the accessible portion of the target population must be delineated. An accessible population might consist of all nurse practitioners in the

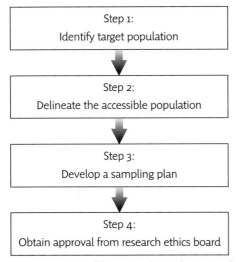

FIG. 12.3   Summary of the general sampling procedures.

province of New Brunswick, all male patients with AIDS admitted to a certain hospital during 2011, all pregnant teenagers in a specific prenatal clinic, or all children with rheumatoid arthritis under care at a specific hospital specializing in the treatment of autoimmune diseases.

Then a sampling plan or a protocol for actually selecting the sample from the accessible population is formulated. The researcher makes decisions about how participants will be approached, how the study will be explained, and who—the researcher or a research assistant—will select the sample. Regardless of who implements the sampling plan, consistency in how it is done is of paramount importance. In reading a research report, you want to find a description of the sample, as well as the sampling procedure, in the study. On the basis of the

appropriateness of what has been reported, you can make judgements about the soundness of the sampling protocol, which, of course, will affect the interpretations of the findings.

Finally, once the accessible population and sampling plan have been established, permission is obtained from the institution's research board, which is commonly referred to as the *research ethics board*. This permission provides free access to the desired population.

When an appropriate sample size and sampling strategy have been used, the researcher can feel more confident that the sample is representative of the accessible population; however, it is more difficult to feel confident that the accessible population is representative of the target population. Are nurse practitioners in New Brunswick representative of all nurse practitioners in Canada? It is impossible to know for sure. Researchers must exercise judgement when assessing typicality. Unfortunately, no guidelines for making such judgements exist, and critiquers have even less basis on which to make such decisions. The best rule to use when evaluating the representativeness of a sample and its generalizability to the target population is to be realistic and conservative about making sweeping claims in relation to the findings.

 Research Hint _____

Remember to evaluate the appropriateness of the generalizations made about the findings of a quantitative study in view of the target population, the accessible population, the type of sampling strategy, and the sample size. In qualitative research, evaluate the transferability of the findings on the basis of the research design and its sampling strategy and size.

APPRAISING THE EVIDENCE

Sample

The criteria for critiquing the sampling technique of a study are presented in the Critiquing Criteria box. You (the reader) and the researcher approach the "Sample" section of a research report with different

perspectives. You need to raise the following two questions:

1. If this study were to be replicated, is enough information available about the nature of the population,

APPRAISING THE EVIDENCE—cont'd

Sample

the sample, the sampling strategy, and the sample size for another investigator to carry out the study?

2. Are the previously mentioned factors appropriate for the particular research design, and, if not, which factors require modification, especially if the study is to be replicated?

Sampling is considered to be one important aspect of the methodology of a research study. Thus, data pertaining to the sample usually appear in the "Methodology" section of the research report. The sampling content presented should reflect the outcome of a series of decisions based on sampling criteria appropriate to the design of the study, as well as the options and limitations inherent in the context of the investigation. The following discussion highlights several sampling criteria that you should consider when you evaluate the merit of a sampling strategy in relation to a specific research study.

Initially, the parameters or attributes of the study population should clearly specify to what population the findings may be generalized. In general, the target population of the study is not specifically identified by the researcher, but the nature of it is implied in the description of the accessible population, the sample, or both. For example, if a researcher states that 100 participants were randomly selected from a population of men and women older than 65 and with a diagnosis of COPD who were treated in a respiratory rehabilitation program at a particular hospital during 2011, you can specifically evaluate the parameters of the population. The demographic characteristics of the sample (e.g., age, gender, diagnosis, ethnicity, religion, and marital status) should also be presented in either a tabular or a narrative summary because they provide further explication about the nature of the sample and enable you to evaluate the sampling procedure more accurately. For example, in their study on Quebec nurse educators' beliefs about teaching smoking cessation in undergraduate nursing education, Lepage and associates (2015) presented detailed data summarizing demographic variables of importance. These data are reproduced as follows:

Descriptive statistics revealed that 80.6% of the participants are affiliated with college-level programs, while 19.4% are with university-level programs. There were 16 regions of Quebec represented in the sample: 79.1% were teachers, 5.4% were professors, and 15.4% were lecturers. (Lepage et al., 2015, p. 381)

This example illustrates how a detailed description of the sample both provides a frame of reference for the study population and sample and generates questions to be raised. When this demographic sample information is available, you are able to evaluate the sampling strategy and the impact on the findings. Also helpful is the researcher's rationale for having elected to study one type of population versus another. For example, why did Lepage and associates (2015) use only nurse educators in Quebec in their study?

In a research study in which a nonprobability sampling strategy is used, it is particularly important to fully describe the population and the sample in terms of who the study participants were, how they were chosen, and the reason they were chosen. If these criteria are adhered to, the degree of heterogeneity or homogeneity of the sample can be determined. The use of a homogeneous sample minimizes the amount of sampling error introduced, a problem particularly common in nonprobability sampling.

Next, the defined representativeness of the population should be examined. Probability sampling is clearly the ideal sampling procedure for ensuring the representativeness of a study population. Use of random selection procedures (e.g., simple random, stratified random, cluster, or systematic sampling strategies) minimizes the occurrence of conscious and unconscious biases that affect the researcher's ability to generalize about the findings from the sample to the population. You should be able to identify the type of probability strategy used and determine whether the researcher adhered to the criteria for a particular sampling plan. In experimental and quasiexperimental studies, you must also know whether or how the participants were assigned to groups. If the criteria have not been followed, you have a valid reason for being skeptical about the proposed conclusions of the study.

Random selection is the ideal in establishing the representativeness of a study population; more often,

Continued

APPRAISING THE EVIDENCE—cont'd

Sample

however, realistic barriers (e.g., institutional policy, inaccessibility of participants, lack of time or money, and current state of knowledge in the field) necessitate the use of nonprobability sampling strategies. Many important research problems that are of interest to nurses do not lend themselves to experimental design and probability sampling, particularly qualitative research designs. A well-designed, carefully controlled study with a nonprobability sampling strategy can yield accurate and meaningful findings that make a significant contribution to nursing's scientific body of knowledge. As the critiquer, you must ask a philosophical question: "If it is not possible or appropriate to conduct an experimental or quasiexperimental investigation with the use of probability sampling, should the study be abandoned?" The answer usually suggests that it is better to perform the investigation and be fully aware of the limitations of the methodology than not to acquire the potential knowledge. The researcher is always able to move on to subsequent studies that either replicate the initial study or entail the use of more stringent design and sampling strategies to refine the knowledge derived from a nonexperimental study.

The greatest difficulty in nonprobability sampling stems from the fact that not every element in the population has an equal chance of being represented in the sample. Therefore, some segment of the population will probably be systematically underrepresented. If the population is homogeneous with regard to critical characteristics, systematic bias will not be an important problem. Few of the attributes that researchers are interested in, however, are sufficiently homogeneous to render sampling bias an irrelevant consideration.

Next, the sampling plan's suitability to the research design should be evaluated. In experimental and quasiexperimental designs, some form of random selection or random assignment of participants to groups is used (see Chapter 10). In critiquing the report, you evaluate whether the researcher adhered to the principles of random selection and assignment. Lack of adherence to such principles compromises the representativeness of the sample and the external validity of the study.

The following are questions that you might pose in relation to this issue:

- Has a random selection procedure (e.g., a table of random numbers) been identified?
- Has the appropriate random sampling plan been selected? In other words, has a proportional stratified sampling plan been selected instead of a simple random sampling plan in a study in which three distinct occupational levels appear to be critical variables for stratification?
- Has the particular random sampling plan been carried out appropriately? In other words, if a cluster sampling strategy was used, did the sampling units logically progress from the largest to the smallest?

Random sampling should not be regarded as a perfect method of obtaining a representative sample. Sometimes, bias is inadvertently introduced even when random selection is used. In many nonexperimental designs, nonprobability sampling strategies are used. For such studies, you can ask whether a nonexperimental design and a related nonprobability sampling plan were most appropriate. Sometimes, if the researchers had used another type of design or sampling plan, they could have constructed a stronger study that would have produced findings that were more generalizable and more reliable. In critiquing, however, you are rarely in a position to know what factors entered into the decision to plan one type of study rather than another.

You should then determine whether the sample size is appropriate and its size is justifiable. The researcher usually indicates in a research article how the sample size was determined; a similar indication is also seen commonly in doctoral dissertations. The method of arriving at the sample size and the rationale should be briefly mentioned. For example, a researcher may state the following:

A power analysis was performed to test for difference of means with a two-tailed t-test, and a power of 0.80 with an alpha of 0.05. For a large effect size (0.70), a sample size of 33 was needed. (Forman, Currie, Lauck, et al., 2015, p. 562)

In Wing, Regan, and Laschinger's (2013) study on the influence of empowerment and incivility on the mental health of new graduates, a power

APPRAISING THE EVIDENCE—cont'd

Sample

analysis was conducted, and it was determined that a minimum sample size of 66 respondents was needed for a moderate effect size (.15; alpha = .05; power = .80). (p. 636)

The importance of such examples lies in understanding that this type of statement meets the criteria stated at the beginning of the paragraph and should be evident in the research report. Other considerations with regard to sample size, especially when the sample size appears to be small or inadequate and no rationale is stated for the size, are as follows:

- How will the sample size affect the accuracy of the results?
- Are any subsets or cells of the sample overrepresented or underrepresented?
- Are any of the subsets so small as to limit meaningful comparisons?
- Has the researcher examined the effect of attrition on the results?
- Has the researcher recognized and identified any limitations posed by the size of the sample?

Essentially, these criteria necessitate that you carefully scrutinize several important elements pertaining to sample size that have implications for the generalizability of the findings. Keep in mind that in reports of qualitative studies, neither the predetermining nor the method of determining the sample size will be discussed. Rather, the sample size depends on the methodology used and is a function of data saturation (see Chapter 8).

With qualitative research designs, you apply criteria related to sampling strategies that are relevant for a particular type of qualitative study. In general, sampling strategies are purposive because the study of specific phenomena in their natural setting is emphasized; any participant belonging to a specified group is considered to represent that group. For example, in the qualitative study by MacDonald and associates (2015; see Appendix A), the specified group was Mi'kmaq women. The researchers' goal was to understand their experiences related to Pap screening.

Finally, the "Sample" section of the research report should provide evidence that the rights of human participants have been protected. You will evaluate whether permission was obtained from an institutional research ethics board that reviewed the study with regard to maintaining ethical research standards (see Chapter 6). For example, the research ethics board examines the research proposal to determine whether the introduction of an experimental procedure may be potentially harmful and therefore undesirable. You also need to examine the report for evidence of the participants' informed consent, as well as protection of their confidentiality or anonymity. Research studies that do not demonstrate evidence of having met these criteria are highly unusual. Nevertheless, you will want to be certain that ethical standards that protect sample participants have been maintained.

Many factors must be considered when you critique the "Sample" section of a research report. The type and appropriateness of the sampling strategy become crucial elements in the analysis and interpretation of data, in the conclusions derived from the findings, and in the generalizability of the findings from the sample to the population. As stated earlier in this chapter, the major purpose of sampling is to increase the efficacy of a research study by representing the particular population so that not every element need be studied, while producing the findings that can be generalized from the sample to the population. You must demonstrate that the sampling strategy used provided a valid basis for the findings and their generalizability.

CRITIQUING CRITERIA

1. Have the sample characteristics been completely described?
2. Can the parameters of the study population be inferred from the description of the sample?
3. To what extent is the sample representative of the population as defined?
4. Are criteria for eligibility in the sample specifically identified?
5. Have sample delimitations been established?
6. Would it be possible to replicate the study population?

Continued

CRITIQUING CRITERIA—cont'd

7. How was the sample selected? Is the method of sample selection appropriate?
8. What kind of bias, if any, is introduced by this method?
9. Is the sample size appropriate? How is it substantiated?
10. Does the researcher indicate that the rights of participants have been ensured?

11. Does the researcher identify the limitations in generalizability of the findings from the sample to the population? Are those limitations appropriate?
12. Is the sampling strategy appropriate for the design of the study and level of evidence provided by the design?

13. Does the researcher indicate how replication of the study with other samples would provide increased support for the findings?

CRITICAL THINKING CHALLENGES

■ A research classmate asks the instructor the following question: "Why isn't it better to study an entire population of patients with lung cancer instead of using the research technique of sampling?" How would you answer this question? Include examples that will help the student see your point of view.

■ In the report of a quasiexperimental study, the researchers indicated that they used a convenience sample with random assignment. How is this possible? Would they have used a nonprobability or a probability sample? If you agree that this is a legitimate sampling technique, present both the advantages and the disadvantages; if you disagree, indicate your rationale.

■ Your research class is having a debate on probability sampling versus nonprobability sampling with regard to desirability and feasibility. You are assigned to present the advantages of nonprobability sampling in nursing research. What arguments would you use?

■ Discuss the principle of "larger is better" and its relationship to network sampling and the sample size of qualitative studies. Include in your discussion the concept of data saturation and the use of computer technology.

■ Your research classmate is arguing that a random sample is always better, even if it is small and represents only one site. Another student is arguing that a very large convenience sample representing multiple sites can be very significant. Which classmate would you defend, and why?

KEY POINTS

- Sampling is a process in which representative units of a population are selected for study. Researchers select representative segments of the population because selecting entire populations of interest to obtain accurate and meaningful information is rarely feasible or necessary.
- Researchers establish eligibility criteria; these are descriptors of the population and provide the basis for inclusion into a sample. Eligibility criteria can include age, gender, socioeconomic status, level of education, religion, and ethnicity.
- The researcher must identify the target population (i.e., the entire set of cases about which the researcher would like to make generalizations). Because of pragmatic constraints, however, the researcher usually uses an accessible population (i.e., one that meets the population criteria and is available).
- A sample is a set of elements that make up the population.
- A sampling unit is the element or set of elements used for selecting the sample. The foremost criterion in evaluating a sample is the representativeness or congruence of characteristics with the population.
- Sampling strategies consist of nonprobability and probability sampling.
- In nonprobability sampling, the elements are chosen by nonrandom methods. Types of

nonprobability sampling include convenience, quota, and purposive sampling.

- Probability sampling is characterized by the random selection of elements from the population. In random selection, each element in the population has an equal and independent chance of being included in the sample. Types of probability sampling include simple random, stratified random, cluster, and systematic sampling.
- Sample size is a function of the type of sampling procedure being used, the degree of precision required, the type of sample estimation formula being used, the heterogeneity of the study attributes, the relative frequency of occurrence of the phenomena under consideration, and the cost.
- Criteria for selecting a sample vary according to the sampling strategy. Systematic organization of the sampling procedure minimizes bias. The target population is identified, the accessible portion of the target population is delineated, permission to conduct the research study is obtained, and a sampling plan is formulated.
- In critiquing a research report, you evaluate the sampling plan for its appropriateness in relation to the particular research design.
- The completeness of the sampling plan is examined with regard to the potential replicability of the study. In critiquing, you evaluate whether the sampling strategy is the strongest plan for the particular study under consideration.
- An appropriate systematic sampling plan will maximize the efficiency of a research study. It will increase the accuracy and meaningfulness of the findings and enhance the generalizability of the findings from the sample to the population.

FOR FURTHER STUDY

Go to Evolve at http://evolve.elsevier.com/Canada/LoBiondo/Research for the Audio Glossary and Appendix Tables that provide supplemental information for Appendix E.

REFERENCES

Babenko-Mould, Y., Iwasiw, C., Andrusyszyn, M. A., et al. (2012). Effects of clinical practice environments on clinical teacher and nursing student outcomes. *Journal of Nursing Education, 51*(4), 217–225.

Cossette, S., Frasure-Smith, N., Robert, M., et al. (2012). A pilot randomized trial of a smoking cessation nursing intervention in cardiac patients after hospital discharge. *Canadian Journal of Cardiovascular Nursing, 22*(4), 16–26.

Cummings, G., Raymond-Seniuk, C., Lo, E., et al. (2013). Factors influencing job satisfaction of oncology nurses over time. *Canadian Oncology Nursing Journal, 23*(3), 162–171.

Dahlke, S. A., & Baumbusch, J. (2015). Nursing teams caring for older adults. *Journal of Clinical Nursing, 24*, 3177–3185.

El-Masri, M. M., Omar, A., & Groh, E. M. (2015). Evaluating the effectiveness of a nurse practitioner-led outreach program for long-term care homes. *Canadian Journal of Nursing Research, 47*(3), 39–55.

Forman, J., Currie, L., Lauck, S., et al. (2015). Exploring changes in functional status while waiting for transcatheter aortic valve implantation. *European Journal of Cardiovascular Nursing, 14*(6), 560–569.

Fox, M. T., Sidani, S., & Brooks, D. (2010). Differences in sleep complaints in adults with varying levels of bed days residing in extended care facilities for chronic disease management. *Clinical Nursing Research, 19*(2), 181–202.

Freeman, M., Beaulieu, L., & Crawley, J. (2015). Canadian nurse graduates considering migrating abroad for work: Are their expectations being met in Canada? *Canadian Journal of Nursing Research, 47*(4), 80–96.

Graziotti, A. L., Hammond, J., Messinger, D. S., et al. (2012). Maintaining participation and momentum in longitudinal research involving high-risk families. *Journal of Nursing Scholarship, 44*(2), 120–126.

Green, T., Demchuk, A., & Newcommon, N. (2015). Aggressive surgical interventions for severe stroke: Impact on quality of life, caregiver burden and family outcomes. *Canadian Journal of Neuroscience Nursing, 37*(2), 15–25.

Hawkins, M., & Rodney, P. (2015). A precarious journey: Nurses from the Philippines seeking RN licensure and employment in Canada. *Canadian Journal of Nursing Research, 47*(4), 97–112.

Hertzog, M. A. (2008). Consideration in determining sample sizes for pilot studies. *Research in Nursing & Health, 32*, 180–191.

Im, E., Chang, S. J., Ko, Y., et al. (2012). A national Internet survey on midlife women's attitudes toward physical activity. *Nursing Research, 61*(5), 342–352.

Jansen, L., McWilliam, C. L., Forbes, D., et al. (2013). Social-interaction knowledge translation for in-home management of urinary incontinence and chronic care. *Canadian Journal of Aging, 32*(4), 392–404.

Koopman, W. J., LeBlanc, N., Fowler, S., et al. (2016). Hope, coping, and quality of life in adults with myasthenia gravis. *Canadian Journal of Neuroscience Nursing, 38*(1), 56–64.

Laschinger, H. K. S., Read, E., Wilk, P., et al. (2014). The influence of nursing unit empowerment and social capital on unit effectiveness and nurse perceptions of patient care quality. *Journal of Nursing Administration, 44*(6), 347–352.

Lepage, M., Dumas, L., & Saint-Pierre, C. (2015). Teaching smoking cessation to future nurses: Quebec educators' beliefs. *Western Journal of Nursing Research, 37*(3), 376–393.

MacDonald, C., Martin-Misener, R., Steenbeek, A., et al. (2015). Honouring stories: Mi'kmaq women's experiences with Pap screening in Eastern Canada. *Canadian Journal of Nursing Research, 47*(1), 72–96.

Mackenzie, G., Ireland, S., Moore, S., et al. (2013). Tailored interventions to improve hypertension management after stroke or TIA—Phase II (TIMS II). *Canadian Journal of Neuroscience Nursing, 35*(1), 27–34.

Morse, J. M. (1994). Designing funded qualitative research. In N. K. Denzin & Y. S. Lincoln (Eds.), *Handbook of qualitative research* (pp. 220–235). Thousand Oaks, CA: Sage.

Newman, K., Doran, D., & Nagle, L. M. (2014). The relation of critical care nurses' information-seeking behavior with perception of personal control, training, and non-routineness of the task. *Dynamics, 25*(1), 13–18.

O'Byrne, P., Bryan, A., Hendriks, A., et al. (2014). Social marginalization and internal exclusion: Gay men's understandings and experiences of community. *Canadian Journal of Nursing Research, 46*(2), 57–79.

O'Keefe-McCarthy, S., McGillion, M., Nelson, S., et al. (2014). Content validity of the Toronto Pain Management Inventory–Acute Coronary Syndrome Version. *Canadian Journal of Cardiovascular Nursing, 24*(2), 11–18.

Ostry, A., Maggi, S., Hershler, R., et al. (2010). Mental health differences among middle-aged sawmill workers in rural compared to urban British Columbia. *Canadian Journal of Nursing Research, 42*(3), 84–100.

Palys, T. (2008). Purposive sampling. In L. M. Given (Ed.), *The Sage encyclopedia of qualitative research methods* (Vol. 2, pp. 697–698). Los Angeles: Sage.

Rajacich, D., Kane, D., Lafreniére, K., et al. (2014). Male RNs: Work factors influencing job satisfaction and intention to stay in the profession. *Canadian Journal of Nursing Research, 46*(3), 94–109.

Ridout, J., Aucoin, J., Browning, A., et al. (2014). Does perioperative documentation transfer reliability? *Computers, Informatics, Nursing, 32*, 37–42.

Salami, B., Nelson, S., McGillis-Hall, L., et al. (2014). Workforce integration of Philippine educated nurses who migrate to Canada through the live-in caregiver program. *Canadian Journal of Nursing Research, 46*(4), 65–82.

Sandelowski, M. (1995). Sample size in qualitative research. *Research in Nursing & Health, 18*, 179–183.

Sawatzky, R. G., Ratner, P. A., Richardson, C. G., et al. (2012). Stress and depression in students: The mediating role of stress management self-efficacy. *Nursing Research, 61*(1), 13–21.

Wing, T., Regan, S., & Laschinger, H. K. S. (2013). The influence of empowerment and incivility on the mental health of new graduate nurses. *Journal of Nursing Management, 23*, 632–643.

Wong, C. A., Laschinger, H. K. S., & Cziraki, K. (2014). The role of incentives in nurses' aspirations to management roles. *Journal of Nursing Administration, 44*, 362–367.

CHAPTER 13

Data-Collection Methods

Susan Sullivan-Bolyai | Carol Bova | Mina D. Singh

LEARNING OUTCOMES

After reading this chapter, you will be able to do the following:

- Define the types of data-collection methods used in nursing research.
- List the advantages and disadvantages of each of these methods.
- Compare how specific data-collection methods contribute to the strength of evidence in a research study.
- Critically evaluate the data-collection methods used in published nursing research studies.

KEY TERMS

biological measurement	intervention fidelity	physiological measurement
closed-ended item	interview	questionnaire
concealment	Likert-type scale	reactivity
consistency	measurement	records or available data
debriefing	objective	scale
external criticism	open-ended item	scientific observation
internal criticism	operational definition	social desirability
intervention	operationalization	systematic

STUDY RESOURCES

(e) Go to Evolve at http://evolve.elsevier.com/Canada/LoBiondo/Research for the Audio Glossary and Appendix Tables that provide supplemental information for Appendix E.

QUANTITATIVE DATA COLLECTION

NURSES USE ALL OF THEIR SENSES when collecting data from the patients to whom they provide care. Nurse researchers also have many ways to collect information about their research participants. Both the data collected when they perform patient care and the data collected for the purpose of research are objective and systematic. **Objective** means that the data must not be influenced by the person who collects the information, and **systematic** means that the data must be collected in the same methodical way by each person involved in the collection procedure. The methods that researchers use to collect information about participants are the identifiable and repeatable operations that define the major variables being studied.

Operationalization is the process of translating the concepts of interest to a researcher into observable and measurable phenomena. For example, in their study on the Nursing Competence Self-Efficacy Scale, Kennedy, Tomblin-Murphy, Martin-Misener, and colleagues (2015) used Pajares and Urdan's (2006) definition of self-efficacy as "having confidence in one's capability to succeed in a specific context or given situation."

This purpose of this chapter is to familiarize you with the various ways in which researchers collect information from and about participants. The chapter provides nurse readers with the tools for evaluating the selection, use, and practicality of the various ways to collect data.

MEASURING VARIABLES OF INTEREST

To a large extent, the success of a study depends on the quality of the data-collection methods chosen and employed. Researchers have many types of methods available for collecting information from participants in research studies. **Measurement** is a term used in quantitative research and is the assignment of numbers to objects or events according to rules; determining which measurement to use in a particular investigation may be the most difficult and time-consuming step in the study design. In addition, nurse researchers have an array of quality instruments with adequate reliability and validity (see Chapter 14). This aspect of the research process necessitates painstaking effort from the researcher. Thus, the process of evaluating and selecting the available tools to measure variables of interest is crucial for the potential success of the study. In this section, the selection of measures and the implementation of the data-collection process are discussed. An algorithm that influences a researcher's choice of data-collection methods is diagrammed in the Critical Thinking Decision Path.

Information about phenomena of interest to nurses can be collected in many different ways. Nurses are interested in the biological and physical indicators of health (e.g., blood pressure and heart rate), but they are also interested in complex psychosocial questions presented by patients. Psychosocial variables, such as anxiety, hope, social support, and self-concept, may be measured by several different techniques, such as observation of behaviour, self-reports of feelings, or self-reports about attitudes in interviews or questionnaires. To study variables of interest, researchers also may use data that have already been collected for another purpose, such as records, diaries, or other media.

Selection of the data-collection method begins during the literature review. As noted in Chapter 5, one purpose of the literature review is to provide clues about instrumentation. As the literature review is conducted, the researcher begins to explore how previous investigators defined and operationalized variables similar to those of interest in the current study. The researcher uses this information to define conceptually the variables to be studied. Once a variable has been defined conceptually, the researcher returns to the literature to define the variable operationally—that is, describe how a concept is measured and what instruments are used to capture the essence of the variable. This **operational definition** translates the conceptual

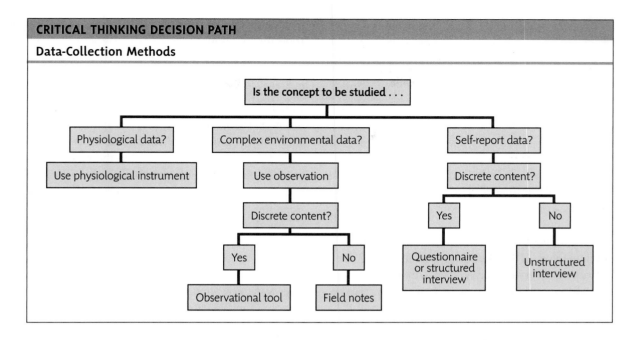

CRITICAL THINKING DECISION PATH

Data-Collection Methods

Is the concept to be studied . . .

- Physiological data?
  - Use physiological instrument

- Complex environmental data?
  - Use observation
    - Discrete content?
      - Yes
        - Observational tool
      - No
        - Field notes

- Self-report data?
  - Discrete content?
    - Yes
      - Questionnaire or structured interview
    - No
      - Unstructured interview

definition into behaviours or verbalizations that can be measured for the study. In this second literature review, the researcher searches for measurement instruments that might be used "as is" or adapted for use in the study. If instruments are available, the researcher must obtain the author's permission for their use.

The following examples illustrate the relationship of conceptual and operational definitions. Stress research is of interest to researchers from many disciplines, including nursing. Definitions of stressors may be psychological, social, or physiological. If researchers are interested in studying stressors, they must first define what they mean by the concept of "stressor," both conceptually and operationally. Quality-of-life research is popular with researchers from many disciplines, including nursing. Definitions of quality of life may be related to health functioning, life satisfaction, or well-being.

Quality of life may also be interpreted in a general way (well-being) or be related specifically to a type of illness. Therefore, if researchers are interested in studying quality of life, they

need first to define what they mean by the concept of "quality of life." For example, Thomas, Elliott, Rao, and colleagues (2012) defined quality of life as including the four domains of physical, social, emotional, and functional well-being measured by the FACT-G, which is commonly used in cancer studies. If another researcher disagreed with this definition or was more interested in the quality of life of people with another specific illness or the quality of life of children, a different instrument might be more appropriate.

Sometimes no suitable measuring device exists, and so the researcher must then decide how important the variable is to the study and whether a new device should be constructed. The construction of new instruments for data collection that have reasonable reliability and validity (see Chapter 14) is a difficult task. If no suitable measuring device exists, the researcher may decide not to study a variable, or the researcher may decide to invest time and energy in instrument development. Either decision is acceptable, depending on the goals of the study and the goals of the researcher.

Research Hint

Remember that the researcher may not always present complete information about the way the data were collected, especially when established tools were used. To learn about the tool that was used, the reader may need to consult the original article that described the use or development of the tool.

Whether the researcher uses available methods or creates new ones, once the variables have been operationally defined in a manner consistent with the aims of the study, the population to be studied, and the setting, the researcher decides how the data-collection phase of the study will be implemented. This decision concerns how the instruments for data collection will be given to the participants. Consistency is the most important issue in this phase.

Consistency in data collection means that the method used to collect data from each participant in the study is exactly the same or as close to the same as possible. Consistency can minimize the bias introduced when more than one person collects the data. Data collectors must be carefully trained and supervised. To ensure consistency in data collection, sometimes referred to as **intervention fidelity** (Santacroce, Maccarelli, & Grey, 2004), researchers must train data collectors in the methods to be used in the study so that each data collector acquires the information in the same way. Information about how to observe, ask questions, and collect data often is included in a kind of "cookbook" protocol or manual for the research project. A researcher needs to spend time developing the protocol and training data collectors to gather data systematically and reliably. Comments about their training and the consistency with which they collected data for the study should be provided by the researcher. An index of agreement called the *kappa statistic* is used to measure interrater agreement, where researchers will indicate the range of agreement expressed as a percentage of agreement among raters or observers or as a coefficient

of agreement that considers the element of chance (coefficient kappa).

An example of intervention fidelity is given in the study by Carpenter, Burns, Wu, and associates (2013), in which they designed an intervention to improvement symptoms in menopausal women. To ensure that there was standardization in the intervention, they used standardized delivery of treatment packets, trained the staff, maintained logs if unblinding occurred, and followed up with each participant to ensure that they understood the treatment instructions.

Another example of the importance of training data collectors appears in the study by Berman, Mason, Hall, and associates (2014), on women who had a previous traumatic labour experience and were now in the second trimester of pregnancy. The researchers prepared all research assistants on building rapport, active listening, probing for clarification, responding to disclosures and distress, and supporting the women's well-being.

Evidence-Informed Practice Tip

It is difficult to place confidence in a study's findings if the data-collection methods are not consistent.

TYPES OF DATA-COLLECTION METHODS

In general, data-collection methods can be divided into the following five types: *physiological measurements, observational methods, interviews* and *questionnaires,* and *records or available data.* Each method has a specific purpose, as well as certain advantages and disadvantages inherent in its use. In the following sections, these data-collection methods are discussed, along with their respective uses and problems.

Physiological or Biological Measurements

In everyday practice, nurses collect physiological data about patients, such as their temperature, pulse rate, blood pressure, blood glucose level, urine specific gravity, and pH of bodily fluids.

Such data are frequently useful to nurse researchers. Because physiological variables, such as cardiac output and blood pressure, can be measured in several different ways, researchers need to measure these outcomes at similar intervals and in similar ways for all participants of the study. An example of a study using a physiological variable is that by Héon, Goulet, Garofalo, and colleagues (2016; see Appendix D), who compared the production of breast milk in two groups of mothers of preterm infants: those receiving an additional supportive intervention and those receiving usual care. The physiological variable of breast milk was the outcome variable and was for lipid concentration.

Physiological measurement and biological measurement involve the use of specialized equipment to determine the physical and biological status of participants. Frequently, such measurements also require specialized training. These measurements can be *physical,* such as weight or temperature; *chemical,* such as blood glucose level; *microbiological,* as with cultures; or *anatomical,* as in radiological examinations. What distinguishes these measurements from others used in research is that special equipment is needed to make the observation. A researcher can say, "This participant feels warm," but to determine how warm the participant is requires the use of a sensitive instrument: a thermometer.

The advantages of using physiological data-collection methods include their objectivity, precision, and sensitivity. Such methods are generally considered to yield objective findings because unless a technical malfunction occurs, two readings of the same instrument taken at the same time by two different nurses are likely to yield the same result. Because such instruments are intended to measure the variable being studied, they offer the advantage of being precise and sensitive enough to pick up subtle variations in the variable of interest. Also, the deliberate distortion of physiological information by a participant in a study is highly unlikely to occur.

Physiological measurements are not without inherent disadvantages, however. Some instruments, if not available through a hospital, may be quite expensive to obtain and use. In addition, the accurate use of such instruments often necessitates specialized knowledge and training. Another problem with physiological measurements is that simply by using them, the variable of interest may be changed. Although some researchers think of these instruments as being nonintrusive, the presence of some types of devices might change the measurement. For example, the presence of a heart rate monitoring device might make some patients anxious and thereby increase their heart rate. In addition, nearly all types of measuring devices are affected in some way by the environment. Even a simple thermometer can be affected by the participant's drinking something hot or cold immediately before the temperature is taken. Thus, when assessing studies that use physiological measurements you need to consider whether the researcher controlled such environmental variables in the study. Finally, a physiological way to measure the variable of interest may not exist. On occasion, researchers try to force a physiological parameter into a study in an effort to increase the precision of measurement. If the device does not measure the variable of interest, however, the validity of the device's use is suspect.

Observational Methods

Although observing the environment is a normal part of living, scientific observation places a great deal of emphasis on the objective and systematic nature of the observation. The researcher is not merely watching what is happening but is watching with a trained eye for certain specific events. **Scientific observation** fulfills the following four conditions:

1. The observations undertaken are consistent with the study's specific objectives.
2. A standardized and systematic plan exists for the observation and the recording of data.

3. All of the observations are checked and controlled.
4. The observations are related to scientific concepts and theories.

Observation is particularly suitable as a data-collection method in complex research situations that are best viewed as total entities and that are difficult to measure in parts, such as studies dealing with the nursing process, parent–child interactions, or group processes (see Practical Application box for an example). In addition, observational methods can be the best way to operationalize some variables of interest in nursing research studies, particularly individual characteristics and conditions, such as traits and symptoms; verbal and nonverbal communication behaviours, activities, and skill attainment; and environmental characteristics.

Practical Application

Baumbusch, Dahlke, and Phinney (2014) conducted a critical ethnographic study to understand the role of families in institutional-based care work for older adults. They made observations over different times of the day and different days of the week. They observed day-to-day informal routines and formal activities. These observations took place when family members were interacting with their relatives and staff. Field notes were made of all observations. The researchers also collected data through in-depth interviews, reviewing institutional data and policies. All data were analyzed in an iterative process.

Observational methods can also be distinguished by the role of the observer. This role is determined by the amount of interaction between the observer and the people being observed. Each of the following four basic types of observational roles is distinguishable by the amount of concealment or intervention implemented by the observer:

1. Concealment without intervention
2. Concealment with intervention
3. No concealment without intervention
4. No concealment with intervention

These methods are illustrated in Figure 13.1; examples are given later. **Concealment** refers to a study method in which participants do not know that they are being observed; through **intervention,** the observer provokes actions from those who are being observed.

Observational studies commonly involve no concealment and no intervention. In this case, the researcher obtains informed consent from the participant to be observed and then simply observes the participant's behaviour.

When a researcher is concerned that the participants' behaviour will change as a result of being observed (reactivity), the type of observation most commonly employed is that of concealment without intervention. In this case, the researcher watches the participants without their knowledge of the observation and does not provoke them into action. Often, such concealed observations involve the use of hidden television cameras,

		Concealment	
		Yes	No
Intervention	Yes	Researcher hidden An intervention	Researcher open An intervention
	No	Researcher hidden No intervention	Researcher open No intervention

FIG. 13.1 Types of observational roles in research.

audio recordings, or one-way mirrors. Concealment without intervention is often used in observational studies of children. You may be familiar with rooms with one-way mirrors through which a researcher can observe the behaviour of the occupants of the room without being observed by them. Such studies allow the observation of children's natural behaviour and are often used in developmental research. Observing participants without their knowledge may violate assumptions of informed consent; therefore, researchers face ethical problems with this type of approach. However, researchers sometimes have no other way to collect such data, and the data collected are unlikely to have negative consequences for the participant. In these cases, the disadvantages of the study are outweighed by the advantages. Furthermore, the problem of consent is often handled by informing participants after the observation and allowing them the opportunity to refuse to have their data included in the study and to discuss any questions they might have. This process is called **debriefing.**

When the observer is neither concealed nor intervening, the ethical question is not a problem. Here, the observer makes no attempt to change the participants' behaviour and informs them that they are to be observed. Because the observer is present, this type of observation allows a greater depth of material to be studied than if the observer is separated from the participants by an artificial barrier, such as a one-way mirror. In a commonly used observational technique, the researcher functions as part of a social group to observe the participants. For example, in their study, Pauly, McCall, Browne, and colleagues (2015; see Appendix C) used unconcealed observation, with the nurses and patients giving full consent for participation in the study. The problem with this type of observation, however, is **reactivity** (also referred to as the Hawthorne effect; see Chapter 9), or the distortion created when the participants change behaviour because they know they are being observed.

No concealment with intervention is used when the researcher is observing the effects of an intervention introduced for scientific purposes. Because the participants know they are participating in a research study, few problems with ethical concerns occur, but reactivity is a problem with this type of study.

Concealed observation with intervention involves staging a situation and observing the behaviours that are evoked in the participants as a result of the intervention. Because the participants are unaware of their participation in a research study, this type of observation has fallen into disfavour and is rarely used in nursing research.

Observational methods may be structured or unstructured. Unstructured observational methods are not characterized by a total absence of structure but rather usually involve collecting descriptive information about the topic of interest. In unstructured observations, the observer keeps field notes that record the activities, as well as the observer's interpretations of these activities. Field notes are usually not restricted to any particular type of action or behaviour; rather, they are intended to depict a social situation in a more general sense.

Another type of unstructured observation is the use of stories or anecdotes, which usually focus on the behaviours of interest and frequently add to the richness of research reports by illustrating a particular point. In the study by MacDonald, Martin-Misener, Steenbeek, and associates (2015; see Appendix A), in-depth interviews were conducted for women to share their stories about their attitudes, beliefs, and experiences related to Pap screening, and field notes were made and incorporated into the data set of the exploration of the topic.

The use of structured observations without a standardized tool involves specifying in advance what behaviours or events are to be observed and preparing forms for record keeping, such as categorization systems, checklists, and rating scales.

Whichever system is employed, the observer watches the participant and then marks on the recording form what was seen. In both cases, the observations must be similar among the observers (see the earlier discussion and Chapter 14 for an explanation of interrater reliability). Thus, observers need to be trained to be consistent in their observations and ratings of behaviour.

Evidence-Informed Practice Tip _____

When you read a research report that uses observation as a data-collection method, you will want to note evidence of consistency across data collectors through use of internal consistency reliability data in quantitative research and credibility in qualitative research. When that evidence is present, you can have greater confidence in the results.

Scientific observation has several advantages as a data-collection method. The main advantage is that observation may be the only way for the researcher to study the variable of interest. For example, what people say they do is often not what they really do. Therefore, if the study is designed to obtain substantive findings about human behaviour, observation may be the only way to ensure the validity of the findings. In addition, no other data-collection method can match the depth and variety of information that can be collected with the techniques of scientific observation. Such techniques are also flexible in that they may be used in both experimental and nonexperimental designs and in laboratory and field studies.

Research Hint _____

Sometimes researchers carefully train observers or data collectors, but the research report does not address this training. The limitations on length of research reports often prevent the inclusion of certain information. Readers can often assume that if reliability data are provided, then appropriate training occurred.

As with all data-collection methods, observation also has its disadvantages. Earlier in this chapter, the problems of reactivity and ethical concerns were mentioned with regard to concealment and intervention. In addition to these problems, data obtained by observational techniques are vulnerable to the bias of the observer. Emotions, prejudices, and values can influence the way that behaviours and events are observed. In general, the more the observer needs to make inferences and judgements about what is being observed, the more likely it is that distortion will occur. Thus, in judging the adequacy of observational methods, you will need to consider how observational tools were constructed and how observers were trained and evaluated.

Interviews and Questionnaires

Participants in a research study often have information that is important to the study and that can be obtained only by asking the participants. Such questions may be asked through the use of interviews and questionnaires. For both, the purpose is to ask participants to report data for themselves, but each method has unique advantages and disadvantages. The **interview** is a method of data collection in which a data collector questions a participant verbally. Interviews may be face to face or performed over the telephone, Skype, or other electronic means and may consist of open-ended or closed-ended questions. In contrast, the **questionnaire** is an instrument designed to gather data from individuals about knowledge, attitudes, beliefs, and feelings. Survey research relies almost entirely on questioning participants with either interviews or questionnaires, but these methods of data collection can also be used in other types of research.

No matter what type of study is conducted, the purpose of questioning participants is to seek information. This information may be of either direct interest, such as the participant's age, or indirect interest, such as when the researcher uses a combination of items to estimate the degree to which the respondent has a particular trait or characteristic. An intelligence test is an example of how individual items are combined with several others to develop an overall scale of intelligence. When items of indirect interest on a survey or questionnaire are combined to obtain an overall score, the measurement tool is called a **scale.**

The investigator determines the content of an interview or questionnaire from the literature review (see Chapter 5). When evaluating interviews and questionnaires, you should consider the content of the scale, the individual items, and the order of the items. The basic standard for evaluating the individual items in an interview or questionnaire is that the item must be clearly written so that the intention of the question and the nature of the information sought are clear to the respondent. The only way to know whether the questions are understandable to the respondents is to pilot test them in a similar population. It is also critical not to rely on only the instrument developer's reports of reliability and validity (see Chapter 14). A pilot test allows researchers to test the reliability and validity for their unique sample rather than relying only on previously reported results.

Although each questionnaire item must consist of only one question or concept, be free of suggestions, and be worded with correct grammar, such items may be either open-ended or closed-ended. An **open-ended item** is used when the researcher wants the participants to respond in their own words or when the researcher does not know all of the possible alternative responses. A **closed-ended item** is a question that the respondent may answer with only one of a fixed number of alternative responses. Many scales use a fixed-response format called a Likert-type scale. A **Likert-type scale** is a list of statements for which responses are varying degrees of agreement or opinion—for example, whether respondents "strongly agree," "agree," "disagree," or "strongly disagree." Sometimes finer distinctions are given, or a neutral category (e.g., "no opinion") may be provided. The use of the neutral category, however, sometimes creates problems because it is

often the most frequent response and is difficult to interpret. Fixed-response items also can be used for questions requiring a "yes" or "no" response or when the interview or questionnaire has categories, as with income.

Evidence-Informed Practice Tip ____

Scales used in nursing research should have evidence of adequate reliability and validity so that readers feel confident that the findings reflect what the researcher intended to measure (see Chapter 14).

Figure 13.2 shows a few items from a fictional survey of pediatric nurse practitioners. The first items are taken from a list of similar items, and they are both closed-ended and of a Likert-type format. Note that respondents are asked to choose how strongly they agree with each item. In using these questions in the survey, respondents are forced to choose from only these answers because it is thought that these will be the only responses. The only possible alternative response is to skip the item, leaving it blank.

Sometimes researchers have no idea or only a limited idea of what the respondent will say, or researchers want the answer in the respondent's own words, as with the second (open-ended) set of items. In this situation, respondents may also leave the item blank but are not forced to make a particular response.

Interviews and questionnaires are commonly used in nursing research. Both are strong approaches to gathering information for research because they enable the researcher to approach the task directly. In addition, both can elicit certain kinds of information, such as the participants' attitudes and beliefs, that would be difficult to obtain without asking the participant directly.

All methods that involve verbal reports, however, share a problem with accuracy. Often, it is impossible to know whether what the researcher is told is indeed true. For example, people are known to respond to questions in a way that

Closed-Ended (Likert-Type Scale)
A. How satisfied are you with your current position?
     1. Very satisfied
     2. Moderately satisfied
     3. Undecided
     4. Moderately dissatisfied
     5. Very dissatisfied
B. To what extent do the following factors contribute to your current level of positive satisfaction?

	Not at all	Very little	Somewhat	Moderate amount	A great deal
1. % of time in patient care	1	2	3	4	5
2. Type of patients	1	2	3	4	5
3. % of time in educational activity	1	2	3	4	5
4. % of time in administration	1	2	3	4	5

Closed-Ended
A. On average, how many patients do you see in one day?
     1. 1 to 3
     2. 4 to 6
     3. 7 to 9
     4. 10 to 12
     5. 13 to 15
     6. 16 to 18
     7. 19 to 20
     8. More than 20
B. How would you characterize your practice?
     1. Too slow
     2. Slow
     3. About right
     4. Busy
     5. Too busy

Open-Ended
A. Are there incentives that the Canadian Nurses Association ought to provide for members that are not currently being provided?

_____
_____
_____
_____
_____

FIG. 13.2 Examples of closed-ended and open-ended questions.

makes a favourable impression. This response style is known as **social desirability,** which can be regarded as resulting from two factors: self-deception and other-deception.

Neyerhof (2006) has discussed the two main modes of coping with social desirability bias. The first mode is aimed at the detection and measurement of social desirability bias and is represented by two methods: the use of social desirability scales and the rating of item desirability. The second mode is aimed at preventing or reducing social desirability bias and is represented by the following methods: forced-choice items, the randomized response technique, the bogus pipeline, self-administration of the questionnaire, the selection of interviewers, and the use of proxy participants. Neyerhof found that no one method excelled completely and suggested that a combination of prevention and detection methods is the best strategy to reduce social desirability bias.

Questionnaires and interviews also have some specific purposes, advantages, and disadvantages. Questionnaires are useful tools when the purpose is to collect information. If questionnaires are too long, however, respondents are not likely to complete them. Questionnaires are most useful when the set of questions to be asked is finite and the researcher can be assured of the clarity and specificity of the items. Face-to-face techniques or interviews are most appropriate when the researcher may need to clarify the task for the respondent or is interested in obtaining more personal information from the respondent. Telephone interviews allow the researcher to reach more respondents than do face-to-face interviews and provide more clarity than do questionnaires.

Research Hint

Remember that sometimes researchers make trade-offs when determining the measures to be used. For example, if a researcher wants to learn about an individual's attitudes regarding practice, and practicalities preclude using an interview, a questionnaire may be used instead.

Pauly and colleagues (2015; see Appendix C) used both unconcealed observations and in-depth interviews to understand what constitutes culturally safe care for people who use illicit drugs. Both the nurses and patients were asked questions about their experiences in giving and receiving care, their understanding of comfort and safety, and their experiences of health care settings and any barriers and enablers in providing and receiving care (p. 124). Two researchers conducted 275 hours of unconcealed observations to gain an understanding of the various contexts under which nurses provide care to persons who use illicit drugs. This use of multiple measures provides a more complete picture than the use of just one measure.

When determining whether to use interviews or questionnaires, researchers often face difficult choices. The final decision is based on the instruments available and their relative costs and benefits.

Both face-to-face and telephone interviews have some advantages over questionnaires. The rate of response to interviews is almost always better than that to questionnaires, which helps eliminate bias in the sample (see Chapter 12). Respondents seem to be less likely to hang up the telephone or to close the door in an interviewer's face than to throw away a questionnaire. Another advantage of the interview is that some people—such as young children, people with visual impairments, and people who are illiterate—cannot fill out a questionnaire but can participate in an interview. With an interview, the data collector knows who is giving the answers. When questionnaires are mailed, for example, anyone in the household could be the person who supplies the answers.

Interviews also allow for some safeguards to be built into the interview situation. Interviewers can clarify misunderstood questions and observe the level of the respondent's understanding and cooperativeness. In addition, the researcher has strict control over the order of the questions. With questionnaires, the respondent can answer questions in any order. Changing the order of the questions can sometimes change the response.

Finally, interviews allow for richer and more complex data to be collected. The interview questioning can be open-ended or closed-ended; in either case, interviewers can probe to understand why a respondent answered in a particular way. In the qualitative study by Vandenberg and Kulig (2015), semi-structured interviews were conducted to compare and contrast the understanding and decision-making process of nonimmunizing mothers' and health care providers' perceptions of these mothers. The questions for the mothers centred around their knowledge of childhood immunization, sources of immunization, and decision making, whereas the questions for the health care providers were about perceptions of the mother's role, and patient–clinician relationship.

Interviews can also be conducted in a group setting, called a *focus group interview,* which may include about six to eight participants. Bottorff, Haines-Saah, Oliffe, and colleagues (2014) used a semi-structured interview schedule to guide focus group discussions to engage youth in discussing the merits and limitations of a variety of sample messages related to smoking and breast cancer and in generating ideas to guide youth-friendly message development and delivery media. Eight semi-structured focus groups were held outside school hours in community locations over a period of 4 months. Two focus groups were held with each of the following groups: First Nations and Métis girls, non-Indigenous girls, First Nations and Métis boys, and non-Indigenous boys. The aim was to capture diversity of opinion within each subgroup and to meet target participant numbers. These small-group interviews allowed the participants to freely explain and share information individually and collectively. Agreement and disagreement among participants may be elicited, which allows the researchers to obtain specific information from a number of participants efficiently and simultaneously.

Questionnaires are much less expensive to administer than interviews because interviews may require the hiring and training of interviewers. Thus, if a researcher has a fixed amount of time and money, a larger and more diverse sample can be obtained with questionnaires. Questionnaires also provide complete anonymity, which may be important if the study deals with sensitive issues. Finally, the fact that no interviewer is present assures the researcher and the reader that no interviewer bias will occur. Interviewer bias occurs when the interviewer unwittingly leads the respondent to answer in a certain way. This problem is especially pronounced in studies with unstructured interview formats. A subtle nod of the head, for example, could lead a respondent to change an answer to correspond with what he or she perceives that the researcher wants to hear.

For instance, Borycki, Sangster-Gormley, Schreiber, and associates (2014) used surveys to collect data about electronic-record adoption and use among nurse practitioners in British Columbia. To reach a large sample, save time, and reduce the labour costs of interviewing participants, letters including a link to the online survey were mailed.

In another study, McInnis-Perry, Weeks, and Stryhn (2013) mailed questionnaires to 8,880 community-dwelling adults age 65 and over in the Maritimes to investigate age and gender differences in emotional and informational social support insufficiency. The questionnaire packets for those interested in participating contained a cover letter from the researchers, an informed consent form, the survey, and a reply envelope.

Records or Available Data

All of the data-collection methods discussed thus far concern the ways that nurse researchers gather new data to study phenomena of interest. Not all studies, however, require a researcher to acquire new information. Existing information can sometimes be examined in a new way to study a problem. The use of records and available data is sometimes considered to be primarily the concern of historical research, but hospital records, care plans, and existing data sources (e.g., the census) are frequently used for collecting information. What sets these studies apart from a literature review is that these available data are examined in a new way and not merely summarized; they also answer specific research questions.

Records or available data, then, are forms of information that are collected from existing materials, such as hospital records, historical documents, or audio or video recordings, and are used to answer research questions in a new manner. For example, Carriere, Carriere, Ayas, and associates (2014) conducted a retrospective chart review to determine the proportion of postcardiac patients who achieved the adequate hypothermic temperature within 4 hours or less. The use of available data has certain advantages. Because the data-collection step of the research process is often the most difficult and time consuming, the use of available records often produces a significant saving of time. If the records have been kept in a similar manner over time, analysis of these records allows examination of trends over time. In addition, the use of available data decreases problems of reactivity and response set bias. The researcher also does not have to ask individuals to participate in the study.

However, institutions are sometimes reluctant to allow researchers access to their records. If the records are kept so that an individual cannot be identified, access for research purposes is usually not a problem. Also, the Privacy Act, a federal law, protects the rights of individuals who may be identified in records, which would be a violation of anonymity.

One problem that affects the quality of available data concerns survival of records. If the records available are not representative of all of the possible records, the researcher may have a problem with bias. Often, because researchers have no way to tell whether the records have been saved in a biased manner, they need to make an intelligent guess as to their accuracy. For example, a researcher might be interested in studying socioeconomic factors associated with the suicide rate. These data frequently are underreported because of the stigma attached to suicide, and so the records would be biased. Recent interest in computerization of health records has led to an increase in the discussion about the desirability of access to such records for research. At this time, how much of such data will continue to be readily available for research without consent is unclear.

Another problem is related to the authenticity of the records. The distinction of primary and secondary sources is as relevant in this discussion as it was in the discussion of the literature review to determine the source of the work (see Chapter 5). A book, for example, may have been ghost-written, but all credit was accorded to the known author. The researcher may have a difficult time ferreting out these subtle types of biases.

Lastly, existing records may be missing a significant amount of data. For example, years of education may be recorded on only a portion of the sample records. Nonetheless, records and available data constitute a rich source of data for study.

ONLINE AND COMPUTERIZED METHODS OF DATA COLLECTION

With the fast-paced progression of the Internet and computer technology, many researchers are using online data collection. The information obtained can be quantitative or qualitative, closed-ended or open-ended. This method of data collection can take the form of Web-based surveys or data input directly into microcomputers. For example, Freeman, Beaulieu, and Crawley (2015) collected data through a Web-based self-report survey in their study exploring job values and expectations of baccalaureate nursing students who indicated they were emigrating for work abroad for their first job.

Many online survey tools, such as Survey-Monkey or QuestionPro, are available; a survey can be downloaded quickly and the results obtained for a small fee. The advantages of this method are that it is anonymous and inexpensive; respondents can fill out the survey in their own time; a large number of participants can be accessed; respondent time is reduced; data-collection time is reduced; duplicate responses can be identified; and, for the researcher, implementation is time efficient. The disadvantages are that not everyone has access to a computer or is computer literate, the response rates may be low, and a large amount of data may be missing.

Computerized data collection can be accomplished through the use of laptop computers or electronic tablets or smartphones. Researchers can input their data directly into these handheld microcomputers. The data can then be transferred to a larger computer for analysis.

Evidence-Informed Practice Tip

A critical evaluation of any data-collection method includes evaluating the appropriateness, objectivity, consistency, and credibility of the method employed.

CONSTRUCTION OF NEW INSTRUMENTS

As already mentioned in this chapter, researchers sometimes cannot locate an existing instrument or method with acceptable reliability and validity to measure the variable of interest. This situation is often the case when part of a nursing theory is tested or when the effect of a clinical intervention is evaluated. For example, Carter, Dobbins, Peachey, and associates (2014) developed and tested a survey tool to ascertain the information needs and knowledge-dissemination preferences of acute-care administrators with respect to advanced practice nursing. (see Chapter 14).

Instrument development is complex and time consuming, however. It consists of the following steps:
- Defining the construct to be measured
- Formulating the items (questions)
- Assessing the items for content validity
- Developing instructions for respondents and users
- Pretesting and pilot testing the items
- Estimating reliability and validity

Defining the construct (concepts at a higher level of abstraction) to be measured requires that the researcher develop an expertise in the construct, which necessitates an extensive review of the literature and of all tests and measurements that deal with related constructs. The researcher uses all this information to synthesize the available knowledge so that the construct can be defined.

Once the construct is defined, the individual items for measuring the construct can be developed. The researcher will develop many more items than are needed to address each aspect of the construct or subconstruct. A panel of experts in the field evaluates the items so that the researcher is assured that the items measure what they are intended to measure (content validity; see Chapter 14). Eventually, the number of items is decreased because some items will not elicit the intended information and will be dropped. In this phase, the researcher needs to ensure consistency both among the items and in testing and scoring procedures.

Finally, the researcher administers or pilot tests the new instrument by applying it to a group of people who are similar to those who will be studied in the larger investigation. The purpose of this analysis is to determine the quality of the instrument as a whole (reliability and validity) and the ability of each item to discriminate individual respondents (variance in item response). The researcher also may administer a related instrument to see whether the new instrument is sufficiently different from the older one.

It is important that researchers who invest significant time in tool development publish their results. For example, Kennedy and associates (2015) were interested in measuring nursing students' self-efficacy for practice competence. From their literature review, Kennedy and associates determined that no suitable instrument was available to measure this concept related to practice. They devised their draft instrument of 66 items by using the competency documents developed by other researchers and the College of Registered Nurses of Nova Scotia. To ensure reliability and validity, they took the following steps: (1) content and face validation by an in-depth assessment of competency documents; (2) two-step review by a panel of experts for content validity; (3) assessment by student readers; (4) construct validity; (5) a factor analysis to determine clusters of variables linked to form specific domains of practice; and (6) a reliability analysis of the final 22 items that produced Cronbach's alphas between 0.75 and 0.84. This type of research serves not only to introduce other researchers to the tool but also to ultimately enhance the field, inasmuch as the ability to conduct meaningful research is limited only by the ability to measure important phenomena.

Research Hint

Determine whether a newly developed survey or questionnaire was pilot tested to obtain preliminary evidence of reliability and validity.

QUALITATIVE DATA COLLECTION

In qualitative research, data collection is more flexible and may evolve over the course of the study. Some of the data-collection methods outlined previously are also used in qualitative research, such as observations and semi-structured interviews. In addition, other methods, such as focus groups and photovoice, are used.

Focus Groups

A focus group is an interview of about five to eight people on the topic of interest. The interviewer has predetermined questions with probes, in the event that the group is not forthcoming with information. The setting for this interview is usually a neutral one. Most qualitative researchers use voice recorders so that they can be sure that they have captured what the participant says. This reduces the need to write things down and frees up the researchers to listen fully. Interview recordings are usually transcribed verbatim and then listened to for accuracy. In a research report, investigators describe their procedures for collecting the data, such as obtaining informed consent, all the steps from initial contact to the end of the study visit, and how long each interview or focus group lasted or how much time the researcher spent "in the field" collecting data.

Photovoice

Photography has been used in research since the 1950s, as photographs provide a permanent record of events and activities. In the early 1990s, Dr. Caroline Wang developed *photovoice*, an innovative approach used in participatory action research (Wang, 1999) in which interviews are stimulated and guided by photographs. These photographs empower members of marginalized groups to work together to "identify, represent and enhance their community through a specific photographic technique" (Wang & Burris, 1997). They also aid in breaking down barriers between researchers and participants. Participants use photographs, which act as prompts, to help others to see their world, and stories are told while discussing the photographs; this can be empowering to the individual. Photovoice requires that community members take on multiple roles, such as photographer, key informant, and co-researcher.

Duffy (2015) used photovoice to better understand the livelihood of single mothers after leaving an abusive relationship. Through photos and stories, these women related their arduous journey while creating a life for their children

APPRAISING THE EVIDENCE

Data-Collection Methods

Evaluating the adequacy of data-collection methods from written research reports is often problematic for new nursing research readers. Because the tool itself is not available for inspection, you may not feel comfortable judging the adequacy of the method without seeing it. However, you can ask questions to judge the method chosen by the researcher. These questions are listed in the Critiquing Criteria box.

In all studies, data-collection methods should be clearly identified. The conceptual and operational definitions of each important variable should be present in the report. Sometimes it is useful for the researcher to explain why a particular method was chosen. For example, if the study dealt with young children, the researcher may explain that a questionnaire was deemed to be an unreasonable task, and so an interview was chosen.

Once you have identified the method chosen to measure each variable of interest, you should decide whether the method used was the best way to measure the variable. For example, if a questionnaire was used, you might wonder why the researcher decided not to use an interview. Also consider whether the method was appropriate to the clinical situation. Does it make sense to interview patients in the recovery room, for example?

Once you have decided whether all relevant variables are operationalized appropriately, you can begin to determine how well the method was carried out. For studies involving physiological measurement, determine whether the instrument was appropriate to the problem and not forced to fit it. The rationale for selecting a particular instrument should be given. For example, it may be important to know that the study was conducted under the auspices of a manufacturing firm that provided the measuring instrument. In addition, the researcher should have made provisions to evaluate the accuracy of the instrument and the skill level of the people who used it.

Several considerations are important when you read studies that involve observational methods. Who were the observers, and how were they trained? Is there any reason to believe that different observers perceived events or behaviours differently? Remember that the more inferences the observers are required to make, the more likely it is that observations will be biased. Also, consider the problem of reactivity: In any observational situation, it is possible that the mere presence of the observer will cause the participant to change the behaviour in question. Of importance is not that reactivity could occur but the extent to which reactivity could affect the data. Finally, consider whether the observational procedure was ethical. You need to consider whether the participants were informed that they were being observed, whether any intervention was performed, and whether the participants had agreed to be observed.

Interviews and questionnaires should be clearly described to allow the reader to decide whether the variables were adequately operationalized. Sometimes the researcher will reference the original report about the tool, and you may wish to read this study before deciding whether the method was appropriate for the current study. Also, the respondents' task should be clear. Thus, the researcher should have made provisions for the participants to understand both their overall responsibilities and the individual items of the interview or questionnaire. The following questions must be considered: Who were the interviewers in the interview situation? Does the researcher explain how they were trained to decrease any interviewer bias?

Available data, such as medical records, are subject to internal and external criticism. **Internal criticism** concerns the evaluation of the worth of the records and refers primarily to the accuracy of the data. The researcher should present evidence that the records are genuine. **External criticism** is concerned with the authenticity of the records. Are the records really written by the first author? The researcher may have a biased sample of all of the possible records in the problem area, which may have a profound effect on the validity of the results.

Once you have decided that the data-collection method used was appropriate for the problem and the procedures were appropriate for the population studied, the reliability and validity of the instruments themselves need to be considered. These characteristics are discussed in Chapter 14.

CRITIQUING CRITERIA

1. Is the framework for research clearly identified?

DATA-COLLECTION METHODS
1. Are all of the data-collection instruments clearly identified and described?
2. Is the rationale for their selection given?
3. Is the method used appropriate for the problem being studied?
4. Were the methods used appropriate for the clinical situation?
5. Are the data-collection procedures similar for all participants?
6. Were efforts made to ensure intervention fidelity through the data-collection protocol?

PHYSIOLOGICAL MEASUREMENT
1. Is the instrument used appropriate for the research problem and not forced to fit it?
2. Is a rationale given for why a particular instrument was selected?
3. Is there a provision for evaluating the accuracy of the instrument

and the skill of the people who used it?

OBSERVATIONAL METHODS
1. Who conducted the observation?
2. Were the observers trained to minimize any bias?
3. Was an observational guide provided?
4. Were the observers required to make inferences about what they saw?
5. Is there any reason to believe that the presence of the observers affected the behaviour of the participants?
6. Were the observations performed according to the principles of informed consent?

INTERVIEWS/FOCUS GROUPS
1. Is the interview schedule described adequately enough for you to know whether it covers the purpose of the study?
2. Is it clear that the participants understood the task and the questions?

3. Who were the interviewers, and how were they trained?
4. Is any interviewer bias evident?

QUESTIONNAIRES
1. Is the questionnaire described well enough for you to know whether it covers the purpose of the study? Is evidence provided that participants were able to perform the task?
2. Is it clear that the participants understood the questionnaire?
3. Are the majority of the items appropriately closed- or open-ended?

AVAILABLE DATA AND RECORDS
1. Are the records used appropriate for the problem being studied?
2. Are the data examined in such a way as to provide new information and not summarize the records?
3. Has the author addressed questions of internal and external criticism?
4. Is there any indication of selection bias in the available records?

CRITICAL THINKING CHALLENGES

- Physiological measurements are objective, precise, and sensitive. Discuss factors that might influence their validity and feasibility.
- A student in research class asks why nurses who participate in a clinical research study in the role of a data collector or who perform a "treatment intervention" need to be trained. What important factors or rationale would you offer to support the establishment of interrater reliability?
- Observation is a data-collection method used frequently in nursing research. Discuss the factors that make nurses perfect potential candidates for this role and the disadvantages of using this method.
- Studies often use a survey to collect data. How can researchers increase their return rate for the survey, and how do they determine whether the survey return is adequate?

KEY POINTS

- Data-collection methods are described as being both objective and systematic. The data-collection methods of a study provide the operational definitions of the relevant variables.
- Types of data-collection methods include physiological measurements, observational methods, interviews, questionnaires, and records or available data. Each method has advantages and disadvantages.
- Physiological measurements are the methods in which technical instruments are used to collect data about patients' physical, chemical, microbiological, or anatomical status. These methods are suited to studying how to improve the effectiveness of nursing care. Physiological measurements are objective, precise, and sensitive, but they may be

very expensive and may distort the variable of interest.

- Observational methods are used in nursing research when the variables of interest deal with events or behaviours. Scientific observation requires preplanning, systematic recording, controlling the observations, and determining the relationship to scientific theory. This method is best suited to research problems that are difficult to view as part of a whole. Observers may be required to perform or not perform interventions, and their activity may be concealed or obvious.

- Observational methods have several advantages: (1) they provide flexibility to measure many types of situations, and (2) they enable a great depth and breadth of information to be collected.

- Observation has disadvantages as well: (1) data may be distorted as a result of the observer's presence (reactivity), (2) concealment requires the consideration of ethical issues, and (3) data from observations may be biased by the person who is doing the observing.

- Interviews are data-collection methods commonly used in nursing research. Items on interview schedules may be of direct or indirect interest. Participants may be asked either open-ended or closed-ended questions. The form of the question should be clear to the respondent, free of suggestion, and grammatically correct.

- Questionnaires, or surveys, are useful when the number of questions to be asked is finite. The questions need to be clear and specific. Questionnaires are less costly and less time consuming to administer to large groups of participants, particularly if the participants are geographically widespread. Questionnaires also can be completely anonymous and prevent interviewer bias.

- Interviews are most appropriate when a large response rate and an unbiased sample are important because the refusal rate for interviews is much lower than that for questionnaires. Interviews enable the participation of people who cannot use a questionnaire, such as children and people who are illiterate. An interviewer can clarify and maintain the order of the questions for all participants.

- Records or available data are also an important source of research data. The use of available data may save the researcher considerable time and money in conducting a study. This method reduces problems with both reactivity and ethical concerns. However, records and available data are subject to problems of availability, authenticity, and accuracy.

- A critical evaluation of data-collection methods should emphasize the appropriateness, objectivity, and consistency of the method employed.

FOR FURTHER STUDY

(e) Go to Evolve at http://evolve.elsevier.com/Canada/LoBiondo/Research for the Audio Glossary and Appendix Tables that provide supplemental information for Appendix E.

REFERENCES

Baumbusch, J., Dahlke, S., & Phinney, A. (2014). Clinical instructors' knowledge and perceptions about nursing care of older people. *Nursing Education in Practice*, *14*, 434–440.

Berman, H., Mason, R., Hall, J., et al. (2014). Laboring to mother in the context of past trauma: The transition to motherhood. *Qualitative Health Research*, *24*(9), 1253–1264.

Borycki, E., Sangster-Gormley, E., Schreiber, R., et al. (2014). Electronic record adoption and use among nurse practitioners in British Columbia. *Canadian Journal of Nursing Research*, *46*(1), 44–65.

Bottorff, J. L., Haines-Saah, R., Oliffe, J. L., et al. (2014). Designing tailored messages about smoking and breast cancer: A focus group study with youth. *Canadian Journal of Nursing Research*, *46*(1), 66–86.

Carpenter, J. S., Burns, D., Wu, J., et al. (2013). Strategies used and data obtained during treatment fidelity monitoring. *Nursing Research*, *62*, 59–65.

Carriere, S. A., Carriere, K., Ayas, N., et al. (2014). Barriers to achieving a time-to-target temperature goal in post-cardiac arrest patients treated with mild therapeutic hypothermia. *Dynamics, 25*(4), 27–32.

Carter, N., Dobbins, M., Peachey, G., et al. (2014). Knowledge transfer and dissemination of advanced practice nursing information and research to acute-care administrators. *Canadian Journal of Nursing Research, 46*(2), 10–27.

Duffy, L. (2015). Achieving a sustainable livelihood after leaving intimate partner violence: Challenges and opportunities. *Journal of Family Violence, 30*, 403–417.

Freeman, M., Beaulieu, L., & Crawley, J. (2015). Canadian nurse graduates considering migrating abroad for work: Are their expectations being met in Canada? *Canadian Journal of Nursing Research, 47*(4), 80–96.

Héon, M., Goulet, C., Garofalo C., et al. (2016). An intervention to promote breast milk production in mothers of preterm infants. *Western Journal of Nursing Research, 385*(5), 529–552.

Kennedy, E., Tomblin-Murphy, G., Martin-Misener, R., et al. (2015). Development and psychometric assessment of the Nursing Competence Self-Efficacy Scale. *Journal of Nursing Education, 54*(10), 550–558.

MacDonald, C., Martin-Misener, R., Steenbeek, A., et al. (2015). Honouring stories: Mi'kmaq women's experiences with Pap screening in Eastern Canada. *Canadian Journal of Nursing Research, 47*(1), 72–96.

McInnis-Perry, G., Weeks, L. E., & Stryhn, H. (2013). Age and gender differences in emotional support and informational social support insufficiency for older adults in Atlantic Canada. *Canadian Journal of Nursing Research, 45*(4), 50–68.

Neyerhof, A. J. (2006). Methods of coping with social desirability bias: A review. *European Journal of Psychology, 15*, 263–280.

Pajares, F., & Urdan, T. (Eds.). (2006). *Self-efficacy beliefs in adolescents*. Greenwich, CT: Information Age Publishing.

Pauly, B., McCall, J., Browne, A. J., et al. (2015). Toward cultural safety: Nurse and patients perceptions of illicit substance use in a hospitalized setting. *Advances in Nursing Science, 38*(2), 121–135.

Santacroce, S. J., Maccarelli, L. M., & Grey, M. (2004). Intervention fidelity. *Nursing Research, 53*, 63–66.

Thomas, M. L., Elliott, J. E., Rao, S. M., et al. (2012). A randomized clinical trial of education or motivational-interviewing–based coaching compared to usual care to improve cancer pain management. *Oncology Nursing Forum, 39*(1), 39–49.

Vandenberg, S. Y., & Kulig, J. C. (2015). Immunization rejection in Southern Alberta: A comparison of the perspectives of mothers and health professionals. *Canadian Journal of Nursing Research, 47*(2), 81–96.

Wang, C. (1999). Photovoice: A participatory action research strategy applied to women's health. *Journal of Women's Health, 8*(2), 185–192.

Wang, C., & Burris. M. A. (1997). Photovoice: Concept, methodology, and use for participatory needs assessment. *Health Education and Behaviour, 24*(3), 369–387.

CHAPTER 14

Rigour in Research

Geri LoBiondo-Wood | Judith Haber | Mina D. Singh

LEARNING OUTCOMES

After reading this chapter, you will be able to do the following:

- Discuss the purposes of reliability and validity.
- Define reliability.
- Discuss the concepts of stability, equivalence, and homogeneity as they relate to reliability.
- Compare the estimates of reliability.
- Define validity.
- Compare content validity, criterion-related validity, and construct validity.
- Discuss how measurement error can affect the outcomes of a research study.
- Identify the criteria for critiquing the reliability and validity of measurement tools.
- Use the critiquing criteria to evaluate the reliability and validity of measurement tools.
- Discuss the purpose of credibility, auditability, and fittingness.
- Apply the critiquing criteria to evaluate the rigour in a qualitative report.
- Discuss how evidence related to research rigour contributes to clinical decision making.

KEY TERMS

alpha coefficient
alternate-form reliability
auditability
chance error
Cohen's kappa
concurrent validity
constant error
construct validity
content validity
contrasted-groups approach
convergent validity
credibility
criterion-related validity
Cronbach's alpha
divergent validity

equivalence
error variance
face validity
factor analysis
fittingness
homogeneity
hypothesis-testing approach
internal consistency
interrater reliability
item-to-total correlation
known-groups approach
Kuder-Richardson (KR-20)
    coefficient
multitrait-multimethod
    approach

observed test score
parallel-form reliability
predictive validity
random error
reliability
reliability coefficient
rigour
split-half reliability
stability
systematic error
test-retest reliability
validation sample
validity

STUDY RESOURCES

ⓔ Go to Evolve at http://evolve.elsevier.com/Canada/LoBiondo/Research
for the Audio Glossary and Appendix Tables that provide supplemental
information for Appendix E.

IN BOTH QUANTITATIVE AND QUALITATIVE RESEARCH, the purpose is to collect trustworthy data that can be used for analyses to make generalizations about the population and that are transferable to other groups. Because findings need to be generalizable and transferable, measurement of nursing phenomena is a major concern of nursing researchers, and rigour is strived for. **Rigour** refers to the strictness with which a study is conducted to enhance the quality, believability, or trustworthiness of the study findings. Rigour in quantitative research is determined by measurement instruments that validly and reliably reflect the concepts of the theory being tested, so that conclusions drawn from a study will be valid and will advance the development of nursing theory and evidence-informed practice. Thus, psychometric assessments are designed to obtain evidence of the quality of these instruments—that is, their reliability and validity.

Issues of reliability and validity are of central concern to the researcher, as well as to you as the critiquer of research. From either perspective, the measurement instruments that are used in a research study must be evaluated. Many new constructs are relevant to nursing theory, and a growing number of established measurement instruments are available to researchers. However, researchers often face the challenge of developing new instruments and, as part of that process, establishing the reliability and validity of those tools.

In qualitative research, rigour is ascertained by credibility, auditability, and fittingness. The growing importance of measurement issues, tool development, and related issues (e.g., reliability and validity, qualitative rigour) is evident in issues of the *Journal of Nursing Measurement,* *Canadian Journal of Nursing Research, International Journal of Qualitative Methods,* and other nursing research journals. In this chapter, concepts related to quantitative rigour are discussed first, followed by factors that contribute to the trustworthiness of qualitative research.

When you read quantitative research studies and reports, you must assess the reliability and validity of the instruments used in each study to determine the soundness of the selection of these instruments in relation to the concepts or variables under investigation. The appropriateness of the instruments and the extent to which reliability and validity are demonstrated have a profound influence on the findings and on the internal and external validity of the study. Invalid measures produce invalid estimates of the relationships between variables, thus affecting internal validity. The use of invalid measures also leads to inaccurate generalizations to the populations being studied, thus affecting external validity and the ability to apply or not apply research findings in clinical practice. Thus, the assessment of reliability and validity is an extremely important skill to develop for critiquing nursing research.

Regardless of whether a new or already developed measurement tool is used in a research study, evidence of reliability and validity is crucial. Box 14.1 identifies several Internet resources that you can use to access and evaluate the reliability and validity of the measurement instruments used in research studies.

RELIABILITY

People are considered reliable when their behaviour is consistent and predictable. Likewise, the **reliability** of a research instrument is the extent to which the instrument yields the same results on repeated measures. Reliability, then, is concerned with consistency, accuracy, precision, stability, equivalence, and homogeneity. Concurrent with questions of validity, or after these questions are answered, the researcher and you, as the critiquer, ask how reliable the instrument is.

A reliable measure can produce the same results if the behaviour is measured again by the same scale. Reliability, then, refers to the proportion of

accuracy to inaccuracy in measurement. In other words, if researchers use the same or comparable instruments on more than one occasion to measure behaviours that ordinarily remain relatively constant, the researchers would expect similar results if the tools are reliable.

The three main attributes of a reliable scale are stability, homogeneity, and equivalence. The **stability** of an instrument refers to the instrument's ability to produce the same results with repeated testing. The **homogeneity,** or **internal consistency,** of an instrument means that all of the items in a tool measure the same concept or characteristic. An instrument is said to exhibit **equivalence** if the tool produces the same results when equivalent or parallel instruments or procedures are used. Each of these attributes and the means to estimate them are discussed here. Before these are discussed, however, an understanding of how to interpret reliability is essential.

Interpretation of the Reliability Coefficient

Because all of the attributes of reliability are concerned with the degree of consistency between scores that is obtained at two or more independent times of testing, these attributes often are expressed in terms of a correlation coefficient. The **reliability coefficient,** or **alpha coefficient,** expresses the relationship between the error variance, true variance, and the observed score, and it ranges from 0 to 1. A correlation of 0 indicates no relationship, and thus the error variance is high. When the error variance in a measurement instrument is low, the reliability coefficient is closer to 1. The closer to 1 the coefficient is, the more reliable the tool is. For example, suppose that a reliability coefficient of a tool is reported to be .89. This number indicates that the error variance is small and the tool has little measurement error. But if the reliability coefficient of a measure is reported to be .49, the error variance is high, and the tool has a problem with measurement error. For a tool to be considered reliable, a level of .70 or higher should be reported, although the intended purpose of the instrument needs to be considered if lower levels are accepted.

The interpretation of the reliability coefficient depends on the proposed purpose of the measure. Seven major tests of reliability can be used to calculate a reliability coefficient, depending on the nature of the tool: *test-retest reliability, parallel-* or *alternate-form reliability, item-to-total correlation, split-half reliability, Kuder-Richardson coefficient, Cronbach's alpha,* and *interrater reliability.* These tests are discussed as they relate to the attributes of stability, homogeneity, and equivalence (Box 14.2). In critiquing research reports, you should be aware that no single best way exists to assess reliability in relation to these attributes and that the researcher's method should be consistent with the aim of the research.

Stability

An instrument is thought to be stable or to exhibit stability when repeated administration of the instrument yields the same results. Researchers are concerned with an instrument's stability because they expect the instrument to measure a concept consistently over a period of time. Measurement over time is important in a longitudinal study because in that type of research, an instrument is used on several occasions. Stability is also a consideration when a researcher is conducting an intervention study that is designed to effect a change in a specific variable. In this case, the instrument is administered once and then again after the alteration or change intervention has been completed. The tests that are used to estimate stability are test-retest reliability and parallel- or alternate-form reliability.

Test-Retest Reliability

Test-retest reliability is the stability of the scores of an instrument when it is administered more than once to the same participants under similar conditions. Scores from repeated testing are compared. This comparison is expressed by a correlation coefficient, usually a Pearson *r* (see Chapter 16). The interval between repeated administrations varies and depends on the concept or variable being measured. For example, if the variable that the test measures is related to developmental stages in children, the interval between test administrations should be short. The amount of time over which the variable was measured should also be recorded in the report.

An example of an instrument that was assessed for test-retest reliability is O'Keefe-McCarthy, McGillion, Nelson, and associates' (2014) Prodromal-Symptoms Screening Scale. Test-retest reliability was assessed at approximately a 2-week interval, and a high test-retest reliability coefficient ($r = .81$, $p < .01$) was obtained. The interval was adequate (2 weeks between testing), and coefficients exceeded .80 and were thus very good (Nunnally & Bernstein, 1994).

Parallel- or Alternate-Form Reliability

Parallel-form reliability is applicable and can be tested only if two comparable forms of the same instrument exist. **Parallel-form reliability,** or **alternate-form reliability,** is like test-retest reliability in that the same individuals are tested more than once within a specific interval, but in the assessment of parallel-form reliability, a different form of the same test is given to the participants

---

BOX **14.2**

MEASURES USED TO TEST RELIABILITY

STABILITY

Test-retest reliability
Parallel- or alternate-form reliability

HOMOGENEITY

Item-to-total correlation
Split-half reliability
Kuder-Richardson (KR-20) coefficient
Cronbach's alpha

EQUIVALENCE

Parallel- or alternate-form reliability
Interrater reliability

on the second testing. Parallel forms or tests contain the same types of items that are based on the same domain or concept, but the wording of the items is different. The development of parallel forms is desired if the instrument is intended to measure a variable for which a researcher believes that "testwiseness" will be a problem; that is, respondents might recognize the test items and try to answer them in the same way as previously, instead of spontaneously.

For example, in their randomized controlled trial, Budin, Hoskins, Haber, and colleagues (2008) compared the differential effect of a phase-specific standardized educational video intervention with that of a telephone counselling intervention on physical, emotional, and social adjustment in women with breast cancer and their partners. Because repeated measures over the four data-collection points—coping with the diagnosis, recovering from surgery, understanding adjuvant therapy, and ongoing recovery—were used, it was appropriate to use two alternative forms of the Partner Relationship Inventory (Hoskins, 1988) to measure emotional adjustment in partners. Each item on one scale (e.g., "I am able to tell my partner how I feel") is paired with one item on the second form (e.g., "My partner tries to understand my feelings"), and the responses should therefore be consistent.

Practically speaking, developing alternative forms of an instrument is difficult because of the many issues of reliability and validity. If alternative forms of a test exist, they should be highly correlated if they are to be considered reliable.

 Research Hint_____

When a longitudinal design with multiple data-collection points is being conducted, look for evidence of test-retest reliability or parallel-form reliability.

Homogeneity, or Internal Consistency

Another attribute related to reliability of an instrument is the homogeneity with which the items within the scale reflect or measure the same concept. In other words, the items within the scale are correlated with, or complementary to, each other, and the scale is *unidimensional*. A unidimensional scale measures one concept, such as exercise self-efficacy. A total score is then used in the analysis of data.

When Babenko-Mould, Iwasiw, Andrusyszyn, and associates' (2012) Empowering Teaching Behaviours Questionnaire–Student (ETBQ-S) was tested for homogeneity, the reliability (alpha) coefficients for the subscales ranged from .74 to .96 with an overall reliability of .89. In exceeding .70, the reliability coefficient provided sufficient evidence of the internal consistency of the instrument. Homogeneity can be assessed with one of four methods: item-to-total correlation, split-half reliability, Kuder-Richardson coefficient, or Cronbach's alpha.

 Research Hint_____

When the characteristics of a study sample differ significantly from those of the sample in the original study, check to see whether the researcher has re-established the reliability of the instrument with the current sample.

Item-to-Total Correlation

The **item-to-total correlation** is a measure of the relationship between each scale item and the total scale. When item-to-total correlations are calculated, a correlation for each item on the scale is generated (Table 14.1). Items that do not achieve a high correlation may be deleted from the instrument. In a research study, the lowest and highest item-to-total correlations are typically reported; the other correlations are usually not reported unless the study is a methodological investigation. An example of an item-to-total correlation report is illustrated in the study by McQueen, Montelpare, and Dennis (2013), who tested the reliability and validity of the Breastfeeding Self-Efficacy Scale. In that study, the item-to-total correlations ranged between .65 and .81 According to Nunnally and Bernstein (1994), these results are

TABLE 14.1	
EXAMPLES OF ITEM-TO-TOTAL CORRELATIONS FROM COMPUTER-GENERATED DATA	
ITEM	**ITEM-TO-TOTAL CORRELATION**
1	.5069
2	.4355
3	.4479
4	.4369
5	.4213
6	.4216

acceptable because the minimal mandatory correlation should be greater than .30.

Grassley, Spencer, and Bryson (2013) conducted a study to develop and test the psychometric properties of the Supportive Needs of Adolescents Breastfeeding Scale. Cronbach's alpha was .83 for the 20-item scale. Two items with corrected item-to-total correlations of .31 and .27 were eliminated. The item-to-total correlation of the final 18 items ranged from .35 to .55. For items on the same subscale, an item-to-total correlation of .30 to .70 is considered sufficient (deVellis, 2012).

Split-Half Reliability

Split-half reliability involves dividing a scale into halves and making a comparison. The halves may be, for example, odd-numbered and even-numbered items or a simple division of the first from the second half, or items may be randomly grouped into halves that will be analyzed opposite one another. Split-half reliability provides a measure of consistency in terms of sampling the content. The two halves of the test or the contents in both halves are assumed to be comparable, and a reliability coefficient is calculated. If the scores for the two halves are approximately equal, the test may be considered reliable.

The Spearman-Brown formula is one method of calculating the reliability coefficient. In a test

of the Worry Interference Scale, a seven-item self-report measure was developed to assess the degree to which respondents believe that thoughts about breast cancer are interfering with daily functioning. The measure is embedded within a larger questionnaire that is also used to assess perceived risk, intention to undergo genetic testing, and frequency of worry about getting breast cancer. The Worry Interference Scale items concern disruptions in sleep, work, concentration, relationships, having fun, feeling sexually attractive, meeting family needs, and reproductive decisions. Ibrahim (2002) computed a Spearman-Brown split-half reliability and found a reliability coefficient that ranged from .83 to .92 for the first four items and from .75 to .83 for the other items. Split-half reliabilities of at least .75 are considered internally consistent.

Kuder-Richardson Coefficient

The **Kuder-Richardson (KR-20) coefficient** is the estimate of homogeneity used for instruments that have a dichotomous response format. A *dichotomous response format* is one in which the answer to a question should be either "yes" or "no" or either "true" or "false." The technique yields a correlation that is based on the consistency of responses to all items of a single form of a test that is administered once.

For example, in an investigation of the effectiveness of a randomized support group intervention for women with breast cancer, breast cancer knowledge was assessed with a 25-item true/false questionnaire developed for the study. Items were obtained from the American Cancer Society's (2010) publication *Cancer Facts and Figures* and were categorized as follows: knowledge of risk factors for developing breast cancer (10 items; e.g., "Most women diagnosed with breast cancer have at least one known risk factor for the disease"); symptoms of breast cancer (5 items; e.g., "Women who have breast cancer never experience any symptoms of the disease"); side effects of treatment (3 items; e.g., "A common side effect of radiation is sunburn-like symptoms"); treatment efficacy (4 items; e.g., "For women with small tumours that may not have spread outside the breast, having either a mastectomy or lumpectomy with axillary lymph node dissection results in the same overall life expectancy"); and methods of treatment (3 items; e.g., "Hormone treatment is used only for premenopausal women"). Because the scale was a binary format (true/false), the Kuder-Richardson reliability for the entire scale was calculated at .75, which is acceptable, having exceeded the minimum acceptable score of .70; however, the magnitude of the correlation is not robust.

Cronbach's Alpha

The fourth and most commonly used test of internal consistency is Cronbach's alpha. **Cronbach's alpha** is a test of internal consistency in which each item in the scale is simultaneously compared with the others, and a total score is then used to analyze the data. Many tools used to measure psychosocial variables and attitudes have a Likert-type scale response format (Figure 14.1),

which is very suitable for testing internal consistency. In a Likert-type scale format, the participant responds to a question on a scale of varying degrees of intensity between two extremes. The two extremes are anchored by responses ranging from, for example, "strongly agree" to "strongly disagree" or from "most like me" to "least like me." The points between the two extremes may range from 1 to 5 or 1 to 7. Participants are asked to circle the response that most closely represents what they believe. Examples of reported Cronbach's alpha for various studies are given in Box 14.3.

Figure 14.1 displays examples of items from a tool in which a Likert-type scale format was used to develop a nurses' perception of clinical reasoning instrument (Liou, Liu, Tsai, et al., 2015). The psychometric properties of Kennedy, Tomblin-Murphy, Martin-Misener, and colleagues' (2015) Nursing Competence Self-Efficacy Scale were tested for internal consistency and construct validity. The testing revealed that there were four separate domains: proficiency, altruism, prevention, and leadership, as illustrated in Table 14.2. Cronbach's

---

Directions: Please read each item and circle the number that best describes your current performance. There is no right or wrong answer.
5 = Strongly agree, 4 = Agree, 3 = Neutral, 2 = Disagree, 1 = Strongly disagree

1. I know how to collect an admitted patient's health information quickly.	5	4	3	2	1
2. I can apply proper assessment skills to collect a patient's current health information.	5	4	3	2	1
3. I can identify abnormalities from the collected patient information.	5	4	3	2	1
4. I can identify a patient's health problems from the abnormal information collected.	5	4	3	2	1
5. I can recognize possible early signs or symptoms when a patient's health deteriorates.	5	4	3	2	1
6. I can explain the mechanism and development associated with the early signs or symptoms when a patient's health deteriorates.	5	4	3	2	1
7. I can accurately prioritize and manage any identifiable patient problems.	5	4	3	2	1
8. I can correctly explain the mechanism behind a patient's problems.	5	4	3	2	1
9. I can set nursing goals properly for the identified patient problems.	5	4	3	2	1
10. I can provide appropriate nursing intervention for the identified patient problems.	5	4	3	2	1
11. I am knowledgeable of each nursing intervention provided.	5	4	3	2	1
12. I can identify and communicate vital information clearly to the doctors based on the patient's current condition.	5	4	3	2	1
13. I can anticipate the prescription ordered by the doctor according to the patient information provided.	5	4	3	2	1
14. I can accurately evaluate and identify whether a patient's condition is improved.	5	4	3	2	1
15. I know the follow-up steps to take if the patient's condition does not improve.	5	4	3	2	1

FIG. 14.1 Example of a Likert-type scale response format.
From Liou, S. R., Liu, H. C., Tsai, H. M., et al. (2015). The development and psychometric testing of a theory-based instrument to evaluate nurses' perception of clinical reasoning competence. *Journal of Advanced Nursing, 72*(3), 707–717. Copyright © 2015 John Wiley & Sons Ltd.

EXAMPLES OF REPORTED CRONBACH'S ALPHA

"Inter-item correlation coefficients were reviewed for redundancy ($r > .85$) among items. Item-to-total correlation coefficients $> .30$ and alpha coefficient $\geq .70$ supported the TSC [Therapeutic Self-Care] measure's internal consistency reliability" (Sidani & Doran, 2014, p. 20).

"For the ETBQ-S [Empowering Teaching Behaviours Questionnaire], Cronbach's alpha reliability coefficients for subscales ranged from .74 to .96 with an overall reliability of .89" (Babenko-Mould et al., 2012, p. 7).

"Internal consistency for survey responses in hospital using Cronbach's alpha was 0.95" (McQueen et al., 2013, p. 66).

"The estimated Cronbach's alpha for the revised 22-item NCSES [Nursing Competence Self-Efficacy Scale] with the study population was high (.919)" (Kennedy, et al., 2015, p. 554).

alpha exceeded 70 for each domain, thereby providing sufficient evidence of the internal consistency of the instrument.

Research Hint

If a research article provides information about the reliability of a measurement instrument but does not specify the type of reliability, it is probably safe to assume that internal consistency reliability was assessed with Cronbach's alpha.

TABLE **14.2**

CRONBACH'S ALPHA SCORES FOR THE FOUR DOMAINS OF THE NURSING COMPETENCE SELF-EFFICACY SCALE

OPTIONS	CRONBACH'S ALPHA
Proficiency	.79
Altruism	.85
Prevention	.78
Leadership	.75

Adapted from Kennedy, E., Tomblin-Murphy, G., Martin-Misener, R., et al. (2015). Development and psychometric assessment of the Nursing Competence Self-Efficacy Scale. *Journal of Nursing Education, 54*(10), 550–558. Copyright © 2009 Wiley Periodicals, Inc.

Equivalence

Equivalence is either the consistency or agreement among observers who use the same measurement tool or the consistency or agreement between alternative forms of a tool. An instrument is thought to demonstrate equivalence when two or more observers have a high percentage of agreement about a certain behaviour or when alternative forms of a test yield a high correlation. Two methods to test equivalence are interrater reliability and alternate- or parallel-form reliability.

Interrater Reliability

Some measurement instruments are not self-administered questionnaires but instead are direct measurements of observed behaviour that must be systematically recorded. Such instruments must be tested for **interrater reliability** (the consistency of observations between two or more observers with the same tool). To accomplish interrater reliability, either two or more individuals should make an observation or one observer should observe the same behaviour on several occasions. The observers should score their observations with regard to the definition and operationalization of the behaviour to be observed.

When the research method of direct observation of a behaviour is required, consistency (or reliability) of the observations among all observers is extremely important. Interrater reliability concerns the reliability (or consistency) of the observer, not the reliability of the instrument. Interrater reliability is expressed either as a percentage of agreement between scorers or as a correlation coefficient of the scores assigned to the observed behaviours.

In a study by deMan-van Ginkel, Gooskens, Schepers, and colleagues (2012) that investigated the reliability, validity, and clinical utility of the nine-item patient health questionnaire (PHQ-9) and the two-item PHQ-2 patient health questionnaires in stroke patients in a clinical setting, interrater reliability was established based on the sum score level of the PHQ-9 and the PHQ-2, which showed similar results (ICC [intraclass correlation] = .98, 95% CI [confidence interval] [.96, .99]) demonstrating very good interrater reliability. Another type of interrater reliability is Cohen's kappa, a coefficient of agreement between two raters that is considered to be a more precise estimate of interrater reliability. **Cohen's kappa** expresses the level of agreement that is observed beyond the level that would be expected by chance alone. A Cohen's kappa of .80 or better is generally assumed to indicate good interrater reliability. A Cohen's kappa of .68 allows tentative conclusions to be drawn when lower levels of reliability are acceptable (McDowell & Newell, 1996). In her study on metacognitive factors that affect student nurses' use of point-of-care technology in clinical settings, Kuiper (2010) established interrater reliability (.70 to .90) to determine consistency in order to reflect self-regulated learning processes in journal prompts.

 Evidence-Informed Practice Tip _____

Interrater reliability is important for minimizing bias.

Parallel- or Alternate-Form Reliability

Parallel- or alternate-form reliability was described in the discussion of stability (see pp. 307–308). Use of parallel forms is thus a measure of stability and equivalence. The procedures for assessing equivalence through the use of parallel forms are the same.

VALIDITY

Validity refers to whether a measurement instrument accurately measures what it is intended to measure. To be valid, an instrument must first be reliable; without reliability, the instrument cannot have validity. However, reliability, although necessary, is not a sufficient condition for validity. Internal and external validity of a study are discussed in Chapter 9.

For example, a valid instrument that is intended to measure anxiety does so; it does not measure another construct, such as stress. A reliable measure can consistently rank participants on a given construct (e.g., anxiety), but a valid measure correctly measures the construct of interest. A measure can be reliable but not valid. Suppose that a researcher wanted to measure anxiety in patients by measuring their body temperatures. The researcher could obtain highly accurate, consistent, and precise temperature recordings, but such a measure would not be a valid indicator of anxiety. Thus, the high reliability of an instrument is not necessarily congruent with evidence of validity. A valid instrument, however, is reliable. If an instrument is erratic, inconsistent, and inaccurate, it cannot validly measure the attribute of interest.

The three major kinds of validity—content, criterion-related, and construct validity—vary according to the kind of information provided and the investigator's purpose. In critiquing research articles, you will want to evaluate whether sufficient evidence of validity is present and whether the type of validity is appropriate to the design of the study and instruments used in the study. The sample that provides the initial data for determining the reliability and validity of a measurement tool is termed a **validation sample.**

 Evidence-Informed Practice Tip _____

Selecting measurement instruments that have strong evidence of validity increases the reader's confidence in the study findings—that the researchers actually measured what they intended to measure.

Content Validity

Content validity is the degree to which the content of the measure represents the universe of content—that is, the domain of a given construct. The universe of content provides the framework and basis for formulating the items that will adequately represent the content. When an investigator is developing a tool and issues of content

Practical Application

Kennedy and colleagues (2015) reported on the item selection process and evaluation of the content validity of the Nursing Competence Self-Efficacy Scale for baccalaureate students. Items were developed through the use of several sources: review of entry to practice documents within Nova Scotia, literature review, and an expert panel. Content validity was measured by a panel of experts through the use of a content validity questionnaire. A content validity index was calculated to determine the relevance of each indicator and panel members' agreement with the scales. Kennedy at al. (2015) sought content validity for the Nursing Competence Self-Efficacy Scale by including an expert panel in a two-step assessment of items for potential inclusion. Then, student readers reviewed the instrument for clarity and ease of interpretation.

validity arise, the concern is whether the measurement tool and the items it contains are representative of the universe of content that the researcher intends to measure. The researcher begins by defining the concept and identifying the dimensions that are the components of the concept. The items that reflect the concept and its dimensions are formulated (see Practical Application box for an example).

When the researcher has completed this task, the items are submitted to a panel of judges considered to be experts on this concept. Researchers typically request that the judges indicate their level of agreement with the scope of the items and the extent to which the items reflect the concept under consideration.

A subtype of content validity is **face validity,** which is a rudimentary type of validity in which the instrument intuitively gives the appearance of measuring the concept. To establish face validity, colleagues or participants are asked to read the instrument and evaluate the content in terms of whether it appears to reflect the concept that the researcher intends to measure. This procedure may be useful in the tool development process in terms of determining the readability and clarity of the content. Face validity, however, should in no

way be considered a satisfactory alternative to other types of validity. In the development of the ETBQ-S, Babenko-Mould and associates (2012) established face validity by using a panel of nursing professors familiar with the empowerment process model they were using to build the questionnaire. The panel agreed that the items within each subscale represented the specific categories and empowerment as a whole.

Evidence-Informed Practice Tip ____

When face validity and content validity, the most basic types of validity, are the only types of validity reported in a research article, you, as a research consumer, cannot appraise the measurement tools as having strong psychometric properties; thus, you would lack confidence in the usefulness of the study findings.

Criterion-Related Validity

Criterion-related validity is the degree of relationship between the participant's performance on the measurement tool and the participant's actual behaviour. The criterion is usually the second measure, which is used to assess the same concept being studied.

Two types of criterion-related validity are concurrent and predictive. **Concurrent validity** is the degree of correlation of two measures of the same construct administered at the same time. A high correlation coefficient indicates agreement between the two measures. **Predictive validity** is the degree of correlation between the measure of the concept and a future measure of the same concept. Because of the passage of time, the correlation coefficients are likely to be lower for predictive validity studies.

For example, in a study by Sherman, Haber, Hoskins, and colleagues (2012) investigating the effects of psychoeducation and telephone counselling on the physical, emotional, and social adjustment of women with early-stage breast cancer, criterion-related validity was supported by correlating amount of distress experienced (ADE) scores, measured by the Breast Cancer Treatment

Response Inventory (BCTRI), and total scores from the Symptom Distress Scale ($r = .86$; $p < .000$). An example of predictive validity appears in the study of Babenko-Mould and colleagues (2012), who assessed the psychometric properties of the ETBQ-S scale. The researchers assessed the predictive validity of this scale by analyzing the extent to which students' perceptions of clinical teachers' use of Empowering Teaching Behaviour (ETB) scores (criterion) predicted overall students' structural empowerment between the ETBQ-S and the Conditions of Work Effectiveness-II-ED (Siu, Laschinger, & Vingilis, 2005) instrument. Predictive validity was confirmed, as nursing students' scores on all ETB predicted their structural empowerment scores.

Construct Validity

Construct validity is the extent to which a test measures a theoretical construct or trait. To establish this type of validity, the researcher attempts to validate a body of theory underlying the measurement and testing of the hypothesized relationships. Empirical testing confirms or fails to confirm the relationships that would be predicted among concepts and, as such, provides more or less support for the construct validity of the instruments measuring those concepts. Establishing construct validity is a complex process, often involving several studies and approaches. The following approaches are discussed in this section: hypothesis-testing, convergent and divergent, contrasted-groups, and factor-analytical.

In their study, McQueen and associates (2013) assessed construct validity by factor analysis and hypothesizing that women who had previously breastfed an infant would have higher self-efficacy than primiparous and multiparous women who had never breastfed.

Hypothesis-Testing Approach

When the **hypothesis-testing approach** is used, the investigator uses the theory or concept underlying the measurement instrument to validate the instrument. The investigator accomplishes this task first by developing hypotheses about the behaviour of individuals with varying scores on the measure; then by gathering data to test the hypotheses; and, finally, on the basis of the findings, by making inferences about whether the rationale underlying the instrument's construction is adequate to explain the findings. Hypothesis-testing approaches include convergent validity, divergent validity, and known-groups validity.

For example, McQueen and colleagues (2013) used a hypothesis testing approach to establish the Breastfeeding Self-Efficacy Scale-Short Form (BSEF-SF). Construct validity was tested positively on the basis of two hypotheses: (1) women who had previously breastfed would have higher breastfeeding self-efficacy than those who had not, and (2) women who had depressive symptoms would have lower breastfeeding self-efficacy.

Convergent and Divergent Approaches

Two strategies for assessing construct validity are convergent and divergent approaches.

Convergent validity exists when two or more tools that are intended to measure the same construct are administered to participants and are found to be positively correlated. A correlational analysis (i.e., a test of relationship; see Chapters 11 and 16) determines whether the measures are positively correlated, in which case convergent validity is said to be supported.

Williams, Dixon, Van Ness, and associates (2011) developed and tested the Determinants of Meditation Practice Inventory (DMPI), an instrument used to capture barriers to meditation use. They used two validated instruments to test convergent validity: the Big Five Inventory (BFI), which is a personality inventory, and the Caregiver Reactions Assessment (CRA), which is a burden measure. The authors hypothesized that participants with high-perceived burden (as measured by the CRA) and high neuroticism personality trait (as measured by the BFI) would identify a high number of barriers to meditation (as measured by the DMPI). The BFI and CRA were significantly and positively correlated with the DMPI.

In contrast to convergent validity, the calculation of **divergent validity** requires measurement approaches that differentiate one construct from others that may be similar. Sometimes researchers search for instruments that measure the opposite of the construct. If the divergent measure is negatively related to other measures, the measure's validity is strengthened.

As an example, Melnyk, Oswalt, and Sidora-Arcoleo (2014) assessed the psychometric properties of scores on the Neonatal Intensive Care Unit Parental Beliefs Scale (NICU PBS) in a sample of mothers and fathers of preterm infants receiving intensive care. The NICU PBS is a rating instrument designed to assess parental beliefs about their premature infant and their role during hospitalization. For convergent and divergent (discriminant) validity assessment, correlation analysis of the Time 1 data was used for assessment of the NICU PBS with maternal demographic characteristics (age, education, employment status), mental health, stress, pregnancy history variables (gravidity, high-risk status, subsequent pregnancy in 12 months), and baby outcome variables (Clinical Risk Index for Babies [CRIB] scores, birth weight, NICU length of stay). Higher total PBS scores were associated with younger maternal age, lower education, lower income, receipt of Medicaid, minority status, mothers' employment, no biological father in the study, higher gravidity, having had another child in the past 12 months, shorter NICU length of stay, and lower stress, anxiety, and depression.

A specific method of assessing convergent and divergent validity is the **multitrait-multimethod approach.** Similar to the divergent validity approach just described, this method, proposed by Campbell and Fiske (1959), also involves examining the relationships between instruments that are intended to measure the same construct and between those that are intended to measure different constructs. A variety of measurement strategies, however, are used. In other words, this approach is a type of validation in which more than one method is used to assess the accuracy of an instrument. For example, anxiety could be measured by the following:

- Administering the State-Trait Anxiety Inventory
- Recording blood pressure readings
- Asking the participant about anxious feelings
- Observing the participant's behaviour

The results of one of these measures should then be correlated with the results of each of the others in a multitrait-multimethod matrix (Waltz, Strickland, & Lenz, 1991).

The use of multiple measures of a concept decreases systematic error. The use of a variety of data-collection methods (e.g., self-report, observation, interview, and collection of physiological data) also diminishes the effect of systematic error.

Contrasted-Groups Approach

In the **contrasted-groups approach** (sometimes called the **known-groups approach**) to the development of construct validity, the researcher identifies two groups of individuals expected to score extremely high or extremely low in the characteristic being measured by the instrument. The instrument is administered to both groups, and the differences in scores are examined. If the instrument is sensitive to individual differences in the trait being measured, the mean performance of these two groups should differ significantly, and evidence of construct validity would be supported. A *t* test or analysis of variance is used to statistically measure the difference between the two groups.

Factor-Analytical Approach

A final approach to assessing construct validity is **factor analysis.** This procedure gives the researcher information about the extent to which a set of items measures the same underlying construct or the same dimension of a construct. In factor analysis, the researcher assesses the degree to which the individual items on a scale truly cluster around one or more dimensions. Items designed to measure the same dimension should load on the same factor; those designed to measure differing dimensions should load on different factors (Nunnally & Bernstein, 1994).

A factor analysis also indicates whether the items in the instrument reflect a single construct or several constructs. Several factors may be identified in a set of data. The study must have a large sample size in order to conduct a factor analysis. Nunnally and Bernstein (1994) recommended 10 observations for each variable. Thus, to develop the factor structure and reliability of the Nursing Competence Self-Efficacy Scale, Kennedy and associates (2015) used 252 students to test 22 items.

Research Hint

When validity data about a study's measurement instruments are not included in a research article, you cannot determine whether the intended concept is being captured by the measurement tool. Before you use the results, check the instrument's validity by reviewing the original source.

Evidence-Informed Practice Tip

When the tools used in a study are presented, note whether the sample used to develop the measurement instruments is similar to your patient population.

The Critical Thinking Decision Path will help you assess the appropriateness of the type of validity and reliability selected for use in a particular research study.

Researchers may be concerned about whether the scores that were obtained for a sample of participants were consistent, true measures of the behaviours, and thus an accurate reflection of the differences between individuals. The extent of variability in test scores that is attributable to error rather than a true measure of the behaviours is the **error variance.**

An **observed test score** that is derived from a set of items consists of the true score plus error (Figure 14.2). The error may be either chance (random) error or systematic error.

A **chance error** or a **random error** is an error that is difficult to control (e.g., a respondent's anxiety at the time of testing). These errors are unsystematic and are not predictable; thus, they cannot be corrected. However, awareness of the sources of these errors may help the researcher minimize their effect on measurement accuracy. These sources are as follows:

1. Transient human conditions, such as hunger, fatigue, health, lack of motivation, and anxiety, which are often beyond the awareness and control of the examiner.

2. Variations in the measurement procedure, such as misplacement of the blood pressure cuff, not waiting for a specific time period before taking the blood pressure, or placing the arm randomly in relation to the heart while measuring blood pressure; changing the wording of interview questions between administrations; or environmental factors, such as the presence of others while data are being obtained, a cold room, or discomfort with the researcher (who is part of the environment).

3. Errors in data processing, such as coding errors and incorrect inputting into the computer.

Chance errors affect an individual's observed score, so that the person's observed score may be higher than his or her true score, whereas another person's observed score may be lower than his or her true score. Instruments that are free of chance errors are considered reliable. A **systematic error**

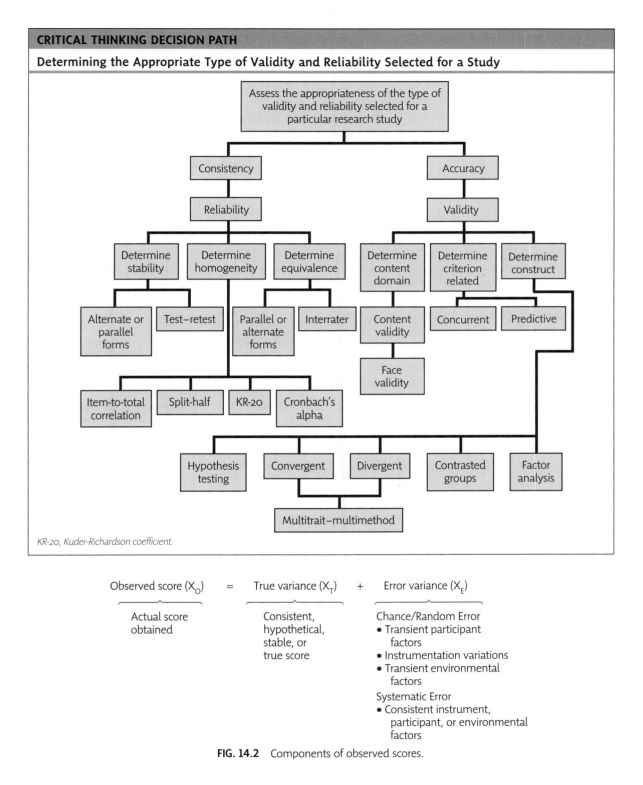

CRITICAL THINKING DECISION PATH

Determining the Appropriate Type of Validity and Reliability Selected for a Study

Assess the appropriateness of the type of validity and reliability selected for a particular research study

Consistency

Accuracy

Reliability

Validity

Determine stability

Determine homogeneity

Determine equivalence

Determine content domain

Determine criterion related

Determine construct

Alternate or parallel forms

Test–retest

Parallel or alternate forms

Interrater

Content validity

Concurrent

Predictive

Face validity

Item-to-total correlation

Split-half

KR-20

Cronbach's alpha

Hypothesis testing

Convergent

Divergent

Contrasted groups

Factor analysis

Multitrait–multimethod

KR-20, Kuder-Richardson coefficient.

Observed score (X_O)	=	True variance (X_T)	+	Error variance (X_E)
Actual score obtained		Consistent, hypothetical, stable, or true score		Chance/Random Error • Transient participant factors • Instrumentation variations • Transient environmental factors Systematic Error • Consistent instrument, participant, or environmental factors

FIG. 14.2 Components of observed scores.

or a **constant error** is a measurement error that is attributable to relatively stable characteristics of the study population that may bias their behaviour, cause incorrect instrument calibration, or both. Such error has a systematic biasing influence on the participants' responses and thereby influences the validity of the instruments. Level of education, socioeconomic status, social desirability, response pattern, or other characteristics may influence the validity of the instrument by altering the measurement of the "true" responses in a systematic way. For example, a participant who wants to please the investigator may constantly answer items in a socially desirable way, thus making the estimate of validity inaccurate.

Systematic error also occurs when an instrument is improperly calibrated. Consider a scale that consistently gives a person's weight at 1 kg less than the actual body weight. The scale could be quite reliable (i.e., capable of reproducing the precise measurement), but the result is consistently invalid. Systematic error is considered part of the true score. The multimethod-multitrait approach is one method of decreasing systematic error. The validity of an instrument is the extent to which it is free of both chance errors and systematic errors.

The amount of detail about reliability and validity varies considerably among research articles. When the focus of a study is tool development, psychometric evaluation—including extensive reliability and validity data—is carefully documented and appears throughout the article rather than briefly in the "Instruments" section, as in other research studies.

RIGOUR IN QUALITATIVE RESEARCH: CREDIBILITY, AUDITABILITY, AND FITTINGNESS

As in quantitative research, the basic approach to ensure rigour in qualitative research is methodical research design, data collection, interpretation, and communication. Qualitative researchers seek to achieve two goals: (1) to account for the method and the data, which must be independent so that another researcher can analyze the same data in the same way and make the same conclusions, and (2) to produce a credible and reasoned explanation of the phenomenon under study. Thus, this rigour in qualitative methodology is judged by unique criteria appropriate for the research approach and is called *trustworthiness*. Credibility, auditability, and fittingness are some of the scientific criteria for trustworthiness proposed for qualitative research studies by Lincoln and Guba (1985). Although these criteria are not new, they still capture the rigorous spirit of qualitative inquiry and are reasonable for evaluation. The meanings of credibility, auditability, and fittingness are briefly explained in Table 14.3. Guba and Lincoln (1994) added authenticity, as a criterion for qualitative rigour.

TABLE **14.3**

CRITERIA FOR JUDGING SCIENTIFIC RIGOUR: CREDIBILITY, AUDITABILITY, FITTINGNESS	
CRITERIA	**CHARACTERISTICS**
Credibility	Truth of findings as judged by participants and others within the discipline. For example, you may find the researcher returning to the participants to share interpretation of findings and query accuracy from the perspective of the persons living the experience.
Auditability	Accountability as judged by the adequacy of information leading the reader from the research question and raw data through various steps of analysis to the interpretation of findings. For example, you should be able to follow the reasoning of the researcher step by step through explicit examples of data, interpretations, and syntheses.
Fittingness	Faithfulness to the everyday reality of the participants, described in enough detail so that others in the discipline can evaluate importance for their own practice, research, and theory development. For example, you will know enough about the human experience being reported that you can decide whether it "rings true" and is useful for guiding your practice.

Credibility

Credibility is a characteristic of qualitative research that refers to the accuracy, validity, and soundness of data. It is similar to internal validity in qualitative research. The methods to ensure credibility are prolonged engagement, persistent observation, peer debriefing, and member checks (Lincoln, 1995). In prolonged engagement and persistent observation, the researchers spend sufficient time with the study's participants to check for discrepancies in responses. Peer debriefing is conducted with experts in the field, whose probing questions and review about the research can assist the researchers in improving trustworthiness in the data. Member checking verifies the accuracy of participants' responses by asking the study participants to review the themes and narratives to determine whether the researchers accurately described their experiences (Lincoln & Guba, 1985).

Triangulation, crystallization, and searching for disconfirming evidence through negative case analyses are also used to ensure credibility and confirmability. In Chapter 7, triangulation—the cross-checking and verification of data through the use of different information sources, such as a variety of data sources, investigators, theoretical models, and research methods—and crystallization in both qualitative and mixed method research are discussed. Triangulation is viewed as offering completeness to naturalistic inquiry (Tobin & Begley, 2004).

Auditability and Fittingness

Engaging in an inquiry audit establishes both the auditability and the fittingness of the data. **Auditability** is the characteristic of a qualitative study, developed by the investigator's research process, that allows another researcher or a reader to follow the thinking or conclusions of the investigator. **Fittingness** is the degree to which study findings are applicable outside the study situation and the degree to which the results are meaningful to individuals not involved in the research. The audit trail was proposed by Guba (1981) to allow external auditors to follow the trail of qualitative data gathering and has been described by Lincoln and Guba (1985) as "the most important trustworthiness technique available to the naturalistic" (p. 283). The audit trail involves reviewing all documents relating to the study, such as research protocol, memos and correspondences, research tools, and field notes.

Authenticity

Authenticity refers to fairness in the presentation in that all value conflicts, differences, and views of the participants are noted in the analysis. The reader is able to understand the moods and experiences of the participants while reading the thematic analyses (Guba & Lincoln, 1994).

See the Practical Application boxes for examples of establishing rigour in qualitative research.

Ethnographers keep track of changes in their ideas, beliefs, and values as they are engaged in the research.

> **Practical Application**
>
> In an illustration of how rigour is ascertained, MacDonald, Martin-Misener, Steenbeek, and associates (2015) (see Appendix A) conducted a qualitative study to identify Mi'kmaq women's experiences with Pap screening. MacDonald and associates established trustworthiness in the data by engaging in a variety of methods. For credibility, they used verbatim quotations to illustrate findings, member checking, presenting their preliminary findings to some participants, and requesting participants' views on the accuracy of interpretation. The women then changed some of the titles of the themes and subthemes and offered explanations from an Indigenous perspective for why the titles were or were not appropriate. In addressing the study's generalizability, the authors stated that "women under 21 years of age and women who had never had Pap screening were excluded from the study; therefore, the findings may not be transferable to their experiences or perspectives" (p. 90).

> ## Practical Application
>
> Pauly, McCall, Browne, et al. (2015) (see Appendix C) incorporated several strategies to ascertain rigour. They explored the nurses' and patients' perceptions of illicit drug use in a hospital setting. Credibility was established through the transcription of the interviews, field notes, immersion of the researchers by being participant observers, triangulating data from multiple sources, and reading the data multiple times. Multiple researchers read and coded the data independently, leading to confirmability. To strengthen confirmability, the authors involved nurse and peer advisory groups in the interpretation of the data. Applicability/fittingness and transferability were achieved by presenting to audiences who found resonance in the findings. Because the three criteria of credibility, fittingness, and auditability were met, confirmability was achieved.

APPRAISING THE EVIDENCE

Reliability and Validity

Reliability and validity are two crucial aspects in the critical appraisal of a measurement instrument. The reviewer evaluates an instrument's level of reliability and validity, as well as how they were established. In a research report, the reliability and validity for each measure should be presented. If these data have not been presented, the reviewer must seriously question the merit and use of the tool and the study's results. Criteria for critiquing reliability and validity are presented in the Critiquing Criteria box.

If reliable and valid questionnaires are not used in a study, the results cannot be credible. As a critiquer, you have an ethical responsibility to question the reliability and validity of instruments used in research studies and to examine the findings in view of the quality of the instruments used and the data presented. The following discussion highlights key areas related to reliability and validity that should be evident in a research article.

Appropriate reliability tests should have been performed by the developer of the measurement tool and should then have been included by the current user in the research report. If the initial standardization sample and the current sample have different characteristics, the reader would find either (1) that a pilot study for the present sample would have been conducted to determine whether the reliability was maintained or (2) that a reliability estimate was calculated for the current sample. For example, if the standardization sample for a tool that measures "satisfaction in an intimate heterosexual relationship" comprises undergraduate college students and if an investigator plans to use the tool with married couples, the reliability of the tool should be established with the latter group.

The investigator determines which type of reliability procedure is used in the study, depending on the nature of the measurement tool and how it will be used. For example, if the instrument is to be administered twice, you might determine that test-retest reliability should have been used to establish the stability of the tool. If an alternate form of the instrument has been developed for use in a repeated-measures design, evidence of alternate-form reliability should be presented to determine the equivalence of the parallel forms.

If the degree of internal consistency among the items is relevant, an appropriate test of internal consistency should be presented. In some instances, more than one type of reliability is presented, but you should determine whether all are appropriate. For example, the Kuder-Richardson formula implies that a single right or wrong answer exists, which makes use of the coefficient inappropriate with scales that provide a format of three or more possible responses. In such cases, another formula is applied, such as Cronbach's alpha.

Another important consideration is the acceptable level of reliability, which varies according to the type of test. Coefficients with reliability of .70 or higher are desirable. The validity of an instrument is limited by its reliability; in other words, less confidence can be placed in scores from tests with low-reliability coefficients.

Satisfactory evidence of validity is probably the most difficult determination for you as reviewer. This aspect of measurement is most likely to fall short of meeting the required criteria. Validity studies are time consuming and complex, and researchers sometimes settle for presenting minimal validity data.

APPRAISING THE EVIDENCE—cont'd

Reliability and Validity

Therefore, you should closely examine the item content of a tool when you evaluate its strengths and weaknesses and try to find conclusive evidence of content validity. In the body of a research article, however, it is unusual to have more than a few sample items available for review. Thus, you should determine whether the appropriate assessment of content validity was used to meet the researcher's goal.

Such procedures provide assurance that the tool is psychometrically sound and that the content of the items is consistent with the conceptual framework and the construct definitions. Construct validity and criterion-related validity are two of the more precise statistical tests of whether the tool measures what it is intended to measure. Ideally, an instrument should provide evidence of content validity, as well as criterion-related or construct validity, before a reviewer invests a high level of confidence in the tool.

You should also expect to see the strengths and weaknesses of instrument reliability and validity presented in the "Discussion," "Limitations," or "Recommendations" section, or in all of these sections, of a research article. In this context, the reliability and validity might be discussed in relation to other tools devised to measure the same variable. The relationship of the study's findings to the strengths and weaknesses in instrument reliability and validity is another important discussion point.

Finally, the researcher should propose recommendations for improving future studies in relation to instrument reliability and validity. For example, in the "Implications for Future Research and Practice" section of a report about developing and validating the Nursing Competence Self-Efficacy Scale, Kennedy and associates (2015) noted that they will be conducting a replication of this initial psychometric assessment with a larger sample to support the factor structure in the study.

Collegial dialogue is also an approach to evaluating the merits and shortcomings of an existing instrument, as well as a newly developed one, that is reported in the nursing literature. Such an exchange promotes the understanding of methodologies and techniques of reliability and validity, stimulates the acquisition of a basic knowledge of psychometrics, and encourages the exploration of alternative methods of observation and the use of reliable and valid tools in clinical practice.

CRITIQUING CRITERIA

QUANTITATIVE STUDIES

1. Was an appropriate method used to test the reliability of the tool?
2. Is the reliability of the tool adequate?
3. Was an appropriate method used to test the validity of the instrument?
4. Is the validity of the measurement tool adequate?
5. If the sample from the developmental stage of the tool was different from the current sample, were the reliability and validity recalculated to determine whether the tool is still adequate?
6. Have the strengths and weaknesses of the reliability and validity of each instrument been presented?
7. Are the strengths and weaknesses of the research appropriately addressed in the "Discussion," "Limitations," or "Recommendations" sections of the report?

QUALITATIVE STUDIES

1. Do the participants recognize the data as their own?
2. Is evidence provided that the researcher's interpretation accurately represented the participant's meaning?
3. Can the reader follow the researcher's thinking?
4. Have other professionals confirmed the researcher's interpretation?
5. Can the findings be applicable to outside the study situation?
6. Are the results meaningful to individuals not involved in the research?
7. Do the conclusions, implications, and recommendations give the reader a context in which to use the findings?
8. Do the conclusions reflect the study's findings?

CRITICAL THINKING CHALLENGES

- Discuss the three types of validity that must be established before a reviewer invests a high level of confidence in the tool. Include examples of each type of validity.
- What are the major tests of reliability? Is it necessary to establish more than one measure of reliability for each instrument used in a study? Which do you think is the most essential measure of reliability? Include examples in your answer.
- Is it possible to have a valid instrument that is not reliable? Is the reverse possible? Support your answer with instruments you might use in the clinical setting with your patients.
- What are some ways in which credibility, auditability, and fittingness can be evaluated?
- How do you think the concept of evidence-informed practice has changed research utilization models? Is the review of the literature the same when a research proposal is developed as it is when the steps of research utilization or an evidence-informed practice protocol is implemented? Support your position.

KEY POINTS

- Reliability and validity are crucial aspects of conducting and critiquing research.
- Validity refers to whether an instrument measures what it is purported to measure. It is a crucial aspect of evaluating a tool.
- Three types of validity are content validity, criterion-related validity, and construct validity.
- The choice of a validation method is important and is made by the researcher on the basis of the characteristics of the measurement device in question and its use.
- Reliability refers to the ratio between accuracy and inaccuracy in a measurement device.
- The major tests of reliability are test-retest reliability, parallel- or alternate-form reliability, split-half reliability, item-to-total correlation, the Kuder-Richardson coefficient, Cronbach's alpha, and interrater reliability.

- The selection of a method for establishing reliability depends on the characteristics of the tool, the testing method that is used for collecting data from the standardization sample, and the kinds of data that are obtained.
- Credibility, auditability, and fittingness are criteria for judging the scientific rigour of a qualitative research study.

FOR FURTHER STUDY

Go to Evolve at http://evolve.elsevier.com/Canada/LoBiondo/Research for the Audio Glossary and Appendix Tables that provide supplemental information for Appendix E.

REFERENCES

American Cancer Society. (2010). *Cancer facts and figures.* Atlanta, GA: Author.

Babenko-Mould, Y., Iwasiw, C., Andrusyszyn, M. A., et al. (2012). Nursing students' perceptions of clinical teachers' use of empowering teaching behaviours: Instrument psychometrics and application. *International Journal of Nursing Education Scholarship, 9*(1), 1–16.

Budin, W., Hoskins, C. N., Haber, J., et al. (2008). Education, counselling, and adjustment among patient and partners: A randomized clinical trial. *Nursing Research, 57*, 199–213.

Campbell, D., & Fiske, D. (1959). Convergent and discriminant validation by the matrix. *Psychological Bulletin, 53*, 273–302.

de Man-van Ginkel, J. M., Gooskens, F., Schepers, V. P. M., et al. (2012). Screening for post-stroke depression using the patient health questionnaire. *Nursing Research, 61*(5), 333–341.

DeVellis, R. (2012). *Scale development: theory and applications: Theory and application* (3rd ed.). Thousand Oaks, CA: Sage.

Grassley, J. S., Spencer, B. S., & Bryson, D. (2013). The development and psychometric testing of the Supportive Needs of Adolescents Breastfeeding Scale. *Journal of Advanced Nursing, 69*(3), 708–716.

Guba, E. G. (1981). Criteria for assessing the trustworthiness of naturalistic enquiries. *Educational Communication and Technology Journal, 29*, 75–91.

Guba, E., & Lincoln, Y. (1994). Competing paradigms in qualitative research. In N. Denzin & Y. Lincoln (Eds.), *Handbook of qualitative research* (pp. 105–117). Thousand Oaks, CA: Sage.

Hoskins, C. N. (1988). *Partner relationship inventory.* Palo Alto, CA: Consulting Psychologists Press.

Ibrahim, S. E. R. (2002). Rates of adherence to pharmacological treatment among children and adolescents with attention deficit hyperactivity disorder. *Human Psychopharmacology, 17,* 225–231.

Kennedy, E., Tomblin-Murphy, G., Martin-Misener, R., et al. (2015). Development and psychometric assessment of the Nursing Competence Self-Efficacy Scale. *Journal of Nursing Education, 54*(10), 550–558.

Kuiper, R.-A. (2010). Metacognitive factors that impact student nurse use of point of care technology in clinical settings. *International Journal of Nursing Education Scholarship, 7*(1), Article 5.

Lincoln, Y. S. (1995). Emerging criteria for qualitative and interpretive research. *Qualitative Inquiry, 3,* 275–289.

Lincoln, Y. S., & Guba, E. G. (1985). *Naturalistic inquiry.* New York: Sage.

Liou, S. R., Liu, H. C., Tsai, H. M., et al. (2015). The development and psychometric testing of a theory-based instrument to evaluate nurses' perception of clinical reasoning competence. *Journal of Advanced Nursing, 72*(3), 707–717.

MacDonald, C., Martin-Misener, R., Steenbeek, A., et al. (2015). Honouring stories: Mi'kmaq women's experiences with Pap screening in Eastern Canada. *Canadian Journal of Nursing Research, 47*(1), 72–96.

McDowell, I., & Newell, C. (1996). *Measuring health: A guide to rating scales and questionnaires.* New York: Oxford University Press.

McQueen, K. A., Montelpare, W. J., & Dennis, C. L. (2013). Breastfeeding and Aboriginal women: Validation of the Breastfeeding Self-Efficacy Scale-Short Form. *Canadian Journal of Nursing Research, 45*(2), 58–75.

Melnyk, B. M., Oswalt, K. L., & Sidora-Arcoleo, K. (2014). Validation and psychometric properties of the Neonatal Intensive Care Unit Parental Beliefs Scale. *Nursing Research, 63*(2), 279–289.

Nunnally, J. C., & Bernstein, I. H. (1994). *Psychometric theory* (3rd ed.). New York: McGraw-Hill.

O'Keefe-McCarthy, S., McGillion, M., Nelson, S., et al. (2014). Content validity of the Toronto Pain Management Inventory–Acute Coronary Syndrome Version. *Canadian Journal of Cardiovascular Nursing, 24*(2), 11–18.

Pauly, B., McCall, J., Browne, A. J., et al. (2015). Toward cultural safety: Nurse and patients perceptions of illicit substance use in a hospitalized setting. *Advances in Nursing Science, 38*(2), 121–135.

Sherman, D. W., Haber, J., Hoskins, C. N., et al. (2012). The effect of psychoeducation and telephone counseling on the adjustment of women with early-stage breast cancer. *Applied Nursing Research, 25,* 3–16.

Sidani, S., & Doran, D. I. (2014). Development and validation of a self-care ability measure. *Canadian Journal of Nursing Research, 46*(1), 11–25.

Siu, H., Laschinger, H. K. L., & Vingilis, E. (2005). The impact of problem-based learning on students' perception of empowerment in nursing educational settings. *Journal of Nursing Education, 44,* 459–468.

Tobin, G. A., & Begley, C. M. (2004). Methodological rigour within a qualitative framework. *Journal of Advanced Nursing, 48,* 388–396.

Waltz, C., Strickland, O., & Lenz, E. (1991). *Measurement in nursing research* (3rd ed.). Philadelphia: F. A. Davis.

Williams, A. L., Dixon, J., Van Ness, P. H., et al. (2011). Determinants of Meditation Practice Inventory: Development, content validation and initial psychometric testing. *Alternative Therapies in Health and Medicine, 17*(5), 16–23.

CHAPTER 15

Qualitative Data Analysis

Cherylyn Cameron

LEARNING OUTCOMES

After reading this chapter, you will be able to do the following:

- Describe the processes of qualitative data analysis.
- Outline the steps common to qualitative data analysis.
- Describe how data are reduced to meaningful units (themes).
- Describe the process of identifying themes and categories and the relationships between them.
- Assess the validity of a data analysis from a study.

KEY TERMS

codes	data analysis	thematic analysis
coding	data display	themes
constant comparative	data reduction	
method	member checking	

STUDY RESOURCES

e Go to Evolve at http://evolve.elsevier.com/Canada/LoBiondo/Research for the Audio Glossary and Appendix Tables that provide supplemental information for Appendix E.

AS DISCUSSED IN EARLIER CHAPTERS, QUALITATIVE analysis is not an analysis of the statistical tests used in the study but an analysis of the qualitative text. The text includes transcripts of interviews, narratives, documents, media such as newspapers and movies, and field notes. Qualitative researchers collect enormous amounts of data, which must be managed carefully: more than 150 pages of transcript can result from 25 interviews. To add to the complexity of qualitative data analysis, many researchers take different approaches to analysis. This chapter expands on the discussion in Chapter 8, in which the analysis of data was introduced in the context of several qualitative research traditions, such as phenomenology, grounded theory, ethnography, and case study.

AUDIO RECORDING INTERVIEWS

As discussed in Chapter 7, qualitative researchers gather data from a variety of sources, including interviews, observations, narrative, and focus groups (Merriam & Tisdell, 2016; Streubert & Carpenter, 2011). Interviews are the most common source and serve as the primary source of data for many qualitative research projects. For example, Pauly, McCall, Browne, and colleagues (2015) interviewed 34 people in a private setting and audio recorded the meeting. Although some researchers believe that a recording device inhibits the free flow of discussion, Seidman (2013) and other authors have found that most participants and interviewers forget about the presence of the device. Consequently, most researchers record interviews and then transcribe them verbatim into written text. Some researchers may consider summarizing or paraphrasing the spoken words (Seidman, 2013), but this is not commonly practised. Most researchers wish to use the original words from the participants so that the researcher's own interpretations and personal biases are not juxtaposed with the participant's thoughts. The presence of the original words allows the reader to check the authenticity of the data. New researchers may transcribe the recording into text

themselves; however, most researchers use a transcriptionist. It is recommended that the researcher spot-check interviews to ensure accuracy of the transcription (Streubert & Carpenter, 2011).

DATA MANAGEMENT

The open nature of qualitative inquiry typically results in the collection of more data than required. Glesne (2011) refers to the sheer volume of the data collected as "fat data." Consequently, researchers must be methodical in their organization and management of the data. Some researchers will organize all of these data by hand, but fortunately, computer software simplifies the storage and retrieval of data. In addition, researchers are also required to develop a decision or audit trail, which necessitates the tracking of the participants, the original audio recordings, and original and photocopied documents. Moreover, all of the data must be kept secure to maintain confidentiality.

Computer software to organize and retrieve data is referred to as computer-assisted qualitative data analysis software (CAQDAS). There are many computer programs to choose from, such as ATLAS.ti, Ethnograph, HyperRESEARCH, Inspiration, QSR NVivo, QSR XSight, and C-I-SAID. SPSS and SAS software, commonly used in quantitative data analysis, can also be applied for use in qualitative data analysis, particularly in mixed-methods research design. When choosing software, researchers have to understand what their needs are to determine the best fit. Meadows and Dodendorf (1999) have categorized computer programs into the following three types:

1. Code-and-retrieve programs, which assist in organizing and grouping data (e.g., Data Collector)
2. Theory builders, which move to a different level of data organization by connecting themes and categories (e.g., QSR NVivo)
3. Conceptual network builders, which incorporate graphics with theory-building capabilities (e.g., Inspiration)

Unlike computer programs used with quantitative data, these programs do not analyze data. Data analysis and interpretation remain largely the task of the researcher. In other words, CAQDAS cannot "think for the researcher" (Glesne, 2011, p. 207). However, using computer programs for orderly organization and grouping of data facilitates the researcher's job of analysis and interpretation.

The researcher needs to test software to determine which program will be the most useful one. Often, this process is one of trial and error before the most appropriate computer program is found. Most websites allow the downloading of a demonstration trial for a short time. Reviewing online tutorials (e.g., http://www.qsrinternational.com/industry/nvivo-in-education) can also assist the researcher in selecting the most appropriate software. Although learning new software is very time consuming, the benefits of using computerized software outweigh the time spent researching and learning about it (Streubert & Carpenter, 2011). All data must be backed up and stored in multiple places, such as a cloud storage site. Lost data cannot be replaced easily.

OVERVIEW OF DATA ANALYSIS

"**Data analysis** is the process used to answer the research question" (Merriam & Tisdell, 2016, p. 202). When does data collection end and data analysis begin? This is a controversial area of qualitative research because not all researchers agree on whether data collection should be completed before analysis begins or whether the two processes ought to take place concurrently. Many researchers believe that the stages of data collection and data analysis should be integrated (Denzin & Lincoln, 2000; Merriam & Tisdell, 2016; Miles, Huberman, & Saldaña, 2014; Streubert & Carpenter, 2011), whereas others believe that these stages should be separate (Seidman, 2013). Therefore, the researcher needs to identify the process used.

As mentioned previously, many researchers begin a preliminary analysis as the material accumulates. Typically, the qualitative researcher transcribes all of the interviews, field notes, and observations as they are collected. As each piece of data is transcribed, researchers begin a preliminary

analysis during which they determine what additional data need to be collected.

The overall goal of qualitative data analysis is to make meaning out of massive amounts of text or data, and many methods for analysis are available. Patton (2002) encouraged researchers to do their "very best with . . . full intellectual capacity to fairly represent the data and communicate what the data reveal given the purpose of study" (p. 433). As described earlier, qualitative analysis is not a linear process; rather, it is cyclical, transformative, reciprocal, and iterative. Miles and colleagues (2014, p. 10) have identified some common features among different approaches to qualitative data analysis:

- Affixing codes or themes to a set of field notes, interview transcripts, or documents
- Sorting and shifting though these coded materials to identify similar phrases, relationships between variables, patterns, themes, distinct differences between subgroups, and common sequences
- Isolating these patterns and processes, and commonalities and differences, and taking them out to the field in the next wave of data collection
- Noting reflections of other remarks in the margins
- Gradually elaborating a small set of assertions, propositions, and generalizations that cover the consistencies discerned in the database
- Confronting those generalizations with a formalized body of knowledge in the form of constructs or theories

Guidelines such as these are useful, but they serve only as recommendations. Each qualitative study is unique and is reliant on the creativity, intellect, style, and experience of the researcher.

During the data analysis phase, all researchers fully immerse themselves in the data over a period of weeks to months. This process requires constant reading and rereading of the text until an understanding of what the data convey is reached (Streubert & Carpenter, 2011). Many researchers also listen to the recorded interviews several times to increase their understanding and to remember the emotive component. Using an electronic or digital player is helpful during this intense period of immersion. For example, during the interviews in Cameron's (2005) study, some participants were very emotional as they relived their experiences; the transcribed text did not reflect the emotions. Observations written by the researcher can capture these important elements. An important part of the data analysis is the interplay between data gathering or questioning and verifying what is heard and understood. Researchers continue to ask whether what they understood before is still relevant after subsequent interviews, observations, and reading of related documents. This "cyclic nature of questioning and verifying is an important aspect of data collection and analysis" (Streubert & Carpenter, 2011, p. 46).

Miles et al. (2014) refer to three discrete stages of data analysis: data reduction, data display, and conclusion drawing and verification (Figure 15.1). Many of the common methods used in nursing research fit into this general view of qualitative analysis.

Data Reduction

According to Miles et al. (2014), **data reduction** is "the process of selecting, focusing, simplifying, abstracting, and transforming the data that appear in written-up field notes or transcriptions" (p. 10). This process is ongoing as data are collected. Initially, the data can be organized into meaningful clusters of data by grouping related or similar data. Often, these clusters or groups of data are labelled as **themes,** or structured meaning units of data that occur frequently in the text. **Thematic analysis**—the process of recognizing and recovering the emergent themes—is an important aspect of organizing data. In the qualitative tradition, as van Manen (1997) states, "grasping and formulating a thematic understanding is not a rulebound but a free act of 'seeing' meaning" (p. 79).

Glesne (2011) describes several methods to help researchers discover the meanings embedded in data. The first method is to write memos or keep a reflective journal during the data-collection stage, which allows researchers to record thoughts about the data as these thoughts occur. Analytical files are developed to sort data into general categories, such as interview questions, people, and places, as well as useful quotations from the interviews and relevant quotations from the literature. These files help organize researchers' thoughts and those of others.

Next, Glesne (2011) recommends the development of rudimentary coding schemes. Coding, as Denzin and Lincoln (2000) describe it, "is the heart and soul of whole-text analysis" (p. 780). **Coding** is a progressive marking, sorting, resorting, and defining and redefining of the collected data. Coding allows researchers to transform the "unstructured and messy data to ideas about what is going on in the data" (Richards & Morse, 2007, p. 133).

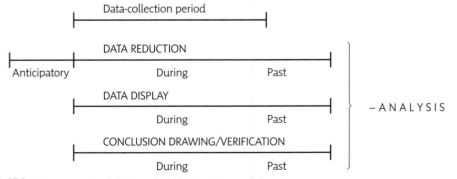

FIG. 15.1 Components of data analysis: Interactive model.
From Miles, M. B., Huberman, A. M., & Saldaña, J. (2014). *Qualitative data analysis: A methods sourcebook* (3rd ed.). Thousand Oaks, CA: Sage (Display 1.1, p. 14).

Evidence-Informed Practice Tip ____

"Coding is nothing more than assigning some sort of shorthand designation to various aspects of your data so you can easily retrieve specific pieces of data" (Merriam & Tisdell, 2016, p. 199).

Last, Glesne (2011) recommends that researchers write themselves monthly field reports as a way of systematically reviewing the progress and determining the next steps. Aside from helping researchers keep track of their progress and communicate progress with other members of the research team, monthly summaries often result in new insights and new ways of approaching the research.

Denzin and Lincoln (2000) provide an overview of the fundamental steps in the coding of data: sampling, identifying themes, building codebooks, and marking texts. Richards and Morse (2007) describe three types of coding: descriptive, topic, and analytic. Researchers use some or all of these steps when coding. *Descriptive coding* helps the researcher keep track of factual knowledge (e.g., gender). In *topic coding,* used most commonly, the data are grouped together by topic "to reflect on all the different ways people discuss particular topics, to seek patterns in their responses, or to develop dimensions of that experience" (Richards & Morse, 2007, p. 134). As the categories become more complicated, the topic coding becomes analytic. *Analytic coding* is more theoretical and leads to the development of themes. Although coding may sound complicated to you, remember that this process is evolutional, and it varies from project to project and from researcher to researcher. For example, many researchers conducting narrative inquiry do not use coding, data reduction, and some of the other commonly used methods of data analysis. Moreover, remember that meanings are waiting to be discovered, not imposed on the data.

Miles et al. (2014) describe the process of coding taking place in two steps. The first is described as *first cycle coding,* in which the data are assigned to data chunks. In Saldaña's 2013 manual on coding, over 25 types of coding are described. Three foundational types of first cycle coding include the following:

- Descriptive coding: labels are assigned, composed as a short phrase or word
- In vivo coding: short phrases or words are drawn from the participants' own language
- Process coding: "ing" is used to describe observations or actions (e.g., knowing)

The next step, finding themes, is the most exciting step of the process, which occurs during and after data collection. These themes or basic units of analysis can be entire texts (e.g., interview transcripts, responses to surveys), grammatical segments (words, phrases, sentences, paragraphs), formatting units (rows, pages), or clusters of texts that reflect a single theme. Most researchers try to divide data into units of analysis that do not overlap with others. Researchers approach this step in a variety of ways; for example, experts in grounded theory recommend that the researcher read the text line by line. Miles et al. (2014) describe this phase as second cycle coding: pattern codes. While the first cycle summarized chunks of data, in this second cycle the first-cycle codes are organized into a smaller number of categories, themes, or constructs.

The coding process itself is analysis (Miles et al., 2014). Glesne (2006) has stated that coding is as simple as identifying "what is important and giving it a name (code)" (p. 154). **Codes** are simply tags or labels that are assigned to the themes; often, the code itself is only one to four words long. Major codes may exist along with subcodes. Codes evolve during the analysis; more may be added, and others may be blended together. They mean something to the researcher and are not typically included in the research study. As the coding and themes are fine-tuned and finalized, much of the analysis is completed.

The next step is to build codebooks by organizing codes into lists, composed of either words or numbers that are used by the researcher. Then the text is marked, whereby the codes are assigned to the units of text. During this process, the researcher is immersed in the data, which results in new insights and interpretations.

Richards and Morse (2007) describe two primary steps to data analysis: categorizing and conceptualizing: "Categorizing is how we understand and come to terms with the complexity of data in everyday life" (p. 155). Coding is one method for categorizing the data: however, other researchers in qualitative studies can think about data without coding. Many studies do not extend beyond categorizing if their research goal is to describe "what is going on" in a specific phenomenon. Conceptualizing moves up the ladder of abstraction (see Chapter 2) to build frameworks of concepts or theory. It is a process of forming theoretical definitions to "make sense" or organize the data. Phenomenology, ethnography, and grounded theory are all methods that necessitate conceptualization. In Table 15.1, the differences in the methods of abstraction are described by means of the following questions:

- When does abstraction occur?
- Where does abstraction come from?
- How is abstraction done?
- What analytical outcome is being sought?

Some researchers explicitly describe the process of data analysis. For example, Wuest, Merritt-Gray, Berman, and colleagues (2002) describe the data analysis of grounded theory with an example of an earlier study by Wuest (2001) on women's caring. Wuest read each field note, transcript, or document line by line while asking herself two questions: "What is this a conceptual indicator of?" and "What is going on here?" (Wuest et al., 2002). Codes were assigned to each grouping of data, from sentences to paragraphs to whole pages (Table 15.2). The codes (time for self, social interaction, and cultivating the marital relationship) were eventually grouped together into a single category: "replenishing."

TABLE **15.1**

DOING ABSTRACTION IN THREE DIFFERENT METHODS

METHOD	WHEN DOES ABSTRACTION OCCUR?	WHERE DOES ABSTRACTION COME FROM?	HOW IS ABSTRACTION DONE?	WHAT ANALYTICAL OUTCOME IS BEING SOUGHT?
Phenomenology	Not until one has the data: previous ideas and knowledge are bracketed	Themes and meanings in accounts, texts	Deep immersion, focus, thorough reading	To describe the essence of a phenomenon
Ethnography	Prior knowledge of site, situation; understanding develops during field research	Knowledge of social and economic setting; observation and learning from the setting	Rich description; combination of qualitative and quantitative patterning, coding, comparing, reviewing field notes	To identify themes and patterns; to explain and account for a social and cultural situation
Grounded theory	Abstraction is from the data, but can be informed by previously derived theories	Categories derived from data (observations or line-by-line analysis of texts); constant comparison with other situations or settings	Theoretical sensitivity; seeking concepts and their dimensions; open coding, dimensionalizing, memo writing, diagramming	To identify a core category and theory grounded in data

From Morse, Janice M.; Richards, Lyn. (2007). *Readme First for a User's Guide to Qualitative Methods*, p. 159. SAGE Publications Inc.

TABLE **15.2**

CODE ASSIGNMENTS AS DESCRIBED BY WUEST AND COLLEAGUES

CODE	TEXT EXAMPLE
Time for self	I steal an hour during the day.
Social interaction	I work not only for the money but to get out . . . for the social contacts.
Cultivating the marital relationship	So, after I get the kids to bed, I usually go downstairs and sit with him [partner] for an hour.

From Wuest, J., Merritt-Gray, M., Berman, H., et al. (2002). Illuminating social determinants of women's health using grounded theory. *Health Care International, 23,* 794–808.

In the study by Seneviratne, Mather, and Then (2009), data were gathered from field notes that were based on observations in the naturalistic setting and on interviews. The researchers analyzed the field notes and discovered three main themes. The researchers then kept returning to the field for further observations to cross-check their findings. Thorne, Armstrong, Harris, and associates (2009) used a semistructured interview guide for the first face-to-face meeting to interview participants. The initial analysis identified themes to guide the subsequent bimonthly interviews that took place for up to two years. Through this constant comparative analysis process, the emerging themes were clarified with each interview.

Cameron (2003) analyzed the transcripts of interviews with 13 participants about their experiences transferring from a college to a university in a collaborative baccalaureate nursing program. She identified an initial set of themes at three points: as they emerged while she transcribed the interviews, after she relistened to the recorded interviews, and after a reading and a rereading of the transcripts. Differences, similarities, contradictions, and gaps in the data were noted as she returned to the original material to confirm the findings. As a result of highlighting the students' stories, 29 subthemes emerged. From these, six major themes surfaced. Table 15.3 shows the coding scheme used to code the transcripts, and

TABLE **15.3**

CAMERON'S (2005) CODING SCHEME

MAJOR THEME	SUBTHEME	CODE
Academic shock	Workload	AS-Work
	Underprepared	AS-Uprep
	Curriculum	AS-C
	Unfulfilled promises	AS-prom
	Academic shock	AS
Professional transformation	Hospital to community	PT-H to C
	Practice to theory	PT-P to T
	Professionalization	PT-prof
Geographic relocation	Financial	GR-Fin
	Time and commuting	GR-T/C
	University structure	GR-US
	Campus size	GR-Size
	University culture	GR-Cul
	Guinea pigs	GR-GP
Transition stress	Self-doubt	TS-SD
	Going back	TS-GB
	Family and personal responsibility	TS-F
		TS-R
	Rumours	TS-E
	Emotions	
What social life?	Separation	S-sep
	Loneliness	S-L
	Bonding	S-B
Adaptation	Supports	A-Supp
	Personal attributes	A-P
	Learning the ropes	A-L
	Satisfaction	A-Sat
	Personal change	A-C
	Recommendations— college	A-RC
	Recommendations— university	A-RU

From Cameron, C. (2005). Experiences of transfer students in a collaborative baccalaureate nursing program. *Community College Review, 33*(2), 22–44. SAGE Publications Inc.

Table 15.4 shows how one small section of the text was coded to validate the themes after the data had been collected.

Data Display

The second major step in data analysis is the data display. Miles et al. (2014) define **data display** as "a visual format that presents information

TABLE 15.4

SAMPLE CODING

TEXT	CODE
"The first week of school?—Going out of my mind—coming home and crying. It was the expectations, they seem to be going on and on about these expectations that they were expecting of us. I don't think the information that was given to us was, I don't think was clarified properly or they didn't say it in a way to us that made us want to do it. It was . . . I felt very intimidated by the way they were talking to us by the expectations . . . you are going to do this and this and this . . . starting next week. I'm just in there—going out of my mind . . . . I don't know if I am going to be able to do this and it was again the self-doubt. It was . . . I don't think I'm going to be able to handle this. I want to go back to my college. And I remember me and my friends were just outside of our class and we were just like . . . this is unbearable and a couple of my friends wanted to call the college to see if they could get back in and . . . I knew if I could just last this week and last through a month . . . then I will see . . . Because I wasn't going to give up, just then. But it was definitely an eye opening experience. It wasn't at all what I expected. The professors were great but they just, it was too much information during that one week of the orientation."	TS-E

AS-Work

AS-Uprep

TS-SD
AS-Uprep
TS-GB

TS-E

A-P

AS-Uprep

AS-Work |

From Cameron, C. (2005). Experiences of transfer students in a collaborative baccalaureate nursing program. *Community College Review, 33*(2), 22–44. SAGE Publications Inc.

systematically so the user can draw conclusions and take needed action" (p. 108). This display helps the researcher understand the data and can be in the form of graphs, flowcharts, matrices, or any other visual representation. Like the rest of the analysis, the data display changes as more is known about the phenomenon under study. For example, MacDonald, Martin-Misener, Steenbeek, et al. (2015) identified five themes and 13 subthemes to describe Mi'kmaq women's experiences with Pap screening (Figure 15.2) *Finding our* way described how women were finding their way by taking care of their health. The second theme, *Our understanding and perceptions of Pap screening*, revealed how the Aboriginal women's beliefs, experiences, and feelings about Pap screening were shaped through a cultural lens of thinking about body and self. *The impact of history on our health and our health-care experiences* focused on the historical, social, political, and economic factors that affect their accessing of Pap screening. The fourth theme, *Encounters with health-care providers: making a difference on our path to Paps*, described the impact of interactions with health care providers on accessing Pap screens. *The health-care system is complicating our going for Paps* included a subtheme describing issues around confidentiality and privacy (see Figure 15.2).

Although many researchers use figures and charts as part of their data display, profiles or vignettes can also display what is to be learned from the participant's experience. Vignettes of the participant's experience can summarize what was learned from each participant and can then be shared with each participant for validation (Seidman, 2013). This narrative form transforms the text into a story—a compelling way of sharing meaning.

For example, Cameron (2003) studied the lived experience of transfer students in a collaborative nursing program and, as part of the mixed-methods design, interviewed 13 students. Vignettes were developed for each interview participant who, in turn, selected a pseudonym that had personal meaning. The vignette was shared with each participant, who then had the opportunity to change or modify the description. An example of one vignette is as follows:

Zion, a young minority student, immigrated to Canada as a child. She attended college directly after graduating from high school. She chose the collaborative program

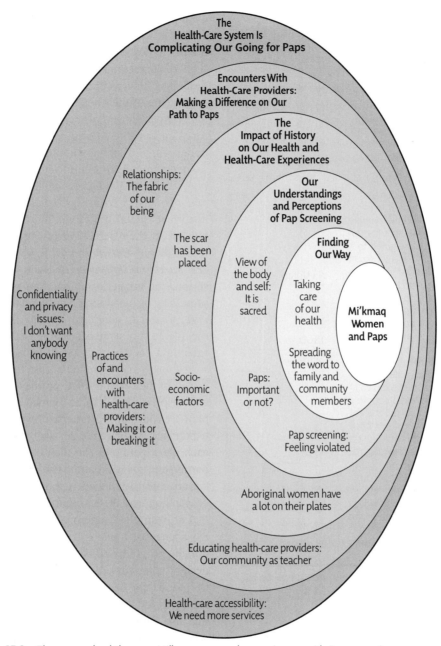

FIG. 15.2 Themes and subthemes: Mi'kmaq women's experiences with Pap screening.
From MacDonald, C., Martin-Misener, R., Steenbeek, A., & Browne, A. (2015). Honouring stories: Mi'kmaq women's experiences with Pap screening in Eastern Canada. *Canadian Journal of Nursing Research*, 47(1), 72–96. SAGE Publications Inc.

because she was aware that the degree would be mandatory for nursing in the future and her mother felt that nursing, as a career choice, was perfect. During the college portion she struggled academically as she was commuting four hours per day. However, through perseverance, she managed to achieve a "B" average in her second year at college and was admitted to the university portion of the program. Zion rated her transition as fairly difficult. Her primary concern was financial and resulted in the delay of purchase of textbooks and course materials. The ensuing stress led to a breakdown in class. With the intervention of a professor, she stuck it out. Now in the final days of her first year at the university, Zion reflects that she settled in by February and at that point realized that she would not quit and could make it. Driving Zion is her determination and to be a good example for other minority students living below the poverty line. Her motto is "I don't let circumstances determine my outcome." Zion reports that this transition has made her stronger, more self-confident, and that overall she will be a better nurse. (Cameron, 2003, p. 120)

Rich descriptions, such as those found in vignettes or direct quotations, enliven the data and give meaning to people's experiences. Most qualitative research includes selected quotations to illustrate the themes and to provide readers with the opportunity to understand and validate the themes chosen by the researcher. For example, Pooler (2014) chose the following quotation to describe the theme of *have to stop* in her study on the lived experience of patients with moderate to severe chronic obstructive pulmonary disease (COPD) or asthma.

When I go to the doctor, my wife drops me off and parks the van. And I'll go into the hospital. Generally just inside the door there's some wheelchairs sitting around in there. Most times is what I've done is I'll grab one of them as a walker. But the last couple of times that I've been there, there hasn't been one. So just walking from the front door to the elevator, I have to stop. I get halfway! I don't have a choice but to stop. Completely. Whatever I'm doing I gotta, I have to stop. (p. 7)

As another example of rich description, Table 15.5 includes selected quotations from participants to support the themes emerging from MacDonald et al.'s (2015) study.

When the data are presented, the most important consideration for the research is to ensure that the presentation supports the findings and relays what needs to be known (Streubert & Carpenter, 2011). The purpose of the study determines how the story is told. If the method is descriptive phenomenology, the focus is on the description of the lived experiences, whereas in a grounded theory study, the focus is on a more careful description of how the narrative gives rise to the analysis and interpretation, which results in theory development.

Conclusion Drawing and Verification

Conclusion drawing starts at the beginning of data collection but is not finalized until the project is completed. Although qualitative research is inductive, it is tempting to draw conclusions prematurely. The challenge for the researcher is to remain amenable to new ideas, themes, and concepts as they appear.

Conclusion drawing is essentially the description of the relationship between the themes. Richards and Morse (2007) describe this process as "doing abstraction" (p. 158), in which data are moved from categories (codes and themes) to concepts and constructs. As discussed earlier and shown in Table 15.1, the ways of abstracting vary with the type of method. Grounded theory formalizes this stage through the development of models, which lead to theory. Verification occurs as the data are collected; this process can vary from questioning one's own conclusion through the rechecking of the text to verification by colleagues and to finding new cases and applying the model to them. In grounded theory and many other qualitative methods, researchers use the **constant comparative method,** in which new data are compared as they emerge with data previously analyzed.

Miles et al. (2014) have stated that this process of making sense of the data is a skill that all nurses have. People make sense of the world around them by organizing and interpreting it; this skill is applied to drawing and verifying conclusions.

TABLE 15.5

EXAMPLES OF SELECTED QUOTATIONS TO SUPPORT THE THEMES FROM APPENDIX A

THEMES	SUBTHEME	EXAMPLE OF A QUOTATION
Finding our way	Taking care of our health	"I know when my appointments [for Pap screening] are due. Usually I'll remember and I keep track."
	Spreading the word to family and community members	"we learned about it [Pap screening] through word of mouth from family."
Our understanding and perceptions of Pap screening	View of the body and self: It is sacred	"I don't really feel like there's a cultural thing—it's a private area."
	Paps: Important or not	"I don't want to find out that I have cervical cancer. I want to make sure that I don't end up with any kind of disease . . . and if so, [that] they can get it early."
	Pap screening: feeling violated	"Sexual abuse could be a reason for our women [Aboriginal] not to go. It could bring up bad memories from the past."
The impact of history on our health and our health-care experiences	The scar has been placed	"Issues with trusting health-care providers and the health-care system, I think, have been passed on from our history, from our ancestors that attended residential schools . . . They still have power over us, just like they did when we were in residential schools."
	Socioeconomic factors	"We never had a lot of money or education. We didn't know it [Pap screening] was important."
	Aboriginal women have a lot on their plates	"Having a lot on their plates, they do not place themselves at the top of the list for care, particularly when they are single parents or have jobs."
Encounters with health-care providers: making a difference on our path to Paps	Relationships: The fabric of our being	A female health-care provider understands what it is like to be a woman and knows what it is like to experience Pap smear screening."
	Practices of and encounters with health-care providers: Making it or breaking it.	"They generalize [about] us too much. They think we're drunks. You're hung over or something like that. Or . . . pill poppers."
	Educating health care providers: Our community as teacher	"Get educated and trusted in the community, and learn from the community as opposed to just [from] a book . . . I think that maybe if they [came to] study in here [community] for a bit, they would understand us more."
The health-care system is complicating our going for Paps	Confidentiality and privacy issues: I don't want anyone knowing	"I've never actually been there [community health centre] for a Pap test. . . . The reason is [that] I know my results will come back there. I know my file will be there, everything about me—anybody can look at my file. That's why I won't go there."
	Health-care accessibility: We need more services	"We need more services. I like the idea of women's clinics and women's health days that would be accessible for everyone."

Based on MacDonald, C., Martin-Misener, R., Steenbeek, A., et al. (2015). Honouring stories: Mi'kmaq women's experiences with Pap screening in Eastern Canada. *Canadian Journal of Nursing Research, 47*(1), 72–96.

Miles et al. (2014) list the following 13 tactics for drawing meaning from the data (pp. 277–278):

1. Noting patterns and themes (repetitive or recurring patterns among many separate pieces of data)
2. Seeing plausibility (realizing that the finding or conclusion sounds true or makes sense)
3. Clustering (grouping together things that seem to share characteristics)
4. Making metaphors (using a literary device in which different things are compared to make sense of the experience)
5. Counting (noting that something is happening a number of times)
6. Making contrasts or comparisons (comparing sets of things)
7. Partitioning variables (breaking down the themes into smaller units)
8. Subsuming particulars into the general (using a higher level of abstraction)
9. Factoring (generating words [factors] to express common findings)
10. Noting relationships between variables (depicting the relationships between the findings)
11. Finding intervening variables (discerning other variables that may link findings together)
12. Building a logical chain of evidence (validating each of the relationships identified)
13. Making conceptual or theoretical coherence (linking the findings into an overarching "how" and "why" of the phenomenon under study)

Refer to Miles et al. (2014) for more detail about these tactics. Merriam and Tisdell's (2016) text on qualitative research also describes the step-by-step process.

To verify the emergent themes and subthemes, MacDonald et al. (2015) returned to the field to recheck their findings and changed the titles of the themes as advised by the participants. Other researchers can use different methods to validate their themes. For example, Bottorff, Johnson, Moffat, and colleagues (2004) used NVivo to search the data for content related to explanations of nicotine dependence, addiction, lack of control over smoking, and experiences associated with cessation. These data were then subjected to a thematic analysis in which the participants' explanations of addiction were compared. To verify the findings, the research team regularly discussed the analysis and interpretation. Once the initial analysis was complete, secondary analysis took place with a second set of interviews. As a final analysis, further interviews took place with eight selected participants to validate the findings.

No matter what method is used, researchers ask themselves, "What have I learned? How do I understand this, make sense of it and see the connections in it?" (Seidman, 2013). The conclusions drawn are simply to "describe, make contributions and contribute to greater understanding, or at least, more informed questioning" (Glesne, 2011, p. 210). As discussed in Chapter 7, through the processes of reflexivity and bracketing, researchers constantly compare their findings with their own personal beliefs and knowledge to ensure that the analysis reflects the participants' beliefs rather than their own.

SPECIFIC ANALYTICAL PROCEDURES

The processes of data analysis vary according to the type of qualitative research. Table 15.6 summarizes the methods of analysis in qualitative methods, including phenomenology, ethnography, grounded theory, and case study. Excerpts from Canadian studies are included to exemplify the methods.

TRUSTWORTHINESS

As described in Chapter 14, rigour in qualitative research is determined by credibility, auditability, and fittingness as the criteria for evaluation. Trustworthiness is also important for determining the validity of the data interpretation or analysis. To ensure the trustworthiness of their findings, qualitative researchers must ask themselves the following questions (Hollway & Jefferson, 2000):

• What do you notice? The researcher has captured some impressions about the data; however,

TABLE **15.6**

METHODS OF ANALYSIS

TRADITION	METHOD OF ANALYSIS	EXAMPLE
Phenomenology: includes a variety of traditions	• Immersion in the data: listen to recordings, read and reread transcripts • Identify and extract significant statements • Determine relationships among the extracted statements (themes) • Prepare exhaustive description of the phenomenon and the relationships among the themes • Synthesize the themes into a consistent description or statement of the phenomenon under study (essence)	Pooler (2014). "Living with chronic lower pulmonary disease: disruptions of the embodied phenomenological self." Asking what is it like to experience moderate to severe COPD or asthma, Pooler (2014) identified three central themes of slowing down, doing less, and having to stop. For example, a quotation exemplifying the theme of *slowing down* is as follows: "I'll start walking at the same speed as the people I'm with are walking. And I can't sustain it. They don't notice that I'm in trouble. And I have to say to them, 'I'm sorry, but you're going to have to slow down because I can't walk at that speed'" (p. 4).
Ethnography	• Immersion in the data • Identify patterns and themes • Complete a cultural inventory • Interpret the findings • Compare the findings with those in the literature	Pauly et al. (2015). "Toward cultural safety: Nurse and patient perceptions of illicit substance use in a hospitalized setting." Pauly et al. (2015) coded the interviews, field notes, and documents. The data were reviewed to identify patterns of interaction, key concepts, and emerging themes. The emerging themes and data were further conceptualized to higher levels. Each researcher read the data independently, and then with the involvement of advisory groups with expertise in the field, the emergent themes were confirmed.
Grounded theory	• Examine data carefully line by line • Divide data into discrete parts • Compare data for similarities and differences • Compare data with other data continuously in a process: constant comparative method • Cluster codes to form categories • Expand and develop categories or collapse them into one another • Determine relationships between categories	Vandenberg and Kulig (2015). "Immunization rejection in Southern Alberta: A comparison of the perspectives of mothers and health professionals." The authors implemented the main features of grounded theory such as theoretical sampling, concurrent data collection and analysis, comparative methods and the three phases of data coding, memo-writing, and theory generation.
Case study	• Identify unit of analysis (person, family, organization) • Code continuously as data are collected • Find commonalities and themes • Analyze field notes • Review description of themes to identify patterns and connections between them	Maddalena, Bernard, Etowa, et al. (2010): "Cancer care experiences and the use of complementary and alternative medicine at end of life in Nova Scotia's Black communities." In this study, the verbatim-transcribed interviews from seven people were coded manually and individually by four members of the research team. The team met to compare coding and engage in the analysis of the data. Once the team reached consensus, a thematic and discourse analysis was used to further analyze the data. As prevalent themes emerged, each was explored in the context of how culture influenced their experiences during the time from initial diagnosis through interactions with the health system to death and bereavement. With the researchers' etic view of the Black community and culture, the team made sense of the data through the shared historical and cultural experiences of the Black community. Using a discourse analysis approach, the researchers examined each of the themes in terms of their social, political, and historical contexts.

information may be missing. Detailed or thick descriptions of the phenomenon also allow the reader to assess whether the account "rings true."

- Why do you notice what you notice? Researchers must consider their own biases and predispositions as they interpret the data to produce trustworthy interpretations. Many researchers use a journal to document their reflections to monitor their own developing interpretations.
- How can you interpret what you notice? Credibility stems from prolonged engagement and persistent observation. To be able to complete a full interpretation, the researcher must spend a sufficient amount of time in the field to build sound relationships with the participants.
- How can you know that your interpretation is the "right" one? The quickest way to know whether

the interpretation is accurate is through sharing the findings with the participants. This sharing is an integral part of participatory action research, as outlined in Chapter 8, and is referred to in many studies as **member checking.** The researcher is also checking whether the connections between the categories or themes are logical. Inviting other experts to review the data analysis is another option for many researchers. In addition, some researchers analyze their data from several different frameworks (a form of triangulation) to increase the trustworthiness of the data analysis.

Finally, it is important to consider the limitations of the study. Many researchers describe the issues they faced so that readers will understand the research in the proper context (Glesne, 2006).

APPRAISING THE EVIDENCE

Qualitative Data Analysis

The general criteria for critiquing qualitative data analysis are proposed in the Critiquing Criteria box; however, remember that many different approaches to data analysis exist. The data analysis is consistent with the research philosophy, the question, and the design. For example, researchers using grounded theory build a case for substantive theory, explaining the phenomenon under study, whereas a researcher in phenomenological studies is interested in expressing the meaning of the phenomenon itself.

Regardless of the study's research method, several commonalities exist among methods used in qualitative data analysis. For example, analysis is conducted alongside the data collection, and in most cases the two processes are interrelated. Researchers become immersed in the data; they listen over and over to the interviews, read

and reread the transcripts, and spend substantial time in the field. Although the methods may differ, the text is coded to search for themes and categories through a process of data reduction. The emergent themes are then verified through member checking. As themes emerge, logical connections and relationships between the themes are identified to form a whole picture. The results are displayed in such a manner that the reader can understand and validate the conclusions that the researcher has drawn through the use of diagrams, tables, charts, direct quotations from the participants, and rich descriptions of the findings. In summary, qualitative data analysis involves much disparate data and transforms them into a coherent whole or story to provide meaning about the human experience.

CRITIQUING CRITERIA

1. The method of data analysis should be clearly stated.
2. The strategy of data analysis should be appropriate for the methodology of the study.
3. The steps of analysis should be listed for readers to follow.
4. The researcher should provide evidence that his or her interpretation captures the phenomenon under study.
5. The researcher should address the credibility, auditability, and fittingness of the data.

CRITICAL THINKING CHALLENGES

- How do researchers determine whether they have spent enough time with the data?
- Is it important for the researcher to personally transcribe the interviews?
- Why do some researchers reread the literature as themes emerge from the data?
- Often, data analysis takes place as data are collected. How can analysis of the data change the data collection?
- Researchers validate their interpretation of the data through a process of member checking. What happens if the participants indicate that the analysis does not reflect their experience?

- Grounded theorists use the constant comparative method, in which new data are compared with data previously analyzed.
- Member checking is the process of sharing findings with the participants in order to check whether the interpretation of the findings is accurate.

FOR FURTHER STUDY

ⓔ Go to Evolve at http://evolve.elsevier.com/ Canada/LoBiondo/Research for the Audio Glossary and Appendix Tables that provide supplemental information for Appendix E.

KEY POINTS

- Qualitative data are text derived from transcripts of interviews, narratives, documents, media such as newspapers and movies, and field notes.
- Computer software can be used to simplify the storage and retrieval of data.
- Qualitative research data can be managed through the use of computers, but the researcher must interpret the data.
- Data analysis and data collection are parallel processes.
- Qualitative analysis is not a linear process; rather, it is a cyclical and iterative process.
- The three discrete stages of data analysis are data reduction, data display, and conclusion drawing and verification.
- Data are organized into meaningful chunks of data through a clustering of related or similar data and are labelled as themes.
- Coding is the process of progressively marking, sorting, resorting, and defining and redefining the collected data.
- Data display involves the use of graphs, flowcharts, matrices, or any other visual representation to assemble data and to allow for conclusion drawing.

REFERENCES

Bottorff, J. L., Johnson, J. L., Moffat, B., et al. (2004). Adolescent constructions of nicotine addiction. *Canadian Journal of Nursing Research, 38,* 22–39.

Cameron, C. (2003). The lived experience of transfer students in a collaborative baccalaureate nursing program. Unpublished doctoral dissertation, University of Toronto.

Cameron, C. (2005). Experiences of transfer students in a collaborative baccalaureate nursing program. *Community College Review, 33*(2), 22–44.

Denzin, N., & Lincoln, Y. (2000). *Handbook of qualitative research* (2nd ed.). Thousand Oaks, CA: Sage.

Glesne, C. (2006). *Becoming qualitative researchers: An introduction* (3rd ed.). Don Mills, ON: Longman.

Glesne, C. (2011). *Becoming qualitative researchers: An introduction* (4th ed.). Toronto: Pearson.

Hollway, W., & Jefferson, T. (2000). *Doing qualitative research differently: Free association, narrative and the interview method.* Thousand Oaks, CA: Sage.

MacDonald, C., Martin-Misener, R., Steenbeek, A., et al. (2015). Honouring stories: Mi'kmaq women's experiences with Pap screening in Eastern Canada. *Canadian Journal of Nursing Research, 47*(1), 72–96.

Maddalena, V. J., Bernard, W. T., Etowa, J., et al. (2010). Cancer care experiences and the use of complementary and alternative medicine at end of life in Nova Scotia's Black communities. *Journal of Transcultural Nursing, 21*(2), 114–122.

Meadows, L. M., & Dodendorf, D. M. (1999). Data management and interpretation using computers to assist. In B. Crabtree & W. L. Miller (Eds.), *Doing qualitative research* (2nd ed., pp. 195–220). Thousand Oaks, CA: Sage.

Merriam, S. B., & Tisdell, E. J. (2016). *Qualitative research: A guide to design and implementation.* San Francisco: Jossey-Bass.

Miles, M. B., Huberman, A. M., & Saldaña, J. (2014). *Qualitative data analysis: Methods source book* (3rd ed.). Thousand Oaks, CA: Sage.

Patton, M. (2002). *Qualitative research & evaluation methods* (3rd ed.). Thousand Oaks, CA: Sage.

Pauly, B., McCall, J., Browne, A. J., et al. (2015). Toward cultural safety: Nurse and patient perceptions of illicit substance use in a hospitalized setting. *Advances in Nursing Science, 38*(2), 121–135.

Pooler, C. (2014). Living with chronic lower pulmonary disease: Disruptions of the embodied phenomenological self. *Global Qualitative Nursing Research, 1.*

Richards, L., & Morse, J. M. (2007). *Read me first for a user's guide to qualitative methods* (2nd ed.). Thousand Oaks, CA: Sage.

Saldaña, J. (2013). *The coding manual for qualitative researchers* (2nd ed.). New York: Oxford University Press.

Seidman, I. (2013). *Interviewing as qualitative research: A guide for researchers in education and the social sciences* (4th ed.). New York: Teachers College Press.

Seneviratne, C. C., Mather, C. M., & Then, K. L. (2009). Understanding nursing on an acute stroke unit: Perceptions of space, time and interprofessional practice. *Journal of Advanced Nursing, 65*(9), 1872–1881.

Streubert, H. J., & Carpenter, D. (2011). *Qualitative research in nursing: Advancing the humanistic imperative* (5th ed.). Philadelphia: Wolters Kluwer.

Thorne, S., Armstrong, E., Harris, S. R., et al. (2009). Patient real-time and 12 month-retrospective perceptions of difficult communications in the cancer diagnostic period. *Qualitative Health Research, 19*(10), 1383–1394.

Vandenberg, S. Y., & Kulig, J. C. (2015). Immunization rejection in southern Alberta: A comparison of the perspectives of mothers and health professionals. *Canadian Journal of Nursing Research, 47*(2), 81–96.

van Manen, M. (1997). *Researching lived experience.* London, ON: Althouse Press.

Wuest, J. (2001). Precarious ordering: Toward a formal theory of women's caring. *Health Care for Women International, 22*(1–2), 167–193.

Wuest, J., Merritt-Gray, M., Berman, H., et al. (2002). Illuminating social determinants of women's health using grounded theory. *Health Care International, 23,* 794–808.

CHAPTER 16

Quantitative Data Analysis

Susan Sullivan-Bolyai | Carol Bova | Mina D. Singh

LEARNING OUTCOMES

After reading this chapter, you will be able to do the following:

- Differentiate between descriptive and inferential statistics.
- State the purposes of descriptive statistics.
- Identify the levels of measurement in a research study.
- Describe a frequency distribution.
- List measures of central tendency and their use.
- List measures of variability and their use.
- Identify the purpose of inferential statistics.
- Distinguish between a parameter and a statistic.
- Explain the concept of probability as it applies to the analysis of sample data.
- Distinguish between type I and type II errors and their effects on a study's outcome.
- Distinguish between parametric and nonparametric tests.
- List the commonly used statistical tests and their purposes.
- Critically analyze the statistics used in published research studies.

KEY TERMS

alpha
analysis of covariance (ANCOVA)
analysis of variance (ANOVA)
chi-square (χ^2)
confidence interval
correlation
degree of freedom
descriptive statistics
factor analysis
Fisher's exact probability test

frequency distribution
inferential statistics
interval measurement
kurtosis
level of significance (alpha level)
levels of measurement
logistic regression (logit analysis)
mean (M)
measurement
measures of central tendency

measures of variability
median
modality
mode
multiple regression
multivariate analysis of variance (MANOVA)
nominal measurement
nonparametric statistics
nonparametric tests of significance
normal curve
null hypothesis

KEY TERMS—cont'd

odds ratio	power	skew
ordinal measurement	probability	standard deviation
p value	range	standard error of the mean
parameter	ratio measurement	statistic
parametric statistics	sampling error	systematic review
Pearson correlation	scatter plots	*t* statistic
coefficient (Pearson *r*)	scientific hypothesis	type I error
percentile	semiquartile range	type II error
population	(semi-interquartile	Z score
post hoc analysis	range)	

STUDY RESOURCES

ⓔ Go to Evolve at http://evolve.elsevier.com/Canada/LoBiondo/Research for the Audio Glossary and Appendix Tables that provide supplemental information for Appendix E.

STATISTICS ARE USED EXTENSIVELY IN THE nursing and health care literature. Descriptive and inferential statistics are described in the "Methods" section, the "Results" section, or both sections of a research article. Before you become overwhelmed by the complexity of the information, bear in mind that you do not need to be familiar with or to be able to calculate a large number of complex statistical formulas to analyze data. An understanding of which tests are used with which kind of design and which type of data is sufficient. This basic understanding will help you to appraise evidence from a research study, which is essential for informing decisions you make in your practice.

As a reader, you do not analyze the data yourself, but it is important to understand the researcher's challenge in analyzing the data. After carefully collecting data, the researcher is faced with the task of organizing and analyzing the individual pieces of information so that the meaning of study results is clear. The researcher must choose methods of organizing and analyzing the raw data on the basis of the design, the type of data collected, and the hypothesis or question that

was tested. Statistical procedures are used to organize and give meaning to the data.

The "Results" section of a research article contains the data generated from the testing of the hypothesis or research questions. These data are the result of analysis with both *descriptive* and *inferential statistics*. An example of what may be found is as follows: "the durations of breast milk expression/day for mothers in the EG [Experimental Group] at Weeks 4, 5, and 6 were significantly higher than those of mothers in the CG [Control Group]" (Héon, Goulet, Garofalo, et al., 2016, p. 540; see Appendix D). The data in Table 1 of Appendix D (Héon and colleagues') are known as descriptive statistics, which are usually the first set of statistical results in a report or published article.

Descriptive statistics are obtained through descriptive statistical techniques that reduce data to manageable proportions by summarizing and organizing them. These techniques allow researchers to arrange data visually to display meaning and to help in understanding the sample characteristics and variables before the researchers engage in inferential data analyses. In some studies, descriptive statistics may be the only results sought from statistical analysis. Descriptive statistical techniques include **measures of central tendency,** which describe the average member of a sample, such as mode, median, and mean; measures of variability, such as range and standard deviation (SD); and some correlation techniques, such as a **scatter plots,** which are a visual representation of the strength and magnitude of the relationship between two variables.

In contrast to descriptive statistics, inferential statistics allow researchers to estimate how reliably they can make predictions and generalize findings on the basis of the data. **Inferential statistics** are statistical details that combine mathematical processes and logic to test hypotheses about a population with the help of sample data. Through the use of inferential statistics, researchers can draw conclusions that extend beyond the immediate data of the study. An example of inferential statistics is in the study by El-Masri, Omar, and Groh (2015): "an RN was almost 20 times more likely than an NP or an MD to transfer a resident to the ED [emergency department] (OR [odds ratio] = 19.93; 95% CI [confidence interval] 12.37–32.11)" (p. 48).

The purpose of this chapter is to demonstrate how researchers use descriptive and inferential statistics in nursing research studies so that you, as a reader, will be better able to determine the appropriateness of the statistics used and to interpret the strength and quality of the reported findings, their clinical significance, and their applicability to practice. Basic concepts and terminology common in evidence-informed practice publications are presented in Chapter 20. The information in this chapter will help you begin to make sense of the statistics used in research papers.

DESCRIPTIVE STATISTICS

Levels of Measurement

Measurement is the assignment of numbers to variables or events according to rules. Every variable in a research study that is assigned a specific number must be similar to every other variable assigned that number. For example, male participants may be assigned the number 1 and female participants the number 2. The measurement level is determined by the nature of the object or event being measured. **Levels of measurement**—categorization of the precision with which an event can be measured—from low to high are nominal, ordinal, interval, and ratio (Table 16.1). The levels of measurement help determine the type of statistics to be used in analyzing data. The higher the level of measurement, the greater the flexibility the researcher has in choosing statistical procedures. Every attempt should be made to use the highest level of measurement possible so that the maximum amount of information will be obtained from the data. The Critical Thinking Decision Path illustrates the relationship between levels of measurement and appropriate choice of specific descriptive statistics.

In **nominal measurement,** variables or events are classified into categories (see Table 16.1). The categories are mutually exclusive; a variable or an event either has or does not have the characteristic of a particular category. The numbers assigned to each category are nothing more than labels; such numbers do not indicate more or less of a characteristic. Nominal measurement can be used to categorize a sample with regard to such information as gender, hair colour, marital status, or religious affiliation.

El-Masri, Fox-Wasylyshyn, Springer, and colleagues' (2014) study comparing the impact of three types of prostate cancer radiation treatment—brachytherapy, external beam radiotherapy (EBR), and high-dose radiation brachytherapy in combination with EBR—involved nominal measurement. The nominal level of measurement allows the least amount of mathematical manipulation. Most commonly, the frequency of each event is counted, as is the percentage of the total that each category represents.

A variable at the nominal level can also be considered a *dichotomous* or a *categorical* variable. A

TABLE **16.1**

SCALES OF MEASUREMENT

MEASUREMENT LEVEL	DESCRIPTION	EXAMPLE
Nominal (may be dichotomous or categorical)	Variables or events are classified into categories; the categories are mutually exclusive, there is no ranking. Dichotomous variables are mutually exclusive and have two true values: e.g., true/false, male/female. Categorical variables are mutually exclusive and have more than two true values: e.g., marital status may be single, married, divorced, separated, widowed.	Gender Hair colour Marital status Religious affiliation
Ordinal	Sorting on relative rankings of variables or events	High school education and less/more than high school education
Interval	Rank ordering on an attribute such as items on a survey	Highly disagree, disagree, neutral, agree, highly agree
Ratio	Highest level of measurement Absolute zero, so can divide, multiply	A person weighing 100 kg is twice as heavy as one who weighs 50 kg

CRITICAL THINKING DECISION PATH

Descriptive Statistics

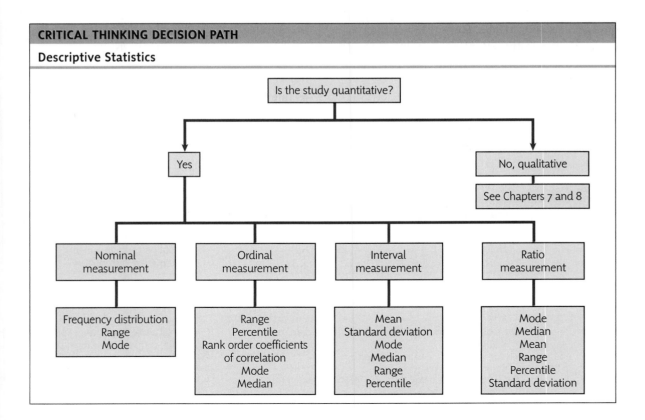

dichotomous nominal variable has only two true values, such as true/false or gender (male/female) (see Table 16.1). Nominal variables that are categorical still have mutually exclusive categories but have more than two true values, such as marital status (single, married, divorced, separated, or widowed). In both cases, the nominal variables are mutually exclusive. The gender variable of the graduate nurses in the study by Wing, Regan, and Laschinger (2013) would be considered a dichotomous nominal variable (male/female).

Ordinal measurement reveals relative rankings of variables or events. The numbers assigned to each category can be compared, and the members of a higher ranked category can be said to have more of an attribute than members of a lower ranked category. The intervals between numbers on the scale are not necessarily equal, and zero is not absolute but arbitrary. For example, ordinal measurement is used to formulate class rankings, in which one student can be ranked higher or lower than another. However, the actual grade point averages of students may differ widely. Another example is ranking individuals by their level of wellness and their ability to carry out activities of daily living. El-Masri and colleagues' (2014) measure of level of education by the two categories of high school education and less/more than high school education is an example of an ordinal variable.

The New York Heart Association's classification of cardiac failure adopted by the Canadian Cardiovascular Society (Arnold, Liu, Demers, et al., 2006) consists of four classifications. Classification I represents little disease or interference with activities of daily living, whereas classification IV represents severe disease and little ability to carry out the activities of daily living independently; however, an individual in class IV cannot be said to be four times sicker than an individual in class I. Forman, Currie, Lauck, and colleagues (2015) used this classification in their study examining changes in functional status while awaiting transcatheter aortic valve implantation. A similar scale based on an individual's current health status is used to classify an individual's risk for adverse effects from anaesthesia.

With ordinal-level data, the amount of mathematical manipulation possible is limited. In addition to what is possible with nominal-level data, medians, percentiles, and rank-order coefficients of correlation can be calculated (Table 16.2). In most cases, ordinal variables in a scale are treated as interval measurements when converted to numerical codes. For example, when patients are asked to rate their level of satisfaction with life as "not satisfied," "satisfied," or "very satisfied,"

TABLE 16.2			
LEVEL OF MEASUREMENT SUMMARY TABLE			
MEASUREMENT	**DESCRIPTION**	**MEASURES OF CENTRAL TENDENCY**	**MEASURES OF VARIABILITY**
Nominal	Classification	Mode	Modal percentage, range, frequency distribution
Ordinal	Relative rankings	Mode, median	Modal percentage, range, frequency, percentile, semiquartile range, frequency distribution
Interval	Rank ordering with equal intervals	Mode, median, mean	Modal percentage, range, percentile, semiquartile range, standard deviation
Ratio	Rank ordering with equal intervals and absolute zero	Mode, median, mean	All

their responses are an ordinal measurement. When their ratings are treated numerically and coded as 1, 2, and 3, respectively, their responses are an interval measurement.

In **interval measurement,** events or variables are ranked on a scale with equal intervals between the numbers. The zero point remains arbitrary and not absolute. For example, interval measurements are used in measuring temperatures on the Fahrenheit scale. The distances between degrees are equal, but the zero point is arbitrary and does not represent the absence of temperature. Test scores also represent interval-level data. The differences between test scores represent equal intervals, but a score of zero does not represent the total absence of knowledge.

In many areas in the social sciences, including nursing, the classification of the level of measurement of intelligence, aptitude, and personality tests is controversial; some researchers regard these measurements as ordinal and others as interval. You need to be aware of this controversy and to examine each study individually in terms of how the data are analyzed. Interval-level data allow more manipulation of data, including the addition and subtraction of numbers and the calculation of means. Because of this additional manipulation, many authorities argue for the higher classification level. The Cortina's Workplace Incivility Scale used by Laschinger (2014) is an example of ordinal measurements but used as an interval measurement (see Appendix B).

In **ratio measurement,** events or variables are ranked on scales with equal intervals and absolute zeros (see Table 16.2). The number represents the actual amount of the property the object possesses. Ratio measurement is the highest level of measurement but is usually achieved only in the physical sciences. Examples of ratio-level data are height, weight, pulse, and blood pressure. All mathematical procedures can be performed with data from ratio scales. Therefore, the use of any statistical procedure is possible as long as it is appropriate for the design of the study.

 Research Hint

Descriptive statistics assist in summarizing the data. The descriptive statistics calculated must be appropriate for both the purpose of the study and the level of measurement.

Frequency Distribution

One of the most basic ways of organizing data is in a frequency distribution. In a **frequency distribution,** the number of times each event occurs is counted, or the data are grouped and the frequency of each group is reported. For example, an instructor reporting the results of an examination could report the number of students receiving each individual grade or could group the grades in ranges and report the number of students who received each group of grades. When reviewing a frequency distribution, symmetry and kurtosis are noted. A distribution can be symmetrical (shaped like a bell) or asymmetrical, where most of the information is to one side, either to the left or the right. **Kurtosis** is the peakedness of the distribution. Table 16.3 shows the results of an examination given to a class of 51 students. The results are reported in two ways. The columns on the left give the raw data tally and the frequency for each grade, whereas the columns on the right give the grouped data tally and grouped frequencies. In research studies, the results are grouped rather than reported individually for each participant.

When data are grouped, the researcher needs to define the size of the group or the interval width so that no score is categorized into two groups and all groups are mutually exclusive. The groupings of the data in Table 16.3 prevent overlap; each score is categorized into only one group. If the grouping had been 70 to 80 and 80 to 90, scores of 80 would have been categorized into two categories. The grouping should allow for a precise presentation of the data without serious loss of information. Very large interval widths lead to loss of data information and may obscure

TABLE **16.3**

FREQUENCY DISTRIBUTION

INDIVIDUAL			GROUP		
SCORE	TALLY	FREQUENCY	SCORE	TALLY	FREQUENCY
90	I	1	>89	I	1
88	I	1	80–89	ⅬⅧ ⅬⅧ ⅬⅧ	15
86	I	1			
84	ⅬⅧ I	6			
82	II	2			
80	ⅬⅧ	5			
78	ⅬⅧ	5	70–79	ⅬⅧ ⅬⅧ ⅬⅧ ⅬⅧ III	23
76	I	1			
74	ⅬⅧ II	7			
72	ⅬⅧ IIII	9			
70	I	1			
68	III	3	60–69	ⅬⅧ ⅬⅧ	10
66	II	2			
64	IIII	4			
62	I	1			
60		0			
58	I	1	<59	II	2
56		0			
54	I	1			
52		0			
50		0			
Total		51	Total		51

Mean, 74.51; standard deviation, +12.1; median, 74; mode, 72; range, 36 (54–90).

patterns in the data. If the test scores in Table 16.3 had been grouped as 40 to 69 and 70 to 99, the pattern of the scores would have been obscured.

Information about frequency distributions may be presented in the form of a table, such as Table 16.3, or in the form of a graph. Figure 16.1 illustrates the most common graph forms: the histogram and the frequency polygon. These two methods are similar in that in both, scores or percentages of occurrence are plotted against frequency. The greater the number of points plotted, the smoother is the resulting graph. The shape of the resulting graph allows for observations that further describe the data.

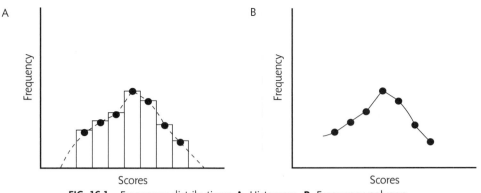

FIG. 16.1   Frequency distributions. **A,** Histogram. **B,** Frequency polygon.

Measures of Central Tendency

Measures of central tendency answer questions such as "What does the average nurse think?" and "What is the average temperature of patients on a unit?" These measures yield a single number that describes the middle of the group and summarizes the members of a sample. In statistics, the three measures of central tendency are the mode, the median, and the mean. Depending on the distribution, these measures may not all give the same answer to the question "What is the average?" Each measure of central tendency has a specific use and is most appropriate for specific kinds of measurement and types of distributions. Of the measures of central tendency, the mean is the most stable and the median the most typical. If the distribution of a sample is symmetrical and unimodal, the mean, median, and mode coincide.

💡 **Research Hint** _____

Measures of central tendency are descriptive statistics that describe the characteristics of a sample.

_____

MODE. The **mode** is the most frequent score or result and can be obtained by inspection of the frequency distribution table or graph. Note that a sample distribution can have more than one mode. The number of modes, or peaks, contained in a distribution is called the **modality** of the distribution. The mode is the type of descriptive statistic most appropriately used with nominal-level data but can be used with all levels of measurement (see Table 16.2). The mode cannot be used for any subsequent calculations and is unstable; in other words, the mode can fluctuate widely from sample to sample from the same population. A change in just one score in Table 16.3 would change the mode from 72.

MEDIAN. The **median** is the middle score: of the other scores, 50% are higher and 50% are lower. The median is not sensitive to extremes in high and low scores; thus, it is a more accurate estimator of central tendency in non-normal distributions. In the series of scores in Table 16.3, the twenty-sixth score is always the median, regardless of how much the high and low scores change. The median is best used when the data are skewed (see the "Normal Distribution" section) and the researcher is interested in the "typical" score. For example, if age is a variable, and if a wide range with extreme scores may affect the mean, it would be appropriate to also report the median. The median is easy to find either by inspection or by calculation and can be used with ordinal or higher data, as shown in Table 16.2.

MEAN. The **mean (M)** is the arithmetical average of all scores and is used with interval- or ratio-level data (see Table 16.2). Most statistical tests of significance refer to the mean, the most widely used measure of central tendency, which is referred to in general conversations as the average. Because the mean is affected by every score, it is affected by extreme scores; however, the larger the sample size, the less effect a single extreme score will have on the mean. For normally distributed populations, the mean is an appropriate measure of central tendency and is generally considered the single best point for summarizing data.

 Research Hint_____

Of the three measures of central tendency, the mean is the most stable, the least affected by extremes, and the most useful for other calculations. The mean can be calculated only with interval- and ratio-level data.

Héon and associates (2016) used a table to describe the sample characteristics in their study that they used to rule out confounding variables. The summary statistics in Appendix D about the sample, comparing the experimental group with the control group, were reported in narrative form; for example, "mothers had an average age of 29.3 years (SD = 5.4; EG: mean = 28.6 ± 5.7; CG; mean = 30.0 ± 5.1)" (p. 537). They did inferential statistics to determine whether there was a difference in ages and found no statistical difference: $p = .419$ (p. 537).

Normal Distribution

The theoretical concept of normal distribution is based on the observation that data from repeated interval or ratio measurements will gather at a midpoint in a distribution, approximating the normal curve illustrated in Figure 16.2. In addition, if the means of a large number of samples of the same interval- or ratio-level data are calculated and plotted on a graph, that curve also approximates the normal curve. This tendency of the means to approximate the normal curve is termed the *sampling distribution of the means*. The mean of the sampling distribution of the means is the mean of the population.

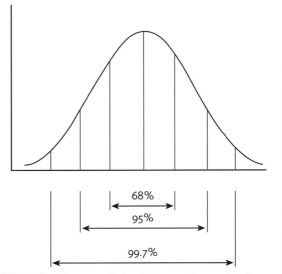

FIG. 16.2 The normal distribution and associated standard deviations.

In visual representations of statistics, the **normal curve** is unimodal and symmetrical about the mean. The mean, median, and mode are equal. An additional characteristic of the normal curve is that a fixed percentage of the scores is located within a given distance of the mean. As shown in Figure 16.2, about 68% of the scores or means are within 1 standard deviation of the mean, 95% within 2 standard deviations of the mean, and 99.7% within 3 standard deviations of the mean.

SKEWNESS. **Skew** is a measure of the asymmetry of a set of scores. Not all samples of data approximate the normal curve. Some samples are nonsymmetrical, and the peak is off centre. For example, worldwide individual income has a positive skew: Most individuals have incomes in the low-to-moderate range and few in the upper range. In a positive skew, the peak of the distribution curve would be to the left of a normal curve, and the mean is to the right of the median. In contrast, age at death in Canada has a negative skew because most deaths occur at older ages. In a negative skew, the peak of the distribution curve would be to the right of a normal curve, and the mean is to the left of the median. Figure 16.3

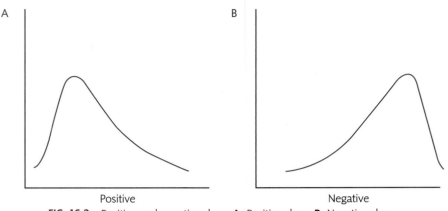

FIG. 16.3   Positive and negative skew. **A,** Positive skew. **B,** Negative skew.

illustrates positive and negative skew. In each diagram, the peak is off centre, and one "tail" of the curve is longer.

If the distribution is skewed, the mean will be pulled in the direction of the long tail of the distribution. With a skewed distribution, all three statistics should be reported. For example, national income in Canada is skewed. The mean wage differs from the median wage because the high salaries greatly outnumber the low salaries.

Evidence-Informed Practice Tip ____

The descriptive statistics for a sample indicate whether the sample data are skewed.

Interpreting Measures of Variability

Variability or dispersion is concerned with the spread of data. **Measures of variability**—statistical procedures that describe the level of dispersion in sample data—answer questions such as "Is the sample homogeneous or heterogeneous?" and "Is the sample similar or different?" If a researcher measures oral temperatures in two samples, one sample drawn from a healthy population and one sample from a hospitalized population, it is possible that the two samples will have the same mean. However, a wider range of temperatures is more likely to be found in the hospitalized sample than in the healthy sample. Measures of variability are used to describe these differences in the dispersion of data. As with

measures of central tendency, the various measures of variability are appropriate to specific kinds of measurement and types of distributions.

Research Hint ____

Descriptive statistics related to variability enable you to evaluate the homogeneity or heterogeneity of a sample.

RANGE. The range is the simplest but most unstable measure of variability. **Range** is the distance between the highest and lowest scores. A change in either of these two scores would change the range. The range should always be reported with other measures of variability. For example, Schneider, Steele, Cadell, and colleagues (2011), who examined differences in psychosocial outcomes between male and female caregivers of children with life-limiting illnesses, found that the range of ages among female caregivers was 22.99 to 68.38 years, whereas the range of ages among the male caregivers was 26.98 to 57.02 years (Table 16.4). Thus, the age range was 45 years among the female caregivers and 30 years among the male caregivers. Range affects the standard deviation, as discussed later. The range in Table 16.4 could easily change with an increase or decrease in the high scores or the low scores with a different sample.

SEMIQUARTILE RANGE. The **semiquartile range (semi-interquartile range)** is the range of the middle 50% of the scores. It is more stable than

TABLE 16.4

DEMOGRAPHIC INFORMATION OF CAREGIVER BY GENDER

VARIABLE	TOTAL (N = 273)			WOMEN (N = 224)			MEN (N = 49)			TEST STATISTIC
	M	SD	RANGE	M	SD	RANGE	M	SD	RANGE	
AGE IN YEARS	41.74	7.61	22.99–68.38	41.19	7.62	22.99–68.38	44.29	7.08	26.98–57.02	$t = -2.61, p = .009$
DIFFICULTY IN MANAGING COSTS	5.71	2.56	1–10	5.90	2.56	1–10	4.92	2.42	1–10	$t = 2.42, p = .016$
HOURS PER WEEK SPENT PROVIDING CARE	62.16	44.72	0–126	68.00	43.88	0–126	37.64	39.97	1.50–126	$t = 4.29, p = .000$
IMPORTANCE OF RELIGION*	3.04	1.03	1–4	3.10	1.01	1–4	2.76	1.09	1–4	$t = 2.16, p = .032$
MARITAL STATUS										$\chi^2 = 12.37, p = .015$
Married or living as married	219	80.2		172	76.8		47	95.9		
Widowed	2	0.7		1	0.4		1	2.0		
Divorced/separated	34	12.5		33	14.7		1	2.0		
Never married	13	4.8		13	5.8		0	0		
Other	5	1.8		5	2.2		0	0		
HIGHEST EDUCATION LEVEL										$\chi^2 = 3.83, p = .429$
Elementary school completed	13	4.8		9	4.1		4	8.2		
High school completed	98	36.2		85	38.3		13	26.5		
College completed	39	14.4		30	13.5		9	18.4		
University degree completed	64	23.6		51	23.0		13	26.5		
Postgraduate degree completed	57	21.0		47	21.2		10	20.4		

	n	%	n	%	n	%	χ^2
SIZE OF COMMUNITY							$\chi^2 = 0.61, p = .737$
Metropolitan area/large city	120	44.0	97	43.3	23	46.9	
Medium city/small city	91	33.3	77	34.4	14	28.6	
Smaller communities	62	22.7	50	22.3	12	24.5	
CURRENT EMPLOYMENT STATUS							$\chi^2 = 59.95, p = .000$
Full-time	114	41.8	70	31.3	44	89.8	
Part-time	38	13.9	37	16.5	1	2.0	
Paid leave	5	1.8	5	2.2	0	0	
Unpaid leave	3	1.1	3	1.3	0	0	
Self-employed	16	5.9	13	5.8	3	6.1	
Not employed	78	28.6	78	34.8	0	0	
Other	19	7.0	18	8.0	1	2.0	
CHANGE IN EMPLOYMENT STATUS							$\chi^2 = 29.05, p = .000$
No	136	50.9	94	43.1	42	85.7	
Yes	131	49.1	124	56.9	7	14.3	
WORK ALLOWS TIME OFF							$\chi^2 = 13.11, p = .001$
No	10	5.2	5	3.4	5	10.4	
Yes completely	110	57.0	93	64.1	17	35.4	
Only partially	73	37.8	47	32.4	26	54.2	
INCOME CHANGED: CHILD'S ILLNESS							$\chi^2 = 5.52, p = 0.19$
No	96	35.3	72	32.1	24	50	
Yes	176	64.7	152	67.9	24	50	

Continued

TABLE 16.4

DEMOGRAPHIC INFORMATION OF CAREGIVER BY GENDER—cont'd

VARIABLE	TOTAL (N = 273)			WOMEN (N = 224)			MEN (N = 49)			TEST STATISTIC
	M	SD	RANGE	M	SD	RANGE	M	SD	RANGE	
AVERAGE HOUSEHOLD INCOME PER YEAR ($)										$U = 3,515.50, p = .001$
<19,999	21	8.0		20	9.2		1	2.2		
20,000–39,999	39	14.8		37	17.0		2	4.3		
40,000–59,999	39	14.8		33	15.1		6	13.0		
60,000–79,999	47	17.8		39	17.9		8	17.4		
80,000–99,999	32	12.1		27	12.4		5	10.9		
100,000–119,999	38	14.4		27	12.4		11	23.9		
120,000–139,999	18	6.8		11	5.0		7	15.2		
140,000–199,999	22	8.3		16	7.3		6	13.0		
≤200,000	8	3.0		8	3.7		0	0		
CURRENT INCOME MEETS NEEDS										$U = 3,999.50, p = .004$
Totally inadequate	10	3.7		10	4.5		0	0		
Not very well	30	11.1		29	13.0		1	2.1		

SD, standard deviation.
*Range. 1 = *not important at all* to 4 = *very important.*
Adapted from Schneider, M., Steele, R., Cadell, S., et al. (2011). Differences on psychosocial outcomes between male and female caregivers of children with life-limiting illnesses. *Journal of Pediatric Nursing, 26*(3), 186–199. p. 6, Copyright 2011, with permission from Elsevier.

the overall range because it is less likely to be changed by a single extreme score. The semiquartile range lies between the upper and lower quartiles; the upper quartile consists of the top 25% of scores, and the lower quartile consists of the lowest 25% of the scores. In Table 16.3, the middle 50% of the scores are between 68 and 78, and the semiquartile range is 10.

PERCENTILE. A **percentile** represents the percentage of scores that a given score exceeds. The median is the fiftieth percentile, and in Table 16.3, it is a score of 74. A score in the ninetieth percentile is exceeded by only 10% of the scores. The zero percentile and the hundredth percentile are usually not used.

STANDARD DEVIATION. The **standard deviation** is the most frequently used measure of variability and is based on the concept of the normal curve (see Figure 16.2). The standard deviation is a measure of average deviation of the scores from the mean and, as such, should always be reported with the mean. The standard deviation accounts for all scores and can be used to interpret individual scores. For the examination in Table 16.3, the mean was 74.51 and the standard deviation was 12.1; thus, a student should know that 68% of the grades were between 85.1 and 61. If the student received a grade of 88, he or she would know that this grade was better than those of most of the class, whereas a grade of 58 would indicate that the student did not do as well as most of the class. Table 2 in Appendix D from the study by Héon and colleagues (2016) reports the mean and standard deviation of the study variables' breast milk expression (BME) scores for both the control and intervention groups. As illustrated in this table, the mean score of volume of BME in millilitres for the control group at Week 1 was 308.7 (SD = 219.8), whereas the mean score for the intervention group was 237.6 (SD = 124.6). This means that 68% of the control group expressed between 88.9 and 528.5 millilitres of breast milk and 68% of the intervention group expressed between 113.0 and 362.2 millilitres. This table allows the reader to inspect the data and see the variation in the data.

The standard deviation is used in the calculation of many inferential statistics. One limitation of the standard deviation is that it is expressed in terms of the units used in the measurement and cannot be used to compare means that have different units. If researchers were interested in the relationship between height measured in centimetres and weight measured in kilograms, it would be necessary to convert the height and weight measurements to standard units, or Z scores. The **Z score** is used to compare measurements in standard units. Each of the scores is converted to a Z score, and then the Z scores are used to examine the relative distance of the scores from the mean. A Z score of 1.5 means that the observation is 1.5 standard deviations above the mean, whereas a score of -2 means that the observation is 2 standard deviations below the mean. By using Z scores, a researcher can compare results from scales that use different measurement units, such as height and weight.

 Research Hint_____

Many measures of variability exist. The standard deviation is the most stable and useful because it provides a visual image of how the scores are dispersed around the mean.

INFERENTIAL STATISTICS

Inferential statistics combine mathematical processes with logic and allow researchers to test hypotheses about a population by using data obtained from probability samples. Statistical inference is generally used for two purposes: to estimate the probability that statistics found in the sample accurately reflect the population parameter and to test hypotheses about a population.

In the first purpose, a **parameter** is a characteristic of a **population**—a well-defined set that has certain specified properties—whereas a **statistic** is a characteristic of a *sample*. Statistics are used to estimate population parameters. Suppose that a researcher randomly selects 100 people with chronic lung disease and use an interval-level scale to study their knowledge of the disease. A mean score of 65 for these participants represents the sample statistic. If the researcher were able to study every participant with chronic lung disease, he or she also could calculate an average knowledge score, and that score would be the parameter for the population. Researchers are rarely able to study an entire population, but inferential statistics provide evidence that allow them to make statements about the larger population from studying the sample.

Both parametric and nonparametric inferential tests can be used in data analyses (Tables 16.5 and 16.6). Parametric statistical models are based on assumptions about the distributions of sample values and parameters; thus, in these models, means and variances are used to test significance. Nonparametric tests are used when populations have non-normal distributions or when researchers wish to explore associations among variables. In these tests, no assumptions about the distribution of the data are made.

The example of the study of patients with lung disease alludes to two important qualifications of how a study must be conducted so that inferential statistics may be used. First, the sample was selected randomly—that is, through the use of probability methods (see Chapter 12). Because you are already familiar with the advantages of probability sampling, you know that in order to make generalizations about a population from a sample, that sample must be representative. All procedures for inferential statistics are based on the assumption that the sample was drawn with a known probability. Second, the scale had to reflect the interval level of measurement. The mathematical operations involved in inferential statistics require this level of measurement. Note that researchers who use nonprobability methods of sampling also use inferential statistics. To compensate for the use of nonprobability sampling methods, researchers use techniques such as sample size estimation through power analysis. The following two Critical Thinking Decision Paths provide algorithms that reflect inferential statistics and that researchers use for statistical decision making.

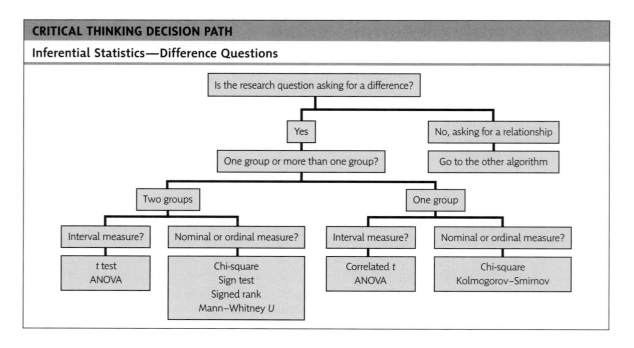

CRITICAL THINKING DECISION PATH

Inferential Statistics—Difference Questions

Is the research question asking for a difference?

Yes → One group or more than one group?

No, asking for a relationship → Go to the other algorithm

Two groups
- Interval measure? → *t* test / ANOVA
- Nominal or ordinal measure? → Chi-square / Sign test / Signed rank / Mann–Whitney *U*

One group
- Interval measure? → Correlated *t* / ANOVA
- Nominal or ordinal measure? → Chi-square / Kolmogorov–Smirnov

CRITICAL THINKING DECISION PATH

Inferential Statistics—Relationship Questions

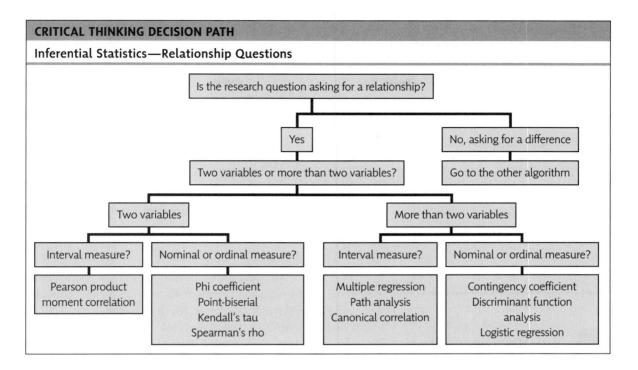

TABLE **16.5**

TESTS OF DIFFERENCES BETWEEN MEANS

LEVEL OF MEASUREMENT	ONE GROUP	TWO GROUPS		MORE THAN TWO GROUPS
		RELATED	INDEPENDENT	
NONPARAMETRIC				
Nominal	Chi-square	Chi-square Fisher's exact probability test	Chi-square	Chi-square
Ordinal	Kolmogorov-Smirnov test	Sign test Wilcoxon matched-pairs test	Chi-square	Chi-square
PARAMETRIC				
Interval or ratio	Correlated *t* test ANOVA (repeated measures)	Correlated *t* test	Independent *t* test	ANOVA
			ANOVA	ANCOVA MANOVA

ANCOVA, analysis of covariance; *ANOVA*, analysis of variance; *MANOVA*, multivariate analysis of variance.

TABLE 16.6		
TESTS OF ASSOCIATION		
LEVEL OF MEASUREMENT	**TWO VARIABLES**	**MORE THAN TWO VARIABLES**
NONPARAMETRIC		
Nominal	Phi coefficient Point-biserial correlation	Contingency coefficient
Ordinal	Kendall's tau Spearman's rho	Discriminant function analysis
PARAMETRIC		
Interval or ratio	Pearson r	Multiple regression Path analysis Canonical correlation

Evidence-Informed Practice Tip

Try to determine whether the statistical test chosen was appropriate for the design, the type of data collected, and the level of measurement.

Hypothesis Testing

The second and most commonly used purpose of inferential statistics is hypothesis testing. Statistical hypothesis testing allows researchers to make objective decisions about the outcome of their study and to answer questions such as "How much of this effect is a result of chance?"; "How strongly are these two variables associated with each other?"; and "What is the effect of the intervention?"

The procedures used to make inferences are based on principles of negative inference. For example, to study the effect of a new educational program for patients with chronic lung disease, the researcher would actually have two hypotheses: the scientific hypothesis and the null hypothesis. The research or **scientific hypothesis** (H₁) is what the researcher believes the outcome of the study will be. In this example,

the scientific hypothesis would be that the educational intervention would have a marked effect on the outcome in the experimental group in comparison with that in the control group. The **null hypothesis** (also called the *statistical hypothesis* or H_0), which is the hypothesis that actually can be tested by statistical methods, would be that no difference exists between the groups. In inferential statistics, the null hypothesis is used to test the validity of a scientific hypothesis in sample data. According to the null hypothesis, no relationship exists between the variables. and any observed relationship or difference is merely a function of chance fluctuations in sampling.

The concept of the null hypothesis is often confusing. An example may help clarify this concept. Sherrard, Duchesne, Wells, and colleagues (2015) used an interactive voice response to follow patients with acute coronary syndrome best practice guidelines and compared this to the usual care offered by the best practice guidelines. On the basis of this hypothesis, Sherrard and colleagues wanted to determine whether the differences found in the dependent variables of medication adherence and adverse effects differed significantly between the intervention group and the control group. The authors had to use the null hypothesis—that no difference would exist between the intervention and control groups—to test the scientific hypothesis. They found a significant improvement in medication adherence and a decrease in unplanned medical visits by the group that received interactive voice response. In other words, the differences between the control and intervention group scores were large enough to conclude that they were unlikely to be caused by chance. Thus, the null hypothesis was rejected.

In another example, Stutsky and Laschinger (2014) explored whether an online learning community would increase perceived leadership practices by nurse educators. Their research hypothesis was that there would be higher levels of perceived leadership practices in the group of nurse educators who were part of an expert-facilitated 12-week online group than in a self-facilitated group. They reported no significant differences between the groups. In other words, the null hypothesis was not rejected, and the differences between the expert-facilitated group and the self-facilitated were not large enough to conclude that they were unlikely to be caused by chance. See information on the interpretation of *p* values in the "Level of Significance" section.

All statistical hypothesis testing is a process of disproof or rejection. It is impossible to prove that a scientific hypothesis is true, but it is possible to demonstrate that the null hypothesis has a high probability of being incorrect. To reject the null hypothesis, therefore, is to show support for the scientific hypothesis, which is the desired outcome of most reports of inferential statistics.

Research Hint

Remember that most samples used in clinical research are samples of convenience, but most researchers use inferential statistics. Although such use violates one of the assumptions of such tests, the tests are robust enough to not seriously affect the results unless the data are skewed in unknown ways.

Probability

The researcher can never *prove* the scientific hypothesis but can show support for it by rejecting the null hypothesis—that is, by showing that the null hypothesis has a high probability of being incorrect. The theory underlying all of the procedures discussed in this chapter is probability theory. Probability is a concept that people talk about all the time, such as the chance of rain, but have a difficult time defining it. The **probability** of an event is the event's long-run relative frequency in repeated trials under similar conditions. In other words, the statistician does not think of the probability of obtaining a single result from a single study but rather of the chances of obtaining the same result from an idealized study that can be carried out many times under

identical conditions. The notion of repeated trials allows researchers to use probability to test hypotheses.

Statistical probability is based on the concept of sampling error. The use of inferential statistics is based on random sampling. However, even when samples are randomly selected, the possibility of errors in sampling always exists. Therefore, the characteristics of any given sample may be different from those of the entire population.

Suppose that a large group of patients with decubitus ulcers is available for study and that researchers wish to learn the average length of time for such ulcers to heal with the usual nursing care. If the researchers studied the entire population, they might obtain an average healing time of 50 days, with a standard deviation of 10 days. Now, suppose that the researchers did not have the money necessary to study all the patients but wished to conduct several consecutive studies of this condition. For this study, the researchers would first select a sample of 25 patients, calculate the mean and standard deviation, and then select the next sample. If this process is repeated many times in different samples, a different mean for each sample would probably result. For example, the researchers might find that one sample's mean might be 50.5 days, the next 47.5, and the next 62.5. The tendency for statistics to fluctuate from one sample to another is known as **sampling error.**

Sampling distributions are theoretical. In practice, researchers do not routinely draw consecutive samples from the same population; they usually compute statistics and make inferences on the basis of data from one sample. However, the knowledge of the properties of the sampling distribution—if these repeated samples are hypothetically obtained—enables the researcher to draw a conclusion on the basis of data from one sample. Such a conclusion is possible because the sampling distribution of the means has certain known properties.

The sampling distribution of the means is shaped like a normal curve, and the mean of the sampling distribution is the mean of the population. As discussed in the earlier "Normal Distribution" section, because the sampling distribution of the means is normal, several other important characteristics are revealed. When scores are normally distributed, 68% of them are between +1 standard deviation and −1 standard deviation, or the probability is 68 per 100 that any one randomly drawn sample mean is within the range of values between +1 standard deviation and −1 standard deviation (see Figure 16.2). In the example described earlier, if only one sample were selected, the chance of finding a sample mean between 40 and 60 would be 68%. The standard deviation of a theoretical distribution of sample means is called the **standard error of the mean.** The word *error* is used because the various means that make up the distribution contain an error in their estimates of the population mean. The error is considered to be standard because it implies the magnitude of the average error, just as a standard deviation implies the average variation from one mean. The *smaller* the standard error, the *less* variable are the sample means and the *more accurate* are those means as estimates of the population value.

Although researchers rarely construct sampling distributions, standard error can be estimated because it bears a systematic relationship to the sample standard deviation and the size of the sample. Thus, increasing the size of the sample will increase the accuracy of estimates of population parameters. It is intuitive that an increase in the size of a sample will decrease the likelihood that one outlying score will dramatically affect the sample mean (see Chapter 12). The other reason that the sampling distribution is so important is that all statistics have sampling distributions. Researchers consult these distributions when making determinations about rejecting the null hypothesis.

 Evidence-Informed Practice Tip ____

Remember that the strength and quality of evidence are enhanced by repeated trials that have consistent findings, thereby increasing the generalizability of the findings and applicability to clinical practice.

Type I and Type II Errors

The researcher's decision to accept or fail to accept (reject) the null hypothesis is based on a consideration of the probability that the observed differences are a result of chance alone. Because data on the entire population are not available, the researcher cannot flatly assert that the null hypothesis is or is not true. Thus, statistical inference is always based on incomplete information about a population, and errors can occur when such inferences are made. These errors are classified as type I and type II.

A **type I error** is the researcher's incorrect decision to reject the null hypothesis (Kline, 2005); that is, the researcher has found that results are statistically significant, but in fact they are not, and has accepted the alternate hypothesis. If, however, the researcher had found that the groups did not differ perhaps because only a few patients had been studied or the design of the study was poor for determining differences, a type II error might occur. In a **type II error**— also known as beta (β)—the results from the sample data lead to the failure to reject the null hypothesis when it is actually false; that is, no statistically significant differences between groups were found but there are indeed real differences. **Power** is the conditional prior probability that the researcher will decide correctly to reject the null hypothesis when it is actually false (Kline, 2005). A standard value of power of .8 is used to conduct power analyses in studies to determine sample size before the study begins. Power and beta are complementary and sum to 1.00. When power is increased, type II error is decreased, and vice versa.

In Campbell-Yeo, Johnston, Joseph, and colleagues' (2015) study on cobedding and recovery time after heel lance in preterm twins, one null hypothesis of the study was that there would be no differences in pain response and time to return to physiological measures between the experimental and control groups. Campbell-Yeo and colleagues reported a significant difference in recovery time; that is, the time was shorter in the cobedding group, mean = 75.6 seconds (SD, 70.0), compared with the usual care group, mean = 142.1 seconds (SD, 138.1, p = .001). If the differences found were truly a function of chance (because this group of participants was unusual in some way) and if the number of participants was too small, a type I error would occur.

The relationship of the two types of errors is shown in Figure 16.4. When you critique a study to determine whether a type I error has occurred (rejecting the null hypothesis when it is actually true), you should consider the reliability and validity of the instruments used. For example, if the instruments did not accurately and precisely measure the intervention variables, the conclusion could be that the intervention made a difference, but, in reality, it did not. It is critical to consider the reliability and validity of all of the measurement instruments reported (see Chapter 14). In a practice discipline, type I errors usually are considered more serious because if a researcher declares that differences exist where none are present, then patient care can potentially be affected adversely. Type II errors (accepting the null hypothesis when it is false) may occur if the sample in the study is too small, thereby limiting the opportunity to measure the *treatment effect,* a true difference between two groups. A larger sample size improves the ability to *detect the treatment effect*—that is, the differences between two groups. If no significant difference is found between two groups with a large sample, this finding provides stronger evidence (than with a small sample) not to reject the null hypothesis.

Level of Significance

The researcher does not know when an error in statistical decision making has occurred. It is possible to know only that the null hypothesis is indeed true or false if data from the total population are available. However, the researcher can control the risk of making type I errors by setting the level of significance before the study begins (a priori). The **level of significance (alpha level)** is the probability of making a type I error—in other words, the conditional probability of rejecting the null hypothesis when it is actually true. **Alpha,** or the level of significance, is considered an a priori probability because it is set before the data are collected, and it is a conditional probability because the null hypothesis is assumed to be true (Kline, 2005). The minimum level of significance acceptable for nursing research is .05. If the researcher sets alpha at .05, the researcher is willing to accept the fact that if the study were done 100 times, the decision to reject the null hypothesis would be wrong in 5 of those 100 trials, only if the null hypothesis is true.

Conclusion of test of significance	REALITY	
	Null hypothesis is true	Null hypothesis is not true
Not statistically significant	Correct conclusion	Type II error
Statistically significant	Type I error	Correct conclusion

FIG. 16.4 Outcome of statistical decision making.

Sometimes the researcher wants to have a smaller risk of rejecting a true null hypothesis; in that case, the level of significance may be set at .01. In this case, the researcher is willing to make the wrong decision only once in 100 trials. The decision as to how strictly the alpha level should be set depends on how important it is not to make an error. For example, if the results of a study are to be used to determine whether a great deal of money should be spent in an area of nursing care, the researcher may decide that the accuracy of the results is so important that an alpha level of .01 is chosen. In most studies, however, alpha is set at .05.

Another concept, the *p* value, is needed to interpret the alpha value. The ***p* value**, or probability value, is the probability of obtaining, from the study data, a test statistic, such as the mean, a result equal to or "more extreme" than what was actually observed, when the null hypothesis is true. The *p* value is different from alpha because it is calculated from the sample data and is considered the *exact level of significance*. Thus, if this exact level of significance is less than the conditional a priori probability of making a type I error (*p* < alpha), then the null hypothesis is rejected, and the result is considered statistically significant at that alpha level. For example, if the alpha is set at .05 and the *p* value is found to be .04, then the results are considered statistically significant.

Whatever level of significance is set, the researcher either rejects or accepts the null hypothesis when comparing the statistical results with the preset alpha. For example, in Stutsky and Laschinger's (2014) study, the null hypothesis regarding participants' perception of their leadership practices was rejected because the variables of the hypothesis were significant at the .05 level or lower; in other words, the *p* values were less than alpha. Héon and colleagues (2016), however, failed to reject the null hypothesis and found that the intervention ability to increase breast milk production was not significantly improved over those of the control group because the *p* values were greater than alpha (see Appendix D).

Perhaps you are thinking that researchers should always use the lowest alpha level possible because it makes sense that they would like to keep the risk of both types of errors at a minimum. Unfortunately, decreasing the risk of making a type I error increases the risk of making a type II error; that is, the stricter the researcher is in preventing the rejection of a true null hypothesis, the more likely the researcher is to accept a false null hypothesis. Therefore, researchers always have to accept more of a risk of one type of error when setting the alpha level.

Another method of determining the level of significance and whether to accept or reject the null hypothesis is called the *critical values method*. In this method, by calculating the estimates of population mean and standard deviation, a range of values is determined from which the researcher can compare the sample mean findings and decide whether to reject the null hypothesis.

Suppose researchers want to know the importance of support groups for caregivers of older adults. They ask 100 caregivers to rate the importance of support groups to them by using an instrument that ranges from 0 (not important at all) to 100 (very important). If Figure 16.2 represents the theoretical distribution for this study (a normal distribution with a mean of 50), 68% of the population would score between 40 and 60, and 95% would score between 30 and 70. Thus, the null hypothesis would be that the mean score for the population of caregivers would be 50, and the scientific hypothesis would be greater or less than 50. After measurements with this sample are completed, the researchers find that the sample mean score is 75. This mean is consistent with the scientific hypothesis, and the researchers can be 95% sure that, most of the time, the sample mean score would fall under this cut-off; thus, they would have confidence in rejecting the null hypothesis. In other words, only 5 of 100 times would they obtain this result by chance alone.

Research Hint

Decreasing the alpha level acceptable for a study increases the chance that a type II error will occur. When a researcher is conducting many statistical tests, the probability that some of the test results will be significant increases as the number of tests increases. Therefore, when a large number of tests are being conducted, many researchers decrease the alpha level to .01.

Practical and Statistical Significance

Statistical significance and practical significance are not the same. When a researcher finds a hypothesis statistically significant, this finding is unlikely to have happened by chance. In other words, if the level of significance has been set at .05, the odds are 95% that the researcher will make the correct conclusion on the basis of the results of the statistical test performed on sample data. The researcher would reach the wrong conclusion only 5 times in 100.

Suppose that a researcher is interested in the effect of loud rock music on the behaviour of laboratory mice. The researcher could design an experiment to study this question and find that loud music makes the mice act strangely. A statistical test suggests that this finding is not the result of chance. However, such a finding may or may not have practical significance, even though the finding has statistical significance. Whereas some authorities would argue that this study might have relevance to understanding the behaviour of teenagers, others would argue that the study has no practical value. Thus, the findings of a study may have statistical significance, but they may have no practical value or significance.

Although researchers should consider the practicality of a problem in the early stages of a research project (see Chapter 3), a distinction between the statistical and practical significance of the findings also should be made in the discussion of the results of a study. Some authorities believe that if the findings are not statistically significant, they have no practical value. In Héon and colleagues' (2016) study, in Appendix D, the research hypothesis was not statistically supported, but nonsupported hypotheses provide as much information about the intervention as do the supported hypotheses. The data allowed Héon and colleagues to return to the previous literature in the area and discern from those findings both statistical and practical significance.

Evidence-Informed Practice Tip

You study the results to determine the effectiveness of the new treatment and the size and clinical importance of the effect.

Tests of Statistical Significance

Tests of statistical significance may be parametric or nonparametric. In most studies in nursing research literature, investigators use parametric tests that have the following three attributes:

1. The estimation of at least one population parameter
2. Measurement at the interval level or higher
3. Assumptions about the variables being studied

One assumption is usually that the variable is normally distributed in the overall population.

In contrast to parametric tests, **nonparametric tests of significance** are not based on the estimation of population parameters, so their assumptions about the underlying distribution are less restrictive. Nonparametric tests are usually applied when the variables have been measured on a nominal or ordinal scale.

Some debate surrounds the relative merits of the two types of statistical tests. The moderate position taken by most researchers and statisticians is that **nonparametric statistics**—also called *distribution-free tests*—are best used when the data cannot be assumed to be at the interval level of measurement or when the sample is small and the normality of the underlying distribution cannot be inferred. If these assumptions can be made, however, most researchers prefer to use **parametric statistics,** which are more powerful and more flexible than nonparametric statistics.

Because stringent assumptions for parametric tests makes them more powerful than nonparametric tests, researchers are able to formulate simple sample statistics, such as the mean and the standard deviation, which enables them to accurately estimate population parameters with standard sampling distributions to obtain probabilities regarding the null hypotheses.

Researchers use many different statistical tests of significance to test hypotheses; however, the procedure and the rationale for their use are similar from test to test. Once the researcher has chosen a significance level and collected the data, the data are used to compute the appropriate test statistic. Each test has a related theoretical distribution that shows the probable and improbable values for that statistic. On the basis of the statistical result and the values in the distribution, the researcher either accepts or rejects the null hypothesis and then reports both the statistical result and its probability. Thus, a researcher may perform a t test, obtain a value of 8.98, and report that it is statistically significant at the $p < .05$ level. This means that in 100 tests, the researcher had five chances to conclude wrongly that this result could not have been obtained by chance.

The likelihood of finding a statistic that is high enough to be statistically significant is increased as the sample size increases. This likelihood is indicated by the degrees of freedom, which are often reported with the statistic and the probability value. Usually abbreviated as df, the **degree of freedom** is the freedom of a score's value to vary depending on the other scores and the sum of these scores; thus, $df = N - 1$. For example, imagine you have four numbers represented by letters ($a, b, c,$ and d) that must add up to a total of x; you are free to randomly choose the first three numbers, but the fourth must be chosen to make the total equal to x, and thus your degree of freedom is 3.

To make statistical inferences from data, many types of tests can be conducted. Tables 16.5 and 16.6 list the tests most commonly used for inferential statistics. The test used depends on the level of the measurement of the variables in question and the type of hypothesis being studied. These statistics test two types of hypotheses: that difference exists between groups (see Table 16.5) and that a relationship exists between two or more variables (see Table 16.6). In addition, many types of regression analyses are available to predict the dependent variable. Simple regression analyses (one independent variable) and multiple regression analyses (several independent variables) are used when the dependent variable is at the interval level or higher. In **logistic regression (logit analysis),** relationships between multiple independent variables and a dependent variable that is binary, ordinal, or polynomial are analyzed.

Research Hint
The use of nonparametric statistics in a study does not mean that the study is useless. The use of nonparametric statistics is appropriate when measurements are not made at the interval level or the variable under study is not normally distributed.

Evidence-Informed Practice Tip
Try to discern whether the test for analyzing the data was chosen because it gave a significant p value. A statistical test should be chosen on the basis of its appropriateness for the type of data collected, not because it gives the answer that the researcher hoped to obtain.

Tests of Differences

The type of test used for any particular study depends primarily on whether the researcher examines differences in one, two, or three or more groups and whether the data to be analyzed are nominal, ordinal, or interval (see Table 16.5). Suppose that a researcher constructs an experimental study with an after-only design (see Chapter 10). What the researcher hopes to determine is that the two randomly assigned groups are different after the introduction of the experimental treatment. If the measurements taken are at the interval level, the researcher would use the *t* test to analyze the data. If the *t* statistic was found to be high enough to be unlikely to have occurred by chance, the researcher would reject the null hypothesis and conclude that the two groups were indeed more different than would have been expected on the basis of chance alone. In other words, the researcher would conclude that the experimental treatment had the desired effect.

Rajacich, Kane, Lafreniere, and colleagues' (2014) study on male RNs and work satisfaction illustrated the use of the *t* statistic. In this study, the *t* test was used to determine differences in sample characteristics and job satisfaction outcome variables by sexual orientation. Participants who identified as gay had higher levels on the McCloskey and Mueller Total Satisfaction Scale than those who identified as heterosexual, $t(366) = -2.51, p = .012$.

 Evidence-Informed Practice Tip ____

Tests of difference are most commonly used in experimental and quasiexperimental designs that provide level II and level III evidence.

PARAMETRIC TESTS. The *t* **statistic** is commonly used in nursing research. This statistic reflects whether two group means are different. Thus, the *t* statistic is used when the researcher has two groups, and the question is whether the mean scores on some measure are more different than would be expected by chance. To use this test, the variables must have been measured at the interval or ratio level, and the two groups must be independent, meaning that nothing in one group helps determine what is in the other group. If the groups are related in some way, as when samples are matched (see Chapter 12), and the researcher also wants to determine differences between the two groups, a paired, or correlated, *t* test would be used.

The *t* statistic illustrates one of the major purposes of research in nursing: to demonstrate that differences exist between groups. Groups may be naturally occurring collections, such as age groups, or they may be experimentally created, such as treatment and control groups. Sometimes a study has more than two groups, or measurements are taken more than once. For example, Rajacich and colleagues (2014) used five groups of male nurses—medical/surgical, emergency room, intensive care/coronary care/operating room/recovery, and psychiatry—to describe and compare scheduling satisfaction. These researchers used **analysis of variance (ANOVA),** a test similar to the *t* test, because there were five groups. Like the *t* statistic, the ANOVA statistic is used to test whether group means differ, but instead of testing each pair of means separately, ANOVA accounts for the variation between groups and within groups. The ANOVA is usually performed with two or more groups by an *F* test rather than multiple pairs of *t* tests (see Practical Application box). If multiple pairs of *t* tests are done, the type I error rate would increase.

When more than two groups are compared over time, a repeated-measures ANOVA is used, because this variation of the ANOVA takes into account the fact that multiple measures at several times affect the potential range of scores. As an example, Hooge, Benzies, and Mannion (2014) evaluated the effects of a parenting program, *Baby and You*, on parenting knowledge, parenting morale, and social support. Data were collected at

> **Practical Application** ▬▬▬▬
>
> Rajacich and associates (2014) investigated environmental work factors in the acute care setting and their influence on male RNs' job satisfaction and intention to stay in the profession. One of their analyses consisted of examining type of hospital unit and scheduling satisfaction. The ANOVA results, $F(4,298) = 3.16$, $p = .014$, indicated that there were differences in satisfaction depending on the type of hospital unit where the male nurses were employed.

baseline and at the end of the 4-week program. Hooge and colleagues used repeated-measures ANOVA to determine whether changes had occurred between the baseline and 4-week collection times.

Another expansion of the notion of ANOVA is **multivariate analysis of variance (MANOVA),** which is also used to determine differences in group means, but only with more than one dependent variable.

POST HOC ANALYSIS. When the decision according to the ANOVA is to reject the null hypothesis, this indicates that at least one of the means is not the same as the other means, as in Rajacich and associates' (2014) study. To determine where the difference in means lies, a **post hoc analysis** is conducted; in this analysis, pairs of means in the main effects and interaction effects are compared to determine whether they are statistically different. Many post hoc analyses are available; the most common include Tukey's Honestly Significant Difference (HSD), the Scheffé analysis, and the Bonferroni analysis. This type of post hoc analysis is also known as *paired comparisons*. In the Rajacich and associates study (2014), post hoc comparisons (Tukey's HSD) revealed that scheduling satisfaction was significantly higher for nurses in the operating room or on medical/surgical units than for those working in intensive care/coronary care.

 Research Hint_____

A research report may not always refer to the test that was done. The reader can find this information by looking at the tables. For example, a table with *t* statistics contains a column for *t* values, and an ANOVA table lists *F* values.

In Freeman, Beaulieu, and Crawley's (2015) study on work expectations and migration of new Canadian nurse graduates, they used paired sample *t* tests to explore differences between the same participants' job expectations for Canada and those for another country. A sample of the findings

indicated that graduates had significantly higher expectations of having their valued job factors met abroad for full-time work ($t = -6.95$, $p < .001$), professional development ($t = -3.02$, $p = .003$), and preferred specialty ($t = -6.7$, $p < .001$), and they were significantly more confident that they would be supported in questioning unsafe and unethical practices ($t = 2.67$, $p = .009$) in Canada.

In other cases, particularly in experimental work, researchers use *t* tests or ANOVA to determine whether random assignment to groups was effective in creating groups that are equivalent before the experimental treatment is introduced. In this case, a researcher wants to show that no difference exists among the groups.

In many cases, researchers check whether groups are different at the beginning of a study or baseline by using the technique of **analysis of covariance (ANCOVA).** ANCOVA also entails measuring differences among group means and helps researchers equate the groups under study on an important variable. For example, El-Masri and associates (2014) explored the effects of three types of radiation therapy on urinary, sexual, and bowel function, bother, and well-being on men with prostate cancer over time. They used the ANCOVA to examine the between-within-group differences in study outcomes, while controlling for baseline scores. They found that the three treatment groups were not significantly different on any of the study outcomes after adjusting for baseline scores.

NONPARAMETRIC TESTS. When data are at the nominal or ordinal level and the researcher wants to determine whether groups are different, the chi-square, another commonly used statistic, is helpful. The **chi-square (χ^2)** is a nonparametric statistic used to determine whether the frequency in each category is different from what would be expected by chance. El-Masri and colleagues (2015) studied whether emergency transfers (yes/no) to hospitals from long-term homes differed by three categories: nurse practitioner (68%), medical doctor (41%), or registered nurse (38.7%); therefore, the chi-square test was performed, and the results were ($\chi^2 = 9.01, p = .34$).

As with the *t* test and ANOVA, if the calculated chi-square is high enough, the researcher would conclude that the frequencies found would not be expected on the basis of chance alone, and the null hypothesis would be rejected. Although this test is robust and can be used in many different situations, it cannot be used to compare frequencies when samples are small and expected frequencies are less than six in each cell. In those instances, **Fisher's exact probability test** is used.

When the data are ranks, or are at the ordinal level, several other nonparametric tests may be used: the Kolmogorov-Smirnov test, the sign test, the Wilcoxon matched-pairs test, the signed-rank test for related groups, the median test, and the Mann-Whitney *U* test for independent groups. Explanation of these tests is beyond the scope of this chapter; readers who desire further information should consult a general statistics book.

In nursing research studies, several different statistical tests are often used. Rajacich and colleagues' (2014) study illustrated the use of several of these statistical tests. They investigated environmental work factors in the acute care setting and their influence on male RNs' job satisfaction and intention to stay in the profession. Although the participants could not be randomly assigned to the group because of the attribute of sexual orientation or type of acute care unit, the researchers needed to determine whether the convenience sampling procedure succeeded in creating equivalent groups. There were no data measured at the nominal level, such as marital status, thus chi-square statistic was not used. For data measured at the interval level, such as the age, hours per week spent providing care, self-esteem, and spiritual involvement and beliefs scales, the *t* test was used. Finally, to test the differences between the two groups, the chi-square

method was used for nominal variables, such as change in employment status and community.

Tests of Relationships

Researchers often are interested in exploring the *relationship* between two or more variables. In such studies, they use statistics that determine the **correlation,** or the degree of association, between two or more variables. Tests of the relationships between variables are sometimes considered to be descriptive statistics when they are used to describe the magnitude and direction of a relationship of two variables in a sample and when the researcher does not wish to make statements about the larger population. Such statistics also can be inferential when they are used to test hypotheses about the correlations that exist in the target population.

In tests of the null hypothesis, no relationship is assumed to exist between the variables. Thus, when a researcher rejects this type of null hypothesis, the conclusion is that the variables are, in fact, related. Suppose that a researcher is interested in the relationship between the age of patients and the length of time it takes them to recover from surgery. As with other statistics discussed, the researcher would design a study to collect the appropriate data and then analyze the data by using measures of association. In this example, age and length of time until recovery can be considered interval measurements. The researcher would use the **Pearson correlation coefficient (Pearson *r*;** also called the *Pearson product-moment correlation coefficient*) in which the calculation reflects the degree of relationship between two interval variables. The distribution of the Pearson *r* enables the researcher to determine whether the value obtained is likely to have occurred by chance. Again, the research reports both the value of the correlation and its probability of occurring by chance.

Correlation coefficients can range in value from -1.0 to $+1.0$ and also can be zero. A zero coefficient means that no relationship exists between the variables. A *perfect positive correlation* is indicated by a coefficient of $+1.0$, and a *perfect negative correlation* by a coefficient of -1.0. The meaning of these coefficients is illustrated by the example from the previous paragraph. If no relationship exists between the age of the patient and the time required for the patient to recover from surgery, the correlation would be zero. However, a correlation of $+1.0$ would mean that the older the patient is, the longer the recovery time is. A negative coefficient would imply that the younger the patient is, the longer the recovery time is. Figure 16.5 illustrates a perfect positive correlation, a perfect negative correlation, and a zero correlation. A correlation value of 0 to .2 is considered extremely weak, a value of .2 to .4 is weak, a value of .4 to .6 is moderate, a value of .6 to .8 is strong, and a value of .8 to 1.0 is very strong (Bluman, 2014).

Of course, relationships are rarely perfect. The magnitude of the relationship is indicated by how close correlation is to the absolute value of 1 (see Practical Application box). Thus, a correlation of $-.76$ is just as strong as a correlation of $+.76$, but the direction of the relationship is opposite. In addition, a correlation of .76 is stronger than a correlation of .32. In testing hypotheses about the relationships between two variables, the researcher considers whether the

> ### Practical Application
>
> An example of a cross-sectional, descriptive, correlational study is that of Creamer, Mill, Austin, and colleagues (2014), who determined how Canadian nurse practitioners rate their levels of therapeutic commitment, role competency, and role support when working with persons with mental health issues. Creamer and colleagues found a significant positive correlation between role support and therapeutic commitment ($r = .357$, $p < .001$).
>
> Boamah and Laschinger (2015) also conducted correlations between two interval variables and found that overall workplace empowerment is significantly related to work engagement ($r = .47$, $p < .01$), and psychological capital ($r = .43$, $p < .01$). All of these variables were measured with validated scales.

magnitude of the correlation is large enough not to have occurred by chance. This is the meaning of the probability value, or the p value, reported with correlation coefficients. As with other statistical tests of significance, the larger the sample is, the greater is the likelihood of finding a significant correlation. Therefore, researchers also report the degrees of freedom associated with the test performed.

Nominal- and ordinal-level data also can be tested for relationships by nonparametric statistics. When two variables being tested are only dichotomous (e.g., male/female; yes/no), the phi coefficient can be used to express relationships. When the researcher is interested in the relationship

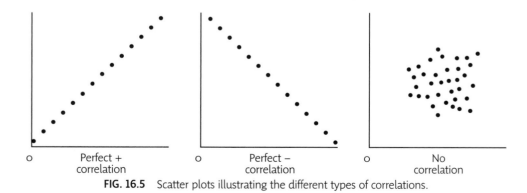

| o | Perfect +
correlation | o | Perfect −
correlation | o | No
correlation |

FIG. 16.5   Scatter plots illustrating the different types of correlations.

between a nominal variable and an interval variable, the point-biserial correlation is used. Spearman's rho is used to determine the degree of association between two sets of ranks, as is Kendall's tau. All of these correlation coefficients may range in value from -1.0 to $+1.0$. These tests are listed in Table 16.6.

Nursing problems are rarely so simple that they can be explained by only two variables. When researchers are interested in studying complex relationships among more than two variables, they use techniques other than those discussed thus far. When researchers are interested in understanding more about a problem than just the relationship between two variables, they often use **multiple regression,** in which the relationship between one dependent variable at the interval level and several independent variables is measured. Multiple regression is the expansion of correlation to include more than two variables and is used when the researcher wants to determine what variables contribute to the explanation of the dependent variable and to what degree.

For example, a researcher may be interested in determining what factors help women decide to breastfeed their infants. A number of variables—such as the mother's age, previous experience with breastfeeding, number of other children, and knowledge of the advantages of breastfeeding—might be measured and then analyzed to determine whether they, separately and together, are predictive of the length of breastfeeding. Such a study would require the use of multiple regression. The results of such a study might help nurses know that a younger mother with only one other child might be more likely to benefit from a teaching program about breastfeeding than would an older mother with several other children.

In reading research reports, you will often see multiple regression techniques described as *forward solution, backward solution,* or *stepwise solution.* These techniques are used in multiple regression to find the smallest group of variables that will account for the greatest proportion of variance in the dependent variable. In the forward solution, the independent variable that has the highest correlation with the dependent variables is entered first, and the next variable is the one that will increase the explained variance the most. In the backward solution, all variables are entered into the solution, and each variable is deleted to determine whether the explained variance drops significantly. The stepwise solution is a combination of the two approaches. In general, all of the approaches yield similar, although not identical, results.

Suppose that the individual who was researching breastfeeding was interested in not just breastfeeding but also maternal satisfaction. *Canonical correlation* is used with more than one dependent variable. If the data are nominal or ordinal, the contingency coefficient or discriminant function analyses are used.

Using multiple regression, Wong, Elliott-Miller, Laschinger, et al. (2015) examined the relationship of front-line managers' personal characteristics, span of control on their job unit, and unit performance outcomes. The overall span of control was a significant predictor of role overload ($\beta = 0.26$), work control ($\beta = -0.23$), and job satisfaction ($\beta = -0.18$). These data allowed them to build on the past research that they had reviewed and to suggest both future descriptive and intervention research, thus moving the data toward evidence-informed practice.

Evidence-Informed Practice Tip

Tests of relationship are usually associated with nonexperimental designs that provide level IV evidence. A strong, statistically significant relationship between variables often provides support for replicating the study, in order to increase the consistency of the findings and provide a foundation for developing an intervention study.

The Use of Confidence Intervals

A **confidence interval** is a range of values, based on a random sample, that is often described with measures of central tendency and measures of association and provides the nurse with a measure of precision or uncertainty about the sample findings. In other words, the confidence interval is an estimated range of values, which is likely to include an unknown population parameter calculated from a given set of sample data.

Typically, investigators record their confidence interval results as a 95% degree of certainty; sometimes, the degree of certainty is recorded as 99%. Today, professional journals often require investigators to report confidence intervals as one of the statistical methods used to interpret study findings. Even when confidence intervals are not reported, they can be easily calculated from study data. The method for performing these calculations is widely available in statistical texts.

Ostry, Maggi, Hershler, and associates (2010) explored whether differences in mental health outcomes were observable between a cohort of sawmill workers living in rural areas and a cohort living in urban places in British Columbia (Table 16.7). The confidence interval helps place the results in context for all patients in the study. The results shown in Table 16.7 demonstrate, for example, that workers who remain at an urban mill have higher odds for neurotic disorder (value greater than 1.0), adjustment reaction, and acute reaction to stress.

 Research Hint _____

When evaluating whether you should spend time reviewing an article, examine the article's tables. The information you need to answer your clinical question should be contained in one or more of the tables.

Harm Studies

The odds ratio in logistic regression can be used in exploring clinical questions of harm, when investigators want to determine whether an individual has been harmed by being exposed to a particular event. In this type of study, investigators select the outcome of interest (e.g., pressure ulcers) and try to determine whether any one factor explains why a patient has or does not have

---

TABLE **16.7**

UNIVARIATE ANALYSES: ODDS RATIOS FOR FOUR MENTAL HEALTH DIAGNOSES AMONG SAWMILL WORKERS, 1994 TO 2001

	MENTAL HEALTH DIAGNOSIS*			
LOCATION	NEUROTIC DISORDER: ICD-9 CODE 300 (N = 6306)	ACUTE REACTION TO STRESS: ICD-9 CODE 308 (N = 4104)	ADJUSTMENT REACTION: ICD-9 CODE 309 (N = 2133)	ANXIETY/DEPRESSION: ICD-9 CODE 311 (N = 7816)
Urban stay	1.14 (1.02–1.27)	1.04 (0.84–1.29)	1.42 (1.08–1.87)	0.99 (0.85–1.15)
Migrate from urban	0.67 (0.48–0.93)	1.19 (0.82–1.72)	0.82 (0.48–1.38)	0.94 (0.73–1.21)
Rural stay	0.94 (0.79–1.11)	0.68 (0.54–0.86)	0.74 (0.55–0.99)	1.04 (0.89–1.21)
Migrate from rural to urban	1.58 (1.28–1.94)	1.69 (1.30–2.19)	1.54 (1.11–2.13)	1.30 (1.09–1.56)
Migrate from urban to rural	0.95 (0.60–0.94)	0.86 (0.66–1.11)	0.63 (0.44–0.99)	0.77 (0.63–0.92)

ICD-9, International Classification of Diseases and Related Health Problems, Ninth Revision (World Health Organization, 1977).
*Numbers in parentheses are 95% confidence intervals.
Adapted from Ostry, A., Maggi, S., Hershler, R., et al. (2010). Mental health differences among middle-aged sawmill workers in rural compared to urban British Columbia. _Canadian Journal of Nursing Research, 42_(3), 84–100. SAGE Publications Inc.

the outcome of interest. The measure of association that best describes the analyzed data is the **odds ratio,** which communicates that one event is likelier to occur than other events. An odds ratio is calculated by dividing the odds in the treated or exposed group by the odds in the control group. Investigators present an odds ratio of factors in study tables; thus, calculation of the odds ratio is rarely necessary. The interpretation of the odds ratio is straightforward and presented in Table 16.8. Note that the null value for the odds ratio is equal to 1.

The use of the odds ratio to describe the probability of an event is illustrated by a study in which investigators sought to test a process evaluation checklist in the documentation of sucrose orders to improve neonatal pain. Yamada, Stevens, Sidani, et al. (2015) found that at the end of the second audit, the odds of documentation of sucrose orders were five times greater compared with the start of the first audit a few months earlier. Harm data, with their measure of probabilities, help nurses identify factors that may or may not contribute to an adverse or beneficial outcome.

Meta-analysis

Meta-analysis is not a type of study design but a research method in which the results of multiple studies (usually randomized controlled trials) are statistically combined to answer focused clinical questions through an objective appraisal of carefully synthesized research evidence (see Chapter 11). People sometimes use the terms *meta-analysis* and *systematic review* interchangeably; however, a meta-analysis is a quantitative analysis used in a systematic review.

Systematic review is the process whereby the investigators evaluate all relevant studies, published and unpublished, on the topic or question (Higgins & Green, 2011). At least two members of the review team independently assess the quality of each study, include or exclude studies on the basis of pre-established criteria, statistically combine the results of individual studies, and present a balanced and impartial summary of the findings that represents a "state-of-the-science" conclusion about the evidence supporting the benefits and risks of a given health care practice.

In the evidence-informed hierarchy, the findings of a systematic review are considered to provide the strongest evidence available to the clinician because they summarize large amounts of information derived from multiple experimental studies of the effect of the same intervention. A methodologically sound systematic review with a rigorous meta-analysis is more likely than an individual study to identify the true effect of an intervention because the meta-analysis limits bias.

In a systematic review, the researcher quantitatively combines the data from the selected experimental studies by using their measures of association (see Table 16.6). An odds ratio is the statistic of choice for use in a meta-analysis. The same interpretation of odds ratio described in Table 16.8 applies to the odds ratios obtained in a meta-analysis.

TABLE **16.8**

INTERPRETATION OF ODDS RATIOS

ODDS RATIO	ADVERSE OUTCOME (E.G., MYOCARDIAL INFARCTION)	BENEFICIAL OUTCOME (E.G., ADHERENCE TO MEDICATION REGIMEN)
<1 (e.g., .375)	Intervention produced better results	Intervention produced worse results
1	Intervention produced no better/worse results	Intervention produced no better/worse results
>1 (e.g., 4.0)	Intervention produced worse results	Intervention produced better results

The usual manner of displaying data from a meta-analysis is by a pictorial representation known as a *blobbogram,* or forest plot, accompanied by a summary measure of effect size in odds ratios. In the meta-analysis depicted in Figure 16.6, the investigators were interested in whether follow-up affects the psychological well-being of women after miscarriage (Murphy, Lipp, & Powles, 2012). The investigators searched the literature for randomized controlled trials in which the participants were females of child-bearing age who experienced a miscarriage, defined as premature expulsion of an embryo or fetus from the uterus up to 23 weeks of pregnancy and weighing up to 500 grams. The investigators found six trials involving 1,001 women that met these criteria. Three trials compared one counselling session with no counselling. There was no significant difference in psychological well-being, including anxiety, grief, depression avoidance, and self-blame. One trial compared three 1-hour counselling sessions with no counselling at 4 and 12 months. Some subscales showed statistical significance in favour of counselling and some in favour of no counselling. The results for two trials were given in narrative form, as data were unavailable for meta-analyses. One trial compared multiple interventions. The other trial compared two counselling sessions with no counselling. Neither study favoured counselling.

Close to the centre of the figure, each trial in the analysis is represented by a horizontal line. The findings from each study are represented as a blob or square (the measured effect) on the vertical line. The size of the blob or square (sometimes just a small vertical line) reflects the amount of information in that study. The width of the horizontal line represents the 95% confidence interval. The vertical line is the line of no effect (odds ratio = 1). When the confidence interval of the result (horizontal line) crosses the line of no effect (vertical line), then the differences in the effect of the treatment are not statistically significant. If the confidence interval does not cross the vertical line, then the study results are statistically significant.

As shown in the blobbogram in Figure 16.6, in the analyses of one counselling session versus no counselling, the studies yielded analysis lines that did cross the line of no effect. Because the analysis lines did cross the line of no effect, these studies have no statistically significant findings. Murphy and colleagues (2012) also provided the numerical equivalent of each blobbogram entry.

Other important information and additional statistical analysis may accompany the blobbogram, such as a test to determine the degree to which the results of each of the individual trials are mathematically compatible (heterogeneity). For more information, refer to a book of advanced research methods.

Advanced Statistics

Sometimes, researchers are interested in even more complex problems. For example, El-Masri and colleagues (2015) conducted an observational prospective cohort study to evaluate the effectiveness of a nurse-practitioner-led outreach program on the health outcomes, emergency department (ED) transfers, and hospital admissions of long-term-care residents. El-Masri and colleagues had a sample size of 311 long-term-care residents with 1,353 observations. The results of the logistic regression revealed that transfers by nurse practitioners were 27% less likely to be non-urgent than transfers by physicians (OR = .73; 95% CI .54–.97). On the basis of a proposed model, the relationships between the independent and dependent variables were tested through logistic regression analysis. Logistic regression is a form of advanced statistics used when a researcher wishes to confirm the relationship of a set of categorical data (data that have a discrete value).

This notion of testing specific relationships in a specific order can be extended further to test hypothesized variables that are made up of several measures. In structural equation modelling, path

Study or Subgroup	One Counselling Session N	Mean (SD)	No Counselling N	Mean (SD)	Std. Mean Difference IV, Fixed, 95% CI	Weight	Std. Mean Difference IV, Fixed, 95% CI
1 Anxiety							
Lee 1996	21	7.4 (5.9)	18	8.1 (6.2)		37.3%	−0.11 [−0.74, 0.52]
Nikcevic 2007	33	5.6 (4.5)	33	7 (4.4)		62.7%	−0.31 [−0.80, 0.17]
Subtotal (95% CI)	**54**		**51**			**100.0%**	**−0.24 [−0.62, 0.15]**
Heterogeneity: Chi^2 = 0.24, df = 1 (P = 0.63); I^2 = 0.0%							
Test for overall effect: Z = 1.21 (P = 0.23)							
2 Depression							
Lee 1996	21	3.2 (4.2)	18	4.8 (7)		36.9%	−0.28 [−0.91, 0.36]
Nikcevic 2007	33	2.8 (4.1)	33	3.7 (3.7)		63.1%	−0.23 [−0.71, 0.26]
Subtotal (95% CI)	**54**		**51**			**100.0%**	**−0.25 [−0.63, 0.14]**
Heterogeneity: Chi^2 = 0.01, df = 1 (P = 0.90); I^2 = 0.0%							
Test for overall effect: Z = 1.21 (P = 0.21)							
3 Grief							
Adolfsson 2006	43	31 (19.2)	45	32.7 (20)		57.2%	−0.09 [−0.50, 0.33]
Nikcevic 2007	33	39.9 (12.4)	33	42 (13.4)		42.8%	−0.16 [−0.64, 0.32]
Subtotal (95% CI)	**76**		**78**			**100.0%**	**−0.12 [−0.43, 0.20]**
Heterogeneity: Chi^2 = 0.05, df = 1 (P = 0.82); I^2 = 0.0%							
Test for overall effect: Z = 0.73 (P = 0.46)							
4 Avoidance							
Lee 1996	21	13.5 (12)	18	11.4 (11.3)		100.0%	0.18 [−0.45, 0.81]
Subtotal (95% CI)	**21**		**18**			**100.0%**	**0.18 [−0.45, 0.81]**
Heterogeneity: not applicable							
Test for overall effect: Z = 0.55 (P = 0.58)							
5 Intrusion							
Lee 1996	21	13.2 (11.3)	18	18.1 (11.5)		100.0%	−0.42 [−1.06, 0.22]
Subtotal (95% CI)	**21**		**18**			**100.0%**	**−0.42 [−1.06, 0.22]**
Heterogeneity: not applicable							
Test for overall effect: Z = 1.30 (P = 0.20)							
6 Difficulty in Coping							
Adolfsson 2006	43	21.7 (13.2)	45	22.9 (15.8)		100.0%	−0.08 [−0.50, 0.34]
Subtotal (95% CI)	**43**		**45**			**100.0%**	**−0.08 [−0.50, 0.34]**
Heterogeneity: not applicable							
Test for overall effect: Z = 0.38 (P = 0.70)							
7 Despair							
Adolfsson 2006	43	20.7 (13.5)	45	20.6 (13.8)		100.0%	0.01 [−0.41, 0.43]
Subtotal (95% CI)	**43**		**45**			**100.0%**	**0.01 [−0.41, 0.43]**
Heterogeneity: not applicable							
Test for overall effect: Z = 0.03 (P = 0.97)							
8 Self Blame							
Nikcevic 2007	33	5.7 (3.6)	33	5.6 (3.2)		100.0%	0.03 [−0.45, 0.51]
Subtotal (95% CI)	**33**		**33**			**100.0%**	**0.03 [−0.45, 0.51]**
Heterogeneity: not applicable							
Test for overall effect: Z = 0.12 (P = 0.91)							
9 Worry							
Nikcevic 2007	33	11.9 (3.3)	33	13.5 (4.1)		100.0%	−0.42 [−0.91, 0.06]
Subtotal (95% CI)	**33**		**33**			**100.0%**	**−0.42 [−0.91, 0.06]**
Heterogeneity: not applicable							
Test for overall effect: Z = 1.71 (P = 0.088)							
Test for subgroup differences: Chi^2 = 4.59, df = 8 (P = 0.80); I^2 = 0.0%							

−2   −1   0   1   2

Favors counselling   Favors no counselling

FIG. 16.6 Comparison 1: one counselling session versus no counselling (at 4 months), outcome 1: psychological well-being. *CI*, confidence interval; *IV*, independent variable; *SD*, standard deviation. Fiona A Murphy, Allyson Lipp, Diane L Powles, "Follow-up for improving psychological well being for women after a miscarriage," *Cochrane Database of Systematic Reviews.* Copyright © 2012 The Cochrane Collaboration. Published by John Wiley & Sons, Ltd.

models made up of variables that are not actually measured are tested. For example, a researcher might study the effects of work-unit structural empowerment and social capital on perceptions of unit effectiveness and nurses' ratings of patient care quality by testing a measurement model (Laschinger, Read, Wilk, et al., 2014).

Another advanced technique often used in nursing research is factor analysis. Factor analysis helps researchers understand concepts more fully and contributes to their ability to measure concepts reliably and validly (see Chapter 14). In **factor analysis,** a large number of variables are grouped into a smaller number of factors to reduce a set of data so that it may be easily described and used; this statistical procedure is used to determine the underlying dimensions or components of a variable. Factor analysis is also used for instrument development and theory development.

In instrument development, factor analysis is used to group individual items on a scale into meaningful factors or subscales. For example, Kennedy, Tomblin-Murphy, Martin-Misener, and colleagues (2015) used factor analysis to refine a new instrument, the Nursing Competence Self-Efficacy Scale. The original scale contained 32 items, and psychometric analyses were performed on the final 22-item version. Factor analysis was used to determine whether the scale measured the concepts that it was intended to measure.

The Use of Statistics

Statistics are used in nursing research to describe the samples of research studies and to test for hypothesized differences or associations in the sample. Knowing the characteristics of the sample of a research study allows the researcher to determine the population for whom the results will be generalized. For example, if a study sample was primarily White with a mean age of 42 years (SD = 2.5), the findings may not be applicable to Punjabi older adults. The cultural, demographic, or clinical factors of an older adult population of a different ethnic group may

contribute to different results. Thus, understanding the descriptive statistics of a study assists in determining the applicability of findings to different practice settings.

Statistics are also used to test hypotheses proposed by the researchers. Inferential statistics used to analyze data (e.g., t test, F test, r coefficient) and the associated significance level (p value) indicate the likelihood that the association or difference found in any study results from chance or because of a true difference between groups. The closer the p value is to zero, the less likely it is for the association or difference of a study to result from chance. Thus, inferential statistics provide an objective way to determine whether the results of the study are likely to be a true representation of reality.

 Evidence-Informed Practice Tip _____
A basic understanding of statistics will improve your ability to assess the effect of the independent variable on the dependent variable and related patient outcomes for your patient population and practice setting.

EXAMPLE OF THE USE AND CRITIQUE OF STATISTICS

The purpose of the study by Héon and colleagues (2016) was to estimate the effects of a breast milk expression education and support intervention on breast milk production in mothers of preterm infants when compared with usual care (see Appendix D). The statement of purpose implies that the investigators were interested in differences between groups; thus, an experimental design that provides level II evidence was appropriate. Therefore, you should expect the analysis to consist of statistical tests in which differences between means were examined, such as t tests or ANOVA.

Héon and colleagues (2016; see Appendix D) adequately described sample characteristics. If the participants who did not complete the study differed from those who completed the study, the findings would be difficult to interpret (i.e., those who completed the program had fewer problems). Dependent variables consisted of duration and frequency of breast milk expression, and volume of breast milk expressed. Héon and colleagues were interested in looking at differences between the participants who received standard care (control group) and those who received the experimental intervention. Various statistical tests were used to examine differences, depending on the level of measurement. Dependent variables calculated at the ratio level were compared in repeated-measures ANOVA.

These tests are appropriate for the study design and the hypotheses because Héon and colleagues (2016) were interested in differences between the two groups. The results for each of the hypotheses were suggestive of differences in some of the outcomes between the two groups. The tables agreed with the text, and the results were understandable to readers. The discussion pointed out limitations to the study. Clear implications for practice were described, and they supported the practical significance of the study. The statistical level of significance was set at .05 and was consistent throughout the article. Therefore, the researchers' statistics were appropriate to the study's purpose, design, method, sample, and levels of measurement.

APPRAISING THE EVIDENCE

Descriptive and Inferential Statistics

Many students who have not had a course in statistics think they cannot critique the statistics of research. However, students should be able to critically analyze the use of statistics even if they do not understand how the numbers presented were derived. What is most important in critiquing this aspect of a research study is that the procedures for summarizing and analyzing the data make sense in view of the purpose of the study (see the Critiquing Criteria box).

Before you decide whether the statistics used make sense, return to the beginning of the study and determine the purpose. Although descriptive statistics are used in all studies to summarize the data obtained, many investigators use inferential statistics to test specific hypotheses. In a report of an exploratory study, it is possible that only descriptive statistics are presented because the purpose is to describe the characteristics of a population.

Just as the hypotheses or research questions should follow from the purpose of a study, so should the hypotheses or research questions suggest the type of analysis that follows. The hypotheses or the research questions should indicate the major variables that are expected to be presented in summary form. Each of the variables in the hypotheses or research questions should be presented in the "Results" section along with appropriate descriptive information.

After you study the hypotheses or research questions, proceed to the "Methods" section. Using the operational definition provided, identify the levels of measurement used to measure each of the variables listed in the hypotheses or research questions. From this information, you should be able to determine the measures of central tendency and variability that should be used to summarize the data. For example, you would not expect to see a mean used as a summary statistic for the nominal variable of gender; gender would probably be reported as a frequency distribution. The means and standard deviations should be provided for measurements performed at the interval level. The sample size is another feature described in the "Methods" section that is helpful for evaluating the researcher's use of descriptive statistics. The larger the sample is, the less chance there is that one outlying score will affect the summary statistics.

If tables or graphs are used, they should agree with the information presented in the text. The tables and charts should be clearly and completely labelled. If the researcher presents grouped frequency data, the groups should be logical and mutually exclusive. The size of the

Continued

Descriptive and Inferential Statistics

interval in grouped data should not obscure the pattern of the data, nor should it create an artificial pattern. Each table and chart should be referred to in the text, but each should add to the text, not merely repeat it. Each table or graph should have an obvious connection to the study.

In reading a table such as Table 16.4, first look at the table title. The title should give an indication of the information in the table. Next, review the column headings. Do these headings follow from the title? Is each heading clear, and are any nonstandard abbreviations explained? Are the statistics contained in the table appropriate to the level of measurement used? In Table 16.4, the column headings follow from the title. Each study variable is listed, along with its mean and standard deviation. Mean and standard deviation are appropriate statistics because these data were regarded as interval-level data.

After you evaluate the descriptive statistics, evaluate the inferential statistical analysis of a research report, beginning with the hypothesis or research question. If the hypothesis or research question indicates that a relationship will be found, you should expect to find indices of correlation. If the study is experimental or quasiexperimental, the hypothesis should indicate that the author is looking for differences between the groups studied, and you would expect to find statistical tests of differences between means that test the effect of the intervention.

As you read the "Methods" section of the article, again consider the level of measurement used to measure the important variables. If the level of measurement is interval or ratio, the statistics will probably be parametric. If the variables are measured at the nominal or ordinal level, however, the statistics used should be nonparametric. Also, consider the sample size and remember that samples need to be large enough to enable the assumption of normality. If the sample is quite small—for example, 5 to 10 participants—the researcher may have violated the assumptions necessary for inferential statistics to be used (see Chapter 12). Thus, the important question is whether the researcher has provided enough justification to use the statistics presented.

Finally, consider the results as they are presented. Enough data should be presented for each hypothesis or research question for you to determine whether the researcher actually examined each one. The tables should

accurately reflect the procedure performed and be in harmony with the text. For example, the text should not say that a test result reached statistical significance, but the tables show that the probability value of the test was higher than .05. If the researcher used analyses that are not discussed in this text, you may want to refer to a statistics text to decide whether the analysis was appropriate for the hypothesis or research question and the level of measurement.

You should critique two other aspects of the data analysis. The study should not read as if it were a statistical textbook. The results should be presented clearly enough that the reader can determine what was done and what the results were. In addition, the author should distinguish between the practical and the statistical significance of the evidence in relation to the findings. Some results may be statistically significant, but their practical importance may be doubtful in terms of applicability to a patient population or clinical setting. In this case, the author should note the deficiency. Alternatively, a research report may be elegantly presented, but the findings do not impress you. Such a feeling may indicate that the practical significance of the study and its findings have not been adequately explained in the report. From an evidence-informed practice perspective, a significant hypothesis or research question should contribute to improving patient care and clinical outcomes.

Note that the critical analysis of a research article's statistical analysis is not conducted in a vacuum. The adequacy of the analysis can only be judged in relation to the other important aspects of the article: the problem, the hypotheses, the research question, the design, the data-collection methods, and the sample. If these aspects of the research process are not considered, the statistics themselves have very little meaning. Statistics can be misleading; thus, the researcher must use the appropriate statistic for the problem. For example, a researcher may use a nonparametric statistic when a parametric statistic is appropriate. Because parametric statistics are more powerful than nonparametric statistics, the result of the parametric analysis may not have been what the researcher expected. However, the nonparametric result might be in the expected direction, and so the researcher reports only that result.

CRITIQUING CRITERIA

1. Were appropriate descriptive statistics used?
2. What level of measurement is used for each major variable?
3. Is the sample size large enough to prevent one extreme score from affecting the summary statistics used?
4. What descriptive statistics are reported?
5. Were these descriptive statistics appropriate to the level of measurement for each variable?
6. Are appropriate summary statistics provided for each major variable?
7. Does the hypothesis indicate that the researcher tested for differences between groups or tested for relationships? What is the level of significance?
8. Does the level of measurement enable the use of parametric statistics?
9. Is the sample size large enough to use parametric statistics?
10. Has the researcher provided enough information for you to decide whether the appropriate statistics were used?
11. Are the statistics used appropriate for the problem, the hypothesis, the method, the sample, and the level of measurement?
12. Are the results for each of the hypotheses presented clearly and appropriately?
13. If tables and graphs are used, do they agree with the text and extend it, or do they merely repeat it?
14. Are the results clear?
15. Is a distinction made between practical significance and statistical significance? How is it made?

CRITICAL THINKING CHALLENGES

- Discuss the ways a researcher might use a computer to analyze data and present the descriptive statistical results of a study.
- What is the relationship between the level of measurement used and the choice of a statistical procedure? How is the level of measurement related to the level of evidence in the study design?
- What type of visual depiction can be used to show the use of correlations? Use examples from clinical practice to illustrate the difference between positive and negative correlations.
- A classmate states that it is ridiculous for the instructor to have students critique the descriptive statistics used in a study when none of the students has taken a statistics course. Would you agree or disagree? Defend your position.
- What assumptions are violated when a clinical research study uses a convenience sample and applies inferential statistics?
- What are the advantages and disadvantages of decreasing the alpha level for a study? What is the relationship between setting an alpha level and type I and type II errors?
- Discuss the parameters for using nonparametric statistics in a study and their effect on the usefulness of applying the evidence provided by the findings in practice.
- A research study's findings are not considered significant at the .05 level; are they deemed to provide evidence that is applicable to practice? Justify your answer.

KEY POINTS

- Descriptive statistics are a means of describing and organizing data gathered in research.
- The four levels of measurement are nominal, ordinal, interval, and ratio. Measurement at each level is performed with appropriate descriptive techniques.
- Measures of central tendency describe the average member of a sample. The mode is the score that occurs most frequently, the median is the middle score, and the mean is the arithmetical average of the scores. The mean is the most stable and useful of the measures of central tendency and, with the standard deviation, forms the basis for many inferential statistics.
- The frequency distribution is depicted in tabular or graphic form and allows calculation or observation of characteristics of the data distribution, including skewness, symmetry, modality, and kurtosis.

- In nonsymmetrical distributions, the degree and direction of the pull of the off-centre peak are described in terms of skew.
- The ranges reflect differences between high and low scores.
- The standard deviation is the most stable and most useful measure of variability. It is derived from the concept of the normal curve. In the normal curve, sample scores and the means of large numbers of samples cluster around the midpoint in the distribution, and a fixed percentage of the scores is within given distances of the mean. This tendency of means to approximate the normal curve is called the *sampling distribution of the means*. A Z score is the standard deviation converted to standard units.
- Because the sampling distribution of the means follows a normal curve, researchers are able to estimate the probability that a certain sample will have the same properties as the total population of interest. Sampling distributions provide the basis for all inferential statistics.
- Inferential statistics allow researchers to estimate population parameters and to test hypotheses about populations from sample data. The use of these statistics allows researchers to make objective decisions about the outcome of the study. Such decisions are based on the rejection or acceptance of the null hypothesis, which is that no relationship exists between the variables.
- If the null hypothesis is supported, then the findings are likely to have occurred by chance. If the null hypothesis is rejected, then a relationship does exist between the variables and is unlikely to have occurred by chance.
- Statistical hypothesis testing is subject to two types of errors: type I and type II.
- A type I error is the researchers' incorrect decision to reject the null hypothesis.
- A type II error occurs when the results from the sample data lead to the acceptance of the null hypothesis when it is actually false; this error is also known as beta (β).

- The researcher controls the risk of making a type I error by setting the alpha level, or level of significance. Unfortunately, reducing the risk of a type I error by reducing the level of significance increases the risk of making a type II error.
- The results of statistical tests are reported to be significant or nonsignificant. For a result to be statistically significant, the probability of occurring must be less than .05 or .01, depending on the level of significance set by the researcher.
- Commonly used parametric and nonparametric statistical tests include tests for differences between means, such as the *t* test and ANOVA, and tests for differences in proportions, such as the chi-square test.
- Tests in which data are examined for the presence of relationships include the Pearson *r*, the sign test, the Wilcoxon matched-pairs test, the signed-rank test, and multiple regression.
- Advanced statistical procedures include path analysis and factor analysis.
- The most important aspect of critiquing statistical analyses is the relationship between the statistics used and the problem, design, and method used in the study. Clues to the appropriate statistical test to be used by the researcher should stem from the researcher's hypotheses. You also should determine whether all of the hypotheses have been presented in the article.
- A basic understanding of statistics will improve your ability to think about the level of evidence provided by the study design and findings and their relevance to patient outcomes for your patient population and practice setting.

FOR FURTHER STUDY

ⓔ Go to Evolve at http://evolve.elsevier.com/ Canada/LoBiondo/Research for the Audio Glossary and Appendix Tables that provide supplemental information for Appendix E.

REFERENCES

Arnold, J. M., Liu, P., Demers, C., et al. (2006). Canadian Cardiovascular Society consensus conference recommendations on heart failure 2006: Diagnosis and management. *Canadian Journal of Cardiology, 22*(1), 23–45.

Bluman, A. J. (2014). *A brief version elementary statistics: A step by step approach.* New York: McGraw-Hill.

Boamah, S., & Laschinger, H. K. S. (2015). Engaging new nurses: The role of psychological capital and workplace empowerment. *Journal of Research in Nursing, 20*(4), 265–277.

Campbell-Yeo, M., Johnston, C. C., Joseph, K. S., et al. (2015). Cobedding and recovery time after heel lance in preterm twins: Results of a randomized trial. *Pediatrics, 130*(3), 500–506.

Creamer, A. M., Mill, J., Austin, W., et al. (2014). Canadian nurse practitioners' therapeutic commitment to persons with mental illness. *Canadian Journal of Nursing Research, 46*(4), 13–32.

El-Masri, M. M., Fox-Wasylyshyn, S. M., Springer, C. D., et al. (2014). Exploring the impact of prostrate cancer radiation treatment on functions, bother, and well-being. *Canadian Journal of Nursing Research, 46*(2), 42–56.

El-Masri, M. M., Omar, A., & Groh, E. M. (2015). Evaluating the effectiveness of a nurse practitioner-led outreach program for long-term care homes. *Canadian Journal of Nursing Research, 47*(3), 39–55.

Forman, J., Currie, L., Lauck, S., et al. (2015). Exploring changes in functional status while waiting for transcatheter aortic valve implantation. *European Journal of Cardiovascular Nursing, 14*(6), 560–569.

Freeman, M., Beaulieu, L., & Crawley, J. (2015). Canadian nurse graduates considering migrating abroad for work: Are their expectations being met in Canada? *Canadian Journal of Nursing Research, 47*(4), 80–96.

Héon, M., Goulet, C., Garofalo, C., et al. (2016). An intervention to promote breast milk production in mothers of preterm infants. *Western Journal of Nursing Research, 38*(5), 529–552.

Higgins, J. P. T., & Green, S. (Eds.). (2011). *Cochrane handbook for systematic reviews of interventions, Version 5.1.0* [updated March 2011]. The Cochrane Collaboration. Retreived from http://handbook.cochrane.org.

Hooge, S. L., Benzies, K. M., & Mannion, C. A. (2014). Effects of a brief, prevention-focused parenting education program for new mothers. *Western Journal of Nursing Research, 36*(8), 957–974.

Kennedy, E., Tomblin-Murphy, G., Martin-Misener, R., et al. (2015). Development and psychometric assessment of the Nursing Competence Self-Efficacy Scale. *Journal of Nursing Education, 54*(10), 550–558.

Kline, R. B. (2005). *Beyond significance testing: Reforming data analysis methods in behavioral research.* Washington, DC: American Psychological Association.

Laschinger, H. K. S. (2014). Impact of workplace mistreatment on patient safety risk and nurse-assessed patient outcomes. *Journal of Nursing Administration, 44*(5), 284–290.

Laschinger, H. K. S., Read, E., Wilk, P., et al. (2014). The influence of nursing unit empowerment and social capital on unit effectiveness and nurse perceptions of patient care quality. *Journal of Nursing Administration, 44*, 347–352.

Murphy, F. A., Lipp, A., & Powles, D. L. (2012). Follow-up for improving psychological well-being for women after a miscarriage (review). *Cochrane Database System Review, 3*, 1–39. Retrieved from https://www.ncbi.nlm.nih.gov/pmc/articles/PMC4164469/.

Ostry, A., Maggi, S., Hershler, R., et al. (2010). Mental health differences among middle-aged sawmill workers in rural compared to urban British Columbia. *Canadian Journal of Nursing Research, 42*(3), 84–100.

Profetto-McGrath, J., Negrin, K., Hugo, K., et al. (2010). Clinical nurse specialists' approaches in selecting and using evidence to improve practice. *Worldviews on Evidence-Based Nursing, 7*(1), 36–50.

Rajacich, D., Kane, D., Lafreniere, K., et al. (2014). Male RNs: Work factors influencing job satisfaction and intention to stay in the profession. *Canadian Journal of Nursing Research, 46*(3), 94–109.

Schneider, M., Steele, R., Cadell, S., et al. (2011). Differences on psychosocial outcomes between male and female caregivers of children with life-limiting illnesses. *Journal of Pediatric Nursing, 26*(3), 186–199.

Sherrard, H., Duchesne, L., Wells, G., et al. (2015). Using interactive voice response to improve disease management and compliance with acute coronary syndrome best practice guidelines: A randomized controlled trial. *Canadian Journal of Cardiovascular Nursing, 25*(1), 10–15.

Stutsky, B. J., & Laschinger, H. K. S. (2014). Developing leadership practices in hospital-based nurse educators in an online learning community. *CIN: Computers, Informatics, Nursing, 32*(1), 43–49.

Wing, T., Regan, S., & Laschinger, H. K. S. (2013). The influence of empowerment and incivility on the mental health of new graduate nurses. *Journal of Nursing Management, 23*, 632–643.

Wong, C. A., Elliott-Miller, P., Laschinger, H. K. S., et al. (2015). Examining the relationships between span of control and manager job and unit performance outcomes. *Journal of Nursing Management, 23*, 156–168.

Yamada, J. Y., Stevens, B., Sidani, S., et al. (2015). Test of a process evaluation checklist to improve neonatal pain practices. *Western Journal of Nursing Research, 37*(5), 581–598.

CHAPTER 17

Presenting the Findings

Geri LoBiondo-Wood | Mina D. Singh

LEARNING OUTCOMES

After reading this chapter, you will be able to do the following:

- Discuss the difference between a study's "Results" section and the "Discussion" section.
- Identify the format of the "Results" section.
- Determine whether both statistically supported and statistically unsupported findings are discussed.
- Determine whether the results are objectively reported.
- Describe how tables and figures are used in a research report.
- List the criteria of a meaningful table.
- Identify the format and components of the "Discussion of the Results" section.
- Determine the purpose of the "Discussion" section.
- Discuss the importance of including the generalizations and limitations of a study in the report.
- Determine the purpose of including recommendations in the study report.
- Discuss how the strength, quality, and consistency of evidence provided by the findings are related to a study's limitations, generalizability, transferability, and applicability to practice.

KEY TERMS

confidence interval	generalizability	recommendations
findings	limitations	transferability

STUDY RESOURCES

ⓔ Go to Evolve at http://evolve.elsevier.com/Canada/LoBiondo/Research for the Audio Glossary and Appendix Tables that provide supplemental information for Appendix E.

THE ULTIMATE GOALS OF NURSING RESEARCH are to develop nursing knowledge and to promote evidence-informed nursing practice, thereby supporting the scientific basis of nursing. From the viewpoint of the research consumer, the analysis of the results, interpretations, and the conclusions that a researcher makes from a study becomes a highly important piece of the research report. After the analysis of the data, the researcher constructs an overall view of the findings, like putting the pieces of a jigsaw puzzle together to view the total picture. This process is analogous to evaluation, the last step in the nursing process. In the final sections of the report, after the statistical procedures have been applied, the statistical or numerical findings are described in relation to the theoretical framework, literature, methods, hypotheses, and problem statements. In qualitative research, after the content analyses have been concluded, the themes are discussed in relation to the literature, problem statements, and a theoretical framework, as appropriate.

The final sections of published research reports are generally titled "Results" and "Discussion," but other topics, such as limitations of findings, implications for future research and nursing practice, recommendations, and conclusions, may be addressed separately or subsumed within these sections. The format of the "Results" and "Discussion" is contingent on the stylistic considerations of the author and the journal. The function of these final sections is to depict all aspects of the research process, as well as to discuss, interpret, and identify the limitations, generalizations, and applicability relevant to the investigation, thereby furthering research-based practice.

The process that both the investigator and you as the research consumer use to assess the results of a study is depicted in the Critical Thinking Decision Path. The goal of this chapter is to introduce the purpose and content of the final sections of a research investigation, in which the data are presented, interpreted, discussed, and generalized. An understanding of what an investigator presents in these sections will help you critically analyze the findings.

FINDINGS

The **findings** of a study are the results, conclusions, interpretations, recommendations, generalizations, and implications for future research and nursing practice, which are separated into two major areas: the results and the discussion of the results. The "Results" section focuses on the thematic results or statistical findings of a study, and the "Discussion" section focuses on the remaining topics. For both sections, as well as all other sections of a report, the same rule applies: The content must be presented clearly, concisely, and logically.

Evidence-Informed Practice Tip ____

Evidence-informed practice is an active process that requires you to consider how, and whether, research findings are applicable to your patient population and practice setting.

Presenting Quantitative Results

In the "Results" section of a research report, the researcher presents the quantitative data or numbers generated by the descriptive and inferential statistical tests or the themes from narratives generated from a content or coding analysis. The results of the data analysis are the foundation for the interpretations or "Discussion" section that follows the results. The "Results" section should then reflect the question being posed or hypothesis tested. The information from each hypothesis or research question should be presented sequentially. The tests used to analyze the data should be identified. If the author does not explicitly state the exact test that was used, then the values obtained should be noted. The researcher typically provides the numerical values of the

CRITICAL THINKING DECISION PATH

Assessing Study Results

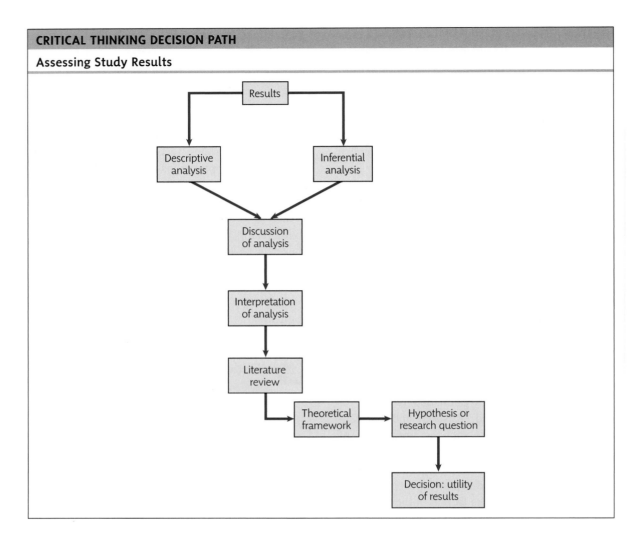

statistics and states the specific test value and probability level achieved (see Chapter 16). Examples of statistical tests and the corresponding statistical values can be found in Table 17.1. An example of a qualitative analysis with themes appears later in this chapter (see Table 17.4).

You should not be intimidated by numbers and symbols. Although these numbers are important, they are only one piece of the whole; the research process is much more important. Whether you superficially understand statistics or have an in-depth knowledge of statistics, you can expect to find the study results clearly stated. Thus, you

EXAMPLES OF REPORTED STATISTICAL RESULTS

STATISTICAL TEST	EXAMPLES OF REPORTED RESULTS
Mean	$M = 118.28$
Standard deviation	$SD = 62.5$
Pearson correlation	$r = .39, p < .01$
Analysis of variance (ANOVA)	$F = 3.59; df = 2, 48; p < .05$
t test	$t = 2.65, p < .01$
Chi-square	$\chi^2 = 2.52, df = 1, p < .05$

df, degrees of freedom.

should note the presence or absence of any statistically significant results. For the conceptual meanings of the numbers found in studies, refer to the discussion in Chapter 16.

Research Hint

In the "Results" section of a research report, the descriptive statistics are generally presented first, followed by the results of each hypothesis or research question tested.

The researcher must present the data for all of the hypotheses posed or research questions asked (e.g., whether the hypotheses were accepted or rejected, supported or not supported). If the data support the hypotheses, you might assume that the hypotheses were proven, but this is not necessarily true. It only means that the hypotheses were supported, and the results suggest that the relationships or differences tested, which were derived from the theoretical framework, were probably logical in that study's sample.

As a novice research consumer, you might also think that if a researcher's hypotheses are not supported statistically or are only partially supported, the study is irrelevant or possibly should not have been published. This is also not true. If the hypotheses are not supported, you should not expect the researcher to bury the work in a file. Reviewing and understanding unsupported hypotheses is as important for a research consumer as it is for the researcher. Information obtained from such studies can often be as useful as data obtained from supported studies.

Unsupported hypotheses can be used to suggest **limitations** (weaknesses) of particular aspects of a study's design and procedures. Data from such studies may suggest that current modes of practice or current theory in an area may not be supported by research and so should be reexamined and researched further. Data help generate new knowledge, as well as prevent knowledge stagnation.

In general, the results are interpreted in a separate section of the report. Sometimes the "Results" section contains not only the results but also the researcher's interpretations, which are more commonly found in the "Discussion" section. Integrating the results with the discussion in a report is the decision of the author or the journal editor. The two sections may be integrated when a study contains several segments that may be viewed as separate subproblems of a major overall problem.

When presenting the results, the investigator should show objectivity. The following quotation gives the appropriate way to express results:

> Analysis of the effect of time was statistically significant for intensity and unpleasantness related to pain ($F = 160.395$, $p < 0.0001$).

Investigators would be accused of lacking objectivity if they stated the results as follows:

> The results were not surprising as we found a significant relationship between effect of time and intensity and unpleasantness, as we expected.

Opinions or reactionary statements to the data in the "Results" section are therefore avoided. Box 17.1 gives examples of objectively stated results.

You should consider the following points when you read a "Results" section:

- The investigators responded objectively to the results in the discussion of the results.
- In the discussion of the results, the investigators interpreted the results, with careful reflection on all aspects of the study that preceded the results.
- The data presented are summarized. Many data are generated, but only the critical summary numbers for each test are presented. Examples of summarized data are the means and standard deviations of age, education, and income. Including all data is too cumbersome. The "Results" section can be viewed as a summary.

EXAMPLES OF OBJECTIVE STATEMENTS IN THE RESULTS SECTION

"Firstly, the correlation between time sums 01 and 02 was found significant with regards to research utilization with a coefficient of $R = 0.86$. Secondly, correlation between time sums 01 and 03 did not yield any significant result at $R = 0.44$. Thirdly, correlation between time sums 02 and 03 was $R = 0.35$, which is not useful to predict research utilization between these two times" (Allard & Jalbert, 2011, p. 171).

"Patients reported that the impact of treatment on survival, urinary function, bowel function, and physician's treatment recommendation were the four factors having the most influence on their treatment decisions" (Davison, Szafron, & Gutwin, 2014, p. 243).

"Women randomized to the intervention group reported significantly greater self-efficacy SEMCD [self-efficacy to manage chronic conditions] in managing their chronic disease at 12 weeks relative to those in the control group (0.8; 95% CI: 0.5, 1.2; $p < 0.001$). The observed difference between groups was moderately large (Cohen's d: 0.48)" (Weinert, Cudney, Comstock, et al., 2014, p. 36).

"Furthermore, nurses who felt better able to measure and track client outcomes expressed more willingness to participate in training activities or seek feedback from colleagues in order to increase their ability to use the device at the point of care" (Doran, Reid-Haughian, Chilcote, et al., 2013, p. 63).

"Clinical instructors also described a more restrictive attitude toward students and clinical placements in addition to challenges around knowledge and perceptions about nursing care of older people. They were able to make progress when they returned to the same unit and gained nurses' trust" (Baumbusch, Dahlke, & Phinney, 2014, p. 438).

DEMOGRAPHICS OF STUDY PARTICIPANTS

	M	SD
Age	42.17	13.01
Years as a registered nurse	16.04	13.57
	n	%
Gender		
Female	298	88.7
Male	37	11.0
Highest education		
Degree	204	60.7
No degree	123	36.6
Unit specialty		
Medical-surgical	124	36.9
Critical care	65	19.3
Maternal child	42	12.5
Mental health	26	7.7
Other (non-acute care)	73	21.7
Employment status		
Full-time	232	69.0
Part-time	82	24.4
Casual	19	5.7

M, mean; *SD*, standard deviation.
From Laschinger, H. K. S. (2014). Impact of workplace mistreatment n patient safety risk and nurse-assessed patient outcomes. *Journal of Nursing Administration, 44*(5), 284–290. http://journals.lww.com/jonajournal/pages/default.aspx

- The data are condensed both in the written text and through the use of tables and figures. Tables and figures facilitate the presentation of large amounts of data.
- Results for the descriptive and inferential statistics for each hypothesis or research question are presented. No data should be omitted even if insignificant.

In the study in Appendix B, Laschinger (2014) developed tables to present the results visually. Table 17.2 lists the demographic descriptive results about the study's participants; Table 17.3 lists the statistics of the variables measured in the study. Tables allow researchers to provide a more visually thorough explanation and discussion of the results. If tables and figures are used, they must be concise. Although the text is the major mode of communicating the results, the tables and figures serve a supplementary but independent role. The role of tables and figures is to report results with details that the investigator does not enter into the text. This does not mean that the content of tables and figures should not be mentioned in the text. The amount of detail that the author uses in the text to describe the specific tabular data varies with the needs of the researcher.

A good table meets the following criteria:
- It supplements and economizes the text.
- It has precise titles and headings.
- It does not repeat the text.

TABLE 17.3

DESCRIPTIVE STATISTICS

STUDY VARIABLE	MEAN	SD	α	1	2	3	4	5	6	7	8	9	10	11
1. Coworker incivility	1.52	0.70	.93											
2. Physician-workplace incivility	1.45	0.56	.85	0.53										
3. Supervisor incivility	1.32	0.51	.88	0.38	0.30									
4. Bullying	1.45	0.59	.89	0.66	0.48	0.57								
5. Quality of care	3.34	0.69	NA	−0.19	−0.23	−0.20	−0.19							
6. Total adverse events	1.98	0.68	.79	0.14	0.17	0.10	0.23	−0.22[a]						
7. Medication errors	1.64	0.76	NA	0.05	0.11	0.02	0.14	−0.17[a]	0.70[a]					
8. Nosocomial infection	1.97	0.98	NA	0.16	0.12	0.05	0.18	−0.09	0.71[a]	0.48[a]				
9. Patient falls	1.80	0.93	NA	0.04	0.05	0.03	0.09	−0.19[a]	0.73[a]	0.47[a]	0.47[a]			
10. Work-related injuries	2.09	0.93	NA	0.09	0.15	0.14	0.18	−0.12[a]	0.76[a]	0.42[a]	0.38[a]	0.45[a]		
11. Patient/family complaints	2.41	1.03	NA	0.17	0.21	0.12	0.26	−0.22[a]	0.73[a]	0.35[a]	0.38[a]	0.39[a]	0.53[a]	
12. Patient safety risk	2.31	1.04	.94	0.21	0.23	0.20	0.33	−0.18[a]	0.16[a]	0.13[a]	0.06	0.09	0.18	0.20

Abbreviation: NA, not applicable.

From Laschinger, H. K. S. (2014). Impact of workplace mistreatment n patient safety risk and nurse-assessed patient outcomes. *Journal of Nursing Administration, 44*(5), 284–290. http://journals.lww.com/jonajournal/pages/default.aspx

Table 17.4 is an example of a table that meets these criteria. This table, which is from the article by Bottorff, Haines-Saah, Oliffe, and associates (2014), lists the study's messaging themes for tailoring messages about smoking and breast cancer to youth. Visualizing the findings of a study is easier if a table clearly summarizes the results, as this table does. Description of each messaging theme's preferences would have taken a lot of space, and the results would have been difficult to visualize. The table developed by the researchers allows you to not only visualize the concepts quickly but also assess the results.

 Research Hint _____

A well-written "Results" section is systematic, logical, concise, and drawn from all of the analyzed data. All that is written in the "Results" section should be geared toward letting the data reflect the testing of the problems and hypotheses. The length of this section depends on the scope and breadth of the analysis.

 Evidence-Informed Practice Tip _____

As you reflect on the results of a study, think about how the results fit with previous research on the topic and the strength and quality of available evidence on which to base clinical practice decisions.

Discussion of the Results

In the final section of the report, the investigator interprets and discusses the results of the study. In the discussion, a skilled researcher makes the data "come alive." The researcher interprets and gives meaning to the numbers in quantitative studies or the concepts in qualitative studies. You may ask how the investigator extracted the meaning that is applied in this section. If the researcher reports properly, the discussion will refer to the beginning of the study, in which a problem statement was identified and independent and dependent variables were related on the basis of a theoretical

TABLE **17.4**

MESSAGING THEMES ON SMOKING AND BREAST CANCER	
GIRLS' MESSAGING PREFERENCES	
NON-ABORIGINAL	**FIRST NATIONS AND MÉTIS**
• Images of activities/contexts popular among girls their age • Promote self-efficacy by offering choice • Real-life stories • Creative/novel images • Include significant others in messages • Promote protecting girlfriends/family members • Minimal written detail	• Images of activities/contexts popular among girls their age • Promote self-efficacy by offering choice • Real-life stories • Creative/novel images • Strategies and advice for avoiding exposure to tobacco • Aboriginal images
BOYS' MESSAGING PREFERENCES	
NON-ABORIGINAL	**FIRST NATIONS AND MÉTIS**
• Images of activities/contexts popular among boys • Humour • Genuine vs. unrealistic/cheesy • Include significant others in messages • Represent masculinity (respect/protect girls)	• Images of activities/contexts popular among boys • Humour • Genuine vs. unrealistic/cheesy • Emphasis on images • Minimal written detail • Use of graphics, such as graffiti • Represent masculinity (respect/protect girls) • Omit stereotypical "sexy" images of girls • Aboriginal images

From Bottorff, J. L., Haines-Saah, R., Oliffe, J. L., et al. (2014). Designing tailored messages about smoking and breast cancer: A focus group study with youth. *Canadian Journal of Nursing Research, 46*(1), 66–86. SAGE Publications Inc.

framework (see Chapter 2) and literature review (see Chapter 5). In this section, the researcher discusses the following:

- The supported and the nonsupported hypotheses
- The limitations, or weaknesses, of a study in view of the design and the sample or data-collection procedures
- How the theoretical framework was supported
- Additional or previously unrealized relationships suggested by the data

Even if the hypotheses are supported, the reviewer should not believe the conclusions to be the final word. Statistical significance is not the endpoint of a researcher's thinking, and low p values may not be indicative of research breakthroughs. Thus, statistical significance in a research study does not always mean that the results of a study are clinically significant. As the body of nursing research grows, so does the profession's ability to critically analyze beyond the test of significance and assess a research study's applicability to practice. Chapter 20 reviews methods for analyzing the usefulness of research findings. Within the nursing literature, discussion of clinical significance and evidence-informed practice has also emerged (Melnyk & Fineout-Overholt, 2011).

As indicated throughout this text, many important pieces in the research puzzle must fit together for a study to be evaluated as a well-done project. Therefore, researchers and reviewers should accept statistical significance with prudence. Statistically significant findings are not the sole means of establishing the study's merit. Remember that accepting statistical significance only means acceptance that the sample mean is the same as the population mean, which may not be true (see Chapter 16).

Another way to assess whether the findings from one study can be generalized is to calculate a confidence interval. A **confidence interval** is an estimated range of values that quantifies the uncertainty of a statistic; that is, it is the probable value range within which a population parameter—for example, the mean—is expected to lie. The width of the confidence interval gives the researcher some idea about the uncertainty surrounding the unknown parameter. A very wide interval may indicate that more data should be collected before definite assertions can be made about the parameter. Confidence intervals are more informative than the simple results of hypothesis tests (in which a researcher rejects the null hypothesis or fails to reject the null hypothesis) because they provide a range of plausible values for the unknown parameter. For example, Sherrard, Duchesne, Wells, and colleagues (2015) used confidence intervals around relative risk to present the effectiveness of an interactive voice response in increased compliance with medication and decreased adverse events for patients with acute coronary syndrome.

The process used to calculate a confidence interval is beyond the scope of this text; references are provided for further explanation (e.g., Bluman, 2014). Other aspects of the study, such as theory, sample, instrumentation, and methods, should also be considered.

When the results do not statistically support the hypothesis, the researcher refers to the theoretical framework and analyzes the earlier thinking process. The results of nonsupported hypotheses do not require that the investigator find fault with each piece of the project. Such a course can become an overdone process. All research has weaknesses. This analysis is an attempt to identify the weaknesses and to suggest the possible or actual problems in the study. At times, the theoretical thinking is correct, but the researcher finds problems or limitations that could be attributed to the tools (see Chapter 14), the sampling methods (see Chapter 12), the design (see Chapters 10 and 11), or the analysis (see Chapters 15 and 16). Therefore, when the hypotheses are not supported, the investigator attempts to find facts rather than fault. The purpose of the discussion, then, is not to show humility or one's technical competence but rather to enable reviewers to judge the validity of the interpretations drawn from the data and the general worth of the study.

In the "Discussion" section, the researcher summarizes all the aspects of the study and refers to the beginning to assess whether the findings support, extend, or counter the theoretical framework of the study. From this point, you can begin to think about clinical relevance, the need for replication, or the germination of an idea for further research study. Finally, you should find the results discussion either in a separate section or subsumed within the "Discussion" section, and it should include generalizability, applicability, and recommendations for future research, as well as a summary or a conclusion.

Generalizability is the extent to which data can be inferred to be representative of similar phenomena in a population beyond the study's sample. Reviewers of research are cautioned not to generalize beyond the population on which a study is based. Rarely, if ever, can one study be a recommendation for action. Beware of research studies that may overgeneralize. An example of making a sweeping generalization is concluding that all patients waiting for cardiac bypass surgery can benefit from preoperative teaching and support when the study sample consisted of only White men, 50 to 70 years of age. Attention must be paid to the "Limitations" section of an article to note what the researchers have considered to affect the generalizability of their study findings. Generalizations that draw conclusions and make inferences within a particular situation and at a particular time are appropriate.

An example of an appropriate generalization is from the study conducted by Creamer, Mill, Austin, et al. (2014), on the therapeutic commitment of Canadian Nurse Practitioners (NPs) to persons with mental illness. From sampling NPs in the two territories and nine provinces, they concluded that the "exclusion of NPs in Quebec, Yukon Territory, and Saskatchewan precludes generalizability of these results to NPs in these jurisdictions" (p. 28). This type of statement is important for reviewers of research. It helps guide thinking in terms of a study's clinical relevance and suggests areas for further research (see Chapter 20).

In a qualitative study, the limitations may be stated differently, as in a study by Dahlke, Phinney, Hall, and colleagues (2015) on orchestrating nursing care for hospitalized older adults: "The theory of orchestrating care is limited because it does not include the perspectives of older adults and other healthcare professionals. Moreover, novice nurses' unique perspectives were not explored in-depth. A grounded theory study can highlight problems and sensitize healthcare providers and policy makers to the complexities of nurses' care for older adults but is not immediately generalizable to other settings" (p. 260)

Presenting Qualitative Results

Transferability is the extent to which findings from one qualitative research study have meaning in other studies with similar situations. Authors must note the issues of a qualitative study to prevent a sweeping transferability of findings, which would lead to misinterpretations of the results. In an example of how the limitations in a qualitative study can affect transferability, Gauthier, Cossette, Ouimette, et al. (2016) conducted a study to pilot an intervention plan to support shared decision making when considering a vascular assist device for patients with advanced heart failure. The researchers noted multiple limitations of the study and that these may affect the transferability of findings. The study included only one cardiac centre. Also, only a few caregivers and patients were included in the study. Lastly, all the study participants were White. One study does not provide all of the answers, nor should it. The final steps of evaluation are critical links to the refinement of practice and the generation of future research. Evaluation of research, like evaluation of the nursing process, is not the last link in the chain but a connection between findings that may serve to improve nursing theory and nursing practice.

In another example regarding transferability, O'Keefe-McCarthy, McGillion, Nelson, and colleagues (2014) conducted a qualitative study to explore the impact of perspectives of nurses and patients diagnosed with acute coronary syndrome (ACS) on the experience of patients with ACS symptoms in a rural emergency department. The researchers noted that an important limitation was the lack of transferability of the findings, for two reasons. First, only one hospital was used. Second, women were not represented among patients in the study, and male RNs were not included among nurses.

 Research Hint

It has been said that a good study is one that raises more questions than it answers. Thus, you should not view a study's limitations, generalizations, and implications of the findings for practice as an investigator's lack of research skills but as the beginning of the next step in the research process.

The final topic that the investigator integrates into the "Discussion" section is the recommendations. The **recommendations** are the investigator's suggestions for the study's application to practice, theory, and further research. These suggestions require the investigator to reflect on the question "What contribution to nursing does this study make?" Box 17.2 provides examples of recommendations for future research and implications for nursing practice. This evaluation places the study in the realm of what is known and what needs to be known before being used. Nursing has grown tremendously over the last century through the efforts of many nursing researchers and scholars.

BOX **17.2**

EXAMPLES OF RESEARCH RECOMMENDATIONS AND PRACTICE IMPLICATIONS

RESEARCH RECOMMENDATIONS

- "It would also be of interest to explore nurses' attitudes to performing and prioritizing routine oral care in care-dependent populations, to further understand the attitudes and barriers to performing preventative care practices over reactive care practices" (Robertson & Carter, 2013, p. 16).
- "However, a study using a larger sample size might allow identification of the particular cardiac diagnoses and treatments that predict the greatest risk of smoking relapse after hospitalization" (Cossette, Frasure-Smith, Robert, et al., 2012, p. 24).
- "Longitudinal studies of both border and non-border regions and cohorts of nursing graduates over time are warranted, to determine whether the expectations of new graduates were indeed met while working in other countries" (Freeman, Beaulieu, Crawley, et al., 2015, p. 93).

PRACTICE IMPLICATIONS

- "Our results have a number of implications for researchers. APN [advanced practice nursing] research designed to clarify the value-added component of APN roles in acute care is indicated" (Carter, Dobbins, Peachey, et al., 2014, p. 23).
- "These findings suggest that a complex interplay of associations between the relational practices of

formal nursing leaders to provide vision, support, staffing resources (Kane, Shamliyan, & Mueller, 2007) and leadership, with the health, competencies, abilities, knowledge, skills and motivation of nurses, are integral to the achievement of better patient outcomes" (Wong, Cummings, & Ducharme, 2013, p. 720).
- "This empirical study showed that unit level nurse staffing and LOS [length of stay] are related, and there is a need for managerial understanding of the complex care process, and importance of well-designed care chains" (Pitkäaho, Partanen, Miettinen, et al., 2016, p. 577).
- "How to eliminate nurses' fear is a crucial issue if the reporting rate is to be increased. Possible nursing management strategies include: (1) introducing reporting systems that guarantee anonymity and carry no potential for sanction, as research has demonstrated that these can double reporting rates (Aasland & Forde, 2005); (2) providing counselling classes in order to diminish fear, enhance nurses' sense of security, and reduce self-incrimination; and (3) offering incentives to encourage reporting and feedback after reporting (Bayazidi, Zarezadeh, Zamanzadeh, et al., 2012)" (Yung, Yu, Chu, et al., 2016, pp. 586–587).

Results and Discussion

The results and the discussion of the results are the researcher's opportunity to examine the logic of the hypothesis or question posed, the theoretical framework, the methods, and the analysis (see the Critiquing Criteria box). This final section requires as much logic, conciseness, and specificity as employed in the preceding steps of the research process.

For quantitative studies, the research consumer should be able to identify statements on the type of analysis that was used and whether the data statistically supported the hypothesis. These statements should be straightforward and not reflect bias. Auxiliary data or serendipitous findings also may be presented. If such auxiliary findings are presented, they should be stated as dispassionately as were the hypothesis data. The statistical test used also should be noted, as well as the numerical value of the data (see Tables 17.1, 17.3, and 17.5). The presentation of the tests, the numerical values found, and the statements of support or nonsupport should be clear, concise, and systematically reported. For illustrative purposes that facilitate readability, the researchers should present extensive findings in tables rather than in the text.

For qualitative studies, the richness of the data should be described. The consumer must also have sufficient detail about the analysis, the coding, the categories of coding or themes, and the level of coding agreement.

The "Discussion" section should interpret the data, gaps, limitations, and conclusions of the study, as well as provide recommendations for further research. Drawing these aspects into the study should give the research consumer an understanding of the relationship between the findings and the theoretical framework. Statements reflecting the underlying theory are necessary, whether or not the hypotheses were supported.

If the findings were not supported, the consumer should—as the researcher did—attempt to identify, without fault finding, possible methodological problems. Finally, a concise presentation of the study's generalizability and the implications of the findings for practice and research should be evident. The last presentation can help the research consumer begin to rethink clinical practice, provoke discussion in clinical settings (see Chapter 20), and find similar studies that may support or refute the phenomena being studied to more fully understand the problem.

CRITIQUING CRITERIA

1. Are the results of each hypothesis presented?
2. Is the information regarding the results concisely and sequentially presented?
3. Are the tests that were used to analyze the data presented?
4. Are the results presented objectively?
5. If tables or figures are used, do they meet the following standards?
   - They supplement and economize the text.
   - They have precise titles and headings.
   - They do not repeat the text.
6. Are the results interpreted in light of the hypotheses and theoretical framework and all of the other steps that preceded the results?
7. If the data are supported, does the investigator provide a discussion of how the theoretical framework was supported?
8. If the data are not supported, does the investigator attempt to identify the study's weaknesses and strengths, as well as suggest possible solutions for the research area?
9. Does the researcher discuss the study's clinical relevance?
10. Are any generalizations made, and, if so, are they within the scope of the findings or beyond the findings?
11. Are any recommendations for future research stated or implied?
12. What is the study's strength of evidence?

TABLE 17.5

RISK FACTORS ASSOCIATED WITH WORK-RELATED VIOLENT INCIDENTS AMONG HEALTH CARE WORKERS IN BRITISH COLUMBIA

VARIABLE: OCCUPATION	NUMBER OF VIOLENT INCIDENTS	RATE (INCIDENTS/100,000 PRODUCTIVE HOURS)	UNADJUSTED RESULTS		ADJUSTED RESULTS (MODEL 2)	
			RISK RATIO	95% CI	RISK RATIO	95% CI
RN	347 (40%)	1.97	6.62	4.63–9.46	6.45	4.37–9.52
LPN	79 (9%)	1.97	10.85	7.23–16.29	8.64	5.56–13.42
Care aide	320 (37%)	3.74	12.55	8.77–17.96	10.05	6.72–15.05

CI, confidence interval; LPN, licensed practical nurse; RN, registered nurse.
Adapted from Kling, R. N., Yassi, A., Smailes, E., et al. (2009). Characterizing violence in health care in British Columbia. *Journal of Advanced Nursing,* 65(8), 1655–1663. © 2009 The Authors. Journal compilation © 2009 Blackwell Publishing Ltd.

CRITICAL THINKING CHALLENGES

■ Defend or refute the following statement: "All results should be reported and interpreted whether or not they support the hypothesis (hypotheses)."

■ What type of knowledge does the researcher draw on to interpret the results of a study?

■ What new knowledge is contributed from the research findings? Are they clinically significant and do they have practice implications?

■ Do you agree or disagree with the statement that a good study raises more questions than it answers? Support your view with examples.

■ How is it possible for readers of research to critique the findings and recommendations of a reported study? How could you use the Internet for critiquing the findings of a study?

■ Now that nursing students and nurses have access to reports of clinical problems (i.e., critiques of multiple studies available on a clinical topic) or critiques of individual studies of a clinical topic published in *Evidence-Based Nursing,* as well as published meta-analyses and meta-syntheses on clinical topics, why is it necessary for them to read and critique research studies on their own? Justify your response.

KEY POINTS

• The analysis of the findings is the final step of a research investigation. In this section, the research consumer will find the results presented in a straightforward manner.

• All results should be reported whether or not they support the hypothesis. Tables and figures may be used to illustrate and condense data for presentation.

• Once the results are reported, the researcher interprets the results. In this presentation, usually titled "Discussion," the consumer should be able to identify the key topics being discussed. The key topics, which include an interpretation of the results, are the limitations, generalizations, implications, and recommendations for future research.

• The researcher draws together the theoretical framework and makes interpretations based on the findings and theory in the section on the interpretation of the results. Both statistically supported and unsupported results should be interpreted. If the results are not supported, the researcher should discuss the results reflecting on the theory, as well as possible problems with the methods, procedures, design, and analysis.

• The researcher should present the limitations or weaknesses of the study. This presentation is important because it affects the study's generalizability. The generalizations or inferences about similar findings in other samples also are presented in light of the findings.

• The research consumer should be alert for sweeping claims or overgeneralizations that a researcher may state. An overextension of the data can alert the consumer to possible researcher bias.

• The recommendations provide the consumer with suggestions regarding the study's application to practice, theory, and future research. These recommendations furnish the reader with a final perspective of the utility of the investigation's findings in practice.

FOR FURTHER STUDY

ⓔ Go to Evolve at http://evolve.elsevier.com/Canada/LoBiondo/Research for the Audio Glossary and Appendix Tables that provide supplemental information for Appendix E.

REFERENCES

Aasland, O. G., & Forde, R. (2005). Impact of feeling responsible for adverse events on doctors' personal and professional lives: The importance of being open to criticism from colleagues. *Quality and Safety in Health Care, 14,* 13–17.

Allard, N., & Jalbert, C. (2011). Towards using evidence in oncology: Identified issues and suggested solutions. *Canadian Oncology Nursing Journal, 21*(3), 169–173.

Baumbusch, J., Dahlke, S., & Phinney, A. (2014). Clinical instructors' knowledge and perceptions about nursing care of older people: A pilot study. *Nurse Education in Practice*, *14*(4), 434–440.

Bayazidi, S., Zarezadeh, Y., Zamanzadeh, V., et al. (2012). Medication error reporting rate and its barriers and facilitators among nurses. *Journal of Caring Sciences*, *1*, 231–236.

Bluman, A. J. (2014). *Elementary statistics: A brief version*. New York: McGraw-Hill.

Bottorff, J. L., Haines-Saah, R., Oliffe, J. L., et al. (2014). Designing tailored messages about smoking and breast cancer: A focus group study with youth. *Canadian Journal of Nursing Research*, *46*(1), 66–86.

Carter, N., Dobbins, M., Peachey, G., et al. (2014). Knowledge transfer and dissemination of advanced practice nursing information and research to acute-care administrators. *Canadian Journal of Nursing Research*, *46*, 10–27.

Cossette, S., Frasure-Smith, N., Robert, M., et al. (2012). A pilot randomized trial of a smoking cessation nursing intervention in cardiac patients after hospital discharge. *Canadian Journal of Cardiovascular Nursing*, *22*(4), 16–26.

Creamer, A. M., Mill, J., Austin, W., et al. (2014). Canadian nurse practitioners' therapeutic commitment to persons with mental illness. *Canadian Journal of Nursing Research*, *46*(4), 13–32.

Dahlke, S. A., Phinney, A., Hall, W. A., et al. (2015). Orchestrating care: Nursing practice with hospitalised older adults. *International Journal of Older People Nursing*, *10*(4), 252–262.

Davison, B. J., Szafron, M., & Gutwin, C. (2014). Using a web-based decision support intervention to facilitate patient–physician communication at prostate cancer treatment discussions. *Canadian Oncology Nursing Journal*, *24*, 241–255.

Doran, D. M., Reid-Haughian, C., Chilcote, A., et al. (2013). A formative evaluation of nurses' use of electronic devices in a home care setting. *Canadian Journal of Nursing Research*, *45*, 54–73.

Freeman, M., Beaulieu, L., Crawley, J., et al. (2015). Canadian nurse graduates considering migrating abroad for work: Are their expectations being met in Canada? *Canadian Journal of Nursing Research*, *47*, 80–96.

Gauthier, M., Cossette, S., Ouimette, M., et al. (2016). Intervention for advanced heart failure patients and their caregivers to support shared decision-making about implantation of a ventricular assist device. *Canadian Journal of Cardiovascular Nursing*, *26*(2), 4–9.

Kane, R. L., Shamliyan, T. A., & Mueller, C. (2007). The association of a registered nurse staffing levels and patient outcomes: Systematic review and meta-analysis. *Medical Care*, *45*(12), 1195–1204.

Laschinger, H. K. S. (2014). Impact of workplace mistreatment on patient safety risk and nurse-assessed patient outcomes. *Journal of Nursing Administration*, *44*(5), 284–290.

Melnyk, B. M., & Fineout-Overholt, E. (2011). *Evidence-based practice in nursing and healthcare: A guide to best practice*. Philadelphia: Lippincott, Williams & Wilkins.

O'Keefe-McCarthy, S. O., McGillion, M., Nelson, S., et al. (2014). Acute coronary syndrome pain and anxiety in a rural emergency department: Patient and nurse perspectives. *Canadian Journal of Nursing Research*, *46*, 80–100.

Pitkäaho, T., Partanen, P., Miettinen, M. H., et al. (2016). The relationship between nurse staffing and length of stay in acute-care: A one-year time-series data. *Journal of Nursing Management*, 571–579.

Robertson, T., & Carter, D. (2013). Oral intensity: Reducing non-ventilator-associated hospital-acquired pneumonia in care-dependent, neurologically impaired patients. *Canadian Journal of Neuroscience Nursing*, *35*(2), 10–17.

Sherrard, H., Duchesne, L., Wells, G., et al. (2015). Using interactive voice response to improve disease management and compliance with acute coronary syndrome best practice guidelines: A randomized controlled trial. *Canadian Journal of Cardiovascular Nursing*, *25*(1), 10–15.

Weinert, C., Cudney, S., Comstock, B., et al. (2014). Computer intervention: Illness self-management/quality of life of rural women. *Canadian Journal of Nursing Research*, *46*(1), 26–43.

Wong, C. A., Cummings, G., & Ducharme, L. (2013). The relationship between nursing leadership and patient outcomes: A systematic review update. *Journal of Nursing Management*, *21*, 709–724.

Yung, H., Yu, S., Chu, C., et al. (2016). Nurses' attitudes and perceived barriers to the reporting of medication administration errors. *Journal of Nursing Management*, *24*, 580–588.

Critiquing Research

RESEARCH **VIGNETTE**

A Program of Research on Smoking Cessation

Joan L. Bottorff, PhD, RN, FCAHS, FAAN
Professor, School of Nursing
Faculty of Health and Social Development
University of British Columbia
Kelowna, British Columbia

I could not have predicted in advance where my program of research would take me. The studies I have conducted in collaboration with my research team evolved over time and took on a new direction as we began to use insights from our research to develop novel interventions. As a nurse with a background in community nursing, I was familiar with the opportunities that nurses have to enhance the health of pregnant and postpartum women and their infants. Becoming aware of a growing body of research indicating that smoking cessation relapse rates during the first 6 months postpartum among women who stopped smoking during pregnancy were between 70 and 90%, other nurse researchers and I initiated the FACET (Families Controlling and Eliminating Tobacco; http://facet.ubc.ca/) research program, which has spanned two decades.

As part of a group of nurse researchers, we began by taking up the challenge to design and evaluate a postpartum smoking relapse prevention intervention that could be delivered by nurses. Although in this clinical trial we found that our intervention showed promise,

we also learned that women often relapsed after our intervention concluded and nursing support was withdrawn. We decided that we needed to learn more about women's experiences of smoking cessation during pregnancy and postpartum to find ways to strengthen our approach. In addition to interviewing women, we interviewed male partners to learn more about couple dynamics influencing women's cessation efforts and how partners supported or undermined women's efforts. The findings of this qualitative research project were fascinating and led us to take an entirely new direction in supporting women's smoking cessation efforts. We learned that many of the women in our study were trying to reduce and quit smoking while their partners continued to smoke. This created a very difficult context in which to quit and, not surprisingly, these women often slipped or relapsed despite their best efforts to quit smoking. We began to wonder why male partners continued to smoke and why women's efforts to quit didn't prompt the men in their lives to also reduce their smoking and quit. A search of the literature produced little information. We found that little attention had been directed to expectant and new fathers' smoking, the exception being that male-partner smoking was an established risk factor

for postpartum smoking relapse. With our curiosity peaked and our questions in hand, we conducted a photovoice project with fathers to see what we could learn.

In this study with expectant new fathers, we learned about the influence of masculinities on smoking patterns, how men construct and justify their continued smoking, and about their intentions and experiences related to quitting. The men were somewhat surprised by our interest in their smoking patterns; they told us that nurses and other health providers don't pay much attention to fathers during pregnancy and postpartum. We were fascinated to learn that, although the men continued to smoke, as fathers they were very interested in quitting and often made attempts to quit. The men began to contemplate quitting smoking when their children came into their lives, and some made attempts to quit. The fathers wanted to be good role models for their children, they wanted to be healthy and fit to keep up with their kids as they grew up, and they wanted to be around to see their children through important life stages (e.g., graduation, getting their first job). This emerging interest in smoking cessation ran counter to dominant gender norms that often position men as uninterested and disengaged from taking care of their health. However, becoming a father is a significant transition period in men's lives. We hypothesized that shifting masculinities related to fatherhood (protector, provider, etc.) created an opening to support men's smoking cessation. It was at this point we decided that we needed to refocus our efforts on expectant and new fathers. We reasoned that supporting fathers' cessation would not only promote men's health and prevent the onset of tobacco-related chronic disease but also support women's cessation efforts and provide smoke-free homes for children. Supporting fathers' cessation was key to promoting family health. Once we realized this, we wondered why we hadn't thought about this before.

With renewed enthusiasm, we began the task of doing something that had not been done before: developing smoking cessation resources tailored specifically for expectant and new fathers. We wanted to develop an approach that would appeal to fathers, draw on our rich qualitative research findings, and take advantage of the evidence base related to smoking cessation. With a Knowledge to Action grant in hand, we shared our findings with groups of fathers who smoked and sought their advice. These sessions were invaluable. Based on men's preferences and suggestions, we launched into developing new resources. We used the "small steps" approach by first developing a motivational booklet, entitled *The Right Times, the Right Reasons. Dads Talk about Reducing and Quitting Smoking*. This booklet includes some of the narratives provided by the fathers in our studies. The messages in the booklet are strengths based; working with graphic designers, we produced a booklet with a masculine look and feel, with strong images of fathers and their children. We have been delighted with the uptake of this booklet. To date, it has been reprinted and distributed in five provinces across Canada.

The next step was to develop a group program to respond to men's desire for a smoking cessation program for fathers where they could help each other quit smoking. We used our research findings to develop *Dads in Gear (DIG)* (http://dadsingear.ok.ubc.ca/), the first smoking cessation program in the world designed specifically for fathers. The DIG group program design is based on three integrated components delivered over an 8-week period: smoking cessation, physical activity, and fathering. In addition to activity-led education and discussion, the program includes friendly competition and social interaction along with positive messaging and promotes autonomous decision making. Based on the success of a pilot study, we proceeded to develop a suite of online resources (e.g., educational materials, videos, quizzes, etc.), a facilitator program manual, and a facilitator training program to enable the program to be delivered by community-based organizations. We are now assessing the feasibility of implementing the program in communities with trained facilitators.

I think this research program fills an important gap in health promotion efforts targeting family health by addressing existing limitations in conventional approaches to engaging men in their health. By promoting autonomy and incorporating a variety of men-friendly hands-on activities, the approaches we have developed encourage fathers to invest in their health on their own terms. We remain excited about continuing this work. We want to adapt the resources we have developed to address the needs of particular groups of fathers (e.g., Indigenous fathers), and we are exploring ways we might use e-health technologies to reach more fathers. This program of research has taught me the importance of being open to the unexpected, of moving beyond description to developing and evaluating new approaches, and of involving potential end-users at each step of the way. It has also taught me that nurses can use research to fill gaps, solve problems, and innovate. ■

CHAPTER 18

Critiquing Qualitative Research

Helen J. Streubert | Cherylyn Cameron

LEARNING OUTCOMES

After reading this chapter, you will be able to do the following:

- Identify the influence of stylistic considerations on the presentation of a qualitative research report.
- Identify the criteria for critiquing a qualitative research report.
- Evaluate the strengths and weaknesses of a qualitative research report.
- Describe the applicability of the findings of a qualitative research report.
- Construct a critique of a qualitative research report.

KEY TERMS

auditability	fittingness	theoretical sampling
credibility	phenomena	trustworthiness

STUDY RESOURCES

ⓔ Go to Evolve at http://evolve.elsevier.com/Canada/LoBiondo/Research for the Audio Glossary and Appendix Tables that provide supplemental information for Appendix E.

NURSES CONTRIBUTE SIGNIFICANTLY TO THE body of health care research. These contributions are evident in nursing, medical, health care, and business journals. Nurse researchers are partnering at an ever-increasing rate with other health care providers to develop, implement, and evaluate a variety of evidence-informed interventions to improve patient outcomes. The methods used to develop evidence-informed practice include quantitative, qualitative, and mixed research approaches. In addition to the increase in the number of research studies and publications, there is also a significant record of externally funded research by nurses that adds to the **credibility**— accuracy, validity, and soundness—of the work. The willingness of private and publicly funded organizations to invest in nursing research attests to its quality and potential for affecting health care outcomes of individuals, families, groups, and communities.

Because the expansion in nursing research and related interventions affects increasing numbers of patients, the evaluation of this research is crucial to improving patients' outcomes. The focus of this chapter is on assessing the quality of qualitative research studies. This chapter demonstrates a set of criteria that can be used to determine the quality of a qualitative research report. Nurses must fully understand how to assess the value of qualitative research, particularly in view of the requirement that nursing practice be evidence informed. According to Straus, Glasziou, Richardson, and colleagues (2011), evidence-informed practice requires the integration of critical appraisal with the "clinical expertise and the patient's unique biology, values, and circumstances" (p. 3).

As a framework for understanding the appraisal of qualitative research as a basis for evidence-informed practice, a published research report, as well as critiquing criteria, is presented. The criteria are then used to demonstrate the process of appraising a qualitative research report.

STYLISTIC CONSIDERATIONS

Qualitative research differs from quantitative research in some very fundamental ways. In qualitative research, investigators seek to discover and understand concepts, phenomena, or cultures. Creswell (2014) stated that "if a concept or phenomenon needs to be explored and understood because little research has been done on it, then it merits a qualitative approach. Qualitative research is especially useful when the researcher does not know the important variables to examine" (p. 20). Jackson, Drummond, and Camara (2007) noted that the primary focus of qualitative research is to understand human beings' experiences in a humanistic and interpretive way (p. 21). In a qualitative study, you should not expect to find hypotheses; theoretical frameworks; dependent and independent variables; large, random samples; complex statistical procedures; scaled instruments; or definitive conclusions about how to use the findings. Because the purpose of qualitative research is to describe or explain concepts, phenomena, or cultures, the report is generally written in a way that allows the researcher to convey the full meaning and complexity of the phenomena or cultures being studied. This narrative includes subjective comments that are intended to depict the depth and richness of the phenomena under study. The goal of the qualitative research report is to describe in as much detail as possible the "insider's," or emic, view of the phenomenon being studied. The emic view is the view of the person experiencing the phenomenon that reflects his or her culture, values, beliefs, and experiences. In reports of qualitative research, the investigator hopes to convey an understanding of what it is like to experience a particular phenomenon or to be part of a specific culture.

One of the most effective ways to convey the emic view is to use quotations that reflect the phenomenon as experienced. For this reason, the qualitative research report has a more conversational tone than a quantitative report. In addition, data are frequently articulated in concepts or phrases, which the researcher calls *themes* (see Chapter 8), as a way of describing large quantities of data in a condensed format.

The richness of the narrative provided in a qualitative research study cannot be shared in its entirety in a journal publication. Page requirements imposed by journals frequently limit research reports to 15 pages. Despite this constraint, investigators in qualitative research need to illustrate the richness of the data and convey to the audience the relationship between the themes identified and the quotes shared. This is essential in order to document the rigour of the research, which is called **trustworthiness,** in a qualitative research study. Of importance is that conveying the depth and richness of the findings of a qualitative study is challenging in a published research report. However, regardless of the page limit, Jackson and associates (2007) suggested that it is the researcher's responsibility to ensure objectivity (use of facts without distortion by personal feeling or bias), ethical diligence (see Chapter 6), and rigour regardless of the method selected to conduct the study. Fully sharing the depth and richness of the data will also help practitioners decide on the appropriateness of applying the findings to their practice.

Some journals, such as *Qualitative Health Research,* are committed to publication of more lengthy reports. Guidelines for publication of research reports are generally listed in each nursing journal or are available from the journal editor. Of importance is that criteria for publication of research reports are not based on a specific type of research method (i.e., quantitative or qualitative). The primary goal of journal editors is to provide their readers with high-quality, informative, timely, and interesting articles. To meet this goal, regardless of the type of research report, editors prefer to publish manuscripts that have scientific merit, present new knowledge, support the current state of the science, and engage their readers. As stated earlier, the challenge in qualitative research

is to meet these editorial requirements within the page limit imposed by the journal of interest.

Nursing journals do not generally offer their reviewers specific guidelines for evaluating qualitative and quantitative research reports. The editors try to ensure that reviewers are knowledgeable in the method and subject matter of the study. This determination is often made, however, on the basis of the reviewer's self-identified area of interest. Research reports are often evaluated in accordance with the ideas or philosophical viewpoints held by the reviewer. The reviewer may have strong feelings about particular types of qualitative or quantitative research methods. Therefore, it is important to clearly state the qualitative approach used and, if appropriate, its philosophical base.

The principles for evaluating different qualitative research approaches are very similar fundamentally. Research consumers are concerned with the plausibility and trustworthiness of the researcher's account of the research and its relevance to current or future theory and practice or both (Horsburgh, 2003). Box 18.1 provides general guidelines for evaluating qualitative research, and Box 18.2 provides guidelines for evaluating grounded theory. The Joanna Briggs Institute in Australia, a research and development organization, lists a number of critical appraisal tools on its website, http://joannabriggs.org/research/critical-appraisal-tools.html, including a Checklist for Qualitative Research, useful for critiquing research articles. For information on specific guidelines for the evaluation of phenomenology, ethnography, grounded theory, and historical and action research, see Streubert and Carpenter (2011). You should review Chapters 7 and 8 in this text before completing this chapter.

APPLICATION OF QUALITATIVE RESEARCH FINDINGS IN PRACTICE

As already stated, one of the purposes of qualitative research is to describe, understand, or explain phenomena. **Phenomena** are events perceived by

BOX 18.1

CRITIQUING GUIDELINES FOR QUALITATIVE RESEARCH

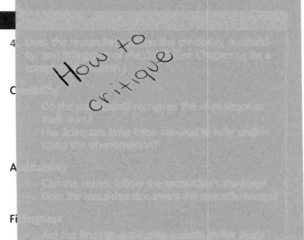

STATEMENT OF THE PHENOMENON OF INTEREST (CHAPTER 4)

1. What is the phenomenon of interest, and is it clearly stated for the reader?
2. What is the justification for using a qualitative method?
3. What are the philosophical underpinnings of the research method?

PURPOSE (CHAPTER 4)

1. What is the purpose of the study?
2. What is the projected significance of the work for nursing?

METHOD (CHAPTER 8)

1. Is the method used to collect the data compatible with the purpose of the research?
2. Is the method adequate for addressing the phenomenon of interest?
3. If a particular approach is used to guide the inquiry, does the researcher complete the study according to the processes described?

SAMPLING (CHAPTER 12)

1. What type of sampling is used? Is it appropriate for the particular method?
2. Are the participants who were chosen appropriate for informing the research?

DATA COLLECTION (CHAPTERS 7, 8, AND 13)

1. Are the data to be collected focused on human experience?
2. Does the researcher describe the data-collection strategies (e.g., interview, observation, field notes)?
3. What are the procedures for collecting the data?
4. Is the protection of human participants addressed?
5. Is saturation of the data described?

DATA ANALYSIS (CHAPTERS 14 AND 15)

1. What strategies are used to analyze the data?
2. Has the researcher reported the data truthfully?
3. Does the researcher describe the steps used for the data analysis?

situation?
- Are the results meaningful to individuals not involved in the research?
- Is the strategy used for analysis compatible with the purpose of the study?

FINDINGS (CHAPTERS 7 AND 17)

1. Are the findings presented within a context?
2. Is the reader able to apprehend the essence of the experience from the report of the findings?
3. Do the researcher's conceptualizations accurately reflect the data?
4. Does the researcher place the report in the context of what is already known about the phenomenon? Was the existing literature on the topic related to the findings?

CONCLUSION, IMPLICATIONS, AND RECOMMENDATIONS (CHAPTER 17)

1. Do the conclusions, implications, and recommendations give the reader a context in which to use the findings?
2. Do the conclusions reflect the study findings?
3. What are the recommendations for future study? Do they reflect the findings?
4. How has the researcher made explicit the significance of the study for nursing theory, research, or practice?

BOX 18.2

CRITIQUING GUIDELINES FOR RESEARCH CONDUCTED WITH THE GROUNDED THEORY METHOD

FOCUS/TOPIC (CHAPTERS 4 AND 8)

1. What is the focus or the topic of the study? What is it that the researcher is studying? Is the topic researchable? Is it focused enough to be meaningful but not too limited so as to be trivial?
2. Has the researcher identified why the phenomenon requires a qualitative format? What is the rationale for selecting the grounded theory approach as the qualitative approach for the investigation?

PURPOSE (CHAPTER 4)

1. Has the researcher made explicit the purpose for conducting the research?

SIGNIFICANCE (CHAPTER 4)

1. Has the researcher described the projected significance of the work for nursing?
2. What is the relevance of the study to what is already known about the topic?

METHOD (CHAPTER 8)

1. In view of the topic of study and the researcher's stated purpose, how does grounded theory methodology help to achieve the stated purpose?
2. Is the method adequate for addressing the research topic?
3. What approach is used to guide the inquiry? Does the researcher complete the study according to the processes described?

SAMPLING (CHAPTERS 8 AND 12)

1. Does the researcher describe the selection process and protection of human participants?
2. What major categories emerged?
3. What were some of the events, incidents, or actions on which these major categories were based?
4. What categories led to theoretical sampling?

DATA GENERATION (CHAPTERS 8 AND 13)

1. Does the researcher describe the data-collection strategies?
2. Have participants been allowed to guide the direction of the inquiry?

3. How did theoretical formulations guide the data collection?

DATA ANALYSIS (CHAPTERS 8 AND 15)

1. Does the researcher describe the strategies used to analyze the data?
   - Has the theoretical construction been checked against the participants' descriptions of the phenomenon?
   - Are the researcher's views and insights about the phenomenon articulated?
   - Has each category that emerged in the theory been described previously in the literature?
2. How does the researcher address the credibility, auditability, and fittingness of the data?
3. Does the researcher clearly describe how and why the core category was selected?

EMPIRICAL GROUNDING OF THE STUDY FINDINGS (CHAPTERS 8 AND 15)

1. Are the concepts grounded in the data?
2. How are the concepts systematically related?
3. Are conceptual linkages described, and are the categories well developed? Do they have conceptual density (in-depth conceptual discussion)?
4. Are the theoretical findings significant? If so, to what extent?
5. Were the data-collection strategies comprehensive, and were analytical interpretations conceptual and broad?
6. Is variation in the interpretations sufficient to allow for applicability in a variety of contexts related to the phenomenon investigated?

CONCLUSIONS, IMPLICATIONS, AND RECOMMENDATIONS (CHAPTERS 8 AND 17)

1. How do the conclusions, implications, and recommendations provide context in which to use the findings?
2. Are the conclusions drawn from the study appropriate? Explain.
3. What are the recommendations for future research?
4. Are the recommendations, conclusions, and implications clearly related to the findings?

From Streubert, H. J., & Carpenter, D. R. (2011). *Qualitative research in nursing: Advancing the humanistic imperative* (5th ed.). Philadelphia: Wolters Kluwer. Adapted from Chiovitti, R., & Prian, N. (2003). Rigour and grounded theory research. *Journal of Advanced Nursing Practice, 44*(4), 427–435; and from Strauss, A., & Corbin, J. (1990). *Basics of qualitative research: Grounded theory procedures and techniques.* Newbury Park, CA: Sage.

the senses and may be experienced emotionally, such as pain and losing a loved one. In addition to clarifying phenomena, qualitative research can give voice to people who have been disenfranchised and whose experiences would have otherwise not been documented (Barbour & Barbour, 2003; Schepner-Hughes, 1992). In qualitative inquiry, unlike quantitative research, prediction and control of phenomena are not the aim. Qualitative results are applied differently than more traditional quantitative research findings. As Barbour and Barbour (2003) stated,

> . . . rather than seeking to import and impose templates and methods devised for another purpose, qualitative researchers and reviewers should look . . . for inspiration from their own modes of working and collaborating and seek to incorporate these, forging new and creative solutions to perennial problems, rather than hoping that these will simply disappear in the face of application of pre-existing sets of procedures. (p. 185)

Therefore, findings may be applicable only in certain circumstances. As Lincoln and Guba (1985) stated, "the trouble with generalizations is that they don't apply to particulars" (p. 110). Thus, in qualitative research, if the investigator studies the pain experience of individuals undergoing bone marrow biopsy, for example, the findings will be applicable only to individuals who are similar to those in the study.

In another example, a study of depression in children with chronic disease should not be viewed as having direct application to adults suffering from chronic disease. The findings must be used within a specific context, or additional studies must be conducted to validate the applicability of the findings across contexts. Hence, nurses who wish to use the findings of qualitative research in their practices must first validate them, either through their own observations or through interaction with groups similar to the original study participants, to determine whether the findings accurately reflect wider experiences.

Evidence-Informed Practice Tip _____

Nurses using qualitative research findings should ask whether the evidence provided in the study enhances their understanding of particular patient care situations.

In qualitative outcome analysis (QOA), researchers can use the findings of a qualitative study to develop interventions and then to test them with selected patients. Morse, Penrod, and Hupcey (2000) described QOA as a "systematic means to confirm the applicability of clinical strategies developed from a single qualitative project, to extend the repertoire of clinical interventions, and evaluate clinical outcomes" (p. 125). Application of knowledge discovered during QOA adds to clinicians' understanding of clinical phenomena because they can select interventions that are based on the patient's expressed experience of a particular clinical phenomenon. QOA is considered a form of evaluation research and, as such, has the potential to add to the literature on evidence-informed practice at either level V or level VI, depending on how the study was designed.

Another use of qualitative research findings is to initiate examination of important concepts in nursing practice, education, or administration. Caring, for example, is considered a significant concept in nursing; therefore, studying its multiple dimensions is important. Using a qualitative approach, Wilkin and Slevin (2004) explored the meaning of caring for critical care nurses. Wilkin and Slevin posited that although caring had been studied extensively, little research had been conducted in the highly technological area of critical care. The authors identified caring in a critical care setting as a "process of competent physical and technical action imbued with affective skills" and confirmed that "to care is human and the capacity to care is affirmed and actualised in caring for the critically ill patient and their relatives" (p. 50).

Wilkin and Slevin's study adds to the existing body of knowledge on caring and extends the current state of nursing science because it was an examination of a specific area of nursing practice and the experience of caring by critical care nurses.

Evidence-Informed Practice Tip ____

Qualitative research studies can be used to guide practice when they are applied within a context. The nurse should ask the following question: "Does this study provide me with a direction for caring for a particular patient group?"

Finally, qualitative research can be used to discover information about phenomena of interest that can lead to instrument development. Usually, qualitative methods are used to direct the development of structured research instruments as part of a larger empirical research project. Instrument development from qualitative research studies is useful to practising nurses because it is grounded in the reality of human experience with a particular phenomenon. For example, after an initial qualitative exploration of the phenomenon, the researcher may develop a survey to collect the data related to specific variables.

CRITIQUING A QUALITATIVE RESEARCH STUDY

CRITIQUE 1

The study "Achieving a Sustainable Livelihood after Leaving Intimate Partner Violence: Challenges and Opportunities" by Lynne Duffy (2015) is critiqued here. The narrative of the article is presented in its entirety and is followed by the critique on pp. 417–419. (From *Journal of Family Violence*, 30, 403–417. © Springer Science+Business Media New York 2015.)

Achieving a Sustainable Livelihood after Leaving Intimate Partner Violence: Challenges and Opportunities

Lynne Duffy
Published online: 1 March 2015
© Springer Science+Business Media New York 2015

ABSTRACT

A community-based research (CBR) study was carried out with single mothers who had left abusive relationships in order to better understand their experiences of finding a sustainable livelihood after experiencing intimate partner violence (IPV). Using the photovoice method and guided by the Sustainable Livelihoods (SL) framework, participants took photographs representing their experiences of violence through their transition to single motherhood and beyond. The findings reported through their photos and stories reveal an often long and arduous journey amidst the complexity of single parenting and the effects of violence. As with many people living on a low income, they incorporated creative strategies to survive and enhance their own and their children's quality of life. Important areas for change are suggested through aspects of the SL framework and primary prevention.

KEYWORDS Lone/single mothers • Violence against women • Sustainable livelihoods framework • Employment • Gender inequality • Photovoice • Community-based participatory research • Visual research

Intimate partner violence (IPV) refers to a pattern of physical, sexual, and/or emotional violence by an intimate partner in the context of coercive control (Tjaden and Thoennes 2000). It is one of the major health and human rights problems of our time with estimates of one in three women affected worldwide (Davis 2002a; World Health Organization [WHO] 2005). Leaving relationships in which they have experienced IPV can push many women into poverty. This lowered economic status results from ongoing physical and mental health effects of IPV, further abuse, debt, and costs of moving away and staying safe (Wuest et al. 2003) with loss of material and fiscal assets. Single mothers have the added challenge of the former partner's continued intrusion through custody, access, and child support conflicts (Wuest et al. 2006). Literature reveals the vulnerability of single mothers after leaving abusive partners, yet, knowledge of women after leaving has often focused on deficits with little known about their strengths or assets, particularly with regards to employment.

While employment itself provides no promise of a living wage, many single mothers want to work to improve their health and quality of life as well as that of their children. We knew little about the livelihood aspirations of women who have left abusive partners, the assets they have and need, and employment strategies they use to sustain their families in the short term and into the future.

GEOGRAPHICAL AND EMPLOYMENT CONTEXT

This study was carried out in the Greater Moncton area of New Brunswick, Canada that includes the three communities of Moncton, Dieppe, and Riverview. In 2011, these two cities and one town had a combined population of 140,500 (Statistics

Duffy, L. *J Fam Viol* (2015) 30: 403. https://doi.org/10.1007/s10896-015-9686-x

Canada 2012). In Moncton in 2006, there were 5,815 single parent families of which 4,845 were female headed (83.3%) and 975 male headed (Statistics Canada 2006). In Canada in 2009, single mothers earned on average $47,700 compared to $65,400 for single fathers (Statistics Canada 2009). Researchers have examined part time employment noting that Canadian women in 2011 chose part time work 20% of the time due to their own illness (3.1%), caring for children (13.3%), and other personal/family responsibilities (3.6%) (Statistics Canada 2011b), whereas the total for men was 6.4%, including 3.6% for their own illness, 1.3% caring for children, and 1.5% for other personal or family responsibilities (Statistics Canada 2011a). In 2010, females in New Brunswick lost an average of 11.2 days due to illness and disability (Statistics Canada 2010b) whereas men lost 7.4 (Statistics Canada 2010a). These statistics show wide gender differences in single household, work, and income patterns and the reasons why women and men might choose part time over full time employment that then impacts their ability to achieve a sustainable livelihood.

STUDY PURPOSES

The overall aim of this inquiry was to explore and describe single mothers' transitions to a sustainable livelihood after leaving an abusive partner. More specifically, to identify their goals for economic sustainability, their strengths and assets in the transition, socio-cultural factors that hinder or facilitate the transition and that increase or decrease their vulnerability, and appropriate supports for achieving a sustainable livelihood.

THEORETICAL FRAMEWORK

The Sustainable Livelihoods (SL) framework includes an upstream antipoverty approach to community economic development, guides the examination of factors that affect people's livelihoods and the relationships between them, and helps identify more appropriate entry points for interventions (Department for International Development DFID 1999; Murray and Ferguson 2002). A livelihood comprises the capabilities, assets, and activities required for a means of living, and is sustainable "when it can cope with and recover from stresses and shocks and maintain or enhance its capabilities and assets" now and in the future (DFID 1999, section 2.4).

An essential characteristic of poverty is a limited ability to accumulate *assets* (Murray and Ferguson 2002). The *Livelihood Assets Pentagon* frames assets as evolving forms of capital that people are able to draw upon to achieve their livelihood goals: *human capital* includes skills, knowledge, health, and ability; *social capital* implies social networks and trust relationships; *physical capital* is infrastructure such as transportation, housing, and information; *financial capital* refers to all financial resources (savings and income); while *natural capital* refers to available natural resources. Natural capital was not included in the study as it was not relevant.

The *Vulnerability Context* includes external factors, largely outside people's control, that have a direct impact on assets and options. Three areas of influence are shocks (economic, health), trends (more contract work, fewer benefits), and seasonality (time-limited work such as farming and fishing, price fluctuations). *Policies, Institutions, and Processes* are social and cultural institutions, organizations, policies, and legislation that control access to capital and influence strategies. *Livelihood Strategies* refer to the dynamic way people undertake various activities to achieve their livelihood outcomes. *Livelihood Outcomes* are people's aspirations with respect to present and future livelihood and could include higher income, increased well-being, food security, and reduced vulnerability (DFID 1999; Murray and Ferguson 2002).

This research was also informed by a feminist perspective that views IPV and socio-economic status (SES) as issues of power, control, and oppression (Varcoe 1996, 2008). Violence against women "does not occur spontaneously but is linked to and embedded in the legal/social mechanisms and systems that inhibit and erode women's equality rights" (Tutty 2006, p. viii).

IPV, EMPLOYMENT, AND THE SL FRAMEWORK

The Vulnerability Context

Within the SL framework, we viewed IPV as a pervasive and unrelenting shock that can escalate over time, forcing many women to leave their partners and abandon homes, belongings, jobs, and social supports (Lutenbacher et al. 2003; Merritt-Gray and Wuest 1995). Unfortunately, the violence often intensifies after leaving, particularly for mothers faced with child custody, visitation, and child support, further increasing their vulnerability by putting their safety at risk (Davies et al. 2009; Fleury et al. 2000; Wuest et al. 2003). IPV also targets women's efforts to establish independence by eroding their sense of competence and ability to trust and interferes with their access to relationships and resources (Ford-Gilboe et al. 2005).

While disclosure of IPV has become more socially acceptable, survivors continue to feel stigmatized with feelings of revictimization when convincing others of their experience (Lempert 1996; Wuest and Merritt-Gray 1999; Wuest et al. 2003) and face many barriers to accessing appropriate services (Kulkarni et al. 2010). Despite this, the process of leaving an abusive relationship can enhance women's sense of control over their lives (Anderson and Saunders 2003).

Livelihood Assets

The asset pentagon is at the center of the model and situated within the vulnerability context. "Assets are both created and destroyed as a result of the shocks, trends, and seasonality of the vulnerability context" (DFID 1999, section 2.3, para 11).

Human Capital

The health impact for survivors of IPV is far reaching and includes both acute and chronic physical and mental health problems. Particularly intrusive and persistent are chronic pain, insomnia, hearing loss, depression, posttraumatic stress disorder symptoms, and bowel disturbances (Campbell 2002; Ford-Gilboe et al. 2006; Humphreys et al. 2010; Plichta 2004; Samuels-Dennis et al. 2010; Wuest et al. 2009). These influence a woman's capacity to labour at home, work, or school and affect relationships with family and friends (Anderson et al. 2003; Canadian Research Institute for the Advancement for Women [CRIAW], 2002; Kimerling et al. 2009; Macy et al. 2005; WHO 2005; Wuest et al. 2003).

Women can become exhausted as a result of the attacks as well as the vigilance needed to survive prolonged IPV (Ford-Gilboe et al. 2005). Additionally, IPV often erodes women's self-efficacy and confidence leading them to question their abilities to be successful. "Employment not only increases a woman's financial well-being but it can also increase her social capital and social networks" (Gibson-Davis et al. 2005, p. 1152) with added gains in "mental respite" and "purpose in life" (Rothman et al. 2007, p. 140). However, an unstable work history, combined with pervasive health problems after leaving, can interfere with women's ability to benefit from employment (Walker et al. 2004). The costs of health care are significantly higher than in non-abused women with increased use of emergency rooms, primary care, and medications that only add to the financial burden (Bonomi et al. 2009).

Social Capital

This refers to social resources that are both a means to achieving livelihood objectives and assisting in coping and recovery from shocks and insecurity (DFID 1999). Social support is seen as a critical protective factor in developing resiliency and other coping skills (Davis 2002b; Staggs et al. 2007). Isolation and control by abusive partners limits women's social connections and leaving often compounds the isolation, especially if the departure requires relocation (Walker et al. 2004). The legacy of IPV and repeated violations of trust complicate the survivor's ability to effectively engage and build meaningful connections with both formal and informal supports (Ford-Gilboe et al. 2005).

Physical Capital

Especially important for single mothers after leaving are safe and secure housing, basic household goods, utilities, transportation, and childcare (Anderson and Saunders 2003); however, many women begin their new life with little or no physical capital. Single mothers with a history of IPV face an additional challenge of needing to be safe from former abusers (Raphael 1999; Tolman and Rosen 2001). Rollins et al. (2012) found clear linkages between housing instability, health, and IPV and noted that unstable housing situations are as important to the development of mental health issues for women after leaving abusive relationships as is the severity of abuse. Leaving is also more difficult in the absence of other physical capital such as timely and accurate information concerning their rights, resources, and eligibility for programs and services (Davis 2002a).

Financial Capital

Even without the vulnerability context of IPV, women-headed households often experience dramatic downward mobility in income and social status following separation and divorce (Davies et al. 2009; Lorenz et al. 1997). Lindhorst et al. (2007) stressed the need for policy makers to recognize the long-term impact of IPV on economic sustainability. Furthermore, Crowne et al. (2011) found that employment instability can continue up to six years after leaving an abusive relationship. Single parents are 1 of 5 high-risk groups for consistent low income in Canada (Human Resources and Skills Development Canada 2008), with 51.6% of women-headed families living in poverty (Canadian Research Institute for the Advancement of Women CRIAW 2005) and 1 in 3 female single parents in New Brunswick living below the poverty line (Advisory Council on the Status of Women 2010).

In order for women to remain out of an abusive relationship, access to economic resources is critical (Anderson and Saunders 2003; Kwesiga et al. 2007; Moe and Bell 2004; Pennington-Zoellner 2009). Recognizing that sustainable employment is an important and socially acceptable way to build financial assets and security, limited structural support for low income single mothers, combined with risks to their own and their children's well-being, may mean that responsible parenting involves a decision to return to social assistance (Bancroft and Vernon 1995; Bell 2003; Mullan-Harris 1996; Scarbrough 2001).

It is evident that the sections of the asset pentagon are very interdependent; a change in one can greatly influence another. This means that a loss in one area could seriously undermine other assets. On the other hand, actions to build or enhance assets can also have positive effects on other forms of capital that could increase women's livelihood sustainability.

Policies, Institutions, and Processes

Women who have left an abusive relationship need a wide range of services to remain free, sustain their families, and deal with the multiple challenges faced by themselves and their children. When positive, these services can be empowering (Anderson et al. 2003; Merritt-Gray and Wuest 1995; Perrin et al. 2011) yet they are often fragmented, poorly coordinated, heavily bureaucratic, vary across sites, and do not deal with women's complex needs in a comprehensive way (Allen et al. 2004; Cole 2001; Kulkarni et al. 2010; Zweig et al. 2002). These shortcomings have "direct consequences for women's safety and well-being" (Allen et al. 2004, p. 1016).

Some workplaces have created provisions such as Employee Assistance Programs (EAPs) and flexible work schedules, yet there is little research on how EAPs respond to IPV (Pollack et al. 2010). With the high costs of IPV to employers in terms of medical expenses, turnover, lost productivity, and absenteeism, workplaces may choose to address the issue by terminating women's employment rather than implementing supportive policy and programs (Moe and Bell 2004; Perrin et al. 2011). Swanberg et al. (2012) found that only about 15% of employers surveyed by the Bureau of Labor Statistics in 2006 had a workplace violence policy relating to domestic violence. Several researchers note the difficulty of single mothers maintaining employment with the high cost, or lack, of structural supports (Butler et al. 2008; Edin and Lein 1997). Within work environments, disclosure of abuse can reduce negative effects and therefore assist in maintaining employment, yet this disclosure is most likely to occur when there is evidence of appropriate employment support (Swanberg et al. 2007).

Livelihood Strategies

Single mothers use various strategies to improve income and quality of life after leaving and, while much is known about the barriers they face, little is known about how they overcome these. Tutty (2006) stressed that education, upgrading, and training programs for women are particularly important in helping them leave especially when the abuser has been the primary family wage earner. Kneipp's (2002) study revealed that lack of health insurance is the main reason women leave work and return to welfare.

Battered women, who experience ongoing harassment after leaving an abusive relationship, may have multiple episodes of short-term, entry-level employment, or underemployment, and with few or no health benefits or job security (Moe and Bell 2004; Staggs et al. 2007; Staggs

and Riger 2005). Strategies used to "break through their current economic ceiling" involve many risks as they enter job retraining, return to school, fight for child support, relocate, or increase their debt load; all requiring a considerable degree of situational stability, self-efficacy, and confidence (Ford-Gilbee et al. 2005, p. 489).

Livelihood Outcomes

Increased well-being and better income are two important outcomes that are relevant to this study, although outcomes are unique for each person. The effects of IPV appear to be serious impediments to employment and self-sufficiency (Butler et al. 2008; Gennetian 2003; Murray and Ferguson 2002; VandeWeerd et al. 2011) while "waged work, increased financial autonomy, educational and vocational development can aid in healing (of IPV) if done in a safe, supportive context (Brush 2000, p. 1044). Paid employment is generally associated with better health and well-being for women (Anderson et al. 2003; Samuels-Dennis 2006). Klumb and Lampert (2004) consolidated 50 years of research on employment and women's health and determined that employed women have improved self-efficacy and social affirmation along with lower mortality rates compared to women who are not employed. It appears that employment may decrease women's vulnerability by enhancing human, social, and financial capital.

METHODS

Photovoice, as one method of community-based research (CBR), was chosen for the way the process involves and engages participants as co-researchers in an active and collaborative process of inquiry. Photovoice is founded on principles of health promotion, education for critical consciousness, feminist theory, and a community-based approach to documentary photography (Wang 1999; Wang and Burris 1997; Wang et al. 1998). Cameras are provided for participants to record everyday life events or representations of the study focus that lead to discussion and reflection on the meaning of the images. The photos and the accompanying stories assist in sharing people's expertise with those who have the power to form and inform policy. The photovoice acronym VOICE stands for *Voicing Our Individual and Collective Experience* and this approach works at a grassroots level to determine what is important to a community.

Recognizing and appreciating the importance of community stakeholders, we were joined by Moncton Head Start (programs for low income families), Moncton's transition house Crossroads for Women, and Support to Single Parents. We were also guided by a Community Advisory Committee, that included representatives of the community partners, others interested or working in areas of poverty reduction, employment, education, or domestic violence as well as two participants from an earlier study with photovoice and single mothers (Duffy 2010). This committee met every six months with the academic researcher and research assistant. Members assisted with recruitment, provided input to the process, and contributed ideas for dissemination.

Ethics and Safety

Approval was obtained from the University of New Brunswick (UNB) Nursing Ethics Committee and the UNB Research Ethics Board. Safety protocols similar to those used by colleagues in previous research with women and IPV were used. Following recruitment and informed consent, participants received training on the SL framework, photovoice method, basic camera skills, and issues of ethics, power, and privacy around community photography. Digital cameras were provided and belonged to the women at the end of the project. In addition, they received a $15.00 honorarium at each meeting with childcare and transportation costs covered. Consent around shared ownership and use of photos was established initially and was ongoing. Participants chose which photos to make public and

were made aware of their rights around withdrawing consent without negative consequences.

Sample

Inclusion criteria included 1) being a single mother living in Greater Moncton, 2) age 18 and older, 3) English speaking, 4) having left an abusive relationship with an intimate partner at least one month ago, 5) having at least one dependent child living with them, and 6) willing to commit to participate for up to two years. Recruitment was through purposive sampling assisted by the three community partners with posters at each site and through their direct contacts with clients individually or in group sessions. The same advertisements were placed in public areas where women in post abuse situations might attend such as Victims Services. Partners received an orientation and recruitment package that included study information, contact permission forms for those who wished to be called, and a contact card to phone directly. As calls were received, the PI or the Research Assistant followed a flow chart to ensure inclusion criteria were met and that participants were fully informed. Safety issues were also reviewed and a one-on-one meeting was held with participants when possible.

Consistent with feminist methodology around representation of diverse perspectives and experiences, the women varied in culture (both Anglophone and Francophone), education (from Grade nine to one participant with a masters degree), age (18 to over 40), time out of relationship (two months to 15 years) and employment. Eight women were working full time, four working part time with two holding more than one part time position, eight were unemployed including two taking upgrading courses, and one on maternity leave. Monthly income ranged from $500 to $4000, with an average of $1368.00 or $16,416 annually. A 2012 provincial report on child poverty noted that a single parent with two children working full time at minimum wage would earn $15,000 below the poverty line (Human Development Council 2012).

Wang (1999) suggests 7 to 10 people as an appropriate photovoice group size. We recruited 20 women who were subsequently divided into two discussion/analysis groups; either a morning group at a partner agency or an evening group at the university to enable attendance. This number allowed for a feasible project in case of attrition.

Data Collection

Monthly photo assignments were based on sections of the SL framework with a one or two page handout prepared for each component that was reviewed at the end of the analysis discussion in preparation for the next month's photo shoot. Participants were asked to photograph and keep field notes on their experiences in each of four areas of livelihood assets (human, physical, social, and financial capital), process and structures, and livelihood outcomes and strategies. Discussions were audio taped and transcribed to document the issues, themes, and stories emerging from the individual and group dialogue. Photographing continued until the participants agreed that the photos accurately represented their issues around the various sections of the SL framework and their recommendations for change.

Data Analysis

In photovoice, analysis is concurrent with data collection. As the women arrived at each meeting that lasted about three hours, their photographs were downloaded from their camera to a computer and projected on a screen. We followed the original three steps of analysis according to Wang and Burris (1997): 1. *Selecting*—Participants choose two or more of their photographs that have the most significant meaning. 2. *Contextualizing*—Participants describe the meaning of their images to group members guided by the photovoice acronym SHOWeD (S—What do you "See" in this photo? H—What is "Happening" here? O—How does this relate to "Our lives"? W—"Why" does this exist? and D—What can

we "Do" to address this issue? Group members could ask questions and add to the discussion, helping to expand meaning and understanding. 3. *Codifying*—Participants identified issues or themes that emerged (Wang et al. 1998) and chose the photos and stories to be made public.

Once the two groups completed their respective photography and analysis sessions, they came together to share and integrate these findings. Through various meetings, the research team (academic researcher, research assistant, and the women) examined the assignment categories (components of the SL framework) and began to consider which photos, from all available, best described their experiences. This resulted in an adaptation of the SL framework we called the Study Process and Outcomes model that describes their journey from IPV, important assets (capital) to their achieving a sustainable livelihood or not, and areas the group decided were priorities for change. Eventually, out of over 1000 photographs, 134 were chosen by the team to represent areas of the model and then a graphic designer integrated captions with photos. Final products for dissemination were developed collaboratively with participants and later with members of the Community Advisory Committee. Over a two and a half year period, each group met 14 times and then worked together for approximately 10 more sessions.

Findings

The findings are presented here according to sections of the Study Process and Outcomes Model along with examples of the photographs. A slide show of all 134 photos with section headings can be viewed at http://www.unb.ca/research/projects/photovoice/phase-two/research-findings.html.

The Vulnerability Context

Participants were clear in how violence had helped define and shape their present life. While IPV was seen as a major "shock" in the Vulnerability Context of the SL framework, the women's vulnerability continued throughout the leaving process and afterwards as they began to care for their families in new contexts and is expressed under the following sections.

IPV

Although this study was with women who had left abusive relationships, all participants stressed the need to begin with the abuse experience. While they used some metaphor and analogy to depict the violence, such as in the photo with the eggshells, four of them thought this wasn't enough and they came together to act out and photograph some of their experiences with a volunteer male "abuser." This was a difficult process of re-living the abuse, but they insisted these pictures were the only way people could really begin to see and understand what they had experienced.

Participants defined abuse as "Anything that takes away our dignity" and used words such as hopelessness, trapped, afraid, a sick feeling that never goes away, and no way out. They described lives filled with fear, threats, intimidation, isolation, control, and cruelty involving physical, emotional, and/or sexual attacks often with a weapon.

Single Parenting

Subsequent to leaving the abusive relationship, the women had experienced and continue to experience high-level demands of single parenting. They are overwhelmed with the responsibility of providing basic needs to a reconstituted family as they also recognize all they are missing due to limited income, such as recreation, travel, understanding, and support from family members and agencies. While struggling for dignity and accessible services, healing needs to occur in order for them and their children to attain some quality of life.

Livelihood Outcomes

The dreams and aspirations of the women include such basic things as a small house, reliable transportation, peace and serenity, safety, ability to adequately care for their children, and enough income to be comfortable. Unfortunately, most of these are out of their reach no matter what they do. This is the result of several things including their level of education and skills, health challenges, the energy and time required for child care and healing from IPV, market trends such as increasing contract and part time work with few if any benefits, and the requirement by many local employers for bilingualism.

Livelihood Strategies

Existing on a limited income, and with sustainable employment only a dream, they did many things to eke out a living. Some of these were income-generating such as making and selling crafts, renting space in their homes, and bartering for goods and services. Many others were income-conserving activities that included keeping old, dilapidated furniture; using food banks and second hand clothing depots; setting goals; budgeting; careful shopping and creative cooking with often nearly bare cupboards; moving back with parents; doing without heat and electricity for periods in the winter; and buying lottery tickets in the hopes of a better life in the future. Several made great sacrifices in order to attend courses and university in hopes of later finding a good job. Others sought social support and networking to improve their asset base, and improving or maintaining their health in order to work and care for their children.

Livelihood Assets

Many aspects of the previous sections relate to forms of capital that are critical to whether one has or is able to achieve a sustainable or unsustainable livelihood. Though sustainability is shown as a dichotomy in the model, in reality it is more a continuum with each person having unique "amounts" of assets at different points in time. As mentioned earlier, these forms of capital, while depicted as separate sections in the SL framework, influence each other and are very much interrelated and overlapping. Therefore, it can be difficult to know which one might have occurred first to influence another.

Human Capital

A major component of this section involves health and wellness with clear connections to financial capital. One photo is of two medicine bottles with the caption *Be Happy*. The photographer described how others told her to "Just take Prozac"—implying that there is an easy way to get over her depression. She recognized at least part of the reason for her depression and asked, "Do they think Prozac is going to pay the bills and put food on the table?" Participants told stories of their attempts to find healing for themselves and their children through appointments with doctors, specialists, and counsellors and the need for frequent testing for chronic illnesses while dealing with inflexible employers not allowing time off for health-related visits. Even if a woman met expected work quotas, she was denied salary increases or promotions because she did not work full time hours. The stress of living with financial uncertainty and daily pressure to meet basic needs means that health is further compromised as is demonstrated in one photo of pills and healthy food that reads: Health and finances are related; Better health and nutrition means less medications.

During the study, the women were encouraged to evaluate strengths as well as challenges. They recognized their strong organizational skills, the growth that had occurred since leaving, and their efforts in continuous learning in order to keep up with rapid change.

Financial Capital

Critical to health, quality of life, and a sustainable future is having stable and adequate income that is properly managed. Long recognized as one of the most important determinants of health, financial security is the most fleeting asset for these women. Healing from the abuse and its many effects while caring for children often results in limited opportunities for full time employment with benefits. In our bilingual province it can be very difficult for a unilingual person to find a full time job, especially when public services require provision in both languages. There are limited opportunities for adults to study language and the cost (in money and time) is beyond what most of the women have.

Social Capital

Another vital area that influences the quality of a transition from IPV to single motherhood is social support. Community agencies are essential for safety, training, building resiliency, and helping with physical resources. However, it was noted that assistance through food banks or soup kitchens is demeaning, as it makes one's poverty public. While faith communities are important and supportive for some, others have reported experiencing judgmental attitudes and were offered help with religious strings attached. Old and new friends often filled the gap when the women had to move away from family and friends to keep safe or when relatives would not accept the reality of the abuse experience. Caring, responsive employees in such areas as police, Victim Services, and the courts made a difference in how these systems were navigated and whether or not the outcomes were positive.

Physical Capital

Transportation and housing emerged as critical assets to well-being and employment. Many working other than regular daytime hours found accessibility limited with bus schedules developed for consumers, not employees. Cost of vehicle repairs, fuel, and insurance also meant that car keys were often left hanging. Finding and keeping a job is nearly impossible without reliable means of transportation. Women who have left abusive relationships also need safe, affordable housing, yet often could only afford substandard accommodations in less than desirable neighbourhoods. Heating and electricity costs also impacted quality of life, particularly given that winter temperatures in this geographic region often stay well below the freezing point for long periods. Furthermore, not having a personal computer limits job searching and preparation of resumes. One positive physical asset is the public library for accessing reading and video materials as well as free Internet.

Opportunities for Change

The following recommendations for change, which emerged from discussions in the combined group, are organized under three categories. While each woman had preferences specific to her personal situation, the following are those that everyone agreed were important. The first two categories are taken from the SL framework: 1) protecting, building, and maintaining livelihood assets and 2) transforming structure and processes. Strategies within these categories often influence each other. For example, obtaining a good job, if available, is difficult without affordable childcare and transportation.

Protecting, Building, and Maintaining Assets

Human Capital

Early teaching and modeling of healthy relationships for males and females; early learning to set boundaries and respect for others' boundaries; raising children with good self-esteem and social intelligence; opportunities for self-development; work-appropriate education and training in official languages; and good physical and emotional health with access to a broad range of affordable western and alternative health services.

Financial Capital

A living wage with benefits for everyone; countering the culture of the working poor who may choose to move from employment to income assistance programs in order to have more benefits; early

education in budgeting and investing; access to savings and pensions to reduce vulnerability to violence and poverty; and, since leaving IPV often involves bankruptcy, access to credit may be needed to start a new life.

Social Capital

Social support and networks include friends, families, neighbours, peer mentors, and caring agencies and institutions. Women are often blamed for leaving abusive relationships and family or friends may not accept that the abuse occurred. Therefore, effective interventions from community agencies are even more critical when more personal level supports are missing.

Physical Capital

Recommendations here focus on accessibility including safe, healthy, and affordable housing and neighbourhoods; reliable and affordable public transport that serves shift workers; recreation for physical and emotional health and healing; and appropriate job training and equipment for sustainable employment.

Transforming Structures and Processes

Along with strengthening personal and physical assets, it is also critical to examine and work for change around many of the larger policies and practices in workplace and government settings.

Business Practices

Workplace support for women experiencing IPV and post abuse assistance including comprehensive employee assistance programs; family friendly and flexible work places; benefits for both part time and full time positions; and equal employment opportunities for men and women.

Laws and Policies

An increase in mental health services and accessibility to alternative health care; sustainable level of employment assistance throughout the healing process; appropriate educational strategies for sustainable employment; laws that promote a living wage for all; enacting pay equity laws and eliminating gender wage gaps; universal day care; and training respectful and caring public employees who do not discriminate.

Legal and Court Services

Access to domestic violence court systems for all with adequate numbers of social workers; continued IPV training for police and other interventionists; and enhanced collaboration between court agencies to ensure seamless and just outcomes of rulings.

Community Resources

A key recommendation involves a single entry point for IPV services along with improved interagency collaboration to avoid duplication and gaps in provision. As the participants spent time together over the two years, they increased their knowledge of resources and often became supports for others, even creating a bartering system and sharing housing. However, it was obvious during their many discussions that each experience of leaving abusive relationships and finding appropriate resources was different and at times seemed to very much depend on "luck" or finding the right person to help. For example, women leaving abusive relationships often require frequent contact with the criminal justice system, which can be complex to navigate as well as lacking in appropriate and timely services (Letourneau et al. 2012). Therefore, while work continues on prevention of societal and family violence, a critical recommendation to mediate effects is for a single entry point for services and resources so that the journey out of IPV is a more effective, efficient, and supportive process for women and their children.

Primary Prevention of Violence

We added this third category of change to our model, noting the critical need for heightened attention on prevention of IPV and other forms of societal violence such as bullying and harassment. More specifically, there is a need to challenge media messages and images that make violence acceptable. A critical area of prevention is eradication of poverty, which is increasingly challenging as the gap between rich and poor widens in most areas of the world. Elimination of all forms of gender inequality is essential to enhancing women's economic and social opportunities.

Limitations

This study was carried out with a group of English-speaking participants due to the language of the academic researcher and therefore excluded women who might only speak French. While some participants were from the Francophone community, their command of English was at a high level, and it is not clear if there would be differences between the two official language groups. Future research should include both groups with comparisons made; as it is always preferable to discuss personal and sensitive topics in one's first language. Women in rural areas were also not included and there may be differences; certainly in access to often centralized resources. The purposeful, yet convenience sampling through the partner agencies meant that women from other cultural groups may not have been reached, such as if we had specifically worked with the local multicultural association.

One challenge was the complexity of the SL framework and finding ways to make it understandable for participants. In addition, the study time frame of over two years, while building community and ownership of the project, presented a long-term commitment. As such, some initial participants were unable to complete the project. Some reasons for this included mental health and addiction issues, changes in interpersonal relationships (i.e., marriage), and new employment responsibilities.

DISCUSSION AND CONCLUSION

This study has offered a unique insight into the transition from IPV to single motherhood by analyzing participant photographs through individual reflections and group dialogue. The SL framework provided a multi-contextual guide for the women to photograph areas important to their experience of IPV, including leaving the abusive relationship, surviving the aftermath, and approaches to poverty reduction (where possible), based on various livelihood outcomes and strategies. One strength in this approach to development is the focus on assets as units of capital. Ford-Gilboe et al. (2009) found that women's personal, economic, and social resources mediated the physical and mental health effects of partner violence after leaving. Far too often, we examine poverty through a deficit lens while Pyles and Bannerjee (2010), who use the language of capabilities, say it is a social justice approach that recognizes each person's entitlement to reach their potential and it is the responsibility of governments to ensure this occurs.

The vulnerability context of the SL framework is an important concept that reminds us of the many environmental issues we often have little control over. In this study, we focused on IPV as a key shock. However, trends are also an important component. High unemployment rates, underemployment, and hiring practices, such as moves to more contract and part time work, also affect ability to achieve a sustainable livelihood. A third aspect of the vulnerability context is seasonality. An example is employment in school systems where workers are without salary for the summer months. Fluctuating food and fuel prices throughout the year are also seasonality factors. Most of us have little control over these except the choice of whether or not to purchase them. Choices are important and the ability to choose wisely is directly related to financial assets. In addition to influencing their family's quality of life, achieving economic security through a sustainable livelihood can also increase women's choices with regards to a romantic partner (Pennington- Zoellner 2009).

This research has revealed the complexity of women's journeys from IPV and the challenges they face while attempting to heal and reconstitute a healthy family system. VandeWeerd et al. (2011) note the intricate relationship between IPV and employment, with women facing a "multiplicity of demographic . . . and mediating factors" as well as many direct and indirect barriers (p. 149). With employers being slow in taking responsibility for addressing IPV, strong and supportive state and national level policies are needed to increase workplace accountability (Swanberg et al. 2012).

Finding and maintaining employment in this complexity, along with societal employment trends, is challenging for all and impossible for some. Riger and Staggs (2004) remind us that in order to understand the various responses and choices women make around employment, we need to focus on multi-level contextual issues, not only individual characteristics, since "women's lives are embedded within an interpersonal and institutional framework" (p. 982). Multi-level actions for change have been suggested that require involvement of governments, communities, workplaces, families, and individuals in the development of societies with zero tolerance of all forms of violence, while mediating the effects of IPV. As identified by the participants in this study, women who have experienced IPV need many supports if they are to have any chance of obtaining a sustainable livelihood and these include affordable housing and child care, sustainable employment with benefits, caring and responsive systems, and safe living and working environments (Bell 2003; Katula 2012; Pyles and Banerjee 2010). Prevention, as part of a comprehensive approach, involves reducing risk factors for violence that include "poverty, stress, substance abuse, depression, and history of child abuse" (Shobe and Dinemann 2008, p. 185).

The physical, emotional, social, and financial costs of IPV to individuals, families, and society, while difficult to measure, are staggering. With violence against women and girls commonly accepted in many societies (WHO 2005), multilevel strategies are needed that normalize non-violence as a way of life for all. An important component of any approach is addressing gender inequality since, "Violence against women is both a consequence and a cause of gender inequality" (WHO 2005, p. viii). Davies et al. (2009) remind us of the need to recognize and address the relationship between abuse and gendered and social inequalities that exist in most of society today. Otherwise we will continue to provide weak and short-term solutions to pervasive, coercive, and dangerous situations for countless women and children.

Acknowledgments Sincere appreciation to the women who participated as co-researchers in this study and taught me so much, as well to our supportive community partners and research assistant, Cathy Kelly.

REFERENCES

Advisory Council on the Status of Women. (2010). *Status report: Women in New Brunswick*. Retrieved May 20, 2012, from http://www.acswcccf.nb.ca/media/acsw/files/english/2010report/Status%20Report%202010%20English.pdf.

Allen, N. E., Bybee, D. I., & Sullivan, C. M. (2004). Battered women's multitude of needs: evidence supporting the need for comprehensive advocacy. *Violence Against Women*, *10*(9), 1015–1035. doi:10.1177/1077801204267377.

Anderson, D. K., & Saunders, D. G. (2003). Leaving an abusive partner: an empirical review of predictors, the process of leaving, and psychological well-being. *Trauma, Violence & Abuse*, *4*(2), 163–191. doi:10.1177/1524838002250769.

Anderson, D. K., Saunders, D. G., Yoshihama, M., Bybee, D. I., & Sullivan, C. M. (2003). Long-term trends in depression among women separated from abusive partners. *Violence Against Women*, *9*(7), 807–838. doi:10.1177/1077801203009007004.

Bancroft, W., & Vernon, S. (1995). *The struggle for self-sufficiency: Participants in the self-sufficiency project talk about work, welfare, and their futures*. Ottawa: SRDC.

Bell, H. (2003). Cycles within cycles: domestic violence, welfare, and low-wage work. *Violence Against Women*, *9*(10), 1245–1262. doi:10.1177/1077801203255865.

Bonomi, A. E., Anderson, M. L., Rivara, F. P., & Thompson, R. S. (2009). Health care utilization and costs associated with physical and nonphysical-only intimate partner violence. *Health Services Research*, *44*(3), 1052–1067. doi:10.1111/j.1475-6773-2009.00957.x.

Brush, L. D. (2000). Battering, traumatic stress, and welfare-to-work transition. *Violence Against Women*, *6*(10), 1039–1065. doi:10.1177/10778010022183514.

Butler, S., Corbett, J., Bond, C., & Hastedt, C. (2008). Long-term TANF participants and barriers to employment: a qualitative study in Maine. *Journal of Sociology and Social Welfare*, *35*(3), 49–69.

Campbell, J. C. (2002). Health consequences of intimate partner violence. *Lancet*, *359*(9314), 1331–1336. doi:10.1016/S0140-6736(02)08336-8.

Canadian Research Institute for the Advancement of Women (CRIAW). (2005). *Violence against women and girls*. Ottawa: Author.

Cole, P. R. (2001). Impoverished women in violent partnerships: designing services to fit their reality. *Violence Against Women*, *7*(2), 222–233. doi:10.1177/10778010122182415.

Crowne, S. S., Juon, H. S., Ensminger, M., Burrell, L., McFarlane, E., & Duggan, A. (2011). Concurrent and long-term impact of intimate partner violence on employment stability. *Journal of Interpersonal Violence*, *26*(6), 1282–1304. doi:10.1177/0886260510368160.

Davies, L., Ford-Gilboe, M., & Hammerton, J. (2009). Gender inequality and patterns of abuse post leaving. *Journal of Family Violence*, *24*, 27–39. doi:10.1007/s10896-008-9204-5.

Davis, R. E. (2002a). Leave-taking experiences in the lives of abused women. *Clinical Nursing Research*, *11*(3), 285–305. doi:10.1177/10573802011003005.

Davis, R. E. (2002b). "The strongest women": exploration of the inner resources of abused women. *Qualitative Health Research*, *12*(9), 1248–1263. doi:10.1177/104973230228248.

Department for International Development (DFID). (1999). *Sustainable livelihoods guidance sheets*. London: Author.

Duffy, L. (2010). Hidden heroines: lone mothers assessing community health using photovoice. *Health Promotion Practice*, *11*(6), 788–797. doi:10.1177/1524839908324779.

Edin, K., & Lein, L. (1997). Work, welfare, and single mothers' economic survival strategies. *American*

Sociological Review, 62(2), 253–266. Retrieved from http://www.jstor/stable/2657303.

Fleury, R. E., Sullivan, C. M., & Bybee, D. I. (2000). When ending the relationship does not end the violence. *Violence Against Women, 6*(12), 1363–1383. doi:10.1177/10778010022183695.

Ford-Gilboe, M., Wuest, J., & Merritt-Gray, M. (2005). Strengthening capacity to limit intrusion: theorizing family health promotion in the aftermath of woman abuse. *Qualitative Health Research, 15*(4), 477–501. doi:10.1177/1049732305274590.

Ford-Gilboe, M., Wuest, J., Varcoe, C., & Merritt-Gray, M. (2006). Developing an evidence-based health advocacy intervention for women who have left an abusive partner. *Canadian Journal of Nursing Research, 38*(1), 147–167.

Ford-Gilboe, M., Wuest, J., Varcoe, C., Davies, L., Merritt-Gray, M., Campbell, J., & Wilk, P. (2009). Modelling the effects of intimate partner violence and access to resources on women's health in the early years after leaving an abusive partner. *Social Science & Medicine, 68*(6), 1021–1029. doi:10.1016/j.socscimed.2001.01.03.

Gennetian, L. A. (2003). Welfare policies and domestic abuse among single mothers: experimental evidence from Minnesota. *Violence Against Women, 9*(10), 1171–1190. doi:10.1177/1077801203255846.

Gibson-Davis, C. M., Magnuson, K., Gennetian, L. A., & Duncan, G. J. (2005). Employment and the risk of domestic abuse among low-income women. *Journal of Marriage and Family, 67*(5), 1149–1168. doi:10.111/j.1741–3737.2005.00207.x.

Human Development Council. (2012). *Child poverty report card.* Saint John: Author.

Humphreys, J., Cooper, B. A., & Miaskowski, C. (2010). Differences in depression, posttraumatic stress disorder, and lifetime trauma exposure in formerly abused women with mild versus moderate to severe chronic pain. *Journal of Interpersonal Violence, 25*(12), 2316–2338. doi:10.1177/0886260509354882.

Katula, S. (2012). Creating a safe haven for employees who are victims of domestic violence. *Nursing Forum, 47*(2), 217–225. doi:10.1111/j.1744-6198. 2012.00278.x.

Kimerling, R., Alvarez, J., Pavao, J., Mack, K. P., Smith, M. W., & Baumrind, N. (2009). Unemployment among women: examining the relationship of physical and psychological intimate partner violence and posttraumatic stress disorder. *Journal of Interpersonal Violence, 24*(3), 450–463. doi:10.1177/0886260508317191.

Klumb, P. L., & Lampert, T. (2004). Women, work, and well-being 1950–2000: a review and methodological

critique. *Social Science & Medicine, 58*(6), 1007–1024. doi:10.1016/S0277-9536(03)00262-4.

Kneipp, S. M. (2002). The relationships among employment, paid sick leave, and difficulty obtaining health care of single mothers with young children. *Policy, Politics & Nursing Practice, 3*(1), 20–30. doi:10.1177/152715440200300104.

Kulkarni, S., Bell, H., & Wylie, L. (2010). Why don't they follow through? intimate partner survivors' challenges in accessing health and social services. *Family & Community Health, 33*(2), 94–105. doi:10.1197/FCH.06013e3181d59316.

Kwesiga, E., Bell, M. P., Pattie, M., & Moe, A. M. (2007). Exploring the literature on relationships between gender roles, intimate partner violence, occupational status, and organizational benefits. *Journal of Interpersonal Violence, 22*(3), 312–326. doi:10.1177/0886260502695381.

Lempert, L. B. (1996). Women's strategies for survival: developing agency in abusive relationships. *Journal of Family Violence, 11*(3), 269–289. doi:10.1007/BF02336945.

Letourneau, N., Duffy, L., & Duffet-Leger, L. (2012). Mothers affected by domestic violence: intersections and opportunities with the justice system. *Journal of Family Violence, 27*(6), 585–596. doi:10.1007/s10896-012-9451-3.

Lindhorst, T., Oxford, M., & Gillmore, M. R. (2007). Longitudinal effects of domestic violence on employment and welfare outcomes. *Journal of Interpersonal Violence, 22*(7), 812–828. doi:10.1177/0886260507301477.

Lorenz, F. O., Simons, R. L., Conger, R. D., Elder, G. H., Johnson, C., & Chao, W. (1997). Married and recently divorced mothers' stressful events and distress: tracing change across time. *Journal of Marriage and Family, 59*(1), 219–232. Retrieved from http://www.jstor.org/stable/353674.

Lutenbacher, M., Cohen, A., & Mitzel, J. (2003). Do we really help? perspectives of abused women. *Public Health Nursing, 20*(1), 56–64. doi:10.1046/j.1525–1446.2003.20108.x.

Macy, R. J., Nurius, P. S., Kernic, M. A., & Holt, V. L. (2005). Battered women's profiles associated with service help-seeking efforts: illuminating opportunities for intervention. *Social Work Research, 29*(3), 137–150. doi:10.1093/swr/29.3.137.

Merritt-Gray, M., & Wuest, J. (1995). Counteracting abuse and breaking free: the process of leaving revealed through women's voices. *Health Care for Women International, 16*(5), 399–412. doi:10.1080/07399339509516194.

Moe, A. M., & Bell, M. P. (2004). Abject economics: the effects of battering and violence on women's work and employability. *Violence Against Women, 10*(1), 29–55. doi:10.1177/1077801203256016.

Mullan-Harris, K. (1996). Life after welfare: women, work, and repeat dependency. *American Sociological Review, 61*(3), 407–426. Retrieved from http://www.jstor.org/stable/2096356.

Murray, J., & Ferguson, M. (2002). *Women in transition out of poverty*. Ottawa: WEDC.

Pennington-Zoellner, K. (2009). Expanding 'community' in the community response to intimate partner violence. *Journal of Family Violence, 24*(8), 539–545. doi:10.1007/s10896-009-9252-5.

Perrin, N. A., Yragui, N. L., Hanson, G. C., & Glass, N. (2011). Patterns of workplace supervisor support desired by abused women. *Journal of Interpersonal Violence, 26*(11), 2264–2284. doi:10.1177/0886260510383025.

Plichta, S. B. (2004). Intimate partner violence and physical health consequences: policy and practice implications. *Journal of Interpersonal Violence, 19*(11), 1296–1323. doi:10.1177/0886260504269895.

Pollack, K., Austin, W., & Grisso, J. A. (2010). Employee assistance programs: a workplace resource to address intimate partner violence. *Journal of Women's Health, 19*(12), 729–733. doi:10.1089/jwh.2009.1495.

Pyles, L., & Banerjee, M. M. (2010). Work experiences of women survivors: insights from the capabilities approach. *Affilia: Journal of Women & Social Work, 25*(1), 43–55. doi:10.1177/0886109909354984.

Raphael, J. (1999). Keeping women poor. In R. Brandwein (Ed.), *Battered women, children, and welfare reform* (pp. 31–43). Thousand Oaks: Sage.

Riger, S., & Staggs, S. L. (2004). Welfare reform, domestic violence, and employment: what do we know and what do we need to know? *Violence Against Women, 10*(9), 961–990. doi:10.1177/1077801204267464.

Rollins, C., Glass, N. E., Perrin, N. A., Billhardt, K. A., Clough, A., Barnes, J., & Bloom, T. L. (2012). Housing instability is as strong a predictor of poor health outcomes as level of danger in an abusive relationship: findings from the SHARE study. *Journal of Interpersonal Violence, 27*(4), 623–643. doi:10.1177/0886260511423241.

Rothman, S., Hathaway, J., Stidsen, A., & de Vries, H. (2007). How employment helps female victims of intimate partner violence: a qualitative study. *Journal of Occupational Health Psychology, 12*(2), 136–143. doi:10.1037/1076-8998.12.2.136.

Samuels-Dennis, J. (2006). Relationship among employment status, stressful life events, and depression in single mothers. *Canadian Journal of Nursing Research, 38*(1), 58–80.

Samuels-Dennis, J., Ford-Gilboe, M., Wilk, P., Avison, W. R., & Ray, S. (2010). Cumulative trauma, personal and social resources, and posttraumatic stress symptoms among income-assisted single mothers. *Journal of Family Violence, 25*(6), 603–617. doi:10.1007/s10896-010-9323-7.

Scarbrough, J. W. (2001). Welfare mothers' reflections on personal responsibility. *Journal of Social Issues, 57*(2), 261. doi:10.1111/0022-4537.00212.

Shobe, M. A., & Dinemann, J. (2008). Intimate partner violence in the United States: an ecological approach to prevention and treatment. *Social Policy & Society, 7*(2), 185–195. doi:10.1017/S1474746407004137.

Human Resources and Skill Development Canada. (2008). *Low income in Canada: 2000–2006 using the Market Basket Measure—October 2008*. Retrieved June 10, 2012, from http://www.hrsdc.gc.ca/eng/publications_resources/research/categories/inclusion/2008/sp-864-10-2008/page08.shtm.

Staggs, S. L., & Riger, S. (2005). Effects of intimate partner violence on low-income women's health and employment. *American Journal of Community Psychology, 36*, 133–145. doi:10.1007/s10464-005-6238-1.

Staggs, S. L., Long, S. M., Mason, G. E., Kirshnan, S., & Riger, S. (2007). Intimate partner violence. social support, and employment in the post-welfare reform era. *Journal of Interpersonal Violence, 22*(3), 345–365. doi:10.1177/0886260506295388.

Statistics Canada. (2006). *Family structure lone parents*. Retrieved March 30, 2012, from http://www40.statcan.gc.ca/l01/cst01/ famil121a-eng.htm.

Statistics Canada. (2009). *Salary lone fathers/mothers*. Retrieved March 30, 2012, from http://www40.statcan.gc.ca/l01/cst01/famil05a-eng.htm.

Statistics Canada. (2010a). *Work lost due to illness (men)*. Retrieved March 30, 2012, from http://www40.statcan.gc.ca/l01/cst01/health47b-eng.htm.

Statistics Canada. (2010b). *Work loss to illness (women)*. Retrieved March 30, 2012, from http://www40.statcan.gc.ca/l01/cst01/health47c-eng.htm.

Statistics Canada. (2011a). *Reasons for part time work (men)*. Retrieved March 29, 2012, from http://www40.statcan.gc.ca/l01/cst01/labor63b-eng.htm.

Statistics Canada. (2011b). *Reasons part time work (women)*. Retrieved March 30, 2012, from http://www40.statcan.gc.ca/l01/cst01/labor63c-eng.htm.

Statistics Canada. (2012). *Population of census metropolitan areas*. Retrieved June 25, 2012, from http://www.statcan.gc.ca/tables-tableaux/sum-som/l01/cst01/demo05a-eng.htm.

Swanberg, J., Macke, C., & Logan, T. K. (2007). Working women making it work: intimate partner violence, employment, and workplace support. *Journal of Interpersonal Violence, 22*(3), 292–311. doi:10.1177/0886260506295387.

Swanberg, J., Ojha, M., & Macke, C. (2012). State employment protection statutes for victims of domestic violence: public policy's response to domestic violence as an employment matter. *Journal of Interpersonal Violence, 27*(3), 587–613. doi:10.1177/0886260511421668.

Tjaden, P., & Thoennes, N. (2000). *Extent, nature, and consequences of intimate partner violence. Findings from the national violence women survey*. Washington: Department of Justice.

Tolman, R. M., & Rosen, D. (2001). Domestic violence in the lives of women receiving welfare: mental health, substance dependence, and economic well-being. *Violence Against Women, 7*(2), 141–158. doi:10.1177/1077801201007002003.

Tutty, L. (2006). *Effective practices in sheltering women leaving violence in intimate partner relationships. Phase II report*. Toronto: YWCA.

VandeWeerd, C., Coulter, M., & Mercado-Crespo, M. (2011). Female intimate partner violence victims and labor force participation. *Partner Abuse, 2*(2), 147–165. doi:10.1891/1946–6560.2.2.147.

Varcoe, C. (1996). Theorizing oppression: implications for nursing research on violence against women. *Canadian Journal of Nursing Research, 28*(1), 61–78.

Varcoe, C. (2008). Inequality, violence, and women's health. In B. S. Bolaria & H. Dickinson (Eds.), *Health, illness, and health care in Canada* (4th ed., pp. 259–282). Toronto: Nelson.

Walker, R., Logan, T. K., Jordan, C. E., & Campbell, J. C. (2004). An integrative review of separation in the context of victimization: consequences and implications for women. *Trauma, Violence & Abuse, 5*(2), 143–193. doi:10.1177/1524838003262333.

Wang, C. (1999). Photovoice: a participatory action research strategy applied to women's health. *Journal of Women's Health, 8*(2), 185–192.

Wang, C., & Burris, M. A. (1997). Photovoice: concept, methodology, and use for participatory needs assessment. *Health Education & Behavior, 24*(3), 369–387. doi:10.1177/109019819702400309.

Wang, C., Wu, K. Y., Zhan, W. T., & Carovano, K. (1998). Photovoice as a participatory health promotion strategy. *Health Promotion International, 13*(1), 75–86. doi:10.1093/heapro/13.1.75.

World Health Organization. (2005). *WHO multi-country study on women's health and domestic violence against women: Summary report of initial results on prevalence, health outcomes and women's responses*. Geneva: Author.

Wuest, J., & Merritt-Gray, M. (1999). Not going back: sustaining the separation in the process of leaving abusive relationships. *Violence Against Women, 5*(2), 110–133. doi:10.1177/1077801299005002002.

Wuest, J., Ford-Gilboe, M., Merritt-Gray, M., & Berman, H. (2003). Intrusion: the central problem for family health promotion among children and single mothers after leaving an abusive partner. *Qualitative Health Research, 13*(5), 597–622. doi:10.1177/1049732303013005002.

Wuest, J., Ford-Gilboe, M., Merritt-Gray, M., & Lemire, S. (2006). Using grounded theory to generate a theoretical understanding of the effects of child custody policy on women's health promotion in the context of intimate partner violence. *Health Care for Women International, 27*(6), 490–512. doi:10.1080/07399330600770221.

Wuest, J., Ford-Gilboe, M., Merritt-Gray, M., Varcoe, C., Lent, B., Wilk, P., & Cambell, J. (2009). Abuse-related injury and symptoms of posttraumatic stress disorder as mechanisms of chronic pain in survivors of intimate partner violence. *Pain Medicine, 10*(4), 739–747. doi:10.1111/j.526.4637.2009.00624.x.

Zweig, J. M., Schlichter, K. A., & Burt, M. R. (2002). Assisting women victims of violence who experience multiple barriers to services. *Violence Against Women, 8*(2), 162–180. doi:10.1177/10778010222182991.

INTRODUCTION TO CRITIQUE 1

The preceding article (Duffy, 2015) is an example of a general qualitative inquiry in which qualitative methods are used without alignment to a particular traditional method, as described in Chapter 7. Although it is a community-based inquiry, it should not be confused with community-based action research (CBAR), as the study focused on discovery, in this case, to better understand the experiences of single mothers who had left abusive relationships and their experiences of finding a sustainable livelihood. The article is critically examined here for its rigour as an action research study, its contribution to nursing, and its usefulness in practice. The criteria listed in Box 18.1 are used to guide the critique.

Title

The title of the article nicely captures the essence of the study; however, the development of an outcomes model is overlooked.

Abstract

The abstract meets the requirements of a good abstract: It contains the background to the study and the method used, and it concludes with the results.

Statement of the Phenomenon of Interest

Duffy (2015) clearly stated the phenomenon of interest in the introduction: "We knew little about the livelihood aspirations of women who have left abusive partners, the assets they have and need, and employment strategies they use to sustain their families in the short term and into the future" (p. 403). The author stated that intimate partner violence is a major health and human rights issue. Further, women who leave these abuse relationships often find themselves compromised financially because of physical and mental health issues, debt, moving costs, and the loss of assets. Because little is known about the challenges they face and the strategies they use to support themselves and their children, the qualitative research method is appropriate.

Purpose

The stated purpose of the research project is "to explore and describe single mothers' transitions to a sustainable livelihood after leaving an abusive partner" (p. 404). The author used the sustainable livelihoods (SL) framework to frame the study and to identify the specific areas to explore. Duffy stated that she specifically wished to identify these women's

- Goals for economic sustainability
- Strengths and assets
- Sociocultural factors
- Appropriate supports

The SL framework was used to identify the factors that affect people's livelihood, such as their vulnerability and assets and relevant public policy.

Method

The method used in the study is described in a section called "Methods." As described earlier, the author used a community-based research method and chose photovoice as the specific means for gathering data and to engage the participants as active collaborators. In public health initiatives from China to California, community people have used photovoice to carry out participatory needs assessment, conduct participatory evaluation, and reach policymakers to improve community health (Wang & Redwood-Jones, 2001). Consistent with community-based research, Duffy used a feminist methodology to ensure that the study included diverse perspectives and experiences. Although implicit in the article, she did not clearly state that she used a constructivist approach, nor that the community-based research design followed many of the tenets of CBAR, including consultation with the community as described in the "Methods" section. The community advisory committee consisted of a diverse group people with experience in poverty reduction, education, domestic violence, and participants from previous studies.

Sampling

The study was carried out in New Brunswick, where the author is a member of the nursing faculty at the University of New Brunswick. The community advisory committee and three community partners assisted with recruitment of participants by posting posters and through direct contacts, either individually or though group sessions. Participants were recruited through purposive sampling. The inclusion criteria included the following: (1) being a single mother living in Greater Moncton, (2) being age 18 or older, (3) English speaking, (4) having left an abusive relationship with an intimate partner at least 1 month ago, (5) having at least one dependent child living with them, and (6) willing to participate for up to 2 years. In qualitative research, the most common type of sampling is purposive or purposeful sampling. According to Streubert and Carpenter (2011), "individuals are selected to participate in qualitative research based on their first-hand experience with a culture, social process, or phenomenon of interest" (p. 28). This ability to describe an experience from one's own perspective is what makes selection purposive. In this study, all participants had experience with intimate partner violence; thus the selection of participants was appropriate.

Data Collection

The primary source of data was a series of monthly photo assignments, participant field notes, and audio recorded discussion about the photos. The participants were given a monthly photo assignment based on the components of the SL framework. For example, they were asked to photograph and keep field notes about their experiences with the livelihood assets such as financial capital—having a stable and adequate income. Most qualitative field researchers document their experiences through field notes; however, it is

unusual to ask participants to document theirs. It was important in this study for the participants to remember clearly what meaning the photo had for them. At monthly meetings the photos were displayed and discussed. The ensuing discussions were audio recorded and transcribed. The participants continued to collect photographs until they determined that their experiences were accurately captured and represented their issues and recommendations related to the SL framework.

Focus groups, or group discussions in this study, are commonly used in qualitative research, and their use was appropriate in this study, although researchers need to be cautious about the development of groupthink, in which one dominant participant can influence other group members (Streubert & Carpenter, 2011). Because the researcher did not identify how she would manage this situation or gather data from other participants through individual interview or observation, this is a potential weakness of the data-collection method.

Ethical approval was sought and received from the nursing ethics committee and the university research ethics board. Given the delicate nature of the study, particular attention was paid to ensuring a safe and ethical environment for the participants. Although this was not explicitly described, the author referred to using safety protocols that had been used in previous research with women and intimate partner violence. This project would have benefited from a more thorough discussion of the process, as the safety protocol is important for the reader to be aware of.

Data Analysis

As in most qualitative research, and particularly photovoice research, the data analysis occurred concurrently with the data collection. The process of analysis followed Wang and Burris's (1997) three steps as follows: (1) selecting—participants select one or two photos that had the most significant meaning for them; (2) contextualizing—participants described the meaning of their images to group members, answering a number of questions, such as "What is happening here?"; and (3) codifying—participants identified the emergent themes and determined which photos and stories should be shared. Finally, the group determined which photos best described experiences that could be assigned to the components of the SL framework. Out of 1,000 photos, eventually 134 were chosen to represent the study.

In general, the measure of rigour in qualitative research is trustworthiness. Trustworthiness includes the concepts of credibility, auditability, and fittingness. It is difficult to determine whether the author of this study addressed the **auditability** (the extent to which another researcher or a reader can follow the method and conclusions drawn by the original researcher[s]) and **fittingness** (how applicable the study findings are to others in similar situations) of the data (see Chapter 14 for a complete discussion). With the long-term engagement of participants over a 2-year period, the depth and quantity of data, and the involvement of a large number of participants, it is clear that this study was a rigorous exploration of the challenges facing women who have left an abusive relationship to realize a sustainable livelihood.

Findings

The author reported her findings clearly and comprehensively. To provide authenticity to the findings, she provided a figure of the Study Process and Outcomes Model with several examples of photos. The 134 photos selected are also available online: http://www.unb.ca/research/projects/photovoice/phase-two/research-findings.html. The photos are a powerful representation of the participants' experiences; the photos enable their voices to be heard in a unique way. The findings are depicted according to the sections of the SL framework. Each of the sections is supported by a thorough discussion of experiences.

Conclusions, Implications, and Recommendations

Duffy's recommendations for change are included in the "Findings" section and are part of the Study Processes and Outcomes Model as they were drawn from the participants themselves. This demonstrates community-based research, in which the participants collaborate in all stages of the research process, including making recommendations. They focused on protecting, building, and maintaining assets; transforming structures and processes; and promoting primary prevention of violence. A specific recommendation was to have a single entry point for services and resources for women leaving abusive relationships. Although the author did not reiterate the recommendations in her discussion and conclusion, she did note that one strength of the study was the focus on assets rather than a poverty deficit model. Although not explicitly stated, this approach can have a more significant impact on developing community support and policy change for vulnerable women and their children. The conclusion could have benefited from a more expansive discussion of the systemic changes that could be made. The author did state that since the study excluded women who were not English speaking and lived in rural areas, a subsequent study to include these potential participants would expand our understanding.

CRITIQUING A QUALITATIVE RESEARCH STUDY

CRITIQUE 2

The study "Immunization Rejection in Southern Alberta: A Comparison of the Perspectives of Mothers and Health Professionals" by Shannon Y. Vandenberg and Judith C. Kulig (2015) is critiqued here. The article is presented in its entirety and is followed by the critique on pp. 430–432. (From *Canadian Journal of Nursing Research, 47*(2), 81–96.)

Immunization Rejection in Southern Alberta: A Comparison of the Perspectives of Mothers and Health Professionals

Shannon Y. Vandenberg, Judith C. Kulig

Qualitative grounded theory was used to compare and contrast the understanding and decision-making process of non-immunizing mothers and health professionals' perceptions of these mothers' understanding and decision-making process. The sample comprised 8 mothers with purposefully unimmunized children under the age of 6 years and 12 health professionals. Semi-structured interviews were conducted and the data generated were analyzed using data immersion, memo-writing, and 3 stages of coding. The mothers and health professionals identified similar, interrelated factors influencing the mothers' decision, categorized into 4 groups: emotions, beliefs, facts, and information. Three primary themes were evident: the health professionals emphasized the influence of religion in decision-making to a greater extent than did the mothers, the meaning of *evidence* appeared to differ for mothers and health professionals, and mothers revealed a mistrust of health professionals. Immunization is a public health issue; collaboration and understanding are necessary to promote positive health outcomes in children.

KEYWORDS: decision-making, mothers, public health, nurse relationships/professional issues

The introduction of vaccines is considered a marvel of modern science and one of the most remarkable successes of public health. According to the World Health Organization (WHO) (2013), two to three million lives are spared annually as a result of immunization, and rates of diseases such as measles, rubella, and polio have decreased by over 95% in Canada since the introduction of vaccines (Gold, 2006). Smallpox, which historically plagued millions of children globally, is now eradicated (Public Health Agency of Canada [PHAC], 2005). Despite the success of immunization, the WHO (2011) specifies that 23 million infants worldwide are not routinely immunized, raising fears that nearly eliminated vaccine-preventable diseases, such as polio, will re-emerge. Currently, measles outbreaks around the globe have highlighted the importance of vaccination. Poor vaccine coverage has led to the resurgence, with 147 reported cases as of February 2015 in the Americas alone (WHO, 2015).

TO IMMUNIZE OR NOT TO IMMUNIZE?

One of the most significant decisions parents make in terms of their child's health is whether to participate in childhood immunization. Austin, Campion-Smith, Thomas, and Ward (2008) and Sturm, Mays, and Zimet (2005) identify factors that influence immunization decision-making: concerns about vaccine safety, risk versus benefit of vaccines, guilt, confusion due to conflicting information, health-care provider attitudes, mistrust of government and health professionals, personal attitudes and beliefs, social norms, media reports, inexperience with vaccine-preventable diseases, and lack of knowledge about immunization. The current literature uses the term *vaccine-hesitant parents* (Sadaf, Richards, Glanz, Salmon, & Omer, 2013), while in this study we also use the term *non-immunizing parents*.

One ongoing challenge is the diversity of populations and their acceptance or rejection of

Shannon Y. Vandenberg, Judith C. Kulig, *Canadian Journal of Nursing Research*, 47(2), 81–96.

immunization. At the site of the present study in southern Alberta, Canada, there exist non-immunizing individuals within cultural or religious groups, including Hutterites, Mennonites, Dutch Reformed, and people adhering to alternative health beliefs (Kulig et al., 2002). According to Matkin, Simmonds, and Suttorp (2014), cultural and religious norms and expectations make it challenging for group members to make informed decisions about immunization.

Over the last decade, southern Alberta has dealt with significant vaccine-preventable disease outbreaks. Pertussis outbreaks have occurred every 3 to 5 years, the most recent outbreaks being in 2009 and 2012 (Matkin et al., 2014). In 2014, outbreaks of measles and pertussis affected a number of communities in Alberta (Matkin et al.), placing avoidable pressure on the health-care system and the economy (Alberta Health and Wellness [AHW], 2007).

According to the Government of Alberta (2012), childhood immunization rates in southern Alberta are slightly lower than in the province as a whole. For instance, in 2010 the percentage of children fully immunized with the measles-mumps-rubella (MMR) vaccine by age 2 was 85.68% for all of Alberta, compared to 83.93% for southern Alberta (Government of Alberta); to achieve effective herd immunity for measles in Alberta, the target is 98% for 2-year-old children to have received one dose of MMR vaccine (Matkin et al., 2014). The immunization rates for all childhood vaccines for 2-year-old children varied among communities in southern Alberta; however, 42.8% of 2-year-olds were unimmunized as of June 2013 (Matkin et al.).

Global, national, and provincial immunization strategies have been drawn up in response to the challenges of low immunization rates, aimed at addressing immunization issues, promoting immunization, and ultimately improving immunization rates (AHW 2007; PHAC, 2005; WHO, 2010). On the whole, health-care professionals (HCPs) have welcomed these strategies as a means to promote health and prevent disease, which is necessary to curb rising health-care costs around the globe (Khorsan, Smith, Hawk, & Haas, 2009).

HCPs, such as physicians, public health nurses (PHNs), and chiropractors, in southern Alberta are impacted by the unique immunization situation there and may be sought for support and advice on the topic of immunization by their patients. Bedford and Lansley (2006) found that 59% of participants in their study in the United Kingdom obtained immunization advice from HCPs. They also found that a trusting relationship with HCPs is crucial in parents' decision whether or not to immunize their children. Similarly, Leask et al. (2008) found that HCPs influence parents in their decision whether or not to immunize their children.

According to Plastow (2006), HCPs are responsible for promoting childhood immunization as well as for providing accurate, evidence-based information to their patients and the general public, while respecting the autonomy and freedom of choice of individuals, as stated in the 2011 *Canadian Charter of Rights and Freedoms*. Childhood immunization falls under public health in Canada (Health Canada, 2009); therefore in many provinces, including Alberta, PHNs deliver the publicly funded immunization programs. The scope of practice of a PHN in Canada involves communicable disease prevention, which consists of planning, coordinating, delivering, and evaluating immunization programs, in addition to being accountable for current knowledge on immunization, skills in administering vaccines, and appropriate therapeutic communication skills (Community Health Nurses of Canada, 2009; Manitoba Health, 1998).

PURPOSE

The purpose of this study was to explore and compare the understanding and decision-making of non-immunizing mothers with the perceptions of HCPs regarding non-immunizing mothers' understanding and decision-making concerning childhood immunization. The study was part of a larger investigation of the topic (Vandenberg, 2013) guided by four research questions: (1) How do mothers develop an understanding of immunization? (2) How does mothers' understanding of immunization influence their decision not to participate in childhood immunization? (3) How do HCPs perceive non-immunizing mothers' understanding of immunization and their decision not to immunize their children? (4) How do the understanding and decision-making process of mothers compare with the perceptions of HCPs regarding childhood immunization?

METHOD

Design

This study took place in southern Alberta with mothers from both rural and urban settings. A qualitative research approach was used, with Straussian grounded theory (Corbin & Strauss, 2008; Glaser & Strauss, 1967) as the research design and symbolic interactionism (Mead, 1934) as the theoretical framework, to explore and compare the perceptions of non-immunizing mothers and HCPs regarding immunization. The selected research design and research questions enabled the participants to openly share their feelings, beliefs, and worldviews.

Symbolic interactionism is a useful perspective for understanding human beings and their behaviours in the world they inhabit and for according their words the greatest importance, which allows for close association with qualitative research (Mead, 1934). Grounded theory is a useful methodology for conceptualizing dimensions of social processes and for considering participants' views, intentions, and actions (Glaser & Strauss, 1967). Straussian grounded theory was chosen because it compels the researcher to assume a position of objective external reality while giving voice to the

participants and acknowledging their worldviews (Corbin & Strauss, 2008).

The main features of grounded theory are theoretical sampling, simultaneous data collection and analysis, comparative methods, three phases of data coding, memo-writing, and theory generation (Ghezeljeh & Emami, 2009; Jeon, 2004), all of which were adhered to in this study. Ethical approval was obtained from the authors' affiliated academic institution and the relevant health-services agency. The *Tri-Council Policy Statement: Ethical Conduct for Research Involving Humans* was followed and hence principles such as confidentiality of documents and information were upheld.

Sample

Eight mothers of children under the age of 6 years who purposefully had not immunized them with routine recommended childhood immunizations according to the Alberta Immunization Schedule were recruited using posters placed at locations frequented by mothers and children, such as health clinics, libraries, and family centres. Also, a notice was placed in a faith-based newsletter outlining the study and inviting interested mothers to contact the first author. Once contact was made with four mothers, snowball sampling was used to make contact with four others. Mothers were specifically chosen, rather than parents, given mothers' intimate, emotional relationship with their children and their involvement in health decision-making.

Twelve HCPs, comprising four PHNs, five chiropractors, two pediatricians, and one specialist physician who had a professional relationship with families, were recruited via formal letter of invitation. Letters were mailed to a wide variety of chiropractors in both rural and urban settings in southern Alberta. A fifth chiropractor was interviewed as a result of one chiropractor in the initial group of four expressing a non-supportive view of immunization; this additional interview allowed for the generation of further information from this perspective.

Although they do not administer vaccines, chiropractors were chosen for the study because the literature suggests that they are consulted by parents for information on childhood immunization (Medd & Russell, 2009; Page, Russell, Verhoef, & Injeyan, 2006). Furthermore, in their study with Alberta chiropractors, Medd and Russell (2009) found that chiropractors did not have a positive view of immunization, and, in another study, Russell, Injeyan, Verhoef, and Eliasziw (2004) found that only 25% of chiropractors advised their patients to immunize and 27% were opposed to immunization.

Letters were mailed to all practising pediatricians in southern Alberta and telephone calls were used to enhance recruitment. PHNs were recruited from both urban and rural settings in southern Alberta. PHNs were chosen because of their direct involvement in delivering the childhood immunization program in Alberta and pediatricians were chosen based on their expert knowledge of pediatric health issues. Additional HCPs who have a role in childhood immunization, such as family physicians, were not recruited because a sufficient sample size was achieved using other groups of providers.

Data Collection and Analysis

Data collection consisted of individual semi-structured interviewing of mothers and HCPs. Interviews were conducted by the first author in a location convenient for the participants. The interviews with mothers focused on knowledge about childhood immunization, experience with HCPs, beliefs and feelings about immunization, sources of information on the subject, and the decision-making process around childhood immunization. Interviews with HCPs concentrated on perceptions of childhood immunization, sources of information on the subject, role in immunization, relationship with non-immunizing mothers, and perceptions about mothers' immunization decision-making process.

Written and oral informed consent was obtained from all participants. Interviews were audio recorded and transcribed verbatim by the first author.

In accordance with grounded theory research, data collection and analysis were carried out concurrently (Strauss & Corbin, 1998). The first author analyzed the data from all of the interview transcripts, field notes, and memos, while the second author analyzed the data from several transcripts. The authors met on several occasions to review the findings and discuss themes and factors. The components of rigour as prescribed by Liamputtong (2013) were ensured in the following ways: credibility was established through the data collection and analysis processes; transferability was achieved by making sure that participants' ideas and perceptions were outlined in considerable detail in the findings; dependability was ensured via proper data management and including details of the data analysis; and confirmability was achieved by means of the two authors independently analyzing and confirming the findings. NVivo software was used in the storing, managing, and analyzing of the data.

Findings

Eight non-immunizing mothers in southern Alberta were interviewed, of whom four were rural residents and four urban. Their ages ranged from 25 to 37 years with a mean age of 30. All but one were married. Their education varied from partial high school to bachelor's degree. Their number of children ranged from two to six. All indicated that they were of Caucasian ethnicity. All mothers specified a religious faith, described as either Christian or Latter Day Saints (Mormon). The first author attempted to recruit mothers from a variety of cultural and religious backgrounds, given the unique demographic situation in southern Alberta; however, mothers of Mennonite,

Hutterite, and First Nations backgrounds did not respond to recruitment efforts.

Twelve HCPs were recruited for the study. Their ages ranged from 29 to 61 years, and there was an even representation of women and men. Length of time as an HCP ranged from less than 1 year to more than 20 years, with a mode length of greater than 20 years. Ten HCPs indicated that they were Caucasian and two identified as of another race.

Mothers described the immunization decision-making process as lengthy, difficult, and complex and indicated that the decision was reached not carelessly but purposefully. They considered the health of their children to be one of the most important matters to them and felt that they were making the decision that was best for their children. Similarly, HCPs realized the difficulty in making decisions regarding the health of children and understood that non-immunizing mothers were doing what they believed would ensure the health of their children. Professionals also acknowledged the importance of the risk-versus-benefit analysis. They knew that mothers weighed the risks of immunization against the risk of disease but felt that the success of immunization programs in keeping vaccine-preventable diseases at bay was not fully appreciated.

Both mothers and HCPs identified a number of interrelated factors that contribute to immunization decision-making, which fall under four themes — *emotions, beliefs, facts, and information* — although the authors acknowledge that the factors discussed below could debatably be placed under multiple themes.

Emotions

Mothers explored a number of emotional factors that had led them to not take part in the universal childhood immunization program. These included fear, negative experiences, guilt, indifference, and social belonging. Comparably, HCPs identified fear and social inclusion as emotional factors in decision-making. HCPs clearly recognized emotional motivation as an important factor.

Mothers discussed fear of the unknown and fear of vaccine effects, in addition to fear resulting from negative experiences with immunization: "I didn't feel secure doing it. To me it was kind of a scary thing." HCPs also found fear to be an integral paralyzing factor that forced mothers to defer to a passive decision, which was to refuse to immunize their children. One PHN said, "They are hearing all these different things — it influences them, because it scares them and it almost paralyzes them to not know what to do . . . they are really quite fearful for their own children."

Mothers also discussed feelings of guilt and the inability to forgive themselves should harm result from immunization: "I think that if I went along with it and something happened, that [it] was my responsibility, just the guilt would be huge." There were feelings of indifference due to the belief that diseases are not as serious as they are thought to be, as a result of tolerable personal experiences with vaccine-preventable diseases. One mother described her experience with chickenpox: "I mean, you go through a couple of days, but it's no big deal really."

Mothers indicated that they felt pressure from family, friends, and religious or cultural groups regarding childhood immunization: "We asked quite a few different people when we were trying to decide whether to immunize or not, like, our friends . . . probably [it was] how the people around me think about immunizations that led to [my] being okay with the decision not to immunize."

HCPs similarly identified social inclusion as an important emotional factor for mothers, who might have grown up in cultural or religious groups where, generationally, immunization was not adhered to and consequently refusing vaccines had become a matter of social or familial inclusion. One PHN said, "Sometimes that informed choice is peer pressure . . . they want to keep their cultural identity . . . there's a tremendous amount of peer pressure."

Beliefs

Mothers identified a combination of religion, natural health beliefs, and mistrust as factors in their decision about immunization. Clearly, religion was a factor: "If my children [were to] get sick, I would consider that . . . God's hand." While all the mothers mentioned a religious affiliation, their affiliations differed. Furthermore, religion was not a predisposing factor in the decision-making process. In contrast, HCPs perceived religious beliefs to be a central influence in southern Alberta for mothers not to immunize their children. However, they generalized non-immunizing mothers into what they viewed as the non-immunizing groups in the region, namely the Hutterites, Mennonites, and Dutch Reformed.

A preference for a natural body free of unnatural substances, such as vaccines, was explored with the mothers. One mother said, "It's more important for me to build up the immune system rather than bombard it with something that could be prevented just by having a stronger immune system." Mothers believed that the body's immune system is designed to ward off vaccine-preventable diseases, a belief that was also held by two HCPs who were unsupportive of childhood immunization.

Mothers openly acknowledged a mistrust of HCPs, pharmaceutical companies, and government, derived from anecdotal information and personal experiences. They believed that HCPs provide biased information, given the role of HCPs in health care, and described government and pharmaceutical companies as being financially motivated to promote vaccines. Comments by two different mothers highlight this perception: "I think HCPs are seen as, well, of course, they are for that [immunization] because that is what HCPs are taught to think, so maybe you discredit it a little bit"; "There's a lot of literature out there how the pharmaceutical companies really push the doctors into pushing vaccines, and they get their perks and their trips."

HCPs knew that the mothers had little trust in them and were aware of the perception that they were financially associated with government and pharmaceutical companies. One chiropractor said, ". . . especially nowadays, distrust of the government and of pharmaceutical companies, and of anyone who has a financial backing in the sales and production of medicine, so that's definitely some powerful, persuasive forces for people to weed through."

Facts

The third theme identified was facts — information that is true or certain. Four factors were placed under this theme: lack of exposure to vaccine-preventable disease, vaccine ingredients, multiple vaccines/antigens, and vaccine ineffectiveness.

Mothers and HCPs acknowledged that immunization programs, on the whole, have been successful at preventing vaccine-preventable diseases and that, consequently, these diseases are no longer considered a threat, making it difficult to appreciate immunization. "It's so easy to forget about it, not think about it," said one mother, "because most of these diseases aren't really a threat immediately . . . it's so easy to put it off, because there's no threat, really. If there is, you don't see it." According to the HCPs, the perceived risk of disease was lower than the perceived risk of vaccine side effects: "Weighing . . . the difference between which one is going to cause harm is sometimes difficult for a parent when you don't see disease."

Vaccine ingredients were a significant obstacle for the mothers, because these were mistakenly associated with harmful chemicals, including mercury, formaldehyde, and animal DNA. Mothers also made reference to the alleged presence of human diploid tissue in vaccines. One mother said, "Over time, all the chemicals and things that have been added, that's what kept us from doing it." HCPs also considered vaccine ingredients to be an impediment to immunization. They expressed concern that mothers believed that vaccines contain various metals and fetal tissue.

The mothers were concerned about the number of recommended childhood vaccines as well as the number of antigens in a specific vaccine, believing that multiple vaccines and/or antigens bombard a child's immature immune system. For instance, they disapproved of vaccines containing multiple antigens, such as the MMR vaccine: "I remember thinking there were an awful lot in the first 2 years . . . it seems like an awful lot to bombard . . . especially because their immune system isn't fully mature yet" Furthermore, mothers were aware of the fact that natural infection with disease provides lifelong immunity whereas immunized children remain susceptible to diseases, as vaccines do not offer absolute protection. In addition, mothers believed that the decline in vaccine-preventable diseases is a result of improvements in personal health and hygiene rather than the introduction of vaccines.

Information

Not knowing and information sources are the two factors included under the final theme. Mothers confessed to having a lack of knowledge about and understanding of vaccines. The mothers admitted that, based on their decision to not immunize their children, they subsequently had not conducted a thorough inquiry into immunization. For this group, information was not viewed as important, as one mother confessed: "I don't really know, because . . . we are flat-out, like, we aren't immunizing, so I've always kind of just pushed it out as fast as they try to give it to me." Comparably, HCPs viewed mothers' understanding across a spectrum, varying from limited understanding to very well informed and educated on the topic.

Mothers indicated they used a variety of information sources for their decision-making, including books, journals, anecdotes, and HCPs, with media and the Internet identified as a key source. Family and friends were seen as an important source. HCPs also indicated that the mothers were a close-knit group and hearsay or informal talk was prevalent. Interestingly, mothers felt that they received conflicting or biased information from HCPs.

Overall, HCPs perceived mothers' sources of information as inaccurate or not evidence-based. However, they acknowledged that it is difficult to locate accurate information given the abundance of information available on the Internet. One chiropractor summarized this view: "It is tough to really sit down and objectively weed through all of it and find the good stuff, so it's . . . a losing situation right from the get-go." The HCPs felt that mothers accessed information that resonated with their emotions on the topic, including sensational media stories, rather than scientific sources, but acknowledged that it is difficult to distinguish between evidence and opinion. In addition, professionals realized that they were only one source of information and that mothers obtained advice from a variety of sources, including other HCPs.

DISCUSSION

This study was limited to a specific geographic area that is home to a number of diverse religious groups. Despite this limitation there are three points worth elaborating on: HCPs and mothers outlined similar factors influencing immunization decision-making, mothers and HCPs understand and define the word "evidence" differently, and the apparent mistrust of HCPs signals a need for greater collaboration among HCPs.

HCPs and mothers outlined a variety of similar, interrelated factors influencing the childhood immunization decision-making process, demonstrating that, overall, HCPs have appropriate insight into nonimmunizing mothers' understanding and decision-making process. However, HCPs placed greater emphasis on religious beliefs as a factor in immunization decision-making, expressing the view that mothers are rejecting immunization for religious reasons, whereas the mothers felt that religiosity was only one factor in their decision. The findings might have been different if mothers had been recruited from a wider range of cultural and religious backgrounds. Downs, de Bruin, and Fischhoff (2008) and Kennedy and Gust (2008) found a similar association between religion and immunization refusal in their studies of parental decision-making around immunization. Additional research may be helpful in exploring the issue among mothers, parents, and HCPs in a larger geographical area with participants from a wider variety of cultural, social, and religious backgrounds.

HCPs indicated that, although the mothers may have appeared to be and considered themselves to be well informed, they were rather misinformed as a result of the unreliable information accessed. The findings suggest that the meaning of *evidence* can be understood very differently by mothers and HCPs. The HCPs acknowledged the difficulty in accessing evidence-based information, particularly on the Internet, as well as the challenges in understanding the material accessed. This finding is consistent with those from previous studies (Betsch, Renkewitz, Betsch, & Ulshofer, 2010; Davies, chapman, & Leask, 2002; Diekema, 2005; Levi, 2007). HCPs should ensure that their practice offers current, evidence-based knowledge about immunization in order to promote informed decision-making among vaccine-hesitant parents (Macdonald, McIntyre, & Barry, 2014), who need to be educated in the importance of immunization and provided with appropriate resources and information.

Research that explores the effectiveness of current immunization campaigns may be fruitful and may help shape the development of more effective education strategies. It would be beneficial to determine if current immunization delivery methods are conducive to positive health outcomes. Trialing of innovative delivery methods would be advantageous and could provide opportunities for evaluation research. For instance, PHNs could administer vaccines in physician clinics and hospitals, as well as in the traditional public health clinic. This could serve to increase immunization uptake and could also yield opportunities to communicate with vaccine-hesitant families who do not access traditional public health clinics.

The mothers' mistrust of HCPs was apparent. Ropeik and Slovic (2003) also found that trust in HCPs was minimal because of HCPs' concern about public protection. Mills, Jadad, Ross, and Wilson (2005) found high levels of public distrust of HCPs. HCPs in the present study were aware of the lack of trust, acknowledging that this could be the result of misperceptions concerning financial motivation for immunization and the information about vaccines that was provided. Immunization is a public health issue, and HCPs across disciplines need to collaborate to address the issue and promote credibility. Furthermore, increased cooperation between mothers and HCPs is necessary to reduce mistrust of HCPs and the information provided by HCPs regarding immunization.

Limitations

There were several limitations to the study. The mothers represented a homogeneous sample from a limited number of cultural and religious groups. Other HCPs, such as family physicians, who also have a role in childhood immunization were not included in the study. Furthermore, the sample size was small and hence the findings may not be generalizable to other geographic areas or to other groups of mothers and HCPs.

CONCLUSION

In this grounded theory study, a number of key themes were constructed from the data, demonstrating that both mothers and HCPs were concerned about the health of children, although there were different conclusions about the meaning of health. Given the current attention centred on vaccine-hesitant parents, understanding their alternative perspectives is becoming increasingly important for both HCPs and the public. Greater understanding will lead to greater collaboration, which can serve to promote positive health outcomes in children now and into the future.

REFERENCES

Alberta Health and Wellness. (2007). *Alberta immunization strategy*. Edmonton: Author. Retrieved December 3, 2014, from http://www.health.alberta.ca/documents/Immunization-Strategy-07.pdf.

Austin, H., Campion-Smith, C., Thomas, S., & Ward, W. (2008). Parents' difficulties with decisions about childhood immunisation. *Community Practitioner*, *81*(10), 32–35.

Bedford, H., & Lansley, M. (2006). Information on childhood immunisation: Parents' views. *Community Practitioner*, *79*(8), 252–255.

Betsch, C., Renkewitz, F., Betsch, T., & Ulshofer, C. (2010). The influence of vaccine-critical Websites on perceiving vaccination risks. *Journal of Health Psychology*, *15*(3), 446–455. doi:10.1177/1359105309353647.

Community Health Nurses of Canada. (2009). *Public health nursing discipline specific competencies version 1.0*. St. John's, NL: Author. Retrieved January 7, 2015, from http://www.chnc.ca/documents/PHNCompetencies FINALEnglish.pdf.

Corbin, J., & Strauss, A. (2008). *Basics of qualitative research: Techniques and procedures for developing grounded theory* (3rd ed.). Thousand Oaks, CA: Sage.

Davies, P., Chapman, S., & Leask, J. (2002). Antivaccination activists on the World Wide Web. *Archives of Disease in Childhood*, *87*(1), 22–26.

Diekema, D. S. (2005). Responding to parental refusals of immunization of children. *Pediatrics*, *115*(5), 1428–1431. doi:10.1542/peds.2005-0316.

Downs, J. S., de Bruin, W. B., & Fischhoff, B. (2008). Parents' vaccination comprehension and decisions. *Vaccine*, *26*(12), 1595–1607. doi:10.1016/j.vaccine.2008.01.011.

Ghezeljeh, T. N., & Emami, A. (2009). Grounded theory: Methodology and philosophical perspective. *Nurse Researcher*, *17*(1), 15–23.

Glaser, B. G., & Strauss, A. L. (1967). *The discovery of grounded theory: Strategies for qualitative research*. Chicago: Aldine.

Gold, R. (2006). *Your child's best shot: A parent's guide to vaccination* (3rd ed.). Ottawa: Canadian Paediatric Society.

Government of Alberta. (2012). *Interactive health data application: Childhood coverage rates (2007–2010)*. Edmonton: Author. Retrieved July 22, 2014, from http://www.ahw.gov.ab.ca/IHDA_Retrieval/select SubCategoryParameters.do.

Jeon, Y. (2004). The application of grounded theory and symbolic interactionism. *Scandinavian Journal of Caring Sciences*, *18*(3), 249–256.

Kennedy, A. M., & Gust, D. A. (2008). Measles outbreak associated with a church congregation: A study of immunization attitudes of congregation members. *Public Health Reports*, *123*(2), 126–134.

Khorsan, R., Smith, M., Hawk, C., & Haas, M. (2009). A public health immunization resource Web site for chiropractors: Discussion of current issues and future challenges for evidence-based initiatives for the chiropractic profession. *Journal of Manipulative and Physiological Therapeutics*, *32*(6), 500–504. doi:10.1016/j.jmpt.2009.06.011.

Kulig, J. C., Meyer, C. J., Hill, S. A., Handley, C. E., Lichtenberger, S. M., & Myck, S. L. (2002). Refusals and delay of immunization within southwest Alberta. *Canadian Journal of Public Health*, *93*(2), 109–112.

Leask, J., Quinn, H. E., Macartney, K., Trent, M., Massey, P., Carr, C., & Turahui, J. (2008). Immunisation attitudes, knowledge and practices of health professionals in NSW. *Australian and New Zealand Journal of Public Health*, *32*(3), 224–229. doi:10.1111/j.1753-6405.2008.00220.x.

Levi, B. H. (2007). Addressing parents' concerns about childhood immunizations: A tutorial for primary care providers. *Pediatrics*, *120*(1), 18–26. doi:10.1542/peds.2006-2627.

Liamputtong, P. (2013). *Qualitative research methods*. Melbourne: Oxford University Press.

Macdonald, G. J., McIntyre, M. A., & Barry, M. A. (October–December, 2014). Immunizing children: Current Canadian health care professional competencies. *SAGE Open*, 1–9, doi:10.1177/2158244014559510.

Manitoba Health. (1998). *The role of the public health nurse within the regional health authority*. Winnipeg: Author. Retrieved January 7, 2015, from http://www.gov.mb.ca/health/rha/docs/rolerha.pdf.

Matkin, A., Simmonds, K., & Suttorp, V. (2014). Measles-containing vaccination rates in southern Alberta. *Canada Communicable Disease Report*, *40*(12). Retrieved June 12, 2014, from http://www.phac-aspc.gc.ca/publicat/ccdr-rmtc/14vol40/dr-rm40-12/dr-rm40-12-surv-2-eng.php.

Mead, G. H. (1934). *Mind, self and society: From the standpoint of a social behaviorist*. Chicago: University of Chicago Press.

Medd, E. A., & Russell, M. L. (2009). Personal and professional immunization behavior among Alberta chiropractors: A secondary analysis of cross-sectional survey data. *Journal of Manipulative and Physiological Therapeutics, 32*(6), 448–452. doi:10.1016/j.jmpt.2009.06.006.

Mills, E., Jadad, A. R., Ross, C., & Wilson, K. (2005). Systematic review of qualitative studies exploring parental beliefs and attitudes toward childhood vaccination identifies common barriers to vaccination. *Journal of Clinical Epidemiology, 58*(11), 1081–1088. doi:10.1016/j.jclinepi.2005.09.002.

Page, S., Russell, M. L., Verhoef, M. J., & Injeyan, H. S. (2006). Immunization and the chiropractor-patient interaction: A western Canadian study. *Journal of Manipulative and Physiological Therapeutics, 29*(2), 156–161.

Plastow, N. A. (2006). Implementing evidence-based practice: A model for change. *International Journal of Therapy and Rehabilitation, 13*(10), 464–469.

Public Health Agency of Canada. (2005). *National immunization strategy: Final report 2003*. Ottawa: Author. Retrieved October 15, 2014, from http://www.phac-aspc.gc.ca/publicat/nis-sni-03/index-eng.php.

Ropeik, D., & Slovic, P. (2003). Risk communication: A neglected tool in promoting public health. *Risk in Perspective, 11*(2), 1–4.

Russell, M., Injeyan, H. S., Verhoef, M. J., & Eliasziw, M. (2004). Beliefs and behaviours: Understanding chiropractors and immunization. *Vaccine, 23*(3), 372–379.

Sadaf, A., Richards, J. L., Glanz, J., Salmon, D. A., & Omer, S. B. (2013). A systematic review of interventions for reducing parental vaccine refusal and vaccine hesitancy. *Vaccine, 31,* 4293–4304.

Strauss, A., & Corbin, J. (1998). *Basics of qualitative research: Techniques and procedures for developing grounded theory* (2nd ed.). Thousand Oaks, CA: Sage.

Sturm, L. A., Mays, R. M., & Zimet, G. D. (2005). Parental beliefs and decision making about child and adolescent immunization: From polio to sexually transmitted infections. *Journal of Developmental and Behavioral Pediatrics, 26*(6), 441–452.

Vandenberg, S. Y. (2013). *Saying no to childhood immunization: Perceptions of mothers and health care professionals in southern Alberta*. Lethbridge, AB: University of Lethbridge.

World Health Organization. (2010). *Global immunization vision and strategy*. Retrieved October 15, 2014, from http://www.who.int/immunization/ givs/en/index.html.

World Health Organization. (2011). *Global immunization vision and strategy*. Retrieved October 15, 2014, from http://www.who.int/immunization/ givs/en/index.html.

World Health Organization. (2013). *Immunization*. Retrieved December 3, 2014, from http://www.who.int/topics/immunization/en/.

World Health Organization. (2015). *Measles*. Retrieved March 22, 2015, from http://www.who.int/csr/don/archive/disease/measles/en/.

INTRODUCTION TO CRITIQUE 2

The preceding article by Vandenberg and Kulig (2015) is an example of a grounded theory study. The article is critically examined here for its rigour as a grounded theory study, its contribution to nursing, and its usefulness in practice. The criteria listed in Box 18.2 are used to guide the critique.

Title

The title of the article concisely captures the essence of the study.

Abstract

The abstract meets the requirements of a good abstract: It contains the background, the method (including the purpose and the sample size), and the findings. The abstract also has a statement about the clinical relevance of the study.

Focus/Topic

The phenomenon of interest is stated clearly in the "Purpose" section of the study. Although the introduction does describe the issues related to immunizations, the focus is not specifically outlined.

Purpose

The purpose is clearly stated in this section. The authors were interested in exploring and comparing the understanding and decision making of nonimmunizing mothers with the perceptions of the health care providers. This is of interest to the authors as child immunization rates in Southern Alberta are slightly lower than in the rest of the province of Alberta.

Significance

The significance of the study is introduced in the introduction, where the lower rate of immunization in Southern Alberta is detailed. A discussion of the potential impact of a lower immunization rate would have strengthened the value of the study.

Method

The method used in this study is clearly identified as grounded theory. Grounded theory is used to explain basic social processes and to develop theory (Streubert & Carpenter, 2011). In this study, the basic social process under study was to compare the understanding and decision making of nonimmunizing mothers with health care providers' perceptions of the mothers' understanding and decision making concerning childhood immunization. The authors implemented the main features of grounded theory, such as **theoretical sampling**, concurrent data collection and analysis, comparative methods, and the three phases of data coding, memo-writing, and theory generation. The grounded theory methodology is appropriate for this study.

Sampling

Vandenberg and Kulig (2015) stated that theoretical sampling was used for data collection, which is appropriate for a grounded theory study. Theoretical sampling begins with an initial sample (chosen purposively) that can shed light on the research study. After initial analysis, the emerging findings lead the researcher to seek other people (or documents) to be interviewed. This evolving process is guided by the emerging theory, hence theoretical sampling (Merriam & Tisdell, 2016). It is not clear in the section describing the sample if, in fact, the method used was theoretical sampling. Initially, four nonimmunizing mothers were recruited who, in turn, recruited others. The initial four mothers were recruited by means of posters placed at locations where mothers might see them. This is an example of purposive and snowball sampling. With purposive or purposeful sampling investigators in qualitative research are able to recruit participants who are knowledgeable about the phenomenon under study; they can provide rich descriptions of their personal experiences. In snowball sampling, a common form of purposive sampling, the number of participants is increased by asking the initial group for referrals to other possible participants who meet the inclusion criteria for the study.

Twelve health care providers were also recruited, by a letter of invitation. The sample consisted of four public health nurses, five chiropractors, two pediatricians, and one specialist physician. The choice of chiropractors is interesting, as they do not normally administer vaccines. But the authors argued that the literature suggests that chiropractors do provide advice to families on childhood immunization. Missing from the sample are family physicians because the sample size was achieved. This is a significant shortcoming of the study, as family physicians are typically the primary health care provider. This limiting of the sample size is not consistent with grounded theory; broader consultation is the norm and there are no limits on sample size.

The authors stated that written and oral consent were provided and research ethics approval was gained from the university and the appropriate health-services agency. These are critical steps to ensuring that participant rights with regard to research are safeguarded.

Data Generation

The primary source of data was semi-structured interviewing of mothers and health care providers. Each interview was audiotaped and transcribed verbatim by the authors. The focus of the interviews differed for the two groups. Mothers were asked about their knowledge of childhood immunizations, experiences with health care providers, sources of information on immunization, and how they made decisions about whether to immunize their children. The interviews with the health care providers focused on their perceptions on and role in immunization, relationship with nonimmunizing mothers, and perceptions regarding the decisions made by nonimmunizing mothers.

Vandenberg and Kulig (2015) did not include the interview questions in the study report. This is typical in grounded theory research, in which the use of interview guides is discouraged because they may be based on preconceived notions that may potentially distort the findings. Glaser (1998) recommended that "adjusted conversational interviewing" (p. 173) replace formal questions, whereas Corbin and Strauss (2008) supported interview guides with open-ended questions and opportunities for open dialogue. The process of collecting field notes and writing memos was not described in the article, although these data-collection methods were referred to in the description of the data analysis.

Data Analysis

True to grounded theory methodology, Vandenberg and Kulig (2015) conducted the data generation and analysis concurrently. Vandenberg, the first author, analyzed all of the data collected from transcripts, fields notes, and memos, whereas Kulig only analyzed the data from several transcripts. They met over several occasions to review the findings and discuss the themes and factors. The authors then identified that they met the rigour criteria of credibility, transferability, dependability, and confirmability. This claim is questionable when only the first author reviewed all of the data. They reported a process of three stages of coding in the "Method" section but did not elaborate on this in the "Data Collection and Analysis" section.

Empirical Grounding of the Study Findings

The main finding in this study is that the mothers and the health care providers identified similar and interrelated factors that influenced the nonimmunizing mothers' decisions. Categorized into four groups of emotions, beliefs, facts, and information, each concept was grounded in the data and supported by specific quotes. Three themes emerged:

- Health care providers felt that religion had a great impact on the mothers' decision to not immunize their children.
- The meaning of *evidence* was different for both groups.

- The mothers were generally distrustful of health professionals.

Although the findings were well described and categorized, the depth of discussion was limited. This is an important health issue and deserves a thorough grounding empirically. Since this was described as part of a larger study, it is hoped that the larger program of study will provide more insight.

Conclusions, Implications, and Recommendations

In the "Discussion" section, the authors reiterated and discussed the three themes. They also described additional research that should be undertaken, with a more diverse sample of participants from a broader geographical area. Although some appropriate recommendations were made to increase immunization uptake, more robust recommendations could have been proposed. The conclusion states that greater understanding will lead to greater collaboration, thus promoting better health outcomes for children.

Evidence-Informed Practice Tip

Qualitative research may generate basic knowledge, hypotheses, and theories to be used in the design of other types of qualitative or quantitative studies. However, qualitative research is not necessarily a preliminary step to another type of research. It is a complete and valuable end in itself.

CRITICAL THINKING CHALLENGES

- Discuss the similarities and differences between the stylistic considerations of reporting a qualitative study versus a quantitative study in a professional journal.
- Are critiques of qualitative studies by consumers of research, in the role of either a student or a practising nurse, valid? Which type of qualitative study is the most difficult for consumers of research to critique? Discuss what assumptions led you to this determination.

- Discuss how nurses would go about incorporating qualitative research in evidence-informed practice. Give an example.

FOR FURTHER STUDY

Go to Evolve at http://evolve.elsevier.com/Canada/LoBiondo/Research for the Audio Glossary and Appendix Tables that provide supplemental information for Appendix E.

REFERENCES

Barbour, R. S., & Barbour, M. (2003). Evaluating and synthesizing qualitative research: The need to develop a distinctive approach. *Journal of Evaluation in Clinical Practice, 9,* 179–186.

Chiovitti, R., & Prian, N. (2003). Rigour and grounded theory research. *Journal of Advanced Nursing Practice, 44*(4), 427–435.

Corbin, J., & Strauss, A. (2008). *Basics of qualitative research* (3rd ed.). Thousand Oaks, CA: Sage.

Creswell, J. W. (2014). *Research design: Qualitative, quantitative and mixed methods approaches* (4th ed.). Thousand Oaks, CA: Sage.

Duffy, L. (2015). Achieving a sustainable livelihood after leaving intimate partner violence: Challenges and opportunities. *Journal of Family Violence, 30,* 403–417.

Glaser, B. G. (1998). *Doing grounded theory: Issues and discussions* (2nd ed.). Mill Valley, CA: Sociology Press.

Horsburgh, D. (2003). Evaluation of qualitative research. *Journal of Clinical Nursing, 12,* 307–312.

Jackson, R. L., Drummond, D. K., & Camara, S. (2007). What is qualitative research? *Qualitative Research Reports in Communication, 8*(1), 21–28.

Lincoln, Y. S., & Guba, E. (1985). *Naturalistic inquiry.* Thousand Oaks, CA: Sage.

Merriam, S. B., & Tisdell, E. J. (2016). *Qualitative research: A guide to design and implementation.* San Francisco: Jossey-Bass.

Morse, J. M., Penrod, J., & Hupcey, J. E. (2000). Qualitative outcome analysis: Evaluating nursing interventions for complex clinical phenomena. *Journal of Nursing Scholarship, 32,* 125–130.

Schepner-Hughes, N. (1992). *Death without weeping: The violence of everyday life in Brazil.* Berkeley: University of California Press.

Straus, S. E., Glasziou, P., Richardson, W. S., et al. (2011). *Evidence-based medicine: How to practice and teach it* (4th ed.). Edinburgh: Churchill Livingstone.

Strauss, A., & Corbin, J. (1990). *Basics of qualitative research: Grounded theory procedures and techniques.* Newbury Park, CA: Sage.

Streubert, H. J., & Carpenter, D. R. (2011). *Qualitative research in nursing: Advancing the humanistic imperative* (5th ed.). Philadelphia: Wolters Kluwer.

Vandenberg, S. Y., & Kulig, J. C. (2015). Immunization rejection in southern Alberta: A comparison of the perspective of mothers and health professionals. *Canadian Journal of Nursing Research, 47*(2), 81–96.

Wang, C. C., & Burris, M. A. (1997). Photovoice: concept, methodology, and use for participatory needs assessment. *Health Education & Behavior, 24*(3), 369–387.

Wang, C. C., & Redwood-Jones, Y. (2001). Photovoice ethics: Perspectives from Flint photovoice. *Health Education and Behavior, 28*(5), 560–572.

Wilkin, K., & Slevin, E. (2004). The meaning of caring to nurses: An investigation into the nature of caring work in an intensive care unit. *Journal of Clinical Nursing, 13*, 50–59.

CHAPTER 19

Critiquing Quantitative Research

Nancy E. Kline | Mina D. Singh

LEARNING OUTCOMES

After reading this chapter, you will be able to do the following:

- Identify the purpose of the critiquing process for a quantitative research report.
- Describe the criteria of each step of the critiquing process for a quantitative research report.
- Evaluate the strengths and weaknesses of a quantitative research report.
- Discuss the implications of the findings of a quantitative research report for nursing practice.
- Construct a critique of a quantitative research report.

KEY TERM

scientific merit

STUDY RESOURCES

ⓔ Go to Evolve at http://evolve.elsevier.com/Canada/LoBiondo/Research
for the Audio Glossary and Appendix Tables that provide supplemental
information for Appendix E.

AS REINFORCED THROUGHOUT EACH CHAPTER of this book, it is important not only to conduct and read research but also to use research for evidence-informed practice. As nurse researchers increase the depth (quality) and breadth (quantity) of research methods from descriptive research designs to randomized clinical trials, the data to support clinical interventions and quality outcomes are becoming more readily available. Each published study, regardless of its design, reflects a *level of evidence,* but the critique of each study covers much more than the level of evidence produced by the design. When you critique a research study, examine each component to determine the merit of the report. Key to the critique is the strength of evidence that each study produces individually and collectively.

This chapter presents critiques of two studies in which research questions were tested with different quantitative designs. The critiquing criteria designed to assist research consumers in judging the relative value of a research report are found at the end of previous chapters. These critiquing criteria have been summarized to create an abbreviated set of questions that will be used as a framework for the two sample research critiques (Box 19.1). These critiques exemplify the process of evaluating reported research for potential application to practice, thus extending the research base for nursing. For clarification, refer to earlier

---

<table>
<tr><td colspan="2">BOX **19.1**</td></tr>
<tr><td colspan="2">**MAJOR CONTENT SECTIONS OF A RESEARCH REPORT AND RELATED CRITIQUING GUIDELINES**</td></tr>
</table>

PROBLEM STATEMENT AND PURPOSE (SEE CHAPTER 4)

1. What is the problem explored in, or the purpose of, the research study?
2. Does the statement about the problem or purpose express a relationship between two or more variables (e.g., between an independent variable and a dependent variable)? If so, what is the relationship? Is it testable?
3. Does the statement about the problem or purpose specify the nature of the population being studied? What is it?
4. What significance of the problem—if any—has the investigator identified?

REVIEW OF THE LITERATURE AND THEORETICAL FRAMEWORK (SEE CHAPTERS 2 AND 5)

1. What concepts are included in the review? Of particular importance, note which concepts are the independent and dependent variables and how they are conceptually defined.
2. Does the literature review make the relationships among the variables explicit or place the variables within a theoretical or conceptual framework? What are the relationships?
3. What gaps or conflicts in knowledge of the problem are identified? How is this study intended to fill those gaps or resolve those conflicts?
4. Are the references cited by the author mostly primary or secondary sources? Give an example of each.
5. What are the operational definitions of the independent and dependent variables? Do they reflect the conceptual definitions?

HYPOTHESES OR RESEARCH QUESTIONS (SEE CHAPTER 4)

1. What hypotheses or research questions are stated in the study? Are they appropriately stated?
2. If research questions are stated, are they used in addition to hypotheses or to guide an exploratory study?
3. What are the independent and dependent variables in the statement of each hypothesis or research question?
4. If hypotheses are stated, is the form of the statement statistical (null) or research?
5. What is the direction of the relationship in each hypothesis, if indicated?
6. Are the hypotheses testable?

SAMPLE (SEE CHAPTER 12)

1. How was the sample selected?
2. What type of sampling method is used in the study? Is it appropriate for the design?
3. Does the sample reflect the population as identified in the problem or purpose statement?
4. Is the sample size appropriate? How is it substantiated?
5. To what population may the findings be generalized? What are the limitations in generalizability?

RESEARCH DESIGN (SEE CHAPTERS 10 AND 11)

1. What type of design is used in the study?
2. What is the rationale for the design classification?
3. Does the choice of design seem logical for the proposed research problem, theoretical framework, literature review, and hypothesis?

Continued

BOX **19.1**

MAJOR CONTENT SECTIONS OF A RESEARCH REPORT AND RELATED CRITIQUING GUIDELINES—cont'd

INTERNAL VALIDITY (SEE CHAPTER 9)

1. Discuss each threat to the internal validity of the study.
2. Does the design have controls at an acceptable level for the threats to internal validity?

EXTERNAL VALIDITY (SEE CHAPTER 9)

1. What are the limits to generalizability in terms of external validity?

RESEARCH APPROACH (SEE CHAPTERS 7 AND 11)

1. Does the research approach fit with the purpose of the study?
2. Is a mixed-methods approach, if used, appropriate for the study?

METHODS (SEE CHAPTER 13)

1. What data-collection methods are used in the study?
2. Are the data-collection procedures similar for all participants?

LEGAL/ETHICAL ISSUES (SEE CHAPTER 6)

1. Have the rights of participants been protected? How?
2. What indications are given that informed consent of the participants was ensured?

INSTRUMENTS (SEE CHAPTER 13)

1. Physiological measurement
   a. Is a rationale given for why a particular instrument or method was selected? If so, what is it?
   b. What provision is made for maintaining the accuracy of the instrument and its use, if any?
2. Observational methods
   a. Who did the observing?
   b. How were the observers trained to minimize bias?
   c. Did the observers have an observational guide?
   d. Were the observers required to make inferences about what they saw?
   e. Is there any reason to believe that the presence of the observers affected the behaviour of the participants?
3. Interviews
   a. Who were the interviewers? How were they trained to minimize bias?
   b. Is there evidence of any interviewer bias? If so, what is it?
4. Questionnaires
   a. What is the type or format of the questionnaires (e.g., Likert-type, open-ended)? Are they consistent with the conceptual definitions?
5. Available data and records
   a. Are the records that were used appropriate to the problem studied?
   b. Were the data used to describe the sample or for hypothesis testing?

RELIABILITY AND VALIDITY (SEE CHAPTER 14)

1. What type of reliability is reported for each instrument?
2. What level of reliability is reported? Is it acceptable?
3. What type of validity is reported for each instrument?
4. Does the validity of each instrument seem adequate? Why?

ANALYSIS OF THE DATA (SEE CHAPTER 16)

1. What level of measurement is used to measure each of the major variables?
2. What descriptive or inferential statistics are reported?
3. Were these descriptive or inferential statistics appropriate for the level of measurement for each variable?
4. Are the inferential statistics used appropriate for the intent of the hypotheses?
5. Does the author report the level of significance set for the study? If so, what is it?
6. If tables or figures are used, do they meet the following standards?
   a. They supplement and economize the text.
   b. They have precise titles and headings.
   c. They do not repeat the text.

CONCLUSIONS, IMPLICATIONS, AND RECOMMENDATIONS

1. If hypothesis testing was done, were the hypotheses supported or not supported?
2. Are the results interpreted in the context of the problem or purpose, hypothesis (see this chapter), and theoretical framework or literature reviewed?
3. What does the investigator identify as possible limitations or problems in the study in relation to the design, methods, and sample?
4. What relevance for nursing practice does the investigator identify, if any?
5. What generalizations are made?
6. Are the generalizations within the scope of the findings or beyond the scope of the findings?
7. What recommendations for future research are stated or implied?

APPLICATION AND UTILIZATION (SEE CHAPTER 20)

1. Does the study appear to be valid? In other words, do its strengths for nursing practice outweigh its weaknesses?
2. Do other studies have similar findings?
3. What risks or benefits are involved for patients if the research findings are used in practice?
4. Is direct application of the research findings feasible in terms of time, effort, money, and legal/ethical risks?
5. How and under what circumstances are the findings applicable to nursing practice?
6. Should these results be applied to nursing practice?
7. Would it be possible to replicate this study in another clinical practice setting?

chapters for detailed presentations of the critiquing criteria and explanations of the research process. The criteria and examples in this chapter are applicable to quantitative studies in which researchers used experimental, quasiexperimental, and nonexperimental research designs that provided levels II, III, and IV evidence.

STYLISTIC CONSIDERATIONS

As an evaluator, you should be aware of several aspects of publishing before you begin to critique research studies. First, different journals have different publication goals, and they target specific professional nursing specialties. For example, the *Canadian Journal of Nursing Research* publishes articles on the conduct or results of research in nursing. The *Canadian Oncology Nursing Journal* also publishes research articles; however, because its emphasis is broader, this journal also contains clinical and theoretical articles relating to knowledge, experience, trends, and policies in oncological nursing. Consequently, the style and content of a manuscript will vary according to the type of journal to which it is being submitted.

Second, the author of a research article prepares the manuscript by using both personal judgement and specific journal guidelines. *Personal judgement* refers to the researcher's expertise that is developed in the course of designing, executing, and analyzing the study. As a result of this expertise, the researcher is in a position to judge which content is most important to communicate to the profession. The decision is a function of the following:

- The research design: experimental or nonexperimental
- The focus of the study: basic or clinical
- The audience to whom the results will be most appropriately communicated

Each journal provides the guidelines for preparing research manuscripts for publication, and usually the following major headings are essential sections of a research manuscript or research report:

- Introduction
- Method
- Results
- Discussion

Depending on the stylistic considerations related to the author's preferences and the journal's requirements, the content included in the research report is specific to each of the sections just mentioned.

Stylistic variations (as factors influencing the presentation of the research study) are very distinct features of a research report and can deter from the focus of evaluating the reported research for **scientific merit**—that is, judging the overall quality or validity of a study. Constructive evaluation is based on objective appraisal of the study's strengths and limitations. This step precedes consideration of the relative worth of the findings for clinical application to nursing practice. Judgements of the scientific merit of a research study are the hallmark of promoting a sound evidence base for quality nursing practice.

CRITIQUE 1

The study "Effects of Incivility in Clinical Practice Settings on Nursing Student Burnout" by Yolanda Babenko-Mould and Heather K. S. Laschinger (2014) is critiqued here. The article is presented in its entirety and is followed by the critique on pp. 449–451 (From *International Journal of Nursing Education Scholarship*, 11(1), 145–154.)

Effects of Incivility in Clinical Practice Settings on Nursing Student Burnout

Yolanda Babenko-Mould and Heather K. S. Laschinger

ABSTRACT

AIMS. To examine the relationship between nursing students' exposure to various forms of incivility in acute care practice settings and their experience of burnout.

BACKGROUND. Given that staff nurses and new nurse graduates are experiencing incivility and burnout in the workplace, it is plausible that nursing students share similar experiences in professional practice settings.

DESIGN AND SAMPLE. A cross-sectional survey design was used to assess Year 4 nursing students' (n=126) perceptions of their experiences of incivility and burnout in the clinical learning environment.

METHODS. Students completed instruments to assess frequency of uncivil behaviors experienced during the past six months from nursing staff, clinical instructors, and other health professionals in the acute care practice setting and to measure student burnout.

RESULTS. Reported incidences of incivility in the practice setting were related to burnout. Higher rates of incivility, particularly from staff nurses, were associated with higher levels of both components of burnout (emotional exhaustion and cynicism).

INTRODUCTION

"Workplace violence is one of the most complex and dangerous occupational hazards facing nurses working in today's health care environment"

Citation Information: International Journal of Nursing Education Scholarship. Volume 11, Issue 1, Pages 145-154, ISSN (Online) 1548-923X, ISSN (Print) 2194-5772, DOI: 10.1515/ijnes-2014-0023, October 2014
International Journal of Nursing Education Scholarship 2014; 11(1): 145-154

(McPhaul & Lipscomb, 2004, p. 1). Incivility is a subtle type of workplace violence and has been classically defined as "low-intensity deviant behavior with ambiguous intent to harm the target, in violation of workplace norms for mutual respect. Uncivil behaviours are characteristically rude and discourteous, displaying a lack of regard for others" (Andersson & Pearson, 1999, p. 457). Increasing patient acuity levels, escalating nursing shortages, and limited programs or regulations to stem incidents of workplace violence in health care practice environments can combine to create a context where incivility may escalate to more harmful forms of workplace violence (Clark & Springer, 2010). Studies in nursing settings have linked nurses' perceptions of workplace violence to negative job and health effects (Laschinger, Leiter, Day, & Gilin, 2009a; Laschinger, Grau, Finegan, & Wilk, 2010; Smith, Andrusyszyn, & Laschinger, 2010) but less is known about nursing students' experiences of incivility and its effects (Clark, 2008; Clark, 2011; Gallo, 2012). Nursing students are a vital resource to the life of the profession, yet there is limited research examining how incivility in nursing education practice settings influences nursing student well-being.

Nursing students are embedded in practice settings where their learning experiences and well-being might be either positively or negatively impacted depending on the 'health' of the workplace. Numerous anecdotal reports of nursing students' exposure to negative workplace behaviours in their clinical learning experiences exist (Foster, Mackie, & Barnett, 2004; Hoel, Giga, & Davidson, 2007). These experiences are stressful for students, undermining their self-confidence and often their emotional health (Bronner, Peretz, & Ehrenfeld, 2003; Fell, 2000; Randle, 2003). Stress can lead to burnout and poor health among nursing students (Deary, Watson, & Hogston, 2003), and the negative health effects of burnout are well documented in the nursing and management literature (Schaufeli, Leiter, & Maslach, 2009). It is not surprising that exposure to these negative interpersonal behaviours in the clinical setting may influence students' career choice (Curtis, Bowen, & Reid, 2007; Hoel et al., 2007). In this time of global critical nursing shortages, it is vital that nursing students, who represent the future workforce, are able to develop and use professional knowledge, skills, and judgments in supportive practice environments. Nursing education practice environments are meant to be settings where students integrate their theoretical and practice-based learning. Such settings should not threaten students' health and wellbeing and lead to premature burnout and possibly decisions to leave the profession.

BACKGROUND

Incivility

In their seminal work on workplace incivility Andersson and Pearson (1999) suggested that unchecked incivility might be a precursor to more severe workplace violence through an upward spiral of incivility. Incivility involves disregarding others' feelings, displaying a lack of regard for one another, and violating workplace norms (Andersson & Pearson, 1999; Pearson & Porath, 2005). Workplace norms consist ". . . of basic moral standards and others that have arisen out of the tradition of that community, including those prescribed by formal and informal organizational policies, rules and procedures" (Andersson & Pearson, 1999, p. 455). Examples of incivility include more covert forms of aggression and violence, such as rude comments, thoughtless acts, and negative gestures (Andersson & Pearson, 1999). Power plays a

central role in incivility; therefore, those of lower status than the instigator are more likely to experience incivility (Pearson & Porath, 2005).

Cortina and Magley (2009) found that 74% of university employees experienced at least once uncivil behaviour in the workplace and employees reported being more distressed when incivility was experienced as coming from the 'top down'. On the other hand, a study of university students revealed that incivility was equally or no less harmful when the perpetrator was a peer or person of authority (Caza & Cortina, 2007). Leiter, Price, and Laschinger (2010) found that supervisor incivility was more strongly related to emotional exhaustion and job turnover than coworker incivility. Interestingly, although supervisor incivility may produce worse outcomes for the staff member, more nurses are experiencing incivility from their co-workers (Laschinger et al., 2009a).

To date, researchers have found that staff nurses' experiences of incivility in the practice setting are associated with job dissatisfaction and higher turnover intentions (Laschinger, et al., 2009a), poor physical health (Gilin Oore, Leblanc, Day, Leiter, Laschinger, Price, & Latimer, 2010), and higher levels of burnout (Laschinger, Finegan, & Wilk, 2009b; Laschinger, Leiter, Day, Gilin Oore, & Mackinnon, 2012; Leiter et al., 2010). Laschinger, et al. (2012) conducted a study of hospital employees' (n=1106) experiences with workplace empowerment, incivility, and burnout and found that of the 612 nurse participants, 47.3% reported severe burnout. Leiter et al., (2010) found that younger nurses (generation X) experienced greater exhaustion, cynicism, turnover intentions, and physical symptoms as a result of incivility than 'Baby Boomer' nurses.

Research with new nurse graduates has linked bullying and incivility in the workplace to burnout, stress, absenteeism, decreased job satisfaction (Boychuk-Duchscher & Cowin 2004; Gustavsson, Hallsten, & Rudman, 2010) and poor mental health (Laschinger, Wong, & Grau, 2013). Given that staff nurses and new nurse graduates are experiencing incivility and burnout in the workplace, it is plausible that nursing students share similar experiences during their learning experiences in professional practice (clinical) settings.

Nursing students experience a wide range of uncivil behaviours throughout their education, both in the classroom and clinical setting. Anthony and Yastik (2011) conducted a qualitative study (n=18) and identified three forms of nursing students' experiences of incivility in the clinical setting, namely: exclusion (students felt they were in the way and nurses did not accept responsibility for them), hostility or rudeness (leading nursing students to question their commitment to nursing), and dismissiveness (nurses often ignored and walked away from students). Ferns and Meerabeay (2009) studied nursing students' experiences of verbal abuse during their clinical learning experiences and discovered that students reported greater abuse from staff nurses than visitors or patients. Marchiondo, Marchiondo, & Lasiter (2010) found that 88% of senior nursing students reported experiencing at least one instance of incivility in their nursing education program. Incivility was highest in the classroom, followed by the clinical setting. In another study by these researchers, nursing students reported being criticised, yelled at, laughed at, threatened, belittled, gossiped about, made to feel incompetent, incapable or stupid as a result of instructors' actions or communication and some suggested nursing students should select a career other than nursing (Lasiter, Marchiondo, & Marchiondo, 2012). Nursing students who experienced bullying and incivility from health care team members reported feeling excluded, dismissed, insignificant, anxious, nervous, and depressed (Anthony & Yastik, 2011; Marchiondo et al., 2010). Alarmingly, one nursing student reported she was still trying "to get over" the experience two years later (Lasiter et al., 2012), suggesting the impact of incivility lasts far beyond the actual incident.

Burnout

The phenomenon of burnout (Maslach, Schaufeli, & Leiter, 2001) is described as a psychological syndrome resulting from prolonged workplace interpersonal stressors (Jackson, Schuler, & Schwab, 1986; Maslach et al., 2001). The three central dimensions include exhaustion (individual stress and depletion of emotional and physical resources), cynicism (depersonalization and negative or detached response to various workplace characteristics), and ineffectiveness (selfevaluation and includes feelings of incompetence and lack of achievement). Exhaustion is central to burnout and is the most widely reported; however, while it is a crucial component of burnout it "fails to capture the critical aspects of the relationship people have with their work" (Maslach et al., 2001, p. 403). Distancing is an immediate reaction to exhaustion; therefore, cynicism is directly linked to exhaustion. More recently, views of burnout focus on the emotional exhaustion and cynicism components of burnout (Bakker, Le Blanc, & Schaufeli, 2005).

Laschinger et al., (2012) found experienced nurses had higher levels of burnout than new nurse graduates, while others suggested younger nurses experienced greater distress (Leiter et al., 2010). Nurse burnout has been linked to higher patient-nurse ratios (Aiken, Clarke, Sloane, Sochalski, & Silber, 2002), authentic leadership (Laschinger et al., 2012), and incivility (Laschinger et al., 2009a; Laschinger et al., 2012; Leiter et al., 2010). Numerous studies have shown that nurses experienced higher levels of exhaustion than cynicism (Laschinger et al., 2009a; Laschinger et al., 2009b; Laschinger et al., 2012), although the two aspects of burnout are strongly correlated (Laschinger et al., 2012).

Nursing student burnout has been related to health problems, lower life satisfaction, and higher turnover (Rudman & Gustavsson, 2012). The issue of burnout among nursing students was being examined as early as 1995 when Beck linked nursing student burnout to poor interpersonal relationships and feelings of irritability and moodiness. Since that time, studies of nursing student burnout have found that burnout rates increase as students progress through educational program (Rella et al., 2008; Rudman & Gustavsson, 2012). Rudman and Gustavsson (2012) found burnout increased from 29.7% in the first year to 41% in the final year. In addition, Rudman and Gustavsson (2012) found that early development of burnout in nursing students was linked to decreased skill mastery, decreased use of research in practice, and higher turnover intentions one year after graduating. This is alarming given the importance of having skilled and informed professional nurses. Additionally, with the current projected nursing shortage, reported turnover intentions of new nurse graduates is concerning. Several studies have linked personality traits to burnout in nursing education (Burisch 2002; Deary et al., 2003; Watson et al., 2008) with mixed results. Burisch (2002) suggest that students' experiences during their nursing education program may be a better predictor of emotional exhaustion then personality traits. Finally, Gibbons (2010) recently noted that final year nursing students who had lower levels of self-efficacy, decreased perceptions of support in practice, and primarily used avoidance coping skills were more likely to be experiencing burnout, in the form of emotional exhaustion and depersonalization, in the clinical practice setting. Negative experiences, such as incivility, are highly concerning and logical precursors of burnout during nursing education, although we could find no research linking these constructs.

PURPOSE

The purpose of this study was to examine the relationship between nursing students' exposure to various forms of incivility in their clinical learning environments and their experience of burnout. We hypothesized that nursing student experiences of incivility from clinical instructors, nursing staff in their clinical learning environments, and from other health professionals are related to their experiences of burnout (emotional exhaustion and cynicism). Thus, it is proposed that increased incidences of incivility are related to increased rates of emotional exhaustion and burnout.

DESIGN AND SAMPLE

A cross-sectional survey design was used to test a theoretical model associating nursing students' perceptions of their experiences of incivility and burnout in the clinical learning environment. One hundred and twenty six baccalaureate nursing students in their fourth year, who were enrolled in a nursing education program in Southwestern Ontario were invited to participate in the study. As an inclusion criterion, only students who had recently completed an acute care clinical practice experience were eligible to participate. Nursing students not in their fourth year of the nursing program, or who had yet to participate in a clinical experience in the year were excluded from participating in the study. The sample size was calculated prior to data collection using the G*Power program. Based on a pre-test post-test design with one-tailed correlational analysis, a power of 0.80 and an alpha of 0.05 it was deemed that 64 participants would be required to detect a small effect size of 0.3. However, given the potential for non-participation, the entire fourth year class of approximately 190 students were recruited to participate in the study.

METHODS
Ethical considerations and data collection

The study was conducted after receiving ethics approval from the institution's Research Ethics Board. There were no known ethical issues associated with the study. One of the researchers attended the final fourth year theory class to distribute the study package to each student. The package consisted of the letter of information, the study demographic form, study instruments, and a gift certificate to a local coffee shop for compensation of students' time. Students were provided with the opportunity to complete and return the package to a researcher within 15 minutes of class time, or to return the package to the researcher's university office. No clinical instructors were present during data collection.

DATA ANALYSIS

Quantitative data from study instrument responses was analyzed using SPSS V19 (IBM). Analysis included: descriptive statistics, Cronbach's alpha reliability analysis, t-tests, and correlational analysis. The study hypotheses were tested using two separate multiple regression analyses.

VALIDITY AND RELIABILITY— INSTRUMENTATION

The Cortina Incivility Scale (CIS) (Cortina & Magley, 2001), was utilized to assess students' perceptions of the frequency of uncivil behaviours experienced during the past six months from nursing staff, clinical instructors, and other health professionals in the clinical learning practice environment. Items are rated on a 5-point Likert scale which ranges from 1 = never to 5 = everyday. Smith et al. (2010) reported acceptable Chronbach alpha reliability (α = .85–89).

The Emotional Exhaustion (EE) and Cynicism (C) subscales of the Maslach Burnout Inventory-General Survey (MBI-GS) (Schaufeli, Leiter, Maslach, & Jackson, 1996) were employed to measure nursing student burnout. Participants are requested to rate how often they have felt a certain way in the practice setting. Ratings are recorded on a 7-point Likert scale where 0 = never and 6 = every day. According to Leiter and Maslach (2004), a score greater than 3 on each subscale is suggestive of burnout. Both studies have demonstrated acceptable reliability and validity across numerous studies (Schaufeli et al., 1996).

TABLE **19C1.1**

PARTICIPANT DEMOGRAPHIC CHARACTERISTICS (N=126)

Variable	M	SD
Age	22.40	3.60

	Frequency	
	N	%
Gender		
Male	3	2.4
Female	123	97.6
Marital Status		
Single	117	92.9
Married	6	4.8
Other	3	2.4
Previous Healthcare Experience		
None	20	15.9
Volunteer Work	11	8.7
Personal Support Worker	34	27.0
High School Co-op	2	1.6
Registered Practical Nurse	2	1.6
Multiple experiences	6	4.8
Other	51	40.5

RESULTS

Demographics

The average age of nursing students in this study was 22.41 years of age (min = 20, max = 44). Three males and 122 females were involved in the study. The majority were single (116), six were married, and three self-identified as 'other'. On average, participants completed six weeks of clinical placement experience in the past six months and worked an average of 11.96 hours per shift. In relation to reporting previous experience in healthcare, 11 had volunteered in a healthcare setting, 34 had been employed as personal support workers, two had participated in a high-school co-op experience, two had been employed as registered practical nurses, and 19 identified as having no previous experience in healthcare (see Table 19C1.1).

TABLE **19C1.2**

MEANS, STANDARD DEVIATIONS, CRONBACH'S ALPHA AND CORRELATION COEFFICIENTS

STUDY VARIABLE	M	SD	α	1.	2.	3.	4.
Incivility							
1. Nurse Incivility	1.83	0.61	.83				
2. Instructor Incivility	1.20	0.55	.94	.13			
3. Healthcare	1.46	0.45	.78	.61*	-.12		
Professionals' Incivility							
Burnout							
4. Emotional Exhaustion	2.91	1.38	.88	.42*	.24*	.18*	
5. Cynicism	1.25	1.15	.86	.29*	.12	.14	.47*

*p < 0.05

DESCRIPTIVE RESULTS

The means and standard deviations for the major study variables are presented in Table 19C1.2. On average, students did not experience high levels of incivility. Incivility from staff nurses in their clinical learning units was highest (M = 1.83, SD = 0.61), followed by incivility from other health professionals and clinical instructors. However, 59% reported experiencing staff nurse incivility 1-2 times per month and 51% experienced incivility from other health professionals at this rate. Clinical instructor incivility was lowest with 15% of students reporting never having experienced incivility from their instructors. Similarly, average burnout levels were moderate but 49.2% reported severe levels of emotional exhaustion according to Maslach, Jackson, and Leiter's (1996) criteria.

Fourth year nursing students' experiences of incivility from nurses, clinical instructors, and other health professionals were significantly related to the emotional exhaustion component of burnout ($r = 0.42$, p < 0.001, $r = 0.24$, p < 0.05, and $r = 0.18$, p < 0.05, respectively). On the other hand, cynicism was significantly associated with students' encounters of incivility from staff nurses ($r = 0.289, p < 0.05$), but not with incivility from clinical instructors or other health professionals. The strongest correlation with both components of burnout was students' incivility experiences with staff nurses in their clinical learning settings (See Table 19C1.2).

Hierarchical multiple regression analyses revealed that incivility experiences from staff nurses, clinical instructors, and other health professionals in the clinical learning environment were significantly related to burnout (after controlling for previous healthcare work experience prior to their educational program). For the emotional exhaustion model, incivility experiences explained 23% of the variance. Both unit staff nurse incivility and clinical instructor incivility towards students were significant independent predictors of students' reported emotional exhaustion ($\beta = .487$ and .193, p < 0.05, respectively). In the cynicism model, the combined sources of incivility, controlling for previous work experience in healthcare explained 9% of the total variance. Staff nurse incivility towards students was the only significant independent predictor of students' reported cynicism ($\beta = .316$, p < .05). Incivility from other health professionals was not a significant predictor of either emotional exhaustion or cynicism.

DISCUSSION

The results provided support to the study hypothesis that nursing students' reported incidences of incivility in the clinical learning environment are related to burnout. Higher rates of incivility, particularly from staff nurses, were associated with higher levels of both components of burnout (emotional exhaustion and cynicism). In this study, all sources of incivility were related to emotional exhaustion, which is concerning given that exhaustion is the core element of burnout. When exhaustion is prolonged, it results in cynicism and personal inefficacy (Maslach & Leiter, 1997). Although staff nurse incivility was also associated with higher cynicism, the effect was not as strong. This may reflect the stage of these students in that their exposure to workplace realities is still limited. Nevertheless, the strong link to emotional exhaustion at this stage of their career is disturbing. Given that almost half of these students reported severe levels of emotional exhaustion, the influence of incivility from staff nurses reported in this study is an important finding and points to an area that must be addressed.

These findings are similar to previous research with new graduate nurses where incivility, primarily attributed from coworkers, was associated with burnout and negative mental health issues (Laschinger et al., 2013). In a comparable study, new graduate nurses' experiences of bullying and burnout were related to access to empowering structures in the practice environment (Laschinger et al., 2010), suggesting that supportive working conditions play an important role in preventing uncivil behaviour. Levels of burnout and incidences of incivility reported by new graduate nurses in Bushell's (2013) study were very similar to those reported by nursing students in this study. Bushell (2013) found that new graduate nurses' experience of co-worker incivility were associated with both emotional exhaustion and cynicism. Budin, Brewer, Chao, and Kovner (2013) found that early career nurses who experienced incidences of verbal abuse from colleagues reported decreased: organizational commitment, job satisfaction, autonomy, and intent to remain in the practice setting. Results from this study with nursing students are in keeping with studies in the general nursing population that have linked co-worker incivility to higher levels of burnout and job dissatisfaction

(Laschinger et al., 2009a). These findings demonstrate the potentially devastating effects of non-supportive colleagues in nursing education environments that threaten students' health and well-being and highlights the need to address incivility in clinical learning settings.

IMPLICATIONS AND RECOMMENDATIONS

If nursing students are already experiencing emotional exhaustion and a sense of detachment in the form of cynicism as an outcome of exposure to workplace incivility, then how might that further impact their professional development as soon-to-be nurses, how will it impact retention rates upon graduation, and what might be the implications for patient care? The rates of incivility experienced by students in the clinical learning environment and the associated levels of burnout in our study are disturbing and could have far reaching implications. Emotional exhaustion might lead to higher rates of student absenteeism from clinical practice, chronic fatigue, decreased mental health, and a decrease in students' ability to focus and concentrate. The cascade effect of a student experiencing chronic fatigue and impaired concentration relates to potential patient safety issues, as well as retention issues upon entering practice after graduation.

The negative effects of exposure to incivility, particularly from staff nurses in their clinical learning environments, which culminate in burnout have serious implications for students' health and well-being. For example, in a qualitative study, Altmiller (2012) found that students who experienced incivility from clinical instructors felt hopeless and fearful, which disrupted their abilities to learn in the practice setting. Nursing students in Clark's (2008) qualitative study reported feeling traumatized, helpless, and upset after having been at the receiving end of uncivil behaviour on the part of a faculty member. When students feel traumatized, might there occur a residual effect that carries forward in regards to students' cognitive, affective, and psychomotor performance during the rest of a clinical practice day or extend through the duration of a clinical course? As Leiter et al. (2010) suggest, when uncivil behaviours in the practice setting become chronic in nature, then nurses might be more apt to consider leaving the profession. Thus, frequent exposure to incivility over the course of their nursing education program may have a negative impact on their career choices before or soon after graduation. Sadly, many nurses can often call to mind instances where they had negative experiences as students in clinical practice where they were berated or belittled by a clinical instructor or nurse. Such memories have the potential to gain traction in one's psyche as a developing professional nurse. However, the implications of such experiences can turn out to be positive, in that students might decide to refuse to ever engage in such behaviours with peers, future nurse colleagues, or in a future role as an educator.

Clearly, issues of incivility and burnout require attention from both educators and students during nursing education programs in a manner that aligns with students' stage of professional development. It is important that students have opportunities during their education to practice how they would respond to real-world scenarios that involved uncivil behaviours. When students have a 'toolbox' of strategies in place, they might feel more confident and competent to deal with incidences of incivility so that they don't progress to stages of exhaustion and burnout. A strengths- based perspective on these issues could enhance students' capacity to understand the varied factors that can contribute to incidents of incivility. Further, developing strong coping and self-care management knowledge and skills might be a way for students to foster trusting, supportive, and collegial relationships in their professional and personal lives (Clark, 2013).

Educators can create learning moments with students as they engage in the process of becoming aware of what civility encompasses and how educators, nurses, and students can contribute to creating and sustaining a culture of civility in the classroom and practice setting (Clark, 2013). Clinical instructors can play a major role in learning about the differences between uncivil behaviours and empowering teaching behaviours so that they are aware of disempowering actions that can negatively impact students' learning and professional development. When educators support students' goal achievement and engage in advocacy behaviours on behalf of students, the potential exists to enhance students' confidence for professional practice (Babenko-Mould, Iwasiw, Andrusyszyn, Laschinger, & Weston, 2012). When clinical instructors become aware of incidences of incivility being perpetuated by staff nurses or other health professionals on students, they have a preventative role to play in taking decisive and reasoned actions to address the issue in order to help create a culture of civility in the practice setting (Clark & Springer, 2010; Vessey & O'Neill, 2011).

It is important for instructors to mobilize supports and resources from the academic setting to help address issues of incivility in students' practice placements; otherwise, the clinical instructor could also be at risk for not feeling as though they can effectively carry out their role (Wiens, 2012). Clinical practice setting co-ordinators also have a key role to play in surveying students' and clinical instructors' experiences of the practice environment in relation to supporting students' learning goals. A database of information could be developed to gain a stronger picture of what practice sites are most conducive for both teacher and student involvement, and why, and which sites might need to be re-evaluated before additional students are sent to the site. In times of placement shortages, the initial reaction might be to preserve all placement sites regardless of student or instructor anecdotal reports. However, nursing education programs have an ethical mandate to ensure students, and instructors, are practicing in areas that don't negatively influence student health or well-being.

STUDY LIMITATIONS

A self-report bias might exist, as students re-ported about their perceptions about their most recent clinical practice experiences. The sample size could be a study limitation, as one nursing program site was sampled from at one point in time. However, the students were responding about experiences they had from a number of acute care practice settings across the Southwest-ern Ontario area, which are teaching hospitals that partner with the academic nursing program.

CONCLUSION

The results of this study provide evidence for the detrimental effects of incivility within nurs-ing student clinical learning environments. All sources of incivility were associated with burn-out, but the influence of incivility from nurses working on clinical learning settings was par-ticularly strong. This is the first study we know of to demonstrate these effects in nursing educa-tion settings and highlight the need for nurse educators to address this serious phenomenon in clinical learning environments. The ethical man-date of advocacy and the underpinning philoso-phy of promoting healthy work environments must always be at the forefront of clinical in-structors' way of being as nurse educators in order to best support students' development as nurses. This approach can go a long way to-wards ensuring that new nurse graduates feel confident in their abilities to practice according to high professional standards and experience satisfying careers. This is particularly important in a time a of an impending nursing workforce shortage worldwide.

REFERENCES

Aiken, L. H., Clarke, S. P., Sloane, D. M., Sochalski, J., & Silber, J. H. (2002). Hospital nurse staffing and pa-tient mortality, nurse burnout and job dissatisfaction. *JAMA, 288*, 1987–1993.

Altmiller, G. (2012). Student perceptions of incivility in nursing education: Implications for educators. *Nursing Education Perspectives, 33*, 15–20. http://dx.doi. org/10.5480/1536-5026-33.1.15.

Andersson, L. M., & Pearson, C. M. (1999). Tit for tat? The spiralling effect of incivility in the workplace. *The Academy of Management Review, 24*, 452–471.

Anthony, M., & Yastik, J. (2011). Nursing students' experience with incivility in clinical education. *Journal of Nursing Education, 50*, 140–144. doi:10/392801484834-20110131-04.

Babenko-Mould, Y., Iwasiw, C., Andrusyszyn, M. A., Laschinger, H. K. S., & Weston, W. (2012). Effects of clinical practice environments on clinical teacher and nursing student outcomes. *Journal of Nursing Educa-tion, 51*, 217–225. doi:10.3928/01484834-20120323-06.

Bakker, A. B., Le Blanc, P. M., & Schaufeli, W. B. (2005). Burnout contagion among intensive care nurses. *Journal of Advanced Nursing, 51*, 276–287.

Beck, C. T. (1995). Burnout in undergraduate nursing students. *Nurse Educator, 20*, 19–23.

Boychuk-Duchscher, J. E., & Cowin, L. (2004). Multi-generational nurses in the workplace. *Journal of Nursing Administration, 34*, 493–501.

Bronner, G., Peretz, C., & Ehrenfeld, M. (2003). Sexual harassment of nurses and nursing students. *Journal of Advanced Nursing, 42*, 637–644.

Budin, W., Brewer, C., Chao, Y. Y., & Kovner, C. (2013). Verbal abuse from nurse colleagues and work environ-ment of early career Registered Nurses. *Journal of Nursing Scholarship, 45*, 308–316. doi:10.1111/ jnu.12033.

Burisch, M. (2002). A longitudinal study of burnout: The relative importance of dispositions and experiences. *Work & Stress, 16*, 1–17. doi:10.1080/02678370110112506.

Bushell, P. (2013). *New graduate nurses' structural em-powerment and their experience of coworker incivility and burnout* (Unpublished doctoral dissertation). Uni-versity of Western Ontario, London, Ontario, Canada.

Caza, B. B., & Cortina, L. M. (2007). From insult to injury: Explaining the impact of incivility. *Basic and Applied Social Psychology, 29*, 335–350.

Clark, C. (2008). Student perspectives on faculty incivil-ity in nursing education: An application of the concept of rankism. *Nursing Outlook, 56*, 4–8.

Clark, C. (2011). Faculty empowerment of students to foster civility in nursing education: A merging of two conceptual models. *Nursing Outlook, 59*, 158–165. doi:10.1016/j.outlook.2010.12.005.

Clark, C. (2013). *Creating and sustaining civility in nursing education*. Indiana: Sigma Theta Tau Interna-tional Honor Society of Nursing.

Clark, C., & Springer, P. J. (2010). Academic nurse leaders' role in fostering a culture of civility in nursing education. *Journal of Nursing Education, 49,* 319–325. doi:10.3928/01484834-20100224-01.

Cortina, L. M., & Magley, V. J. (2009). Patterns and profiles of response to incivility in the workplace. *Journal of Occupational Health Psychology, 14,* 272–288. doi:10.1037/a0014934.

Curtis, J., Bowen, I., & Reid, A. (2007). You have no credibility: Nursing students' experiences of horizontal violence. *Nurse Education in Practice, 7,* 156–163.

Deary, I. J., Watson, R., & Hogston, R. (2003). A longitudinal cohort study of burnout and attrition in nursing students. *Journal of Advanced Nursing, 43,* 71–81.

Fell, L. (2000). Do nurses eat their young? *Kai Tiaki Nursing New Zealand, 6,* 21.

Ferns, T., & Meerabeau, E. (2009). Reporting behaviours of nursing students who have experienced verbal abuse. *Journal of Advanced Nursing, 65,* 2678–2688. doi:10.1111/j.1365-2648.2009.05114.x.

Foster, B., Mackie, B., & Barnett, N. (2004). Bullying in the health sector: A study of bullying of student nurses. *N Z J Employment Relations, 29,* 67–83.

Gallo, V. J. (2012). Incivility in nursing education: A review of the literature. *Teaching and Learning in Nursing, 7,* 62–66. doi:10.1016/j.teln.2011.11.006.

Gibbons, C. (2010). Stress, coping and burnout in nursing students. *International Journal of Nursing Studies, 47,* 1299–1309. doi:10.1016/j.ijnurstu.2010.02.015.

Gilin Oore, D., Leblanc, D., Day, A., Leiter, M. P., Laschinger, H. K. S., Price, S. L., & Latimer, M. (2010). When respect deteriorates: Incivility as a moderator of the stressor-strain relationship among hospital workers. *Journal of Nursing Management, 18,* 878–888. doi:10.1111/j.1365–2834.2010.01139.x.

Gustavsson, J. P., Hallsten, L., & Rudman, A. (2010). Early career burnout among nurses: Modeling a hypothesized process using an item response approach. *International Journal of Nursing Studies, 47,* 864–875. doi:10.1016/j.ijnurstu.2009.12.007.

Hoel, H., Giga, S. I., & Davidsion, M. J. (2007). Expectations and realities of student nurses' experiences of negative behaviour and bullying in clinical placement and the influences of socialization processes. *Health Services Management Research, 20,* 270–278.

Jackson, S. E., Schuler, R. S., & Schwab, R. L. (1986). Toward an understanding of the burnout phenomenon. *Journal of Applied Psychology, 71,* 630–640.

Laschinger, H. K. S., Leiter, M., Day, A., & Gilin, D. (2009a). Workplace empowerment, incivility, and burnout: Impact on staff nurse recruitment and retention outcomes. *Journal of Nursing Management, 17,* 302–311. doi:10.1111/j.1365–2834.00999.x.

Laschinger, H. K. S., Finegan, J., & Wilk, P. (2009b). New graduate burnout: The impact of professional practice environment, workplace civility, and empowerment. *Nursing Economics, 27,* 377–383.

Laschinger, H. K. S., Grau, A. L., Finegan, J., & Wilk, P. (2010). New graduate nurses' experiences of bullying and burnout in hospital settings. *Journal of Advanced Nursing, 66,* 2732–2742. doi:10.1111/j.1365-2648.2010.05420.x.

Laschinger, H. K. S., Leiter, M. P., Day, A., Gilin Oore, D., & Mackinnon, S. P. (2012). Building empowering work environments that foster civility and organizational trust: Testing an intervention. *Nursing Research, 61,* 316–325. doi:10.1097/NNR.0b013e318265a58d.

Laschinger, H. K. S., Wong, C. A., & Grau, A. L. (2013). Authentic leadership, empowerment and burnout: A comparison in new graduates and experienced nurses. *Journal of Nursing Management, 21,* 541–552. doi:10.1111/j.1365-2834.2012.01375.x.

Laschinger, H. K. S., Wong, C. A., Regan, S., Young-Ritchie, C., & Bushell P. (2013). Workplace incivility and new graduate nurses' mental health: the protective role of resiliency. *Journal of Nursing Administration, 43,* 415–421. doi:10.1097/NNA.0b013e31829d61c6.

Leiter, M. P., Laschinger, H. K. S., Day, A., & Gilin Oore, D. (2011). The impact of civility interventions on employee social behaviour, distress, and attitudes. *Journal of Applied Psychology, 96,* 1258–1274. doi:10.1037/a0024442.

Lasiter, S., Marchiondo, L., & Marchiondo, K. (2012). Student narratives of faculty incivility. *Nursing Outlook, 60,* 121–126. doi:10.1016/j.outlook.2011.06.001.

Leiter, M. P., & Maslach, C. (2004). Areas of worklife: A structured approach to organizational predictors of job burnout. In P. L. Perrewe & D. C. Ganster (Eds.), *Research in occupational stress and well-being* (pp. 91–134). Oxford: Elsevier.

Leiter, M. P., Price, S. L., & Laschinger, H. K. (2010). Generational differences in distress, attitudes and incivility among nurses. *Journal of Nursing Management, 18,* 970–980. doi:10.1111/j.1365–2834.2010.01168.x.

Maslach, C., Schaufeli, W. B., & Leiter, M. P. (2001). Job burnout. *Annual Review of Psychology, 52,* 397–422.

Maslach, C., Jackson, S. E., & Leiter, M. P. (1996). *Maslach burnout inventory manual* (3rd ed.). Palo Alto, CA: Consulting Psychologists Press.

Maslach, C., & Leiter, M. P. (1997). *The truth about burnout: How organizations cause personal stress and what to do about it.* San Francisco, CA: Jossey-Bass.

Marchiondo, K., Marchiondo, L. A., & Lasiter, S. (2010). Faculty incivility: Effects on program satisfaction of BSN students. *Journal of Nursing Education, 49*, 608–614. doi:10.3928/01484834-20100524-05.

McPhaul, K., & Lipscomb, J. (September 30, 2004). Workplace violence in health care: Recognized but not regulated. *Online Journal of Issues in Nursing, 9*, Manuscript 6. Retrieved from http://www.nursing-world.org/ojin/topic25/tpc25_6.htm.

Pearson, C. M., & Porath, C. L. (2005). On the nature, consequences and remedies of workplace incivility: No time for "nice"? Think again. *Academy of Management Executive, 19*, 7–18.

Randle, J. (2003). Bullying in the nursing profession. *Journal of Advanced Nursing, 43*, 395–401.

Rella, S., Windwood, P. C., & Lushington, K. (2008). When does nursing burnout begin? An investigation of the fatigue experience of Australian nursing students. *Journal of Nursing Management, 17*, 886–897. doi:10.1111/j.1365-2834.2008.00883.x.

Rudman, A., & Gustavsson, J. P. (2012). Burnout during nursing education predicts lower occupational preparedness and future clinical performance: A longitudinal study. *International Journal of Nursing Studies, 49*, 988–1001. doi:10.1016/j.ijnurstu.2012.03.010.

Schaufeli, W. B., Leiter, M. P., Maslach, C., & Jackson, S. E. (1996). Maslach burnout inventory-general survey. In C. Maslach, S. E. Jackson, & M. P. Leiter (Eds.), *The Maslach burnout inventory-test manual* (3rd ed., pp. 22–26). Palo Alto, CA: Consulting Psychologists Press.

Schaufeli, W. B., Leiter, M. P., & Maslach, C. (2009). Burnout: 35 years of research and practice. *Career Development International, 14*, 204–220. doi:http://dx.doi.org/10.1108/13620430910966406.

Smith, L. M., Andrusyszyn, M. A., & Laschinger, H. K. S. (2010). Effects of workplace incivility and empowerment on newly graduated nurses' organizational commitment. *Journal of Nursing Management, 18*, 1004–1015. doi:10.1111/j.1365-2834.2010.01165.x.

IBM Software. (2012). *SPSS V19*. IBM. http://www-01.ibm.com/software/analytics/spss/products/statistics/downloads.html.

Tatano, C. (1997). Burnout in undergraduate nursing students. *Nurse Educator, 20*, 19–23.

Vessey, J. A., & O'Neill, K. M. (2011). Helping students with disabilities better address teasing and bullying situations: A MASNRN study. *JOSN, 27*, 139–148. doi:10.1177/1059840510386490.

Watson, R., Deary, I., Thompson, D., & Li, G. (2008). A study of stress and burnout in nursing students in Hong Kong: A questionnaire survey. *International Journal of Nursing Studies, 45*, 1534–1542. doi:10.1016/j.ijnurstu.2007.11.003.

Wiens, S. (2012). *Clinical instructors' perceptions of structural and psychological empowerment in academic nursing environments* (Unpublished doctoral dissertation). University of Western Ontario, London, Ontario, Canada.

INTRODUCTION TO CRITIQUE 1

The article "Effects of Incivility in Clinical Practice Settings on Nursing Student Burnout" (Babenko-Mould & Laschinger, 2014) is examined here in terms of its quality and the potential usefulness of the findings for application to nursing practice. The design of this study is level VI, inasmuch as it is a cross-sectional study.

Title

The title of the article captures the essence of the study succinctly.

Abstract

The abstract meets the requirements of a good abstract; it includes aim, background, design and sample, methods, and results.

Problem and Purpose

Babenko-Mould and Laschinger (2014) stated that the overall purpose of the study was "to examine the relationship between nursing students' exposure to various forms of incivility in their clinical learning environments and their experience of burnout" (p. 148); this purpose was met. The significance of the problem was introduced clearly at the beginning of the article in the following statement: "Studies in nursing settings have linked nurses' perceptions of workplace violence to negative job and health effects . . . but less is known about nursing students' experiences of incivility and its effects" (p. 145). This problem statement is very concise, cites several appropriate references, and presents a persuasive argument. In addition, Babenko-Mould and Laschinger specified that "exposure to these negative interpersonal behaviours in the clinical setting may influence students' career choice. . . . It is vital that nursing students . . . are able to develop and use professional knowledge, skills, and judgments in supportive practice environments" (p. 145). This statement adds more credence to the rationale for the research.

Review of the Literature and Definitions

Babenko-Mould and Laschinger (2014) used headings such as "Introduction" and "Background" for sections in which they present the literature review. The formal section of the background guides the reader through two main concepts: (1) the concept of incivility and (2) burnout.

Regarding incivility, the authors reported that incivility has been experienced by university employees, staff nurses, and new nursing graduates. They stated, "given that staff nurses and new graduates are experiencing incivility and burnout in the workplace, it is plausible that nursing students share similar experiences during their learning experiences" (p. 146). The literature review includes studies reporting that nursing students have experienced verbal abuse in their clinical setting and incivility in the classroom. The impact of incivility lasts for years after the event.

The next section, on burnout, outlines the three dimensions of burnout: exhaustion, cynicism, and ineffectiveness. The authors elected not to include ineffectiveness in this study as it focuses on incompetence. In this section, the issue of burnout and its causes and effects was reviewed very well, linking it to incidence among staff nurses and nursing students. The concepts of cynicism and emotional exhaustion were reviewed as they relate to experienced nurses and nursing students. The authors concluded that the gap in research is around the issue of incivility and its relationship to burnout in nursing students. All of the references were apparently primary sources. The literature review provides a logical argument for Babenko-Mould and Laschinger's (2014) study.

Development of a Conceptual Framework

Babenko-Mould and Laschinger (2014) did not use a single conceptual framework for the study. Instead they used relevant concepts from two theories: (1) Andersson and Pearson's (1999) workplace incivility conceptual framework and (2) Maslach and Leiter's (1997) burnout theory.

Hypotheses and Research Question

There was no explicitly stated research question, but the authors hypothesized that nursing students' experiences of incivility from clinical instructors, from nursing staff in their clinical learning environments, and from other health providers are related to their experiences of burnout (emotional exhaustion and cynicism). Thus, the hypothesis is that increased incidences of incivility are related to increased rates of emotional exhaustion and burnout.

Sample

Babenko-Mould and Laschinger (2014) described the sample, which consisted of recruiting about 190 fourth-year baccalaureate nursing students and the final sample size of 126 (a response rate of 66.3% of eligible participants). The inclusion criteria was only fourth-year nursing students who had completed a 12-week acute care experience. Of course, nursing students not in their fourth year was the exclusion criteria. The authors stated that a power analysis was performed and that a sample size of 64 participants was needed for a small effect size of 0.3. Note that each type of statistical test—such as a t test, an analysis of variance (ANOVA), or regression—would have a different sample size.

Research Design

Babenko-Mould and Laschinger (2014) stated that their design was a cross-sectional survey, which was appropriate for this study. Students completed self-report scales on incivility and burnout. They were asked to focus on the 12 weeks of acute care practice they had just completed.

Internal Validity

Although threats to internal validity are germane to experimental research, researchers need to pay attention to factors in a nonexperimental design that may potentially compromise a study. Possible threats to internal validity include acquiescence bias.

External Validity

Generalizability is limited to the sample because the individuals were from a specific geographical area in Canada with one nursing program; thus, generalizing to other populations would be questionable.

Legal/Ethical Issues

Ethical approval was received from an ethics review board at the university; this was necessary before the study could proceed.

Instruments

From the literature review, the authors chose the Cortina Incivility Scale (CIS) to assess students' perception of the frequency of uncivil behaviours experienced during the past 12 weeks from nursing staff, clinical instructors, and other health professionals in the clinical learning environment. The Emotional Exhaustion (EE) and Cynicism© subscales of the Maslach Burnout Inventory–General Survey (MBI-GS) were used to measure student burnout. The authors indicated how the items on each scale are rated.

Reliability and Validity

The CIS and the MBI-GS have acceptable Cronbach's alpha reliability (.85–.93 and .78–.94, respectively).

Analysis of the Data and Findings

The demographic variables mentioned in the article are on a nominal scale of measurement. Gender, marital status, and previous work experiences are measured on a nominal scale. There are no ordinal scale variables.

Descriptive statistics were reported as frequencies in Table 19C1.1 and means and standard deviations in Table 19C1.2 (see pp. 442 and 443); in the text a small amount of repetition of the results highlighted the findings. Correlational and regression analyses at the .05 level of significance were appropriately conducted for obtaining information on the association between the variables.

The answer to the hypothesis lies in the following results. Fourth-year nursing students' experiences of incivility from nurses, clinical instructors, and other health professionals were significantly related to the emotional exhaustion component of burnout ($r = 0.42$, $p < .001$, $r = .24$, $p < .05$, and $r = .18$, $p < .05$, respectively). On the other hand, cynicism was significantly associated with students' encounters of incivility from staff nurses ($r = .289$, $p < .05$), but not with incivility from clinical instructors or other health professionals. The strongest correlation with both components of burnout was students' incivility experiences with staff nurses in their clinical learning settings (see Table 19C1.2).

From the hierarchical multiple regression analyses, incivility experiences explained only 23% of the variance for emotional exhaustion; both staff nurses' incivility and clinical nursing instructor incivility were significant predictors of emotional exhaustion. Staff nurses' incivility was the only predictor of nursing students' cynicism.

Discussion

The findings were explained within the context of previous research, similarities, and differences. The authors concluded that these findings demonstrate the potentially devastating effects of nonsupportive colleagues in nursing education environments that threaten the health and well-being of nursing students, and they stressed the need to address incivility in clinical learning settings.

Implications and Recommendations

Babenko-Mould and Laschinger (2014) discussed the negative implications of burnout for nursing students and made several recommendations for educators to create learning environments for students in which students could become aware of what constitutes incivility and learn to take preventative actions.

Study Limitations

The authors stated that self-report bias and sample size are possible limitations to the study. The issue of one geographical area was ameliorated by stating that the practice settings are in many areas in Southwestern Ontario.

CRITIQUE 2

The study "Effects of an Interdisciplinary Education Program on Hypertension: A Pilot Study" by Thérèse A. Lauzière, Nicole Chevarie, Martine Poirier, et al. (2013) is critiqued here. The article is presented in its entirety and is followed by the critique on pp. 464–466. (From *Canadian Journal of Cardiovascular Nursing*, 23(1),12–19.)

Effects of an Interdisciplinary Education Program on Hypertension: A Pilot Study

Thérèse A. Lauzière, RN, NP, Nicole Chevarie, RN, MN, Martine Poirier, MSc, Anouk Utzschneider, PhD, and Mathieu Bélanger, PhD

ABSTRACT

BACKGROUND: The goal of this pilot study was to examine the effects of a structured interdisciplinary education program on blood pressure, knowledge, anthropometric measures, medication compliance, behavioural risk factors and quality of life.

METHOD: In this quasi-experimental study, participants were assigned to an intervention (n = 21) or a regular care group (n = 19). The intervention group attended four weekly sessions related to hypertension. Anthropometric measures and blood pressure were recorded at baseline, one, three and six months for all participants. Both groups completed questionnaires on knowledge, health-related behaviours and quality of life at these same intervals.

RESULTS: The reduction in systolic blood pressure was greater in the intervention group than in the regular care group (p = 0.05). However, there were no between group differences with regard to the other variables studied.

CONCLUSION: Participation in a structured interdisciplinary education program was associated with a reduction of systolic blood pressure, thus contributing to a risk reduction for cardiovascular disease.

KEY WORDS: hypertension, interdisciplinary, education program, lifestyle, medication adherence

Lauzière, T.A., Chevarie, N., Poirier, M., Utzschneider, A., & Bélanger, M. (2013). Effects of an Interdisciplinary Education Program on Hypertension: A Pilot Study. *Canadian Journal of Cardiovascular Nursing*, 23(1), 12-18.

BACKGROUND

It has been estimated that 19% of Canadian adults 20 to 79 years of age have hypertension (HTN) and that 35% of these are either unaware of their condition (17%), aware but not treated (4%), or not treated to target (14%) (Wilkins et al., 2010). HTN is linked to a 35%-40% increase in risk of cerebral vascular accidents, as well as an increased risk of dementia, cardiovascular, renal and eye diseases (Duron & Hanon, 2010; National Institutes of Health, 2004). A reduction of blood pressure (BP) by 2 mmHg decreases the risk of stroke by 15% and the risk of coronary artery disease by 6% (Madhur, Maron, Riaz, Dreisback, & Harrison, 2012). It is estimated that there is a 90% lifetime risk for developing HTN among the middle aged and elderly (Vasan et al., 2002).

In addressing cardiovascular disease prevention, experts stress the importance of modifying lifestyle and not relying exclusively on pharmacotherapy (Canadian Cardiovascular Congress, 2006). Adoption of a healthy lifestyle has proven to be highly effective to prevent and treat HTN (Bond Brill, 2010). Risk factors for HTN include modifiable behaviours such as high sodium intake, high alcohol consumption, low levels of physical activity, obesity, and smoking (Public Health Agency of Canada, 2010). In developed countries such as Canada, HTN alone is estimated to account for 10% of health care costs (Gaziano, Bitton, Anand, & Weinstein, 2009). This imposes a substantial burden on the health care system and calls for the identification of viable alternatives to our society's heavy reliance on medications. Konrady, Brodskaya, Soboleva and Polunicheva (2001) suggest that the implementation of educational programs including behavioural change components may provide socioeconomic benefits due to the reduction of costs related to treatments.

Previous studies on the effects of educational programs on HTN have demonstrated a reduction in BP among participants (Drevenhorn, Kjellgren, & Bengtson, 2007; Iso et al., 1996; Miura et al., 2004; Wang & Abbott, 1998). Researchers noted an increase in knowledge related to HTN following a structured education program (Cuspidi et al., 2000; Roca et al., 2003). Zernike and Henderson (1998) found that a structured educational program was more efficient to increase patients' knowledge on HTN than the usual approaches of counselling at the bedside or in the office. A meta-analysis demonstrated that multi-faceted approaches are more effective than single strategies in controlling chronic diseases such as HTN (Weingarten et al., 2002). Similarly, Carter, Rogers, Daly, Zheng, and James (2009) reported that the participation of different health professionals, such as nurses and pharmacists, in the provision of education programs is associated with favourable results, including clinic attendance and a better control of HTN.

Patient non-adherence to treatment is also an important factor contributing to inadequate HTN control (Campbell, McKay, & Tremblay, 2008; Uzun et al., 2009). Compliance can, nevertheless, be improved following education (Hadi & Rostami Gooran, 2006) and this translates into better HTN management (Konrady et al., 2001; Morgado, Rolo & Castelo-Branco, 2011) and, subsequently, fewer cardiovascular events (Campbell et al., 2009).

Although Konrady et al. (2001) found no significant improvements in lifestyle following education, Iso et al. (1996) and Dickinson et al. (2006) noted reduced salt intake and alcohol consumption among participants in an education program and this resulted in lowering systolic blood pressure (SBP). Svetkey et al. (2009) found that an intensive intervention related to lifestyle resulted in a significant reduction in BP. Others also found that a reduction in salt (Joffres, Campbell, Manns, & Tu, 2007), fat intake and total energy intake (Miura et al., 2004) was associated with a decrease in SBP. In addition, some demonstrated that an increase in energy expenditure through exercise, as well as activities of daily living also contributed to a reduced SBP (Dickinson et al., 2006; Drevenhorn et al., 2007; Miura et al., 2004). Côté, Moisan, Chabot and Grégoire (2005) found an improvement in quality of life among participants, which they attributed to an increase in physical activity and to a lowered BP.

To our knowledge, no research has yet combined BP, knowledge, body mass index (BMI), waist circumference, medication compliance, lifestyle and quality of life as study outcomes. We designed and piloted an interdisciplinary-led education program aimed at improving knowledge related to the importance of complying with medical prescriptions and adhering to physical activity and dietary recommendations.

PURPOSE

The purpose of this quasi-experimental study was to investigate changes in systolic and diastolic BP, as they relate to participation in an interdisciplinary-led education program on HTN. Secondary study outcomes included changes in knowledge, BMI, waist circumference, medication compliance, lifestyle and quality of life. Therefore, it was predicted that compared to the regular care group, the group exposed to the interdisciplinary education program would present greater improvements in primary and secondary outcomes over a six-month period.

METHODS

Study population

This study was based in a predominantly francophone region of south-eastern New Brunswick, Canada. The target population consisted of men and women aged 20 to 70 years with a BP greater than 140/90 mmHg at the doctor's or nurse practitioner's office on four occasions, or BP readings greater than 135/85 mmHg on four occasions in the community. Participants needed to be fluent in French, to have received no education on HTN or its risk factors beyond information given by their primary care provider, and to be capable to participate in an education program. Diabetic patients and those with cardiovascular or renal disease and pregnant women were excluded, as these conditions could inadvertently influence BP control. Treatment with an antihypertensive medication was not an exclusion criterion.

A systematic sampling approach was used to form our intervention and regular care groups. Individuals were assigned numbers in the order they called or were referred to the study research office. No factor is expected to have influenced the order in which patients were listed. The intervention group consisted of patients assigned to odd numbers and those with even numbers formed the regular care group. Data collection occurred between September 2008 and December 2010. Participants were invited through referral from their family practitioner, a local radio station and flyers placed in pharmacies throughout the community. Twenty-four participants were recruited to the intervention group, whereas the regular care group consisted of 23 members. Due to loss of participants, the final intervention and regular care groups consisted of 21 and 19 participants respectively. The Institutional Research Ethics Review Board reviewed and approved this study prior to its initiation.

Procedures

The intervention consisted of four weekly education sessions of one to two hours duration. At the beginning of the first session, the consent forms were reviewed and signed. Height, weight and BP were measured and BMI was calculated. This session was provided by a nurse practitioner and consisted of an overview of HTN, its risk factors and consequences, and instructions on how to self-monitor BP. In the second session, a dietitian presented Dietary Approaches to Stop Hypertension, otherwise known as the DASH diet (Dietician Canada, 2008). The third session was offered by a physiotherapist who spoke on the benefits of physical activity and provided examples of exercises to be performed. A pharmacist presented the last session, which covered pharmacological options for treating HTN, the potential side effects associated with these medications, and the importance of adhering to pharmacological treatments. All sessions were presented by the same professionals throughout the study. At each session, written materials such as pamphlets and a copy of the visual support for the presentation were provided to the attendees. Participants in the regular care group did not attend education sessions or receive written material during the period of the study, but were offered the sessions and written material at its conclusion.

Sociodemographic information was obtained from all participants at the onset of the study. BP and anthropometric measures (height, weight, waist circumference and BMI) were taken at baseline, one, three and six months of follow-up. The same scale and measuring tape were used throughout the study. BP was measured using a digital BP monitor and the appropriate cuff suited to the individual's arm size. Prior to the BP measurement, subjects were seated for five minutes with both feet on the floor and their left arm resting on a table at heart level.

Three questionnaires were also administered at the same intervals. These included the SF-36 health survey (Version 1.0) to evaluate quality of life, a questionnaire on knowledge related to HTN and its risk factors, and another on lifestyle (diet, physical activity, smoking and alcohol use). The SF-36 has strong psychometrics of reliability and validity (Brazier et al., 1992), and has been shown to be appropriate for hypertensive populations (McHorney, Ware, Lu, & Sherbourne, 1994).

The last two questionnaires were developed for the purpose of this study, based on items found in other validated questionnaires (Barry & Hogan, 2002; Charlton et al., 2007; Aucoin-Gallant, 1998). Five medical experts in the field of HTN were asked to review these, as a means of content validation. The questionnaires were then pre-tested for clarity of items among five lay individuals. More specifically, the questionnaire on knowledge included 20 items with multiple choice answers that covered the definition of HTN (two items), symptoms (two items), treatments (10 items), and risk factors (six items). The questionnaire on lifestyle included 20 multiple choice questions on specific dietary consumption (15 items), frequency of physical activity (one item), tobacco use (one item), alcohol intake (one item) and stress management (two items). Each of these questions was followed by four response options, scored incrementally from 0 to 3 with higher values attributed to healthiest responses. At each encounter, participants were also asked to recall whether they had taken their medications, as prescribed. Data were collected by the same researcher (TL) throughout the study.

Analyses

Potential between-group differences at baseline were investigated with t-tests for continuous scores meeting normality assumptions and with Fisher exact test for other variables. We used multivariable linear regressions to assess if there were differences in the rate of change in the continuous outcomes from baseline to six months between participants exposed to the educational intervention and those exposed to regular care. Because physical activity and knowledge scores were better represented as counts, we used multivariable poisson regressions for these outcomes. Similarly, we used polynomial logistic regressions to assess between-group differences in changes in smoking status and alcohol use over the follow-up period. In each of the regressions, the between-group differences were investigated using interaction terms between time and a dichotomous variable indicating exposure or non-exposure to the educational intervention. In the fully adjusted models, we accounted for age, gender, number of years since diagnosis of HTN, level of education, household income, and employment status. Analyses were conducted within the generalized estimating equation framework to account for non-independence of repeated observations within individuals. We used the SAS statistical package version 9.1 GENMOD procedure (SAS Institute Inc, Cary, NC, USA). Missing values were rare (4.7%) and were considered to be a random occurrence. Through the GENMOD procedure, missing values were, therefore, replaced by regression estimates. Power calculations indicated that the inclusion of 20 participants per group would provide 80% power to detect a between-group difference of 10 mmHg in systolic or diastolic BP change with probability of type I error set at 5%.

RESULTS

This study included 40 hypertensive participants. The 21 participants in the intervention group had higher systolic and diastolic BPs at the onset of the study than participants in the regular care group, but these differences were not statistically significant (Table 19C2.1). In comparison to the regular care group, participants in the intervention group also appeared to be older, to have had their diagnosis of high BP longer, to be heavier, to be less physically active, and to have lower levels of education, but none of these differences were statistically significant. Following statistical adjustments, the baseline between-group difference was only significant for the diastolic BP (Table 19C2.2).

TABLE **19C2.1**

BASELINE CHARACTERISTICS OF PARTICIPANTS

	PARTICIPANTS IN THE REGULAR CARE GROUP N = 19		PARTICIPANTS IN THE INTERVENTION GROUP N = 21		
	MEAN	STD DEV	MEAN	STD DEV	P-VALUE
Systolic blood pressure (mm Hg)	131.1	14.0	139.8	15.6	0.07
Diastolic blood pressure (mm Hg)	79.1	9.4	84.4	8.9	0.07
Age (years)	51.7	9.4	56.6	8.5	0.1
Years since hypertension diagnosis (number)	4.6	4.2	8.0	6.7	0.08
Weight (lbs)	170.7	34.1	179.8	42.4	0.5
Height (cm)	164.4	7.8	164.2	9.8	0.9
Body mass index (kg/m²)	28.8	5.9	30.4	5.8	0.4
Waist circumference (cm)	96.8	13.1	101.6	13.4	0.3
Quality of life (SF36 score range 0–100)	72.3	17.4	77.3	15.4	0.3
Lifestyle (score range: 0–60)	41.9	5.9	41.0	6.0	0.6
Dietary habits (score range: 0–45)	32.4	5.0	31.6	4.7	0.6
	n	%	n	%	
Physical activity (30 minutes/day)					0.4
Always	5	26.3	3	14.3	
Often	9	47.4	7	33.3	
Sometimes	3	15.8	8	38.1	
Never	2	10.5	3	14.3	
Smoking tobacco					0.3
Every day	2	10.5	0	0	
Often	0	0	0	0	
Sometimes	2	10.5	1	4.8	
Never	15	79.0	20	95.2	
Alcohol (> 14 drinks/week for men and > 9/week for women)					0.9
Always	1	5.3	1	4.8	
Often	4	21.1	4	19.1	
Sometimes	6	31.6	8	38.1	
Never	8	42.1	8	38.1	

TABLE **19C2.1**

BASELINE CHARACTERISTICS OF PARTICIPANTS—cont'd

	PARTICIPANTS IN THE REGULAR CARE GROUP N = 19		PARTICIPANTS IN THE INTERVENTION GROUP N = 21		
	MEAN	STD DEV	MEAN	STD DEV	P-VALUE
Knowledge on hypertension (score range: 0–20)					0.6
< 15	0	0	0	0	
15	2	10.5	0	0	
16	0	0	1	4.8	
17	1	5.3	2	9.5	
18	4	21.1	7	33.3	
19	5	26.3	6	28.6	
20	7	36.8	5	23.8	
Sex (# women)	13	68	14	67	1.0
Marital status (# single)	2	10	4	20	0.3
Race (# caucasian)	19	100	21	100	1.0
Education (highest degree obtained)					0.2
High school	3	16	4	19	
College	5	26	11	52	
University	11	58	6	29	
Household income					0.1
< $20,000	0	0	3	17	
$20,000–$49,999	4	21	1	6	
$50,000–$69,999	3	16	6	33	
≥ 70,000$	12	63	8	44	
Employment					0.2
Unemployed	0	0	2	10	
Part time	1	5	4	19	
Retired	3	16	6	29	
Full time	15	79	9	43	

TABLE **19C2.2**

BETA COEFFICIENTS[a] AND 95% CONFIDENCE INTERVALS ESTIMATED IN MULTIPLE LINEAR REGRESSIONS FOR DIFFERENCES BEFORE AND DURING AN INTERDISCIPLINARY EDUCATIONAL PROGRAM ON HTN				
	PARTIALLY ADJUSTED MODELS β (95% CI)	P	FULLY ADJUSTED MODELS β (95% CI)	P
Systolic blood pressure (mm Hg)				
Difference between groups at baseline	-9.3 (-17.2, -1.3)	0.5	-6.4 (-15.9, 3.0)	0.2
Time (1 month)	0.9 (-1.5, 3.3)	0.02	0.7 (-2.0, 3.5)	0.6
Time x Group interaction	-2.0 (-3.6, -0.4)	0.01	-1.8 (-3.5, 0.0)	0.05
Diastolic blood pressure (mm Hg)				
Difference between groups at baseline	-5.0 (-10.1, 0.1)	0.05	-5.6 (-10.2, -0.1)	0.02
Time (1 month)	-0.6 (-2.2, 1.0)	0.5	-1.0 (-2.9, 0.7)	0.2
Time x Group interaction	-0.3 (-1.3, 0.6)	0.5	-0.06 (-1.1, 1.0)	0.9
Weight (kg)				
Difference between groups at baseline	-9.3 (-32.2, 13.6)	0.4	8.5 (-8.3, 25.4)	0.3
Time (1 month)	-0.07 (-1.2, 1.0)	0.9	0.01 (-1.3, 1.3)	1.0
Time x Group interaction	-0.08 (-0.8, 0.6)	0.8	-0.1 (-0.9, 0.7)	0.7
Body mass index (kg/m2)				
Difference between groups at baseline	-1.6 (-5.1, 1.9)	0.4	0.6 (-2.2, 3.3)	0.7
Time (1 month)	-0.08 (-0.3, 0.1)	0.5	-0.06 (-0.3, 0.2)	0.6
Time x Group interaction	0.03 (-0.1, 0.2)	0.6	0.02 (-0.1, 0.2)	0.8
Waist circumference (cm)				
Difference between groups at baseline	-4.4 (-12.4, 3.6)	0.3	2.0 (-4.5, 8.6)	0.5
Time (1 month)	-0.4 (-1.2, 0.3)	0.2	-0.5 (-1.3, 0.4)	0.3
Time x Group interaction	0.2 (-0.2, 0.7)	0.3	0.3 (-0.2, 0.8)	0.3
Lifestyle				
Difference between groups at baseline	-0.3 (-3.8, 3.1)	0.8	-0.7 (-4.3, 2.8)	0.6
Time (1 month)	0.1 (-0.3, 0.6)	0.6	0.1 (-0.4, 0.6)	0.6
Time x Group interaction	0.1 (-0.1, 0.4)	0.3	0.1 (-0.2, 0.5)	0.4

TABLE **19C2.2**

BETA COEFFICIENTS[a] AND 95% CONFIDENCE INTERVALS ESTIMATED IN MULTIPLE LINEAR REGRESSIONS FOR DIFFERENCES BEFORE AND DURING AN INTERDISCIPLINARY EDUCATIONAL PROGRAM ON HTN—cont'd

	PARTIALLY ADJUSTED MODELS β (95% CI)	P	FULLY ADJUSTED MODELS β (95% CI)	P
Quality of life (SF-36)				
Difference between groups at baseline	-4.6 (-13.4, 4.3)	0.3	-5.5 (-14.7, 3.8)	0.2
Time (1 month)	2.0 (-0.2, 4.1)	0.07	2.4 (0.09, 4.7)	0.04
Time x Group interaction	-0.7 (-2.1, 0.7)	0.3	-0.9 (-2.4, 0.6)	0.2
Dietary habits				
Difference between groups at baseline	-0.2 (-3.0, 2.5)	0.9	-0.6 (-3.4, 2.2)	0.7
Time (1 month)	0.01 (-0.4, 0.4)	1.0	-0.05 (-0.5, 0.4)	0.8
Time x Group interaction	0.1 (-0.1, 0.4)	0.3	0.1 (-0.1, 0.4)	0.3

β, regression coefficient; CI, confidence interval; [a]The regression coefficient represents the estimated adjusted difference in the value of the dependent variable (the group receiving regular care is the reference; this group presents higher scores at baseline for all outcomes in the table). In partially adjusted models, independent variables include the baseline value of the outcome, time, and the time-group interaction. Covariates in fully adjusted models additionally include age, sex, number of years since diagnosis of HTN, level of education, household income category, and employment status. The interaction terms present by how much the effect of time differed for the group that received the educational intervention.

Primary study outcomes

Improvement in SBP was greater in the intervention group than in the regular care group (see interaction term in Table 19C2.2). This difference persisted after adjustments for age, number of years since diagnosis of HTN, gender, level of education, household income, and employment status. At the end of the six-month period, the average SBP reduction in the intervention group was 10.8 mmHg greater than the average reduction observed in the regular care group (estimated from the interaction term: -1.8 mmHg per month x six months). No significant improvements were noted for either group with regard to diastolic BP.

Secondary study outcomes

In other linear models, we did not note significant changes in weight, BMI, waist circumference, quality of life, lifestyle, and dietary habits of either group. The physical activity level of both groups appeared to increase throughout the educational program (Poisson regression β estimate and 95% confidence interval: 0.9, -0.01 to 0.2). However, this improvement was not significant once we accounted for potential confounders in the fully adjusted model (0.8, -0.03 to 0.2). Although the frequency of drinking more than 14 and nine alcoholic consumptions per week among men and women respectively decreased for both groups, this decrease was not significant in either group. The smoking status reported by participants and their results on the knowledge assessment did not change significantly during the follow-up period.

Throughout the study, participants from both groups generally reported good compliance with their pharmacological therapy. Reports of missing more than two doses of medication in the past month occurred in only two participants in the regular care group at baseline, one participant in the regular care group at one month, and one participant in the intervention group at six months.

DISCUSSION

In this study, participation in an interdisciplinary educational program was associated with a reduction of SBP. This is in agreement with other studies that showed improvement in BP following structured educational programs (Carter et al., 2009; Drevenhorn et al., 2007; Konrady et al., 2001, Svetkey et al., 2009). In their systematic review, Walsh et al. (2006) examined quality improvement strategies and found that interdisciplinary, team-based care was the only strategy that improved HTN significantly. Several other studies also indicate that educational interventions offered by health care providers from various disciplines result in improved BP control (Carter et al., 2009; Glynn, Murphy, Smith, Schroeder, & Fahey, 2010a; Morgado et al., 2011; Odedosu, Schoenthaler, Vieira, Agyemang, & Ogedegbe, 2012). In Glynn et al.'s review (2010a), it was observed that better BP control was obtained when interventions were directed toward patients rather than toward the physicians.

Participation in the education program was not associated with a demonstrated improvement in HTN-related knowledge. The majority of participants in this study were well educated, thus the questionnaire assessing knowledge about HTN may have been too easy for this group, possibly resulting in an under-estimation of the effect for knowledge improvement. It is also possible that repeating the same questions at every evaluation period led participants in the regular care group to seek answers from external sources. It has been documented that people learn by repetition when completing the same questionnaire on several occasions. This concept of maturation must be acknowledged when considering results of education-based interventions (Boswell & Cannon, 2007). Although we could not find recent studies that examined HTN-related knowledge, Martinez-Amenos, Fernandez Ferre, Mota Vidal, and Alcina Rocasalbas (1990) demonstrated an increase in patient knowledge following an HTN-related education program.

It is well established that a healthy lifestyle, including healthy eating (Svetkey et al., 2009), regular physical activity, moderate alcohol consumption, low sodium intake (Joffres et al., 2007), a smoke-free environment and stress reduction contribute to a reduction in BP and cardiovascular risks (Campbell & Kwong, 2010). Although, in our study, there were no between-group differences at six months, both groups improved their level of physical activity over the follow-up period. Drevenhorn et al. (2007) found that weight reduction and decreased BP were associated with increased exercise. As reported previously, improvements in physical activity can lower SBP by 4 mmHg to 9 mmHg (Madhur et al., 2012) independently of changes in anthropometric measurements (National Institutes of Health, 2004). Despite the lack of structured education, participants in the regular care group did return for regular visits with the nurse practitioner, to have their BP and anthropometric measures evaluated. This heightened attention may have had an impact on the participants' desire and effort to improve their lifestyle. The reported improvements in lifestyles were, nevertheless, not associated with changes in weight, BMI and waist circumference. Longer follow-up and an intervention directed toward weight loss may have led to greater improvements in BP since previous studies show that BP reductions of 5 mmHg-20 mmHg can be expected for every 10 kg of weight loss among overweight patients (Madhur et al., 2012).

Although our study did not demonstrate an improvement in medication adherence, participants reported a high level of compliance with pharmacotherapy throughout the study period. Others have demonstrated that education programs may result in high adherence to antihypertensive treatment, which is associated with better BP control (Morgado et al., 2011) and with a reduction in cardiovascular events (Mazzaglia et al., 2009). Campbell and Kwong (2010) also showed that non-adherence to pharmacotherapy can be prevented and adherence improved through health care professional interventions.

Limitations

Although participants were not allocated randomly to their respective group, the distribution of subjects was the result of chance alone. This said, it is likely that the between-group difference in change in SBP was the result of exposure to the education program (Loiselle & Profetto-McGrath, 2011). Limitations of this study, nevertheless, include the self-report for several of the other components under study. Self-reporting is subject to problems of recall and social desirability bias. However, it is unlikely that either group would have been subject to more of these reporting issues than the other. It should also be noted that the reliability of some of the measure instruments with which no significant change were observed had not been tested. The lack of between-group differences for some outcomes may, therefore, be the result of measures that were not sufficiently sensitive to change. Although unlikely, a potential bias was also introduced because the data collector was not blinded to study group allocation. Finally, although the relatively small sample included in this study provided sufficient statistical power and appropriately served the purpose of pilot-testing the program, it limits the generalizability of the results.

Conclusion

In this study, a simple interdisciplinary education program resulted in a significant reduction in SBP. It is, nevertheless, unclear how the education program led to an improvement in BP, given the potential mediators studied were not associated with significant between-group differences. It is possible that improvements in SBP were the result of an accumulation of small, but non-statistically significant improvements in several mediators. Others have indicated that it is difficult to determine which components of complex interventions

affect changes in BP (Glynn, Murphy, Smith, Schroeder, & Fahey, 2010b). In conclusion, these results suggest that using an interdisciplinary approach to educate patients about HTN may be an effective method to reduce their BP, thus contributing to risk-reduction for cardiovascular disease. Further research is needed to understand what mediates such improvements.

FUNDING SOURCES

The Vitalité Health Network Research Centre provided funds for the development and implementation of this research.

The loan of a Life Source digital blood pressure monitor (UA767-PC) and cuffs were provided by Merck Frosst.

ABOUT THE AUTHORS

Thérèse A. Lauzière, RN, NP, Primary Health Care Nurse Practitioner, Dieppe Medical Centre, Vitalité Health Network

Nicole Chevarie, RN, MN, Clinical Nurse Specialist, Department of Cardiology, Dr. Georges-L.-Dumont University Hospital Centre, Vitalité Health Network

Martine Poirier, MSc, Research Coordinator, Vitalité Health Network Research Centre

Anouk Utzschneider, PhD, Research Officer, Vitalité Health Network Research Centre

Mathieu Bélanger, PhD, Assistant Professor, Department of Family Medicine, Université de Sherbrooke; Director of Research, Centre de Formation Médicale du Nouveau-Brunswick; Epidemiologist, Vitalité Health Network Research Centre.

Address for correspondence: Thérèse Lauzière, NP, Dieppe Medical Centre, 667 Champlain Street, Suite 125, Dieppe, New Brunswick E1A1P6. Phone: 506-862-4215; Fax: 506855-6603; Email: **therese.lauziere@vitalitenb.ca**

REFERENCES

Aucoin-Gallant, G. (1998). Le degré d'intégration des savoirs. In G. Aucoin-Gallant, M. Cormier-Daigle,

Y. Thibeault, M. Dorval, J. D'Astous, & T. Pham-Gia (Eds.), *Étude comparative de deux méthodes de livraison d'un programme d'enseignement en prédialyse. Rapport de recherche*. Moncton, NB: Corporation hospitalière Beauséjour et Université de Moncton.

Barry, D., & Hogan, M. J. (2002). A comparison of responses to a health and lifestyle questionnaire completed before and then after blood pressure screening. *Journal of Exposure Analysis and Environmental Epidemiology*, *12*, 244–251.

Bond Brill, J. (2010). Lifestyle intervention strategies for the prevention and treatment of hypertension: A review. *American Journal of Lifestyle Medicine*, *5*, 346–350.

Boswell, C., & Cannon, S. (2007). Introduction to nursing research: Incorporating evidence-based practice. Sudbury, Massachusetts: Jones & Bartlett.

Brazier, J. E., Harper, R., Jones, N. M., O'Cathain, A., Thomas, K. J., Usher-wood, T., & Westlake, L. (1992). Validating the SF-36 health survey questionnaire: New outcome measure for primary care. *British Medical Journal*, *305*, 160–164.

Canadian Cardiovascular Congress. (2006, October). *Reducing lifetime cardiovascular disease event rates: Emphasizing early risk factor modification and intensive intervention*. Retrieved from www.mednet.ca.

Campbell, N. R. C., Brant, R., Johansen, H., Walker, R. L., Wielgosz, A., Onysko, R. N. G., Sambell, S. P., & McAlister, F. A. (2009). Increases in antihypertensive prescriptions and reductions in cardiovascular events in Canada. *Hypertension: Journal of the American Heart Association*, *53*, 128–134.

Campbell, N., & Kwong, M. M. L. (2010). 2010 Canadian hypertension education program recommendations. *Canadian Family Physician*, *56*, 649–653.

Campbell, N., McKay, D. W., & Tremblay, G. (2008). 2008 Canadian hypertension education program recommendations: An annual update. *Canadian Family Physician*, *54*, 1539–1541.

Carter, B. L., Rogers, M., Daly, J., Zheng, S., & James, P. A. (2009). The potency of team-based care interventions for hypertension. *Archives of Internal Medicine*, *169*, 1748–1755.

Charlton, K. E., Steyn, K., Levitt, N. S., Jonathan, D., Zulu, J., & Nel, J. H. (2007). Development and validation of a short questionnaire to assess sodium intake. *Public Health Nutrition*, *11*(1), 83–94.

Côté, I., Moisan, J., Chabot, I., & Grégoire, J-P. (2005). Health related quality of life in hypertension: Impact of pharmacy intervention program. *Journal of Clinical Pharmacy and Therapeutics*, *30*, 355–362.

Cuspidi, C., Sampieri, L., Macca, V., Fusi, V., Salerno, M., Lonati, L., & Zanchetti, A. (2000). Short and long-term impact of a structured educational program on the patient's knowledge of hypertension. *Italian Heart Journal*, *1*, 839–843.

Dickinson, H. O., Mason, J. M., Nicolson, D. J., Campbell, F., Beyer, F. R., Cook, J. V., & Ford, G. A. (2006). Lifestyle interventions to reduce raised blood pressure: A systematic review of randomized controlled trials. *Journal of Hypertension*, *24*, 215–233.

Dietician Canada. (2008). *Dash diet*. Retrieved from www.dieticians.ca.

Drevenhorn, E., Kjellgren, K. I. & Bengtson, A. (2007). Outcomes of following a programme for lifestyle changes with people with hypertension. *Journal of Clinical Nursing*, *16*, 144–151.

Duron, E., & Hanon, O. (2010). Antihypertensive treatments, cognitive decline, and dementia. *Journal of Alzeimers Disease*, *20*, 903–914.

Gaziano, T. A., Bitton, A., Anand, S., & Weinstein, M. C. (2009). International society of hypertension. The global cost of nonoptimal blood pressure. *Journal of Hypertension*, *27*, 1472–1477.

Glynn, L. G., Murphy, A. W., Smith, S. M., Schroeder, K., & Fahey, T. (2010a). Interventions used to improve control of blood pressure in patients with hypertension. *Cochrane Database of Systematic Reviews*, *3*, 1–90.

Glynn, L. G., Murphy, A. W., Smith, S. M., Schroeder, K., & Fahey, T. (2010b). Self-monitoring and other non-pharmacalogical interventions to improve the management of hypertension in primary care: A systematic review. *British Journal of General Practice*, *60*, e476–488.

Hadi, N., & Rostami Gooran, N. (2006). Effectiveness of a hypertension educational program on increasing medication compliance in Shiraz. *Shiraz E-Medical Journal*, *7*(2), 1–6.

Iso, H., Shimamoto, T., Yokota, K., Sankai, T., Jacobs, D. R., Jr., & Komachi, Y. (1996). Community-based education classes for hypertension control. *Hypertension*, *27*, 968–974.

Joffres, M. R., Campbell, N. R. C., Manns, B., & Tu, K. (2007). Estimate of the benefits of a population-based reduction in dietary sodium additives on hypertension and its related health care costs in Canada. *Canadian Journal of Cardiology*, *23*, 437–443.

Konrady, A. O., Brodskaya, I. S., Soboleva, A. V., & Polunicheva, Y V. (2001). Benefits of the implementation of structured educational program in hypertension management. *Medicine Sciences Monitor*, *7*, 397–402.

Loiselle, C. G., & Profetto-McGrath, J. (2011). Scrutinizing quantitative research design. In D. F. Polit & C. T. Beck (Eds.), Canadian essentials of nursing research (3rd ed., pp. 144–171). Philadelphia: Lippincott, Williams & Wilkins.

Madhur, M. S., Maron, D. J., Riaz, K., Dreisback, A. W., & Harrison, D. G. (2012). *Hypertension treatment & management*. Retrieved from www.emedicine. medscape.com.

Martinez-Amenos, A., Fernandez Ferre, M. L., Mota Vidal, C., & Alcina Rocasalbas, J. (1990). Evaluation of two educative modules in a primary care hypertension programme. *Journal of Human Hypertension, 4*, 362–364.

Mazzaglia, G., Ambrosiomi, E., Alacqua, M., Filippi, A., Sessa, E., Immordino, V., & Mantovani, L. G. (2009). Adherence to hypertensive medication and cardiovascular morbidity among newly diagnosed hypertensive patients. *Circulation, 120*, 1598–1605.

McHorney, C. A., Ware, J. E., Jr., Lu, J. F. R., & Sherbourne, C. D. (1994). The MOS 36-item short-form health survey (SF-36): III. Tests of data quality, scaling assumptions, and reliability across diverse patient groups. *Medical Care, 32*, 40–66.

Miura, S., Yamaguchi, Y, Urata, H., Himeshima, Y., Otsuka, N., Tomita, S., & Saku, K. (2004). Efficacy of a multicomponent program (patient-centered assessment and counseling for exercise plus nutrition [PACE Japan]) for lifestyle modification in patients with essential hypertension. *Hypertension Research, 27*, 859–864.

Morgado, M., Rolo, S., & Castelo-Branco, M. (2011). Pharmacist intervention program to enhance hypertension control: A randomized controlled trial. *International Journal of Clinical Pharmacology, 33*, 132–140.

National Institutes of Health. (2004). *The seventh report of the joint national committee on prevention, detection, evaluation, and treatment of high blood pressure*. Retrieved from http://www.nhlbi.nih.gov.

Odedosu, T., Schoenthaler, A., Vieira, D., Agyemang, C., & Ogedegbe, G. (2012). Overcoming barriers to hypertension control in African Americans. *Cleveland Clinic Journal of Medicine, 79*, 46–56.

Public Health Agency of Canada. (2010). *Report from the Canadian chronic disease surveillance system: Hypertension in Canada, 2010*. Ottawa, ON: Author.

Roca, B., Nadal, E., Rovira, R. E., Valls, S., Consol, L., & Lloria, N. (2003). Usefulness of a hypertension education program. *Southern Medical Journal, 96*, 1133–1137.

Svetkey, L. P., Pollak, K. I., Yancy, W. S., Jr., Dolor, R. J., Batch, B. C., Samsa, G., & Lim, P. (2009). Hypertension improvement project (HIP): Randomized trial of quality improvement for physicians and lifestyle modifications for patients. *Hypertension, 54*, 1226–1233.

Uzun, S., Kara, B., Yokusoglu, M., Arslan, F., Birhan Yilmaz, M., & Karaeren, H. (2009). The assessment of adherence of hypertensive individuals to treatment and lifestyle change recommendation. *Anadolu Kardiyoloji Dergisi, 9*, 102–109.

Vasan, R. S., Beiser, A., Seshadri, S., Larson, M. G., Kannel, W. B., D'Agostino, R. B., & Levy, D. (2002). Residual lifetime risk for developing hypertension in middle-ages women and men: The Framingham heart study. *Journal of American Medical Association, 8*, 1003–1010.

Walsh, J. M. E., McDonald, K. M., Shojania, K. G., Sundaram, V., Nayak, S., Lewis, R., & Goldstein, K. (2006). Quality improvement strategies for hypertension management: A systematic review. *Medical Care, 44*, 646–657.

Wang, C-Y., & Abbott, L. J. (1998). Development of a community-based diabetes and hypertension preventive program. *Public Health Nursing, 15*, 406–414.

Weingarten, S. R., Henning, J. M., Badamgarav, E., Knight, K., Hasselblad, V., Gano, A., Jr., & Ofman, J. J. (2002). Interventions used in disease management programs for patients with chronic illness—which ones work? Meta-analysis of published reports. *British Medical Journal, 325*, 1–8.

Wilkins, K., Campbell, N. R. C., Joffres, M. R., McAlister, F. A., Nichol, M., Quach, S., & Tremblay, M. S. (2010). Blood pressure in Canadian adults. *Health Reports, 21*, 1–10.

Zernike, W., & Henderson, A. (1998). Evaluating the effectiveness of two teaching strategies for patients diagnosed with hypertension. *Journal of Clinical Nursing, 7*, 37–44.

INTRODUCTION TO CRITIQUE 2

The article "Effects of an Interdisciplinary Education Program on Hypertension: A Pilot Study" (Lauzière, Chevarie, Poirier, et al., 2013) is examined in terms of its quality and the potential usefulness of the findings for application to nursing practice. The design of this study was level III, inasmuch as it was a quasiexperimental study.

Title

The title reflects the major purpose of this study.

Abstract

The abstract meets the requirements of thoroughness. It contains the purpose, the method, the research design, the findings, the results, and conclusion.

Problem and Purpose

Lauzière and colleagues (2013) stated that the purpose of the study was to "investigate changes in systolic and diastolic BP [blood pressure], as they relate to participation in an interdisciplinary-led education program on HTN [hypertension]" (p. 13).

The identification of the research problem is very well organized, with an easy flow of the linkages between its elements. Lauzière et al. (2013) outlined the significance of the study by stating, "it has been estimated that 19% of Canadian adults 20 to 79 years of age have hypertension (HTN) and that 35% of these are unaware of their condition (17%) [or] aware and not treated (4%) . . . a reduction of blood pressure (BP) by 2 mm Hg decreases the risk of stroke by 15% and the risk of coronary artery disease by 6%" (p. 12). Next, the authors offered information on cardiovascular disease prevention and the importance of modifying lifestyle and behaviours. The burden on the health care system is stated and the suggestion made that educational programs "may provide socioeconomic benefits."

The authors reviewed research on educational programs and found that "no research has yet combined BP, knowledge, body mass index (BMI), waist circumference, medication compliance, lifestyle and quality of life as study outcomes" (p. 12). This statement adds strength to the rationale for conducting the study.

Review of the Literature and Definitions

The authors combined the literature review with the study background.

Theoretical Framework

There is no theoretical framework, but variables to support the study are clearly articulated. Conceptual definitions of the variables would assist the reader in replicating the study.

Hypotheses and Research Question

Lauzière and colleagues (2013) stated the research hypotheses as follows: "it was predicted that compared to the regular care group, the group exposed to the interdisciplinary education program would present greater improvements in primary and secondary outcomes over a six-month period" (p. 13). The primary outcomes were changes in systolic and diastolic BP, and the secondary outcomes included changes in knowledge, BMI, waist circumference, medication compliance, lifestyle, and quality of life.

No research question was stated, but such a statement could be articulated from the hypotheses as follows: What is the difference in systolic and diastolic BP, knowledge, BMI, waist circumference, medication compliance, lifestyle, and quality of life in the intervention group in comparison with those who receive regular care?

Sample

A systematic sampling approach was used to form the intervention and control groups. Individuals were assigned numbers in the order they were called or referred, then those with odd numbers formed the intervention group, and those with even numbers formed the regular-care group.

The inclusion criteria were men and women aged 20 to 70 years with a BP greater than 140/90 mm Hg at the doctor's or nurse practitioner's office on four occasions or BP readings greater than 135/85 mm HG on four occasions in the community. They had to be fluent in French, to have received no education on HTN or its risk factors beyond information given by their primary care provider, and be capable of participating in an education program. Those excluded were diabetic patients, patients with renal disease or cardiovascular disease, and pregnant women.

Research Design

Lauzière et al. (2013) stated that a quasiexperimental design was used. There were two groups: an intervention group and a regular-care group. This design is consistent with the purpose of the research.

The independent variable was type of group (intervention, regular care). The major dependent variables for this study were systolic and diastolic BP, and the secondary variables were knowledge, BMI, waist circumference, medication adherence, lifestyle, and quality of life. Demographic variables, such as age, number of years since diagnosis of HTN, level of education, household income, employment status, and gender, were used as covariates.

Internal Validity

Lauzière et al. (2013) made no mention of possible threats to internal validity that would inordinately decrease confidence in the results. To rule out measurement effects, the same scale and measuring tape were used throughout the study. BP was measured using a digital BP monitor and the appropriate cuff suited to the individual's size. Prior to BP measurement, subjects were seated for 5 minutes with both feet on the floor and their left arm resting on a table at heart level. The data collection on the three questionnaires was based on self-report measures collected by a researcher, which could have led to social desirability bias or

acquiescence bias, which in turn could have affected the results.

The authors developed two questionnaires: (1) one on knowledge, which consisted of 20 multiple-choice questions, and (2) one on lifestyle, which consisted of 20 multiple-choice questions. They used experts to test for content validity, and the questionnaires were pretested for clarity.

External Validity

Generalizability is limited to the sample because of the effect of lack of random allocation and the small sample size.

Legal/Ethical Issues

Although not explicitly stated, the authors had to have received ethical approval from the health care centre's ethics review board.

Instruments

Lauzière et al. (2013) used several questionnaires that included a number of items and a scoring method. The physiological measures were self-evident.

Reliability and Validity

A description of the reliability and validity of each instrument of the Short Form-36 (SF-36) was provided.

Results

Lauzière et al. (2013) used descriptive statistics to present the baseline characteristics of the two groups; these data are presented in Table 19C2.1, with the p value indicating statistical significance.

A description of the participants' results was also presented in the text (Lauzière et al., 2013, p. 14). Evidence to support the hypotheses was detailed in the text as follows: "improvement in SBP [systolic BP] was greater in the intervention group than in the regular care group" (p. 14), and the hypothesis related to diastolic BP was not supported, as the results were not statistically significant.

Regarding the secondary outcomes, there were no differences.

Discussion

Lauzière et al. (2013) stated that their finding related to the reduction in systolic BP was consistent with other research findings.

They also stated that perhaps the reasons the study showed no improvement in knowledge were that the majority of participants were well educated and the questionnaires were too easy. Also, repeating the same questionnaire at each data-collection point may have led participants to remember the questions and responses. The concept of maturation also could have contributed to no change.

Limitations and Conclusion

Lauzière et al. (2013) discussed the limitation of the sample size self-reporting bias and lack of random allocation. Also, the reliability of the new instruments was not tested. The data collector was not blinded to study group allocation, and this could have affected the results. Lauzière et al. (2013) described the significance of the study: "these results suggest that using an interdisciplinary approach to educate patients about HTN may be an effective method to reduce their BP, thus contributing to risk-reduction for cardiovascular disease. Further research is needed to understand what mediates such improvements" (p. 18).

CRITICAL THINKING CHALLENGES

- Discuss the ways in which the stylistic considerations of a journal affect the researcher's ability to present the research findings of a quantitative study.

- Are critiques of quantitative studies valid when a student or a practising nurse writes them? What level of quantitative study is best for you as a consumer of research to critique? What assumptions did you use to make this determination?
- What is essential for you as a consumer of research to use when you critique a quantitative research study? Discuss the ways you might use Internet resources now or in the future when you critique studies.

FOR FURTHER STUDY

(e) Go to Evolve at http://evolve.elsevier.com/Canada/LoBiondo/Research for the Audio Glossary and Appendix Tables that provide supplemental information for Appendix E.

REFERENCES

Andersson, L. M., & Pearson, C. M. (1999). Tit for tat? The spiraling effect of incivility in the workplace. *Academy of Management Review, 24*(3), 452–471.

Babenko-Mould, Y., & Laschinger, H. K. S. (2014). Effects of incivility in clinical practice settings on nursing student burnout. *International Journal of Nursing Education Scholarship, 11*(1), 145–154.

Lauzière, T. A., Chevarie, N., Poirier, M., et al. (2013). Effects of an interdisciplinary education program on hypertension: A pilot study. *Canadian Journal of Cardiovascular Nursing, 23*(1), 12–19.

Maslach, C., & Leiter, M. P. (1997). *The truth about burnout: How organizations cause personal stress and what to do about it.* San Francisco: Jossey-Bass.

PART SIX

Application of Research: Evidence-Informed Practice

RESEARCH **VIGNETTE**

From Ph.D. to Post-Doctoral Studies: Building a Survivorship Cancer Care Program

Christine Maheu, RN, PhD
Associate Professor
Ingram School of Nursing
McGill University
Montreal, Quebec

My journey in survivorship cancer care research began as funded Ph.D. work, where I focused on patients living with a cancer diagnosis and being at inherited risk for breast and ovarian cancer (BC/OC) (Maheu, 2009a, 2009b; Maheu & Thorne, 2008). The findings from this work facilitated the implementation of a national funded pilot intervention study to help BC and OC patients cope with inconclusive genetic test results. This intervention is now published (Maheu, Meschino, Weiming, et al., 2015) and has been presented at scientific and clinical conferences and has been applied in clinics. Two additional papers were published as part of my post-doctoral studies. The first is a pancreatic cancer risk counselling and screening intervention assessment to mitigate the psychological impact on individuals who are at increased risk for pancreatic cancer from carrying an inherited susceptibility to the disease (Maheu, Vodermaier, Rothenmund, et al., 2010). The second is a co-authored publication on the concepts of stigma in women carrying a cancer genetic mutation (Vodermaier, Esplen, & Maheu, 2010).

Following my post-doctoral work, I aimed to expand my expertise in intervention studies. In 2010, I implemented a pilot intervention study, which was then followed by a randomized controlled trial in 2014, for the study "Cognitive-Existential Intervention to Address Fear of Cancer Recurrence (FCR) in Women with Cancer" (Maheu, Lebel, Courbasson, et al., 2016). The aim of the pilot study was to conduct preliminary testing of a group intervention for FCR in women with BC or OC. The pilot study ended, and the data analysis revealed a large effect size at reducing FCR (Lebel, Maheu, Lefebvre, et al., 2014; Maheu, Lebel, Tomei, et al., 2015). Following the pilot study, funds were received from the Canadian Cancer Society (CCS) to conduct the randomized controlled trial version of the pilot study (2014–2017). The study is ongoing, with the delivery of eight planned cognitive-existential intervention groups, each lasting six sessions.

Fear of cancer recurrence is now getting the recognition and attention it deserves in cancer survivorship care. To this end, in collaboration with international leaders in FCR, I am working in partnership with an international steering committee named "Fear of Recurrence—Special Interest Group (FORWARDS)" to facilitate the implementation of a fear of recurrence research program and future international collaborations. This group is part of a special interest group under the banner of the International Psycho-Oncology Society. There are currently close to 50 international members.

I have had the opportunity to expand my knowledge and skills in cancer survivorship through a Butterfield/Drew Fellowship position, from 2008 to 2015, held with the Cancer Survivorship Program at the Princess Margaret Cancer Centre (Toronto). From the wealth of experience I have gained from the consultative roles, I have been fortunate to obtain funds from the Canadian Partnership Against Cancer (CPAC) to lead the development of a website for cancer survivors on cancer and work (www.cancerandwork.ca). The website is a combined creation of McGill University and the British Columbia Cancer Agency, and the core team works in partnership with de Souza Institute, with contributions from over 40 advisory board members and expert writers. The website includes best practice resources and assessment tools prepared by an interdisciplinary team of experts. It covers a broad range of topics, featuring information, tools, and resources for all parties involved in the return-to-work process (survivors, health care practitioners, and employers), to lend support and assistance to cancer survivors so that they may achieve a successful return to work after cancer. Another crucial project, in partnership with Ipsos Reid, is the development of a national survey of over 13,000 cancer patients to describe their transition needs from end of treatment to 3 years post-treatment. The final goal of this project is to provide recommendations at the policy level. I am very fortunate to be working with leading members in relevant fields of research and with clinicians, knowledge translation experts, knowledge users, and online developers toward engaging future users (cancer survivors, health care providers, employers) of the Cancer and Work website to use, experiment with, and refine the online tools and resources from the website through taking part in workshops, webinars, and live chats.

Through a partnership and engagement with the Pan-Canadian Transition of Care Collaborative Network, my next objectives are to influence the uptake of knowledge and resources and influence policy changes in order to improve the transitions of care between oncology and primary care. Such improvements include more comprehensive patient-centred approaches to care with special attention to the transition process itself; to the physical and psychosocial impact, including fear of cancer recurrence; and to the practical impact, such as with cancer and work.

Overall, my current proposed program of research has expanded significantly. I have gained tremendous experience, knowledge, and recognized expertise in cancer care nursing, psychosocial oncology care, and cancer survivorship. In my new role as director-at-large for Research with the Canadian Association of Nurses in Oncology, my goal is to provide mentorship to nurses to engage in patient-centred care research with the aim of improving cancer care. ▪

REFERENCES

Lebel, S., Maheu, C., Lefebvre, M., et al. (2014). Addressing fear of cancer recurrence among women with cancer: A feasibility and preliminary outcome study. *Journal of Cancer Survivorship*, 8(3), 485–496.

Maheu, C. (2009a). Implications of living with a strong family history of breast cancer. *Canadian Journal of Nursing Research*, 41(2), 100–112.

Maheu, C. (2009b). The search for an explanation: Breast cancer in the context of genetic inheritance. *The Qualitative Report*, 14(1), 129–139.

Maheu, C., Lebel, S., Courbasson, C., et al. (2016). Protocol of a randomized controlled trial of the fear of recurrence therapy (FORT) intervention for women with breast or gynecological cancer. *BMC Cancer*, 16, 291.

Maheu, C., Lebel, S., Tomei, C., et al. (2015). Breast and ovarian cancer survivors' experience of participating in a cognitive-existential group intervention addressing fear of cancer recurrence. *European Journal of Oncology Nursing*, 19(4), 433–440.

Maheu, C., Meschino, W., Weiming, H., et al. (2015). Pilot testing of a psycho-educational telephone intervention for women receiving uninformative BRCA1/2 genetic test results. *Canadian Journal of Nursing Research*, 47(1), 53–71.

Maheu, C., & Thorne, S. (2008). Receiving inconclusive genetic test results: An interpretive description of the BRCA1/2 experience. *Research in Nursing & Health*, 31(6), 553–562.

Maheu, C., Vodermaier, A., Rothenmund, H., et al. (2010). Pancreatic cancer risk counselling and screening: Impact on perceived risk and psychological functioning. *Familial Cancer*, 9(4), 617–624.

Vodermaier, A., Esplen, M. J., & Maheu, C. (2010). Can self-esteem, mastery and perceived stigma predict long-term adjustment in women carrying a BRCA1/2-mutation? Evidence from a multicenter study. *Familial Cancer*, 9(3), 305–311.

CHAPTER 20

Developing an Evidence-Informed Practice

Marita Titler | Cherylyn Cameron

LEARNING OUTCOMES

After reading this chapter, you will be able to do the following:

- Differentiate among conduct of nursing research, research utilization, and evidence-informed practice.
- Describe the steps of evidence-informed practice.
- Identify three barriers to evidence-informed practice and strategies to address each.
- List three sources for finding evidence.
- Describe strategies for implementing evidence-informed practice changes.
- Identify steps for evaluating an evidence-informed change in practice.
- Use research findings and other forms of evidence to improve the quality of care.

KEY TERMS

conduct of research	evidence-informed practice	opinion leaders
dissemination	guidelines	problem-focused triggers
evaluation	knowledge-focused triggers	research utilization
evidence-informed practice	knowledge translation	translation science

STUDY RESOURCES

ⓔ Go to Evolve at http://evolve.elsevier.com/Canada/LoBiondo/Research for the Audio Glossary and Appendix Tables that provide supplemental information for Appendix E.

EVIDENCE-INFORMED HEALTH CARE PRACTICES ARE AVAILABLE for a number of conditions, such as asthma, smoking cessation, heart failure, and management of diabetes. However, these practices are not always implemented in care delivery, and variation in practices abounds (Ward, Evans, Spies, et al., 2006). Availability of high-quality research does not ensure that the findings will be used to affect patient outcomes. Research findings in the United States and the Netherlands suggest that 30% to 40% of patients are not receiving evidence-informed care, and 20% to 25% of patients are receiving unneeded or potentially harmful care (Graham, Logan, Harrison, et al., 2006). The use of evidence-informed practices is now an expected standard in many institutions to prevent nosocomial events such as injury from falls, Foley catheter–associated urinary tract infections, and stages 3 and 4 pressure injuries. However, implementing such evidence-informed safety practices is a challenge and requires use of strategies that address the complexity and systems of care, individual practitioners, senior leadership, and, ultimately, changing health care cultures to be evidence-informed practice environments (Leape, 2005; Melnyk & Fineout-Overholt, 2011).

Conducting research is only the first step in improving practice through the use of research. Because of the gap between discovery and use of knowledge in practice (Melnyk, Gallagher-Ford, Long, et al., 2014; Squires, Graham, Hutchinson, et al., 2015; Titler, 2008), efforts must be concentrated on developing methods to speed translation of research findings into practice. Development and dissemination of evidence-informed practice guidelines are essential steps, but each alone does little to promote knowledge uptake by direct care providers. Melnyk et al. (2014) identified multiple barriers to these steps, including the following:

- The perception that it takes too much time
- A lack of evidence-informed practice knowledge and skills among clinicians
- A focus in health professional education on the research process rather than evidence-informed practice
- Lack of support in organizations
- Lack of evidence-informed practice mentors and appropriate resources
- Resistance from colleagues, managers, and leaders, and physicians

Overcoming such barriers is an active process that is facilitated partly by modelling and imitation of other health care providers who have successfully adopted an innovation, by an organizational culture that values and supports use of evidence, and by localization of the evidence for use in a specific health care setting (Melnyk & Fineout-Overholt, 2011; Rogers, 2003). Understanding and mitigating the barriers will promote the widespread adoption of evidence-informed practice.

Translation of research into practice is a multifaceted, systemic process of promoting adoption of evidence-informed practices in delivery of health care services that goes beyond dissemination of evidence-informed guidelines (Rogers, 2003). **Dissemination** is the communication of research findings; dissemination activities take many forms, including publications, conferences, consultations, and training programs (Adams & Titler, 2010), but promoting knowledge uptake and changing practitioner behaviour requires active interchange with those in direct care (Scott, Plotnikoff, Karunamuni, et al., 2008; Titler, Herr, Brooks, et al., 2009).

Although the science of translation is young, the effectiveness of interventions for promoting adoption of evidence-informed practices is currently being studied, and funding is available to support research in this area (Smith, Williams, Owen, et al., 2008; Stetler, McQuenn, Demkis, et al., 2008).

In addition, more evidence is now available to guide selection of strategies for translating research into practice (Brooks, Titler, Ardery, et al., 2009; Gravel, Légaré, & Graham, 2006; Titler, 2008). This chapter presents an overview of evidence-informed practice, the process of implementing evidence in practice to improve patient outcomes, and a description of translation science.

OVERVIEW OF EVIDENCE-INFORMED PRACTICE

The relationships among conduct, dissemination, and use of research are illustrated in Figure 20.1. **Conduct of research** is the analysis of data collected from a homogeneous group of participants who meet study inclusion and exclusion criteria for the purpose of answering specific research questions or testing specified hypotheses. Research design, methods, and statistical analyses are guided by the state of the science in the area of investigation. Traditionally, conduct of research has included dissemination of findings through research reports in journals and at scientific conferences. In comparison, **research utilization** is the process of using research findings to improve patient care; this process involves implementing sound research-based innovations in clinical practice; dissemination of scientific knowledge; critique of studies; synthesis of research findings; determining applicability of findings for practice;

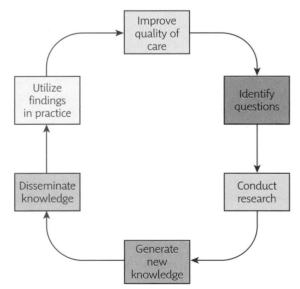

FIG. 20.1 Model of the relationship among conduct, dissemination, and use of research.
(Redrawn from Weiler, K., Buckwalter, K., & Titler, M. (1994). Debate: Is nursing research used in practice? In J. McCloskey & H. Grace (Eds.), *Current issues in nursing* (4th ed.). St. Louis: Mosby.)

developing an evidence-informed standard or guideline; implementing the standard; and evaluating the practice change with respect to staff, patients, and cost/resource utilization (Titler, Kleiber, Steelman, et al., 2001).

Evidence-informed practice is the conscientious and judicious use of current best evidence in conjunction with clinical expertise and patient values to guide health care decisions. As noted in Chapter 1, it is important to differentiate between the terms *evidence-based practice* and *evidence-informed practice*. Evidence-informed practice extends beyond the early definitions of evidence-based practice. Many of the models explored in this chapter refer to evidence-based practice, in as much as they were developed before the use of the term *evidence-informed practice*. The models are still valid and help guide professionals toward actualizing research into best practices. Best evidence includes empirical evidence from systematic reviews, from randomized controlled trials, and from other scientific methods such as descriptive and qualitative research, as well as information from case reports, scientific principles, and expert opinion. When enough research evidence is available, practice should be guided by this evidence, in conjunction with clinical expertise and patients' values. In some cases, however, a sufficient research base may not be available, and health care decision making is derived principally from non-research evidence sources such as expert opinion and scientific principles (Titler et al., 2001). When more research is completed in a specific area, the research evidence must be incorporated into evidence-informed practice. As illustrated in the knowledge generation and use cycle (see Figure 20.1), application of research findings in practice may not only improve quality care but also create new and exciting questions to be addressed through the conduct of research.

The terms *research utilization* and *evidence-informed practice* are sometimes used interchangeably. However, although these two terms are related, they are not one and the same.

Evidence-informed is a broader term that encompasses not only research utilization but also the use of case reports and expert opinion in deciding the practices to be used in health care. If evidence-informed practice is defined as the conscious and judicious use of the current "best" evidence in the care of patients and delivery of health care services, then research utilization is a subset of evidence-informed practice that focuses on the application of research findings.

Use of Evidence in Practice

Nursing has a rich history of using research in practice, pioneered by Florence Nightingale, who used data to change practices that contributed to high mortality rates in hospitals and communities (Nightingale, 1858, 1859, 1863a, 1863b). Although during the early and mid-1900s few nurses built on the solid foundation of research utilization exemplified by Nightingale (Titler, 1994), the nursing profession has provided major leadership for improving care through application of research findings in practice. Today nurses are being prepared as scientists in nursing, leading the way in translation science, and, as a result, the scientific body of nursing knowledge is growing (Estabrooks, Derksen, Winther, et al., 2008; Titler, 2008; Titler et al., 2009). It is now every nurse's responsibility to facilitate the use of nursing knowledge in practice.

Cronenwett (1995) and others have described two forms of using research evidence in practice: conceptual and decision driven (Estabrooks, 2004). Conceptual forms influence the thinking of the health care provider, but not necessarily the action. Exposure to new scientific knowledge occurs, but the new knowledge may not be used to change or guide practice. An integrative review of the literature, formulation of a new theory, or generating of new hypotheses may be the result. Use of knowledge in this way is referred to as *knowledge creep* or *cognitive application*. It is often used by individuals who read and incorporate research into their critical thinking (Weiss, 1980). Decision-driven forms of using evidence in practice encompass application of

scientific knowledge as part of a new practice, policy, procedure, or intervention. In this type of application of research findings, a critical decision is reached to endorse current practice or to change it on the basis of review and critique of studies applicable to that practice. Examples of decision-driven models of using research in practice are the Iowa Model of Evidence-Based Practice to Promote Quality Care (Titler et al., 2001), the Ottawa Model of Research Use (OMRU; Logan & Graham, 1998), the Promoting Action on Research Implementation in Health Services (i-PARIHS) model (Kitson & Harvey, 2016), and the Conduct and Utilization of Research in Nursing (CURN) model (Haller, Reynolds, & Horseley, 1979; Horsley, Crane, Crabtree, et al., 1983).

Multifaceted active dissemination strategies are needed to promote use of research evidence in clinical and administrative health care decision making, and they must address both the individual practitioner's and the organization's perspectives (Titler, 2008). When nurses decide individually what evidence to use in practice, considerable variability in practice patterns results, which can potentially lead to adverse patient outcomes. For example, a solely "individual" perspective of evidence-informed practice would leave the decision about use of pressure injury prevention practices to each nurse. Some nurses may be familiar with the research findings for pressure injury prevention, whereas others may not be. As a result, different nurses may use conflicting practices, especially since shifts change every 8 to 12 hours. From an organizational perspective, policies and procedures are based on research, and then adoption of these practices by nurses is systematically promoted in the organization (Squires, Moralejo, & LeFort, 2007).

Models of Evidence-Informed Practice

Multiple models of evidence-informed practice and translation science are available. Common elements of these models are syntheses of evidence, implementation, evaluation of the effect on patient care, and consideration of the context/setting in which the evidence is implemented. Grol, Bosch, Hulscher, and associates (2007) have provided a summary of models. Included in their summary relevant to quality improvement and implementation of change in health care are cognitive, educational, motivational, social interactive, social learning, social network, and social influence theories, as well as models related to team effectiveness, professional development, and leadership. Additional work by the Improved Clinical Effectiveness through Behavioural Research Group (ICEBeRG) has resulted in the development of a database consisting of planned action models, frameworks, and theories that explicitly describe both the concepts and action steps to be considered or taken. This database was developed from a search of social science, education, and health literature that focused on practitioner or organizational change.

Implementing evidence in practice must be guided by a conceptual model to organize the strategies being used and to clarify extraneous variables (e.g., behaviours and facilitators) that may influence adoption of evidence-informed practices (e.g., organizational size, characteristics of users; ICEBeRG, 2006). Although a thorough review of these models is beyond the scope of this chapter, two models are explored here: the Iowa Model of Evidence-Based Practice to Promote Quality Care and the Ottawa Model of Research Use.

The Iowa Model of Evidence-Based Practice to Promote Quality Care

An overview of the Iowa Model of Evidence-Based Practice to Promote Quality Care, as an example of a practice model, is illustrated in Figure 20.2. This model has been widely disseminated and adopted in academic and clinical settings. Since the original publication of this model in 1994 (Titler, Kleiber, Steelman, et al., 1994), Titler and colleagues have received more than 300 written requests to use the model for publications, presentations, graduate and undergraduate research courses, and clinical research programs. It is an organizational, collaborative model that incorporates conduct of research, use of research evidence, and other types of evidence (Titler et al., 2001). Titler and colleagues adopted the definition of *evidence-based practice* as the conscientious and judicious use of current best evidence to guide health care decisions. Levels of evidence range from randomized controlled trials to case reports and expert opinion.

In this model, knowledge- and problem-focused "triggers" lead staff members to question current nursing practice and whether patient care can be improved through the use of research findings. If, through the process of literature review and critique of studies, staff members find that the number of scientifically sound studies is not sufficient for use as a base for practice, they consider conducting a study. Nurses in practice collaborate with scientists in nursing and other disciplines to conduct clinical research that addresses practice problems encountered in the care of patients. Findings from such studies are then combined with findings from existing scientific knowledge to develop and implement these practices. If research is insufficient for guiding practice, and if conducting a study is not feasible, other types of evidence (e.g., case reports, expert opinion, scientific principles, theory) are used or combined with available research evidence to guide practice. Priority is given to projects in which a high proportion of practice is guided by research evidence. Practice guidelines usually reflect research and nonresearch evidence and therefore are called *evidence-informed practice guidelines*.

An evidence-informed practice guideline is developed from the available evidence. The recommended practices, based on the relevant evidence, are compared with current practice, and a decision is made about the necessity for a practice change. If a practice change is warranted, changes are implemented through a process of planned change. The practice is first implemented with a small group of patients, and it is evaluated. The evidence-informed

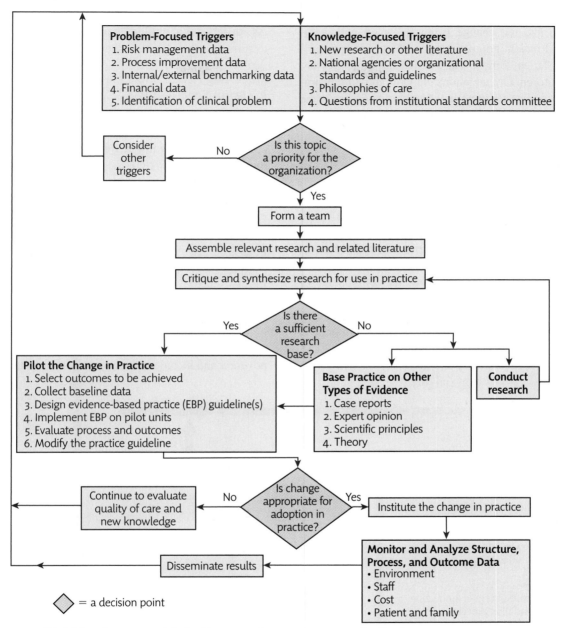

FIG. 20.2 The Iowa Model of Evidence-Based Practice to Promote Quality Care.
(Redrawn from Titler, M. G., Kleiber, C., Steelman, V. J., et al. (2001). The Iowa Model of Evidence-Based Practice to Promote Quality Care. *Critical Care Nursing Clinics of North America, 13*(4), 497–509. Copyright Elsevier 2001.)

practice is then refined on the basis of evaluation data, and the change is implemented with additional patient populations for which it is appropriate. Patient/family, staff, and fiscal outcomes are monitored. Organizational support and administrative support are important factors for success in the use of evidence in care delivery.

The Ottawa Model of Research Use

Logan and Graham (1998) developed the OMRU, a model for interdisciplinary health care research use. The framework was created to "be used by policymakers seeking to increase the use of health research by practitioners, as well as by researchers interested in studying the process by which research becomes integrated into practice" (p. 228). They identified the following six components of research utilization: (1) the practice environment, (2) potential adopters, (3) the evidence-informed innovation, (4) transfer strategies, (5) adoption, and (6) health-related and other outcomes (Figure 20.3). Constant assessment, monitoring, and evaluation

parallel the progression through the components. As barriers are identified, strategies are developed to surmount them and to enhance supports.

Promoting Action on Research Implementation in Health Services (i-PARIHS)

The i-PARIHS model is widely used to introduce knowledge into practice. Kitson and Harvey (2016) spent several years refining the original model, known as PARIHS, into the updated version (i-PARIHS). The aim of this model is to help nurses determine the most appropriate facilitation methods to change practice. The model considers three key elements:

Evidence—the quality and type of evidence
Context—the characteristics of the setting in which the change would occur
Facilitation—the support needed to implement the change into practice

In the newest model, iPARIHS, the *i* stands for *innovation* and includes a practical set of instructions

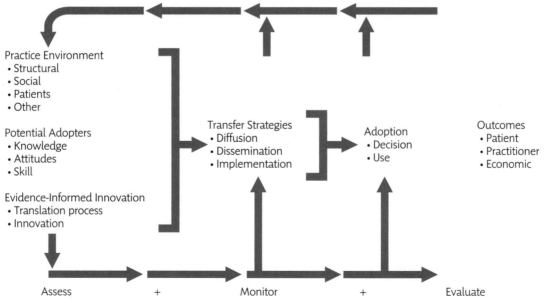

FIG. 20.3 The Ottawa Model of Health Care Research Use.
(Adapted from Logan, J., & Graham, I. (1998). Toward a comprehensive interdisciplinary model of health care research use. *Science Communication, 20*(2), 229. SAGE Publications Inc.)

on how to use the model. Harvey and Kitson (2015) have also developed a clinical resource to facilitate implementation of the PARIHS model.

STEPS OF EVIDENCE-INFORMED PRACTICE

The Iowa Model of Evidence-Based Practice to Promote Quality Care (Titler et al., 2001; see Figure 20.2), in conjunction with Rogers' (1995, 2003) diffusion of innovations model, provides guiding steps in actualizing evidence-informed practice. A team approach is most helpful in fostering a specific evidence-informed practice, with one person in the group providing leadership for the project.

Selection of a Topic

The first step in carrying out an evidence-informed practice project is to select a topic. Ideas for evidence-informed practice come from several sources categorized as problem- and knowledge-focused triggers. **Problem-focused triggers** are research ideas identified by staff through quality improvement, risk surveillance, benchmarking data, financial data, or recurrent clinical problems. For example, the increased incidence of *Clostridium difficile* on a long-term care unit, resulting in increased morbidity, is a problem-focused trigger because it raises concern among hospital staff.

Knowledge-focused triggers are research ideas generated when staff members read research, listen to scientific papers at research conferences, or encounter evidence-informed practice guidelines published by federal agencies or specialty organizations. Examples of such triggers include ideas about pain management, assessing placement of nasogastric and nasointestinal tubes, and use of saline to maintain patency of arterial lines. Sometimes topics arise from a combination of problem- and knowledge-focused triggers, such as the length of bed rest time after femoral artery catheterization. In selecting a topic, nurses must consider how the topic fits with organization, department, and unit priorities in order to garner support from leaders within the organization and the necessary resources to successfully complete the project.

Individuals should work collectively to achieve consensus in topic selection. Working in groups to review performance improvement data, brainstorm about ideas, and achieve consensus about the final selection is helpful. For example, a unit staff meeting may be used to discuss ideas for evidence-informed practice; quality improvement committees may identify several practice areas in need of attention (e.g., urinary tract infections in older patients, reducing the incidence of pressure injuries); an evidence-informed practice task force may be appointed to select and address a clinical practice issue (e.g., pain management); or surveying a panel of experts may be used to prioritize areas for evidence-informed practice. Criteria to consider when a topic is selected are outlined in Box 20.1. Table 20.1 is a helpful chart for selecting a topic.

 Research Hint

Regardless of which method is used to select an evidence-informed practice topic, it is critical that the staff members who will implement the potential practice changes are involved in selecting the topic and view it as contributing significantly to the quality of care.

BOX **20.1**

SELECTION CRITERIA FOR AN EVIDENCE-INFORMED PRACTICE PROJECT

1. The priority of this topic for nursing and for the organization
2. The magnitude of the problem (small, medium, large)
3. Applicability to several or few clinical areas
4. Likelihood of the change to improve quality of care, decrease length of stay, contain costs, or improve patient satisfaction
5. Potential problems associated with the topic and capability to diffuse them
6. Availability of baseline quality improvement or risk data that will be helpful during evaluation
7. Multidisciplinary nature of the topic and ability to create collaborative relationships to effect the needed changes
8. Interest and commitment of staff to the potential topic
9. Availability of a sound body of evidence, preferably research evidence

TABLE **20.1**

TOOL TO USE IN SELECTING A TOPIC* FOR EVIDENCE-INFORMED PRACTICE			
RATING ITEM	TOPIC A	TOPIC B	TOPIC C
Priority for nursing (1 = low; 5 = high)	☐	☐	☐
Priority for organization (1 = low; 5 = high)	☐	☐	☐
Magnitude of the problem (1 = small; 5 = large)	☐	☐	☐
Applicability (1 = narrow; 5 = broad)	☐	☐	☐
Likelihood to improve quality of care (1 = low; 5 = high)	☐	☐	☐
Likelihood to decrease length of stay/contain costs (1 = low; 5 = high)	☐	☐	☐
Likelihood to improve satisfaction (1 = low; 5 = high)	☐	☐	☐
Body of science (1 = little; 5 = multiple studies)	☐	☐	☐
Total	☐	☐	☐

*Each topic should be rated with regard to the scoring criteria and on a 1-to-5 scale. The topic or topics receiving the higher scores should be considered for selection.
Modified from Titler, M. G. (2002). *Toolkit for promoting evidence-based practice.* Iowa City: University of Iowa Hospitals and Clinics, Department of Nursing Services and Patient Care.

Forming a Team

A team is responsible for development, implementation, and evaluation of the evidence-informed practice. The team or group may be an existing committee, such as the quality improvement committee, the practice council, or the research committee. A task force approach also may be used, in which a group is appointed to address a specific practice issue and use research findings or other evidence to improve practice. The composition of the team is directed by the topic selected and should include interested stakeholders in the delivery of care. For example, a team working on evidence-informed pain management should be interdisciplinary and include pharmacists, nurses, physicians, and psychologists. In contrast, a team working on the evidence-informed practice of bathing might include a nurse expert in skin care, assistive nursing personnel, and staff nurses.

In addition to forming a team, key stakeholders who can facilitate the evidence-informed practice project or put up barriers against successful implementation should be identified. A *stakeholder* is a key individual or group of individuals who are directly or indirectly affected by the implementation of the evidence-informed practice. Examples of key stakeholders are nurse managers, nurse educators, researchers, nursing supervisors, chairs of committees or councils that must approve system changes (e.g., policy/procedure revisions; changes in documentation forms), and patients/families. Questions to consider in identification of key stakeholders include the following:

- How are decisions made in the practice areas in which the evidence-informed practice will be implemented?
- What types of system changes will be needed?
- Who is involved in decision making?
- Who is likely to lead and champion implementation of the evidence-informed practice?
- Who can influence the decision to proceed with implementation of an evidence-informed practice?
- What type of cooperation is needed from which stakeholders to be successful?

Use Figure 20.4 to think about the status of key stakeholders and to strategize about interventions to engage various types of stakeholders for your evidence-informed practice project.

STAKEHOLDER INFLUENCE

	High	Low
High	• Can positively affect dissemination and adoption • Need information to gain their buy-in *Strategies:* • Collaborate • Involve and/or provide opportunities where they can be supportive • Encourage feedback • Empower	• Can positively affect dissemination and adoption if given attention • Need attention to maintain buy-in and prevent development of ambivalence *Strategies:* • Collaborate • Encourage feedback • Elicit support via their professional status • Encourage participation, prn • Involve at some level
Low	• Can negatively affect dissemination and adoption • Need great amount of attention and information to obtain and maintain neutrality and work towards buy-in *Strategies:* • Consensus • Build relationships • Detail benefits for them • Involve some (1 or 2) of these individuals on team • Monitor their support	• Least able to influence dissemination and adoption • May have some negative impact • Some attention to obtain neutrality and to work towards buy-in *Strategies:* • Consensus • Build relationships • Involve at some level—team member

(STAKEHOLDER SUPPORT on vertical axis)

Central labels:
- High support / High influence
- High support / Low influence
- Low support / High influence
- Low support / Low influence

FIG. 20.4 Characteristics of stakeholders (resistors and facilitators). (Redrawn from Titler, M. G. (2002). *Toolkit for promoting evidence-based practice.* Iowa City: University of Iowa Hospitals and Clinics, Department of Nursing Services and Patient Care.)

An important early task for the evidence-informed practice team is to formulate the evidence-informed practice question. This helps set boundaries around the project and assists in retrieval of the evidence. A clearly defined question should specify the types of people/patients, interventions or exposures, outcomes, and relevant study designs (Higgins & Green, 2011). For types of people, the team should specify the diseases or conditions of interest, the patient population (e.g.,

age, gender, educational status), and the setting. For example, if the topic for the evidence-informed practice project is pain, the team needs to specify the type of pain (e.g., acute, persistent, cancer), the age of the population (e.g., children, neonates, adults, older adults), and the setting (e.g., inpatient, outpatient, ambulatory care, home care, primary care). For intervention, the types of interventions of interest to the project and the comparison interventions (e.g., standard care, alternative treatments) need to be specified. In the example of pain, the interventions of interest might include pharmacological treatment, analgesic administration methods (e.g., patient-controlled analgesia, epidural, intravenous), pain assessment, nonpharmacological treatment, and patient/family education regarding self-care pain management. For outcomes, the team should select outcomes of primary importance and consider the type of outcome data that will be needed for decision making (e.g., benefits, harm, cost). Outcomes that may be interesting but of little importance to the project should be excluded.

Finally, it is important to consider the types of study designs that are likely to provide reliable data to answer the question, and the team must search for the highest level of evidence available. A similar type of approach to formulating the practice question is PICOT: patient, population, or problem; intervention/treatment; comparison intervention/treatment; outcomes; and time frame (Melnyk & Fineout-Overholt, 2011). This approach is illustrated in Table 20.2.

Evidence Retrieval

Once a topic is selected, relevant research and related literature must be retrieved and should include clinical studies, meta-analyses, integrative literature reviews, and existing evidence-informed practice guidelines. As more evidence is available to guide practice, professional organizations and federal agencies are developing and making available evidence-informed practice guidelines. It is important that these guidelines are accessed as part of the literature retrieval process.

The Agency for Healthcare Research and Quality (AHRQ) sponsors a National Guideline Clearinghouse that makes abstracts of evidence-informed practice guidelines available on its website (http://www.guideline.gov). Other examples of professional organizations that publish evidence-informed practice guidelines are found in Table 20.3. Current best evidence from

TABLE 20.2
PICOT: COMPONENTS OF AN ANSWERABLE, SEARCHABLE QUESTION

Patient population/disease: The patient population or disease of interest, for example:
- Age
- Gender
- Ethnicity
- With certain disorder (e.g., hepatitis)

Intervention or issue of interest: The intervention or range of interventions of interest, for example:
- Therapy
- Exposure to disease
- Prognostic factor A
- Risk behaviour (e.g., smoking)

Comparison intervention or issue of interest: What you want to compare the intervention or issue against, for example:
- Alternative therapy, placebo, or no intervention/therapy
- No disease
- Prognostic factor B
- Absence of risk factor (e.g., nonsmoking)

Outcome: Outcome of interest, for example:
- Outcome expected from therapy (e.g., pressure injuries)
- Risk of disease
- Accuracy of diagnosis
- Rate of occurrence of adverse outcome (e.g., death)

Time: The time involved to demonstrate an outcome, for example:
- The time it takes for the intervention to achieve the outcome
- The time over which populations are observed for the outcome (e.g., quality of life) to occur, given a certain condition (e.g., prostate cancer)

From Melnyk, B. M., & Fineout-Overholt, E. (2011). *Evidence-based practice in nursing and healthcare: A guide to best practice* (2nd ed., p. 30, Table 2-1). New York: Wolters Kluwer.

specific studies of clinical problems can be found in an increasing number of electronic databases (see Table 20.3).

In 1999, the Registered Nurses' Association of Ontario (RNAO) initiated the Nursing Best Practice Guidelines Project to develop practice guidelines for nurses providing patient care. The project had published 50 completed guidelines as of June 2017, with several additional guidelines under development. Each best practice guideline is developed in phases: planning, development, implementation, evaluation, and dissemination.

TABLE 20.3	
SOURCES FOR EVIDENCE-INFORMED PRACTICE GUIDELINES AND STUDIES OF CLINICAL PROBLEMS	
ORGANIZATION	**WEBSITE**
PROFESSIONAL ORGANIZATIONS THAT PUBLISH EVIDENCE-INFORMED PRACTICE GUIDELINES	
American Association of Critical-Care Nurses	http://www.aacn.org
American Pain Society	http://americanpainsociety.org/
Canadian Heart and Stroke Foundation	http://www.strokebestpractices.ca
National Institute for Health and Care Excellence	http://www.nice.org.uk
Registered Nurses' Association of Ontario (RNAO)	http://www.rnao.ca
SOURCES FOR BEST EVIDENCE FROM STUDIES OF CLINICAL PROBLEMS	
American College of Physicians	http://www.acponline.org
Centre for Health Evidence	http://www.cche.net
Cochrane Library	http://www.cochranelibrary.com
Joanna Briggs Institute	http://joannabriggs.org

The topics covered by these guidelines range from smoking cessation to screening for delirium, dementia, and depression in older adults.

The plan for dissemination of the guidelines is threefold. First, the RNAO requested proposals from interested and eligible health care organizations to work in collaboration to plan, implement, and evaluate nursing best practice guidelines and disseminate knowledge from demonstrated experiences with guidelines. Second, the Best Practice Champions Network was established to prepare nurses to disseminate the best practice guidelines in their practices throughout Ontario. Third, the RNAO sponsored 10 demonstration projects for colleges and universities to integrate best practice guidelines into nursing curricula.

The guidelines program now also offers Advanced Clinical/Practice Fellowship (ACPF) for nurses or health care organizations. It is designed to provide registered nurses with a "focused self-directed learning experience to develop clinical, leadership or best practices guideline implementation knowledge and skills, with support from a mentor(s), the organization where the [registered nurse] is employed, and the RNAO. This initiative is aimed at developing and promoting nursing knowledge and expertise, and improving patient care and outcomes in Ontario" (RNAO, 2012, p. 1). The RNAO best practice guidelines are readily available to nurses through an application for personal electronic devices (e.g., BlackBerry, iPhone, and Android). Details are provided at the website: http://rnao.ca/bpg/app.

Another electronic database, Evidence-Based Medicine Reviews (EBMR) from Ovid Technologies (http://www.ovid.com/site/catalog/databases/904.jsp), combines several electronic databases, including the Cochrane Database of Systematic Reviews, Cochrane Database of Methodology Reviews (CDMR), and MEDLINE, plus links to more than 200 full-text journals. EBMR links these databases to one another; if a study on a topic of interest is found on MEDLINE and also has been included in a systematic review in the Cochrane Library, the review also can be readily and easily accessed.

In using these sources, it is important to identify key search terms and to use the expertise of health science librarians in locating publications relevant to the project. Additional information about locating the evidence is in Chapter 5.

Once the literature is located, it is helpful to classify the articles as clinical (nonresearch), integrative research reviews, theory articles, research articles, synthesis reports, meta-analyses, and evidence-informed practice guidelines. Before you read and critique the research, it is useful to read theoretical and clinical articles to have a broad view of the nature of the topic and related concepts and to then review existing evidence-informed practice guidelines. It is helpful to read articles in the following order:

1. Clinical articles, to understand the state of the practice
2. Theory articles, to understand the various theoretical perspectives and concepts that may be encountered when you critique studies
3. Systematic review articles and synthesis reports, to understand the state of the science
4. Evidence-informed practice guidelines and evidence reports
5. Research articles, including meta-analyses

Schemas for Grading the Evidence

There is no consensus among professional organizations or across health care disciplines regarding the best system to use for denoting the type and quality of evidence or for grading schemas to denote the strength of the body of evidence (Atkins, Briss, Eccles, et al., 2005; Guyatt, Oxman, Vist, et al., 2008). For example, the Scottish Intercollegiate Guidelines Network has an extensive method detailed on their website for appraising research and setting forth guideline recommendations (http://www.sign.ac.uk/methodology.html).

The Grading of Recommendations Assessment, Development, and Evaluation (GRADE) Working Group, initiated in 2000, is an informal collaboration of individuals interested in addressing grading schema in health care (http://www.gradeworkinggroup.org). In setting forth practice recommendations, the GRADE system first rates the quality of the evidence as high, moderate, low, or very low and then grades the strength of the evidence as strong or weak (GRADE Working Group, 2004; Guyatt, Oxman, Kunz, et al., 2008a, 2008b; Table 20.4). Their methods are available on their website, with grading software (GRADEpro) available.

The National Guidelines Clearinghouse classifies submitted guidelines according to methods used by developers to accomplish two goals: (1) to assess the quality and strength of the evidence through expert consensus (committee or expert panel method), through subjective review, through weighting according to a rating scheme provided by the developers, or through weighting according to a rating scheme not provided by the developers; and (2) to formulate recommendations through various types of expert consensus (e.g., expert manual method; nominal group technique, consensus development conference) and balance sheets.

The RNAO (2012) guidelines for best practices are based on scientific evidence after a thorough review of the literature. Each of the studies is rated to determine whether it should be included in the guideline. The rating system used for the level of evidence and the grades of recommendation are illustrated in Table 20.4.

Before critiquing research articles, reading relevant literature, and reviewing evidence-informed practice guidelines, an organization or group responsible for the review must agree on methods for noting the type of research, rating the quality of individual articles, and grading the strength of the body of evidence. Users must evaluate which systems are most appropriate for the task being undertaken, the length of time to complete each instrument, and its ease of use. It is also important to decide how the strength of the evidence will be reflected in the guideline.

Critique of Evidence-Informed Practice Guidelines

As the number of evidence-informed practice guidelines proliferate, it becomes increasingly important that nurses critique these guidelines with regard to the methods used for formulating them and consider how they might be used in their practice. Critical areas that should be assessed when evidence-informed practice guidelines are critiqued include the following:

1. Date of publication or release
2. Authors of the guideline
3. Endorsement of the guideline
4. A clear purpose of what the guideline covers and patient groups for which it was designed
5. Types of evidence (research, nonresearch) used in formulating the guideline

TABLE **20.4**

EXAMPLES OF EVIDENCE-INFORMED PRACTICE RATING SYSTEMS

GRADE WORKING GROUP (2004)	REGISTERED NURSES' ASSOCIATION OF ONTARIO (2011)	U.S. PREVENTIVE SERVICES TASK FORCE (2008; HARRIS ET AL., 2001)

STRENGTH OF EVIDENCE/QUALITY OF EVIDENCE

High: Further research is very unlikely to change our confidence in the estimate of effect. Scientific evidence provided by well-designed, well-conducted, controlled trials (randomized and non-randomized) with statistically significant results that consistently support the guideline recommendation.

Moderate: Further research is likely to have an important impact on our confidence in the estimate of effect and may change the estimate.

Low: Further research is very likely to have an important impact on our confidence in the estimate of effect and is likely to change the estimate.

Very Low: Any estimate of effect is very uncertain.

Note: The type of evidence is first ranked as follows:

Randomized trial = high.
Observational study = low.
Any other evidence = very low.

Limitations in study quality, important inconsistency of results, uncertainty about the directness of the evidence, imprecise or sparse data, and high probability of reporting bias can lower the grade of evidence. Expert opinion supports the guideline recommendation because the available scientific evidence did not present consistent results or because controlled trials were lacking. Grade of evidence can be increased if there is (1) strong evidence of association—significant relative risk of >2 (<0.5) based on consistent evidence from two or more observational studies, with no plausible confounders (1); (2) very strong evidence of association—significant relative risk of >5 (<0.2) based on direct evidence with no major threats to validity (2); (3) evidence of a dose response gradient (1); and (4) all plausible confounders would have reduced the effect (1).

LEVELS OF EVIDENCE

Ia: Evidence obtained from meta-analysis or systematic review of randomized controlled trials

Ib: Evidence obtained from at least one randomized controlled trial

IIa: Evidence obtained from at least one well-designed controlled study without randomization

IIb: Evidence obtained from at least one other type of well-designed quasiexperimental study

III: Evidence obtained from well-designed nonexperimental descriptive studies, such as comparative studies, correlation studies, and case studies

IV: Evidence obtained from expert committee reports or opinions and/or clinical experiences of respected authorities

LEVELS OF CERTAINTY REGARDING NET BENEFIT

High: The available evidence usually includes consistent results from well-designed, well-conducted studies in representative primary care populations. These studies assess the effects of the preventive service on health outcomes. This conclusion is therefore unlikely to be strongly affected by the results of future studies.

Moderate: The available evidence is sufficient to determine the effects of the preventive service on health outcomes, but confidence in the estimate is constrained by such factors as the following:

- The number, size, or quality of individual studies
- Inconsistency of findings across individual studies
- Limited generalizability of findings to routine primary care practice
- Lack of coherence in the chain of evidence

As more information becomes available, the magnitude or direction of the observed effect could change, and this change may be large enough to alter the conclusion.

Low: The available evidence is insufficient to assess effects on health outcomes. Evidence is insufficient because of one or more of the following:

- The limited number or size of studies
- Important flaws in study design or methods
- Inconsistency of findings across individual studies
- Gaps in the chain of evidence
- Findings not generalizable to routine primary care practice
- Lack of information on important health outcomes.

More information may allow estimation of effects on health outcomes.

Continued

TABLE **20.4**

EXAMPLES OF EVIDENCE-INFORMED PRACTICE RATING SYSTEMS—cont'd

GRADE WORKING GROUP (2004)	REGISTERED NURSES' ASSOCIATION OF ONTARIO (2011)	U.S. PREVENTIVE SERVICES TASK FORCE (2008; HARRIS ET AL., 2001)
STRENGTH OF RECOMMENDATIONS **Strong:** Confident that the desirable effects of adherence to a recommendation outweigh the undesirable effects. **Weak:** The desirable effects of adherence to a recommendation probably outweigh the undesirable effects, but the developers are less confident. *Note:* Strength of recommendation is determined by the balance between desirable and undesirable consequences of alternative management strategies, quality of evidence, variability in values and preferences, and resource use.	**GRADES OF RECOMMENDATION** A: There is good evidence to recommend the clinical preventive action. B: There is fair evidence to recommend the clinical preventive action. C: The existing evidence is conflicting and does not allow making a recommendation for or against use of the clinical preventive action; however, other factors may influence decision making. D: There is fair evidence to recommend against the clinical preventive action. E: There is good evidence to recommend against the clinical preventive action. I: There is insufficient evidence (in quantity and/or quality) to make recommendations, however other factors may influence decision making.	**GRADES OF RECOMMENDATION** A: The USPSTF recommends the service. There is high certainty that the net benefit is substantial. Practice: Offer or provide this service. B: The USPSTF recommends the service. There is high certainty that the net benefit is moderate or there is moderate certainty that the net benefit is moderate to substantial. Practice: Offer or provide this service. C: The USPSTF recommends against routinely providing the service. There may be considerations that support providing the service in an individual patient. There is at least moderate certainty that the net benefit is small. Practice: Offer or provide this service only if other considerations support the offering or providing the service in an individual patient. D: The USPSTF recommends against the service. There is moderate or high certainty that the service has no net benefit or that the harms outweigh the benefits. Practice: Discourage the use of this service. I: The USPSTF concludes that the current evidence is insufficient to assess the balance of benefits and harms of the service. Evidence is lacking, of poor quality, or conflicting, and the balance of benefits and harms cannot be determined. Practice: Read the clinical considerations section of USPSTF Recommendation Statement. If the service is offered, patients should understand the uncertainty about the balance of benefits and harms.

USPSTF, U.S. Preventive Services Task Force.
From Registered Nurses' Association of Ontario (RNAO). (2011). Rating system described by Canadian Task Force on Preventive Health Care. (CTFPHC). (1997). *Quick tables by strength of evidence.* Available at http://www.canadiantaskforce.ca and http://rnao.ca/sites/rnao-ca/files/storage/related/618_BPG_Falls_summary_revo5.pdf.

6. Types of research included in formulating the guideline (e.g., "We considered only randomized and other prospective controlled trials in determining efficacy of therapeutic interventions.")

7. A description of the methods used in grading the evidence

8. Search terms and retrieval methods used to acquire research and nonresearch evidence used in the guideline

9. Well-referenced statements regarding practice

10. Comprehensive reference list

11. Review of the guideline by experts

12. Whether the guideline has been used or tested in practice and, if so, with what types of patients and in what types of settings

Evidence-informed practice guidelines are principles that help the researcher better understand the evidence base of certain practices, such as guidelines, formulated through the use of rigorous methods, and provide a useful starting point for nurses to understand the evidence base of certain practices. However, more research may have become available since the publication of the guideline, and refinements may be needed. Although information in well-developed, national, evidence-informed practice guidelines is a helpful reference, it is usually necessary to localize the guideline through the use of institution-specific, evidence-informed policies, procedures, or standards before the guideline is applied within a specific setting. A useful tool for critiquing clinical practice guidelines is the AGREE II tool (available at http://www.agreetrust.org/).

As evidence-informed practice guidelines are used more extensively in practice, research is becoming available on whether the utilization of the guidelines results in better patient outcomes. One such study investigated the relationship between the evidence-informed practice and client pain, dyspnea, fall, and pressure ulcer outcomes in the home care setting (Doran, Lefebre, O'Brien-Pallas, et al., 2014). Their results did show an improvement in client outcomes when evidence-informed guidelines (based on the RNAO best practice guidelines) were implemented.

Critique of Research

Critique of each study should involve the same methodology, and the critique process should be a shared responsibility. Methods to make the critique process fun and interesting include the following:

- Using a journal club to discuss critiques performed by each member of the group
- Pairing a novice and expert to do critiques
- Eliciting assistance from students who may be interested in the topic and want experience performing critiques
- Making a class project of critique and synthesis of research for a given topic

Several resources are available to assist with the critique process, including *Evidence-Based Medicine: How to Practice and Teach EBM* and the accompanying compact disc (Straus, Richardson, Glasziou, et al., 2005), and *Evidence-Based Nursing: A Guide to Clinical Practice* (DiCenso, Guyatt, & Ciliska, 2005). If you wish to start your own journal club, refer to Silversides (2011) for practical advice and further references. It takes frequent practice to develop research critique skills.

 Research Hint _____

Keep critique processes simple, and encourage participation by staff members who are providing direct patient care.

Synthesis of the Research

Once studies are critiqued, a decision is made regarding use of each study in the synthesis of the evidence for application in clinical practice. Factors that should be considered for inclusion of studies in the synthesis of findings are overall scientific merit of the study; type (e.g., age, gender, pathological condition) of participants enrolled in the study and their similarity to the patient population to which the findings will be applied; and relevance of the study to the topic of question. For example, if the practice area is prevention of deep venous thrombosis in patients after surgery, a descriptive study with a heterogeneous population of medical patients is not appropriate for inclusion in the synthesis of findings.

To synthesize the findings from research critiques, it is helpful to use a summary table (Table 20.5) in which critical information from studies can be documented. Essential information to include in such a summary is the following:

- Study purpose
- Research questions/hypotheses
- The variables studied
- A description of the study sample and setting
- The type of research design
- The methods used to measure each variable
- Detailed description of the independent variable/intervention tested
- The study findings

TABLE 20.5

EXAMPLE OF A SUMMARY TABLE FOR RESEARCH CRITIQUES

CITATION	PURPOSE AND RESEARCH QUESTION	RESEARCH DESIGN	SAMPLE	INDEPENDENT VARIABLES AND MEASURES	DEPENDENT VARIABLES AND MEASURES	STATISTICAL TESTS	RESULTS	IMPLICATIONS	GENERAL STRENGTHS	GENERAL WEAKNESSES	OVERALL QUALITY OF STUDY*	SUMMARY STATEMENTS FOR PRACTICE

*Use a consistent rating system (e.g., good, fair, poor).

Setting Forth Evidence-Informed Practice Recommendations

On the basis of the critique of evidence-informed practice guidelines and synthesis of research, recommendations for practice are set forth. The type and strength of evidence used to support the practice need to be clearly delineated. Box 20.2 is a useful tool to assist with this activity.

The following are examples of practice recommendation statements:

- "Small, informal group health education classes, delivered in the antenatal period, have a better impact on breastfeeding initiation rates than breastfeeding literature alone or combined with

---

BOX **20.2**

CONSISTENCY OF EVIDENCE FROM CRITIQUED RESEARCH AND APPRAISALS OF EVIDENCE-INFORMED PRACTICE GUIDELINES

1. Are studies replicated with consistent results?
2. Are the studies well designed?
3. Are recommendations consistent among systematic reviews, evidence-informed practice guidelines, and critiqued research?
4. Are risks to the patient identified from evidence-informed practice recommendations?
5. Are benefits to the patient identified?
6. Have cost analysis studies been conducted with regard to the recommended action, intervention, or treatment?
7. Are summary recommendations about assessments, actions, and interventions or treatments available from the research, systematic reviews, and evidence-informed guidelines with an assigned evidence grade?
8. Is one of the following examples of grading the evidence used?
   a. Evidence from well-designed meta-analysis or other systematic reviews
   b. Evidence from well-designed controlled trials, both randomized and nonrandomized, with results that consistently support a specific action (e.g., assessment), intervention, or treatment
   c. Evidence from observational studies (e.g., correlational descriptive studies) or controlled trials with inconsistent results
   d. Evidence from expert opinion or multiple cases

Modified from Titler, M. G. (2002). *Toolkit for promoting evidence-based practice.* Iowa City: University of Iowa Hospitals and Clinics, Department of Nursing Services and Patient Care.

---

formal, noninteractive methods of teaching." (Strength of recommendation = B) (RNAO, 2003, p. 46)

- Older people who have recurrent falls should be offered long-term exercise and balance training. (Strength of recommendation = B) (American Geriatrics Society, British Geriatrics Society, American Academy of Orthopaedic Surgeons, & Panel on Falls Prevention, 2001).
- "Every client should be screened to identify those most likely to be affected by asthma. As part of the basic respiratory assessment, nurses should ask every patient two questions:
  - Have you ever been told by a physician that you have asthma?
  - Have you ever used a puffer or inhaler or asthma medication for breathing problems?" (Strength of recommendation = D) (RNAO, 2004, p. 30).
- Apply dressings that maintain a moist wound environment. Examples of moist dressings include, but are not limited to, hydrogels, hydrocolloids, saline moistened gauze, and transparent film dressings. The pressure injury bed should be kept continuously moist. (Evidence Grade = B) (Colwell, Foreman, & Trotter, 1992; Folkedahl, Frantz, & Goode, 2002; Fowler & Goupil, 1984; Gorse & Messner, 1987; Kurzuk-Howard, Simpson, & Palmieri, 1985; Neill, Conforti, Kedas, et al., 1989; Oleske, Smith, White, et al., 1986; Saydak, 1990; Sebern, 1986; Xakellis & Chrischilles, 1992).

 Research Hint_____

Use of a summary form helps identify commonalities across several studies with regard to study findings and the types of patients to which study findings can be applied. It also helps in synthesizing the overall strengths and weakness of the studies as a group.

Decision to Change Practice

After studies are critiqued and synthesized and evidence-informed practices are set forth, the next step is to decide whether findings are appropriate for use in practice. The following criteria should be considered in making these decisions:

- Relevance of evidence for practice
- Consistency in findings across studies, guidelines, or both
- A significant number of studies, evidence-informed practice guidelines, or both in which sample characteristics are similar to those to which the findings will be applied
- Consistency among evidence from research and other nonresearch evidence
- Feasibility for use in practice
- The risk–benefit ratio (risk of harm; potential benefit for the patient)

Synthesis of study findings and other evidence may result in supporting current practice, making minor practice modifications, undertaking major practice changes, or developing a new area of practice. For example, Madsen, Sebolt, Cullen, and colleagues (2005) used a combination of research findings and expert consultation to derive a guideline that resulted in a change in practice for assessing bowel motility after abdominal surgery in an adult inpatient population. Madsen and colleagues' project resulted in (1) omitting bowel sound assessment as a marker of return of gastrointestinal motility and (2) using return of flatus, first bowel movement, and absence of abdominal distention as primary indicators of return of bowel motility after abdominal surgery in adults.

Development of Evidence-Informed Practice

The next step is to put in writing the evidence base of the practice (Haber, Feldman, Penney, et al., 1994); the grading schema that has been agreed upon should be used. When results of the critique and synthesis of evidence support current practice or suggest a change in practice, a written evidence-informed practice standard (e.g., policy, procedure, guideline) is warranted. This is necessary so that professionals in the organization (1) know that the practices are based on evidence and (2) know which type of evidence (e.g., randomized controlled trial,

expert opinion) was used in developing the evidence-informed standard. Several different formats can be used to document evidence-informed practice changes. The format chosen is influenced by what the document is and how it will be used. Written evidence-informed practices should be part of the organizational policy and procedure manual and should include linkages to the references for the parts of the policy and procedure that are based on research and other types of evidence.

Clinicians (e.g., nurses, physicians, pharmacists) who adopt evidence-informed practices are influenced by the perceived participation they have had in developing and reviewing the protocol (Titler, 2008). It is imperative that once the evidence-informed practice standard is written, key stakeholders have an opportunity to review it and provide feedback to the person or persons responsible for writing it. Focus groups can provide discussion about the evidence-informed standard and identify key areas that may be potentially troublesome during the implementation phase. Key questions that can be used in the focus groups are listed in Box 20.3.

 Research Hint

Use a consistent approach to writing evidence-informed practice standards and referencing the research and related literature.

BOX **20.3**

KEY QUESTIONS FOR FOCUS GROUPS

1. What is needed by (nurses, physicians) to use the evidence-informed practice with patients in units (specify unit)?
2. In your opinion, how will this standard improve patient care in your unit/practice?
3. What modifications would you suggest in the evidence-informed practice standard before you would use it in your practice?
4. What content in the evidence-informed practice standard is unclear? Needs revision?
5. What would you change about the format of the evidence-informed practice standard?
6. What part of this evidence-informed practice change do you view as most challenging?
7. Any other suggestions?

Implementing the Practice Change

If a practice change is warranted, the next steps are to make the evidence-informed changes in practice. This step goes beyond writing a policy or procedure that is evidence informed; it requires interaction among direct care providers to champion and foster evidence adoption, leadership support, and system changes. Rogers's (2003) seminal work on diffusion of innovations is extremely useful for selecting strategies for promoting adoption of evidence-informed practices. Other investigators describing barriers to and strategies for adoption of evidence-informed practices have used Rogers's (2003) model (Gravel et al., 2006; Scott et al., 2008; Thompson, Estabrooks, Scott-Findlay, et al., 2007).

According to this model, adoption of innovations, such as evidence-informed practices, is influenced by the nature of the innovation (e.g., the type and strength of evidence; the clinical topic) and the manner in which it is communicated (disseminated) to members (nurses) of a social system (organization, nursing profession; Rogers, 2003). Strategies for promoting adoption of evidence-informed practices must address these areas within a context of participative, planned change (Figure 20.5). The RNAO (2012) published *Toolkit: Implementation of Best Practice Guidelines* to assist staff in health care settings to successfully integrate the guidelines into clinical practice. The toolkit outlines seven essential components of knowledge translation:

1. Identify the problem: identify, review, select knowledge tools/resources
2. Adapt knowledge tools/resources to local context
3. Assess barriers and facilitators to knowledge use
4. Select, tailor, and implement interventions
5. Monitor knowledge use
6. Evaluate outcomes
7. Sustain knowledge use

Nature of the Innovation/Evidence-Informed Practice

Characteristics of an innovation or evidence-informed practice topic that affect adoption include the relative advantage of the evidence-informed practice (e.g., effectiveness, relevance to the task, social prestige); the compatibility with values, norms, work, and perceived needs of users; and complexity of the evidence-informed practice topic (Rogers, 2003). For example, evidence-informed practice topics that are perceived by users as relatively simple (e.g., influenza vaccines for older adults) are more easily adopted in less time than those that are more complex (e.g., acute pain management for hospitalized older adults).

Strategies to promote adoption of evidence-informed practices related to characteristics of the

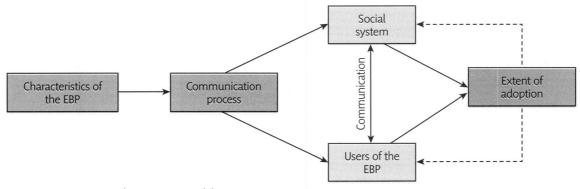

FIG. 20.5 Implementation model.
(Redrawn from Rogers, E. M. (1995). *Diffusion of innovations*. New York: Free Press; and from Titler, M. G., & Everett, L. Q. (2001). Translating research into practice: Considerations for critical care investigators. *Critical Care Nursing Clinics of North America, 13*(4), 587–604.)

topic include practitioner review and "reinvention" of the evidence-informed practice guideline to fit the local context, use of quick reference guides and decision aids, and use of clinical reminders (Doebbeling, Chou, & Tierney, 2006).

An important principle to remember for planning implementation of an evidence-informed practice is that the attributes of the evidence-informed practice topic as perceived by users and stakeholders (e.g., ease of use, valued part of practice) are neither stable features nor sure determinants of their adoption. Rather, it is the interaction among the characteristics of the evidence-informed practice topic, the intended users, and a particular context of practice that determines the rate and extent of adoption (Rogers, 2003).

Studies suggest that clinical systems, computerized decision support, and prompts/quick reference guides that support practice (e.g., decision-making algorithms) have a positive effect on aligning practices with the evidence base (Doebbeling et al., 2006; Titler, Herr, Everett, et al., 2006).

Computerized knowledge management has consistently demonstrated significant improvements in provider performance and patient outcomes (Wensing, Wollersheim, & Grol, 2006). Feldman, Murtaugh, Pezzin, and associates (2005), using a just-in-time email reminder in home health care, demonstrated (1) improvements in evidence-informed care and outcomes for patients with heart failure and (2) reduced pain intensity for cancer patients (McDonald, Pezzin, Feldman, et al., 2005). There is still much to learn about the "best" manner of deploying evidence-informed information through electronic clinical information systems to support evidence-informed care. An example of a quick reference guide is shown in Figure 20.6.

Methods of Communication

Interpersonal communication methods and influence among social networks of users affect adoption of evidence-informed practices (Rogers, 2003). Use of opinion leaders, change champions,

consultation with experts in the field, and education are strategies tested to promote adoption of evidence-informed practices. Education is necessary, and research has demonstrated that attending conferences and in-service programs is effective (Squires, Estabrooks, Gustavsson, et al., 2011).

It is important that staff know the scientific basis and improvements in quality of care anticipated by the changes. Disseminating information to staff needs to be done creatively. A staff in-service may not be the most effective method nor reach the majority of the staff. Although it is unrealistic for all staff to have participated in the critique process or to have read all studies used, it is important that they know the myths and realities of the practice. Staff education must also include ensuring competence in the skills necessary to carry out the new practice.

One method of communicating information to staff is through use of colourful posters that identify myths and realities or describe the essence of the change in practice (Titler et al., 2001). Visibly identifying those who have learned the information and are using the evidence-informed practice (e.g., through wearing buttons, ribbons, pins) stimulates interest in others who may not have internalized the change. As a result, the "new" learner may begin asking questions about the practice and be more open to learning. Other educational strategies such as train-the-trainer programs, webinars, and competency testing are helpful in education of staff.

Several studies have demonstrated that opinion leaders are effective in changing behaviours of health care practitioners (Dopson, FitzGerald, Ferlie, et al., 2010; Doumit, Gattellari, Grimshaw, et al., 2007), especially in combination with educational outreach or performance feedback. **Opinion leaders** are from the local peer group, viewed as a respected source of influence, considered by associates as technically competent, and trusted to judge the fit between the innovation and the local situation (Dobbins,

Use this quick reference guide to help in the assessment of pain:
- Before clients undergo medical procedures or surgeries that can cause pain
- When clients are experiencing pain from recent surgeries, medical procedures, trauma, or other acute illness

General principles for assessing pain in older adults:
- Verify sensory ability (Can the person see you? Hear you?).
- Allow time to respond.
- Repeat questions/instructions as necessary.
- Use printed materials with large type and dark lines.

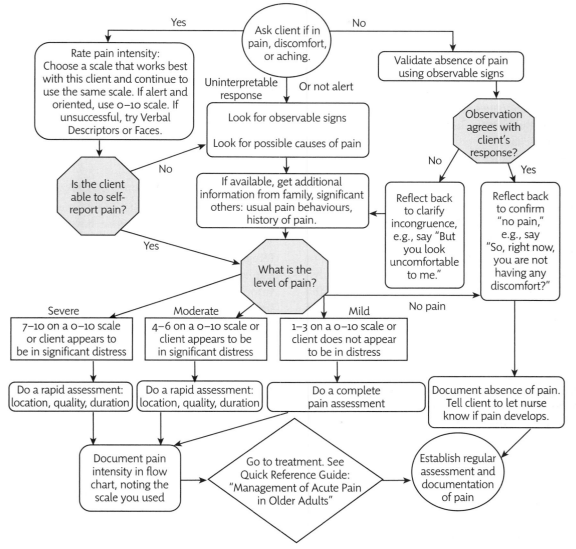

FIG. 20.6 Quick reference guide: Assessment of acute pain in older adults.
(Redrawn from Harris, R. P., Helfan, M., Woolf, S. H., et al. (2001). Current methods of the U. S. Preventive Services Task Force: A review of the process. *American Journal of Preventive Medicine* 20(3S), 21–35; and from Herr, K., Titler, M., Sorofman, B., et al. (2000). Evidence-based guideline: Acute pain management in the elderly. In *From book to bedside: Acute pain management in the elderly* [Grant No. 1 R01 HS10482-01]. Iowa City: University of Iowa.)

Robeson, & Ciliska, 2009; Doumit et al., 2007). The key characteristic of an opinion leader is that he or she is trusted to evaluate new information in the context of group norms. To do this, an opinion leader must be considered by associates as technically competent and a full and dedicated member of the local group (Rogers, 2003).

Social interactions such as "hallway chats," one-on-one discussions, and addressing questions are important yet often overlooked components of translation (Jordan, Lanham, Crabtree, et al., 2009). If the evidence-informed practice that is being implemented is interdisciplinary, discipline-specific opinion leaders should be used to promote the change in practice. Role expectations of an opinion leader are in Box 20.4.

Because nurses prefer interpersonal contact and communication with colleagues rather than Internet or traditional sources of practice knowledge (Estabrooks, Chong, Brigidear, et al., 2005), it is imperative that one or two "change champions" be identified for each patient care unit or clinic where the change is being made so that evidence-informed practices can be enacted by direct care providers (Titler et al., 2006). Staff nurses are some of the best change agents for evidence-informed practice. The change champion believes in an idea; will not take "no" for an answer; is undaunted by insults and rebuffs; and, above all, persists. Conferencing with opinion leaders and change champions periodically during implementation is helpful in addressing questions and providing guidance as needed (Titler et al., 2006).

Additionally, clinical nurse educators can provide one-on-one consultation to staff regarding use of the evidence-informed practice with specific patients, assist staff in troubleshooting issues in application of the practice, and provide feedback on provider performance regarding use of the evidence-informed practice.

Users of the Evidence-Informed Practice

Members of a social system (e.g., nurses, physicians, clerical staff) influence how quickly and widely evidence-informed practices are adopted (Rogers, 2003). Audit and feedback, performance gap assessment (PGA), and trying the evidence-informed practice are strategies that have been tested (Hysong, Best, & Pugh, 2006; Ivers, Jamtvedt, Flottorp, et al., 2012; Jamtvedt, Young, Kristoffersen, et al., 2010; Titler et al., 2006). PGA (baseline practice performance) informs members at the beginning of change about a practice performance and opportunities for improvement. Specific practice indicators selected for PGA are related to the practices that are the focus of the practice change, such as every-4-hour pain assessment for acute pain management (Titler et al., 2006).

The practice of audit and feedback involves ongoing auditing of performance indicators, aggregating data into reports, and discussing the findings with practitioners during the practice change (Ivers et al., 2012; Jamtvedt et al., 2010; Titler et al., 2006). This strategy helps staff know and see how their efforts to improve care and patient outcomes are progressing throughout the implementation process.

BOX 20.4

ROLE EXPECTATIONS OF AN OPINION LEADER

1. Be or become an expert in the evidence-informed practice.
2. Provide organizational or unit leadership for adopting the evidence-informed practice.
3. Implement various strategies to educate peers about the evidence-informed practice.
4. Work with peers, other disciplines, and leadership staff to incorporate key information about the evidence-informed practice into organizational/unit standards, policies, procedures, and documentation systems.
5. Promote initial and ongoing use of the evidence-informed practice by peers.

Modified from Titler, M. G., Herr, K., Everett, L. Q., et al. (2006). *Book to bedside: Promoting and sustaining EBPs in elders* (Final Progress Report to AHRQ, Grant No. 2R01 HS010482-04). Iowa City: University of Iowa College of Nursing.

Social System

Clearly, the social system or context of care delivery matters when implementing evidence-informed practices (Kochevar & Yano, 2006; Rogers, 2003). For example, investigators demonstrated the effectiveness of a prompted voiding intervention for urinary incontinence in long-term care facilities, but sustaining the intervention in day-to-day practice was limited when the responsibility of carrying out the intervention was shifted to facility staff (rather than the investigative team) and required staffing levels in excess of a majority of facility settings (Engberg, Kincade, & Thompson, 2004). This illustrates the importance of embedding interventions into ongoing care processes.

As part of the work of implementing evidence-informed practices, it is important that the social system (e.g., unit, service line, clinic) ensure that policies, procedures, standards, clinical pathways, and documentation systems support the use of the evidence-informed practices (Titler, 2004). Documentation forms or clinical information systems may need revision to support practice changes; documentation systems that fail to readily support the new practice thwart change. For example, if staff members are expected to reassess and document pain intensity within 30 minutes after administration of an analgesic agent, documentation forms must reflect this practice standard. It is the role of leadership to ensure that organizational documents and systems are flexible and supportive of the evidence-informed practices.

A learning organizational culture and proactive leadership that promotes knowledge sharing are important components for building an evidence-informed practice (Lozano, Finkelstein, Carey, et al., 2004) (Figure 20.7). Additional components of a receptive context for evidence-informed practice include the following:
- Strong leadership
- Clear strategic vision
- Good managerial relations

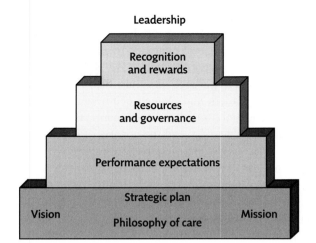

FIG. 20.7 Major building blocks in the process of creating a culture of evidence-informed practice.

- Visionary staff in key positions
- A climate conducive to experimentation and risk taking
- Effective data-capture systems

Leadership support is critical for promoting use of evidence-informed practices and is expressed verbally, and by providing necessary resources, materials, and time to fulfill responsibilities (Stetler, Legro, Wallace, et al., 2006). Senior leadership needs to create an organizational mission, vision, and strategic plan that incorporates evidence-informed practice, implements performance expectations for staff that include evidence-informed practice work, integrates the work of evidence-informed practice into the governance structure of the health care system, demonstrates the value of evidence-informed practices through administrative behaviours, and establishes explicit expectations that nurse leaders will create microsystems that value and support clinical inquiry (Titler, 2002).

In summary, making an evidence-informed change in practice involves a series of action steps in a complex, nonlinear process. The time needed to implement the change depends on the nature of the practice change. Merely increasing staff knowledge about an evidence-informed practice and passive dissemination strategies are not likely to work, particularly in complex health care settings. Strategies that seem to have a positive effect on promoting use of evidence-informed practices include audit and feedback, use of clinical reminders and practice prompts, involvement of opinion leaders and change champions, interactive education, mass media, educational outreach/academic detailing, and the context of care delivery (e.g., leadership, learning, questioning). It is important that senior leadership and those leading evidence-informed practice improvements are aware of change as a process and continue to encourage and teach peers about the change in practice. The new practice must be continually reinforced and sustained or the practice change will be intermittent and soon fade, allowing more traditional methods of care to return.

Evaluation

Evaluation provides an opportunity to collect and analyze data with regard to use of a new evidence-informed practice and then to modify the practice as necessary. It is important that the evidence-informed change is evaluated, both at the pilot testing phase and when the practice is changed in additional patient care areas. The importance of the evaluation cannot be overemphasized; it provides information for performance gap assessment, audit, and feedback, and it provides information necessary to determine whether the evidence-informed practice should be retained, modified, or eliminated. Steps of the evaluation process are summarized in Box 20.5.

Evaluation should include both process and outcome measures. The process component focuses on how the practice change is being implemented. It is important to know if staff are using the practice and implementing the practice as noted in the evidence-informed practice guideline. Evaluation of the process also should note (1) barriers that staff encounter in carrying out the practice (e.g., lack of information, skills, or necessary equipment), (2) differences in opinions among health care providers, and (3) difficulty in

---

BOX 20.5

STEPS OF EVALUATION FOR EVIDENCE-INFORMED PRACTICE

1. Identify process and outcome variables of interest.
   Examples:
   Process variable: For patients older than 65 years, a Braden scale will be completed on admission.
   Outcome variable: Presence/absence of nosocomial pressure injury; if present, determine stage as I, II, III, or IV.
2. Determine methods and frequency of data collection.
   Example:
   Process variable: Chart audit of all patients older than 65 years, 1 day a month
   Outcome variable: Assessment of all patients older than 65 years, 1 day a month
3. Determine baseline and follow-up sample sizes.
4. Design data-collection forms.
   Example:
   Process variable: chart audit abstraction form
   Outcome variable: pressure injury assessment form
5. Establish content validity of data-collection forms.
6. Train data collectors.
7. Assess interrater reliability of data collectors.
8. Collect data at specified intervals.
9. Provide "on-site" feedback to staff regarding the progress in achieving the practice change.
10. Provide feedback of analyzed data to staff.
11. Use data to assist staff in modifying or integrating the evidence-informed practice change.

---

carrying out the steps of the practice as originally designed (e.g., shutting off tube feedings 1 hour before aspirating contents for checking placement of nasointestinal tubes). Process data can be collected from staff and/or patient self-reports, medical record audits, or observation of clinical practice. Examples of process and outcome questions are shown in Table 20.6.

Outcome data are an equally important part of evaluation. The purpose of outcome evaluation is to assess whether the patient, staff, and/or fiscal outcomes expected are achieved. Therefore, it is important that baseline data be used for a preintervention/postintervention comparison (Titler et al., 2001). The outcome variables measured should be those that are projected to change as a result of changing practice. For example, research demonstrates that less restricted family visiting practices in critical

TABLE 20.6

EXAMPLES OF EVALUATION MEASURES

EXAMPLE OF PROCESS QUESTIONS	STRONGLY DISAGREE	DISAGREE	NEITHER AGREE NOR DISAGREE	AGREE	STRONGLY AGREE
1. I feel well prepared to use the Braden Scale with older patients.	1	2	3	4	5
2. Malnutrition increases patient risk for pressure injury development.	1	2	3	4	5

EXAMPLE OF OUTCOME QUESTION

Patient: On a scale of 0 (no pain) to 10 (worst possible pain), how much pain have you experienced over the past 24 hours?   _____ (Pain intensity)

care units result in improved satisfaction with care. Thus patient and family member satisfaction should be an outcome measure that is evaluated as part of changing visiting practices in adult critical care units. Outcome measures should be measured before the change in practice is implemented, after implementation, and every 6 to 12 months thereafter. Findings must be provided to clinicians to reinforce the impact of the change and to ensure that they are incorporated into quality improvement programs. When collecting process and outcome data for evaluation of a practice change, it is important that the data collection tools are user-friendly, short, concise, and easy to complete and have content validity. Focus must be on collecting the most essential data. Those responsible for collecting evaluative data must be trained on data-collection methods and be assessed for interrater reliability. Those individuals who have participated in implementing the protocol can be very helpful in evaluation by collecting data, providing timely feedback to staff, and assisting staff to overcome barriers encountered when implementing the changes in practice.

One question that often arises is how much data are needed to evaluate this change. The preferred number of patients (N) is somewhat dependent on the size of the patient population affected by the practice change. For example, if the practice change is for families of critically ill adult

patients and the organization has 1,000 adult critical care patients annually, 50 to 100 satisfaction responses preimplementation, and 25 to 50 responses postimplementation, at 3 and 6 months should be adequate to look for trends in satisfaction and possible areas that need to be addressed in continuing this practice (e.g., more bedside chairs in patient rooms). The rule of thumb is to keep the evaluation simple, because data often are collected by busy clinicians who may lose interest if the data collection, analysis, and feedback periods are too long and tedious. The evaluation process includes planned feedback to staff who are making the change. The feedback includes verbal and/or written appreciation for the work and visual demonstration of progress in implementation and improvement in patient outcomes. The key to effective evaluation is to ensure that the evidence-informed change in practice is warranted (e.g., will improve quality of care) and that the intervention does not bring harm to patients.

TRANSLATION SCIENCE

Translation science, mentioned previously in this chapter, is the investigation of strategies to increase the rate and extent of adoption and sustainability of evidence-informed practice by individuals and organizations to improve clinical and operational decision making (Eccles & Mittman, 2006; Titler, Everett, & Adams, 2007). It includes research to

(1) understand context variables that influence adoption of evidence-informed practices and (2) test the effectiveness of interventions to promote and sustain use of evidence-informed health care practices. Translation science denotes both the systematic investigation of methods, interventions, and variables that influence adoption of evidence-informed health care practices, as well as the organized body of knowledge gained through such research (Eccles & Mittman, 2006; Rubenstein & Pugh, 2006; Sussman, Valente, Rohrbach, et al., 2006; Titler et al., 2007).

Because translation research is a young science, there are no standardized definitions of commonly used terms (Graham et al., 2006). This is evidenced by differing definitions and the interchanging of terms that, in fact, may represent different concepts to different people. Adding to the confusion is that terminology may vary depending on the country in which the research was conducted (Adams & Titler, 2010). Graham and colleagues (2006) reported identifying 29 terms in nine countries that refer to some aspect of translating research findings into practice. For example, researchers in Canada may use the terms *research utilization, knowledge-to-action, knowledge transfer,* or *knowledge translation* interchangeably, whereas researchers in the United States, the United Kingdom, and Europe may be more likely to use the term *implementation* or *research translation* to express similar concepts (Graham et al., 2006). Kitson and Harvey (2016) state that **knowledge translation** "describes the process by which knowledge moves from where it was first created and refined to where it has to get to in order to make an impact on clinical practice and patient care" (p. 294).

The goals of the Canadian Institutes of Health Research (CIHR) are to not only support the development of new knowledge through research but also ensure that the knowledge is translated into practice. The CHIR define knowledge translation "as a dynamic and iterative process that includes synthesis, dissemination, exchange and ethically sound application of knowledge to improve the health of Canadians, provide more effective health services and products and strengthen the health care system" (CIHR, 2016). The CIHR lists the steps of knowledge to action as follows:

A. Creating Knowledge
   1. Deriving knowledge from primary studies, such as randomized controlled trials (knowledge inquiry)
   2. Synthesizing primary studies to form secondary knowledge, such as systematic reviews or meta-analyses
   3. Generating knowledge tools or products (third-generation knowledge) such as practice guidelines, decision aids, or care pathways based on best available evidence distilled from synthesized knowledge
B. Applying Knowledge
   4. Identifying the problem and identifying, reviewing, and selecting knowledge
   5. Adapting knowledge to local context
   6. Assessing barriers and facilitators to knowledge use
   7. Selecting, tailoring, and implementing intervention to address barriers to knowledge use
   8. Monitoring knowledge use
   9. Evaluating outcome of knowledge use
   10. Developing mechanisms to sustain knowledge use

The CIHR website is an excellent reference for further study on knowledge translation (http://www.cihr-irsc.gc.ca/e/39128.html).

FUTURE DIRECTIONS

Use of research across health care systems for improving the quality of care is essential. As professionals continue to understand the science of nursing and synthesize this science for application in practice, it will become increasingly necessary to test and understand how to best promote the use of this science in daily practice.

Ross-Kerr and Wood (2011) have detailed some future challenges in the research process. Facilitating research utilization in nursing practice is not an easy task, but neither is it an impossible dream.

Some activities that might facilitate the research process include the following:

- Funding key research positions
- Creating institutional infrastructures, including resources needed to access summarized evidence
- Encouraging and assisting nurses to attend practice-based research workshops and conferences
- Providing continuing education courses to assist nurses in critiquing research
- Creating a reward system within the agency for research utilization in practice
- Promoting collaborative efforts between agency personnel and other health care agencies or educational institutions
- Establishing a means for nurses to access research reports relevant to their practice
- Promoting demonstration projects that illustrate the cost-effectiveness of changing from a traditional, intuitively based practice to one that is research based
- Ensuring that research utilization is a role expectation for all nursing positions (management, educational, and clinical) and that it is reinforced in job descriptions, agency policy, and the institution's philosophy of nursing

Diagnosing barriers and planning and implementing strategies to overcome them are challenges. The first challenge is to demonstrate the cost-effectiveness of nursing research and to justify the allocation of resources and personnel to create the necessary infrastructures. The second challenge is to reduce the time gap between when knowledge is developed and when it is used. The third challenge is to create agency infrastructures that will support the transformation of nursing practice from a ritual base to a research base. Efforts to address these challenges require partnerships among practitioners, researchers, administrators, and disciplines (p. 136).

Education of nurses must include knowledge and skills in the use of research evidence in practice. Nurses are increasingly being held accountable for practices informed by scientific evidence. Thus, nurses must integrate into their profession the expectation that all nurses have a professional responsibility to read and use research in their practice and to communicate with nurse scientists the many and varied clinical problems for which a scientific basis for practice does not yet exist.

CRITICAL THINKING CHALLENGES

- Discuss the differences among nursing research, research utilization, and evidence-informed practice. Support your discussion with examples.
- Why would it be important to use an evidence-informed practice model, such as the Ottawa Model of Health Care Research, to guide a practice project focused on justifying and implementing a change in clinical practice?
- You are a staff nurse working on a cardiac step-down unit. Many of your colleagues do not understand evidence-informed practice. How would you help them to understand how evidence-informed practice is relevant to providing optimal care to this patient population?
- What barriers do you see to applying evidence-informed practice in your clinical setting? Discuss strategies to use in overcoming these barriers.

KEY POINTS

- According to the Iowa Model of Evidence-Based Practice to Promote Quality Care, the steps of evidence-informed practice are as follows: selecting a topic, forming a team, retrieving the evidence, grading the evidence, developing an evidence-informed practice standard, implementing the evidence-informed practice, and evaluating the effect on staff, patient, and fiscal outcomes.
- Adoption of evidence-informed practice standards requires education and dissemination to staff and use of change strategies, such as communication with opinion leaders, change champions, a core group, and consultants.
- It is important to evaluate the change. Evaluation provides data for performance gap assessment, audit, and feedback, and provides information necessary to determine whether the practice should be retained.
- Evaluation includes both process and outcome measures.

- It is important for organizations to create a culture of evidence-informed practice. Creating this culture requires an interactive process. To create this culture, organizations need to provide access to information, access to individuals who have skills necessary for evidence-informed practice, and a written and verbal commitment to evidence-informed practice in the organization's operations.
- The terms *research utilization* and *evidence-informed practice* are sometimes used interchangeably. These terms, although related, are not one and the same. *Research utilization* is the process of using research findings to improve practice. *Evidence-informed practice* is a broad term that encompasses the use of not only research findings but also other types of evidence, such as case reports and expert opinion, in deciding the evidence base that informs practice.
- There are two forms of evidence use: conceptual and decision driven.
- There are several models of evidence-informed practice. A key feature of all models is the judicious review and synthesis of research and other types of evidence to develop an evidence-informed practice standard.

FOR FURTHER STUDY

(e) Go to Evolve at http://evolve.elsevier.com/Canada/LoBiondo/Research for the Audio Glossary and Appendix Tables that provide supplemental information for Appendix E.

REFERENCES

Adams, S. L., & Titler, M. G. (2010). Building a learning collaborative. *Worldviews on Evidence-Based Nursing*, 7(3), 165–173.

American Geriatrics Society, British Geriatrics Society, American Academy of Orthopaedic Surgeons, and Panel on Falls Prevention. (2001). Guideline for the prevention of falls in older persons. *Journal of the American Geriatrics Society*, 49, 664–672.

Atkins, D., Briss, P. A., Eccles, M., et al, The GRADE Working Group. (2005). Systems for grading the quality of evidence and the strength of recommendations II: Pilot study of a new system. *BMC Health Services*, 5(1), 25.

Brooks, J. M., Titler, M. G., Ardery, G., et al. (2009). Effect of evidence-based acute pain management practices on inpatient costs. *Health Services Research*, 44(1), 245–263.

Canadian Institutes of Health Research. (2016). *Knowledge translation*. Retrieved from http://www.cihr-irsc.gc.ca/e/29418.html.

Colwell, J. C., Foreman, M. D., & Trotter, J. P. (1992). A comparison of the efficacy and cost-effectiveness of two methods of managing pressure ulcers. *Decubitus*, 6(4), 28–36.

Cronenwett, L. R. (1995). Effective methods for disseminating research findings to nurses in practice. *Nursing Clinics of North America*, 30, 429–438.

DiCenso, A., Guyatt, G., & Ciliska, D. (2005). *Evidence-based nursing: A guide to clinical practice*. St. Louis: Elsevier.

Dobbins, M., Robeson, P., & Ciliska, D. (2009). A description of a knowledge broker role implemented as part of a randomized controlled trial evaluating three knowledge translation strategies. *Implementation Science*, 4, 23.

Doebbeling, B. N., Chou, A. F., & Tierney, W. M. (2006). Priorities and strategies for the implementation of integrated informatics and communications technology to improve evidence-based practice. *Journal of General Internal Medicine*, 21(S2), S50–S57.

Dopson, S., FitzGerald, L., Ferlie, E., et al. (2010). No magic targets! Changing clinical practice to become more evidence based. *Health Care Management Review*, 27(3), 35–47.

Doran, D., Lefebre, N., O'Brien-Pallas, L., et al. (2014). The relationship among evidence-based practice and client dyspnea, pain, falls and pressure ulcer outcomes in the community setting. *Worldviews on Evidence-Based Nursing*, 11(5), 274–283.

Doumit, G., Gattellari, M., Grimshaw, J., et al. (2007). Local opinion leaders: Effects on professional practice and health care outcomes. *Cochrane Database of Systematic Reviews*, (1), CD000125.

Eccles, M. P., & Mittman, B. S. (2006). Welcome to implementation science. *Implementation Science*, 1, 1.

Engberg, S., Kincade, J., & Thompson, D. (2004). Future directions for incontinence research with frail elders. *Nursing Research*, 53(Suppl. 6), S22–S29.

Estabrooks, C. A. (2004). Thoughts on evidence-based nursing and its science: A Canadian perspective. *Worldviews on Evidence-Based Nursing*, 1(2), 88–91.

Estabrooks, C. A., Chong, H., Brigidear, K., et al. (2005). Profiling Canadian nurses' preferred knowledge sources for clinical practice. *Canadian Journal of Nursing Research, 37*(2), 119–140.

Estabrooks, C. A., Derksen, L., Winther, C., et al. (2008). The intellectual structure and substance of the knowledge utilization field: A longitudinal author co-citation analysis, 1945–2004. *Implementation Science, 3*, 49.

Feldman, P. H., Murtaugh, C. M., Pezzin, L. E., et al. (2005). Just-in-time evidence-based e-mail "reminders" in home health care: Impact on patient outcomes. *Health Services Research, 40*(3), 865–885.

Folkedahl, B., Frantz, R., & Goode, C. (2002). *Evidence-based protocol: Treatment of pressure ulcers.* In M. G. Titler (Series Ed.). Iowa City: University of Iowa College of Nursing, Gerontological Nursing Interventions Research Center, Research Dissemination Core (P30 NR03979; PI: T. Tripp-Reimer).

Fowler, E., & Goupil, D. L. (1984). Comparison of the wet-to-dry dressing and a copolymer starch in the management of debrided pressure sores. *Journal of Enterostomal Therapy, 11*(1), 22–25.

Gorse, G. J., & Messner, R. L. (1987). Improved pressure sore healing with hydrocolloid dressings. *Archives of Dermatology, 123*(6), 766–771.

GRADE Working Group. (2004). Grading quality of evidence and strength of recommendations. *British Medical Journal, 328*, 1490–1494.

Graham, I. D., Logan, J., Harrison, M. B., et al. (2006). Lost in knowledge translation: Time for a map? *Journal of Continuing Education in the Health Professions, 26*(1), 13–24.

Gravel, K., Légaré, F., & Graham, I. D. (2006). Barriers and facilitators to implementing shared decision-making in clinical practice: A systematic review of health professionals' perceptions. *Implementation Science, 1*, 16.

Grol, R. P., Bosch, M. C., Hulscher, M. E., et al. (2007). Planning and studying improvement in patient care: The use of theoretical perspectives. *The Milbank Quarterly, 85*(1), 93–138.

Guyatt, G. H., Oxman, A. D., Kunz, R., et al. (2008a). Rating quality of evidence and strength of recommendations: What is "quality of evidence" and why is it important to clinicians? *British Medical Journal, 336*(7651), 995–998.

Guyatt, G. H., Oxman, A. D., Kunz, R., et al. (2008b). Rating quality of evidence and strength of recommendations: Incorporating considerations of resources use into grading recommendations. *British Medical Journal, 336*(7654), 1170–1173.

Guyatt, G. H., Oxman, A. D., Vist, G., et al. (2008). Rating quality of evidence and strength of recommendations GRADE: An emerging consensus on rating quality of evidence and strength of recommendations. *British Medical Journal, 336*(7650), 924–926.

Haber, J., Feldman, H., Penney, N., et al. (1994). Shaping nursing practice through research-based protocols. *Journal of the New York State Nurses Association, 25*(3), 3–8.

Haller, K. B., Reynolds, M. A., & Horsley, J. O. (1979). Developing research-based innovation protocols: Process, criteria, and issues. *Research in Nursing & Health, 2*(2), 45–51.

Harris, R. P., Helfan, M., Woolf, S. H., et al. (2001). Current methods of the US Preventive Services Task Force: A review of the process. *American Journal of Preventative Medicine, 20*(Suppl. 3), 21–35.

Harvey, G., & Kitson, A. (2015). *Implementing evidence-based practice in healthcare. A facilitation guide.* New York: Routledge.

Higgins, J. P. T., & Green, S. (Eds.), (2011). *Cochrane handbook for systematic reviews of interventions 5.1.* Retrieved from http://handbook.cochrane.org/.

Horsley, J. A., Crane, J., Crabtree, M. K., et al. (1983). *Using research to improve nursing practice: A guide.* New York: Grune & Stratton.

Hysong, S. J., Best, R. G., & Pugh, J. A. (2006). Audit and feedback and clinical practice guideline adherence: Making feedback actionable. *Implementation Science, 1*, 9.

ICEBeRG. (2006). Designing theoretically informed implementation interventions: The Improved Clinical Effectiveness through Behavioural Research Group. *Implementation Science, 1*, 4.

Ivers, N., Jamtvedt, G., Flottorp, S., et al. (2012). Audit and feedback: Effects on professional practice and healthcare outcomes. *Cochrane Database of Systematic Reviews*, (6), CD000259.

Jamtvedt, G., Young, J. M., Kristoffersen, D. T., et al. (2010). Audit and feedback: Effects on professional practice and health care outcomes (Review). *Cochrane Database of Systematic Reviews*, (7), CD000259.

Jordan, M. E., Lanham, H. J., Crabtree, B. F., et al. (2009). The role of conversation in health care interventions: Enabling sensemaking and learning. *Implementation Science, 4*, 15.

Kitson, A. L., & Harvey, H. (2016). Methods to succeed in effective knowledge translation in clinical practice. *Journal of Nursing Scholarship, 48*(3), 294–302.

Kochevar, L. K., & Yano, E. M. (2006). Understanding health care organization needs and context: Beyond performance gaps. *Journal of General Internal Medicine, 21*, S25–S29.

Kurzuk-Howard, G., Simpson, L., & Palmieri, A. (1985). Decubitus ulcer care: A comparative study. *Western Journal of Nursing Research*, 7(1), 58–79.

Leape, L. L. (2005). Where the rubber meets the road. In *Advances in patient safety: From research to implementation, Vol. 3: Implementation issues* (AHRQ pub no 05-0021-3). Rockville, MD: Agency for Healthcare Research and Quality.

Logan, J., & Graham, I. (1998). Toward a comprehensive interdisciplinary model of health care research use. *Science Communication*, 20(2), 229.

Lozano, P., Finkelstein, J. A., Carey, V. J., et al. (2004). A multisite randomized trial of the effects of physician education and organizational change in chronic-asthma care. *Archives of Pediatric & Adolescent Medicine*, 158, 875–883.

Madsen, D., Sebolt, T., Cullen, L., et al. (2005). Why listen to bowel sounds? Report of an evidence-based practice project. *American Journal of Nursing*, 105, 40–49.

McDonald, M. V., Pezzin, L. E., Feldman, P. H., et al. (2005). Can just-in-time, evidence-based "reminders" improve pain management among home health care nurses and their patients? *Journal of Pain Symptom Management*, 29(5), 474–488.

Melnyk, B. M., & Fineout-Overholt, E. (2011). *Evidence-based practice in nursing and healthcare: A guide to best practice* (2nd ed.). New York: Wolters Kluwer.

Melnyk, B. M., Gallagher-Ford, L., Long, L. E., et al. (2014). The establishment of evidence-based practice competences for practicing registered nurses and advanced practice nurses in real-world clinical settings: Proficiencies to improve healthcare quality, reliability, patient outcomes, and costs. *Worldviews on Evidence-Based Nursing*, 11(1), 5–15.

Neill, K. M., Conforti, C., Kedas, A., et al. (1989). Pressure sore response to a new hydrocolloid dressing. *Wounds*, 1(3), 173–185.

Nightingale, F. (1858). *Notes on matters affecting the health, efficiency, and hospital administration of the British Army*. London: Harrison and Sons.

Nightingale, F. (1859). *A contribution to the sanitary history of the British Army during the late war with Russia*. London: John W. Parker and Sons.

Nightingale, F. (1863a). *Notes on hospitals*. London: Longman, Green, Roberts, and Green.

Nightingale, F. (1863b). *Observation on the evidence contained in the statistical reports submitted by her to the Royal Commission on the Sanitary State of the Army in India*. London: Edward Stanford.

Oleske, D. M., Smith, X. P., White, P., et al. (1986). A randomized clinical trial of two dressing methods for the treatment of low-grade pressure ulcers. *Journal of Enterostomal Therapy*, 13(3), 90–98.

Registered Nurses' Association of Ontario (RNAO). (2003). *Breastfeeding best practice guidelines for nurses*. Retrieved from http://rnao.ca/bpg/guidelines/breastfeeding-best-practice-guidelines-nurses.

Registered Nurses' Association of Ontario (RNAO). (2004). *Adult asthma care guidelines for nurses: Promoting control of asthma*. Retrieved from http://rnao.ca/bpg/guidelines/adult-asthma-care-guidelines-nurses-promoting-control-asthma.

Registered Nurses' Association of Ontario (RNAO). (2012). *Toolkit: Implementation of best practice guidelines* (2nd ed.). Toronto, ON: Author.

Rogers, E. (1995). *Diffusion of innovations*. New York: Free Press.

Rogers, E. M. (2003). *Diffusion of innovations* (5th ed.). New York: Free Press.

Ross-Kerr, J. C., & Wood, M. J. (2011). *Canadian nursing: Issues and perspectives* (5th ed.). Toronto, ON: Elsevier.

Rubenstein, L. V., & Pugh, J. A. (2006). Strategies for promoting organizational and practice change by advancing implementation research. *Journal of General Internal Medicine*, 21, S58–S64.

Saydak, S. J. (1990). A pilot test of two methods for the treatment of pressure ulcers. *Journal of Enterostomal Therapy*, 17(3), 139–142.

Scott, S. D., Plotnikoff, R. C., Karunamuni, N., et al. (2008). Factors influencing the adoption of an innovation: An examination of the uptake of the Canadian Heart Health Kit (HHK). *Implementation Science*, 3, 41.

Sebern, M. D. (1986). Pressure ulcer management in home health care: Efficacy and cost effectiveness and moisture vapor permeable dressing. *Archives of Physical Medicine and Rehabilitation*, 67(10), 726–729.

Silversides, A. (2011). Journal clubs: A forum for discussion and professional development. *Canadian Nurse*, 107(2), 18–23.

Smith, J. L., Williams, J. W., Owen, R. R., et al. (2008). Developing a national dissemination plan for collaborative care for depression: QUERI Series. *Implementation Science*, 3, 59. doi:10.1186/1748-5908-3-59.

Squires, J. E., Estabrooks, C. A., Gustavsson, P., et al. (2011). Individual determinants of research utilization by nurses: A systematic review update. *Implementation Science*, 6(1), 1–20.

Squires, J. E., Graham, I. D., Hutchinson, A. M., et al. (2015). Identifying the domains of context important to implementation science: A study protocol. *Implementation Science*, 10(135), 1–9.

Squires, J. E., Moralejo, D., & LeFort, S. M. (2007). Exploring the role of organizational policies and procedures in promoting research utilization in registered nurses. *Implementation Science, 2*, 17.

Stetler, C. B., Legro, M. W., Wallace, C. M., et al. (2006). The role of formative evaluation in implementation research and the QUERI experience. *Journal of General Internal Medicine, 21*, S1–S8.

Stetler, C. B., McQuenn, L., Demkis, J., et al. (2008). An organizational framework and strategic implementation for system-level change to enhance research-based practice: QUERI Series. *Implementation Science, 3*, 30.

Straus, S. E., Richardson, W. S., Glasziou, P., et al. (2005). *Evidence based medicine: How to practice and teach EBM* (3rd ed.). Philadelphia: Churchill Livingstone.

Sussman, S., Valente, T. W., Rohrbach, L. A., et al. (2006). Translation in the health professions: Converting science into action. *Evaluation and the Health Professions, 29*(1), 7–32.

Thompson, D. S., Estabrooks, C. A., Scott-Findlay, S., et al. (2007). Interventions aimed at increasing research use in nursing: A systematic review. *Implementation Science, 2*, 15.

Titler, M. G. (1994). Critical analysis of research utilization (RU): An historical perspective. *American Journal of Critical Care, 2*(3), 264.

Titler, M. G. (2002). *Toolkit for promoting evidence-based practice.* Iowa City: University of Iowa Hospitals and Clinics, Department of Nursing Services and Patient Care.

Titler, M. G. (2004). Methods in translation science. *Worldviews on Evidence-Based Nursing, 1*, 38–48.

Titler, M. G. (2008). The evidence for evidence-based practice implementation. In R. Hughes (Ed.), *Patient safety and quality—An evidence-based handbook for nurses.* Rockville, MD: Agency for Healthcare Research and Quality.

Titler, M. G., Everett, L. Q., & Adams, S. (2007). Implications for implementation science. *Nursing Research, 56*(Suppl. 4), S53–S59.

Titler, M. G., Herr, K., Brooks, J. M., et al. (2009). A translating research into practice intervention improves management of acute pain in older hip fracture patients. *Health Services Research, 44*(1), 264–287.

Titler, M. G., Herr, K., Everett, L. Q., et al. (2006). *Book to bedside: Promoting & sustaining EBPs in elders* (Final Progress Report to AHRQ, Grant No. 2R01 HS010482-04). Iowa City: University of Iowa College of Nursing.

Titler, M. G., Kleiber, C., Steelman, V. J., et al. (1994). Infusing research into practice to promote quality care. *Nursing Research, 43*(5), 307–313.

Titler, M. G., Kleiber, C., Steelman, V. J., et al. (2001). The Iowa Model of Evidence-Based Practice to Promote Quality Care. *Critical Care Nursing Clinics of North America, 13*(4), 497–509.

U.S. Preventive Services Task Force. (2008). *U.S. Preventive Services Task Force grade definitions.* Retrieved from http://www.uspreventiveservicestaskforce.org/uspstf/grades.htm.

Ward, M. M., Evans, T. C., Spies, A. J., et al. (2006). National Quality Forum 30 safe practices: Priority and progress in Iowa hospitals. *American Journal of Medical Quality, 21*(2), 101–108.

Weiss, C. H. (1980). Knowledge creep and decision accretion. *Science Communication, 1*(3), 381–404.

Wensing, M., Wollersheim, H., & Grol, R. (2006). Organizational interventions to implement improvements in patient care: A structured review of review. *Implementation Science, 1*(2).

Xakellis, G. C., & Chrischilles, E. A. (1992). Hydrocolloid versus saline gauze dressings in treating pressure ulcers: A cost-effectiveness analysis. *Archives of Physiotherapy and Medical Rehabilitation, 73*(5), 463–469.

RESEARCH **VIGNETTE**
Social Support Needs of Older Adults

Gloria McInnis Perry, BScN, MScN, DNSc
Associate Professor
School of Nursing
University of Prince Edward Island
Charlottetown, Prince Edward Island

As Canada's population ages, there will be increased numbers of older adults with mental illnesses and problems (Mental Health Commission of Canada, 2013). There are many opportunities and challenges that have an impact on the mental health and well-being of older adults. These can include personal growth and development and free time to develop new skills, pick up old interests, and nurture old and new social relationships. In later life, challenges may include the adjustment to normal and abnormal changes in physical health and functioning, coping with a chronic illness or illnesses, adjusting to the loss of social connections such as with family and friends, transitioning into retirement, coping with a reduced income, coping with transportation issues, and confronting the sense of one's own mortality. Assisting older adults in these challenges becomes paramount for all nurses. Moreover, understanding the present state of older adults' social relationships, specifically relationships that provide the opportunity to participate in meaningful activities that promote mental health and well-being, is imperative. Mental health promotion and mental illness prevention are a responsibility of all nurses, with specific responsibility for the geropsychiatric–mental health nurse.

As a clinical nurse specialist in geropsychiatric nursing, I found myself working with a significant number of older adults who were experiencing major depression, anxiety disorders, and substance abuse. Upon a more thorough assessment, I began to realize that a majority of these older adults were expressing strong, painful feelings of loneliness that were largely due to more recent changes in their personal social relationships. What was even more concerning was that most older adults had little involvement with their adult children. I found this phenomenon to be of great interest and concern, so in graduate school I undertook an assignment that required me to complete a concept analysis on the phenomenon of loneliness. During my research of the literature, I soon discovered that this concept was often incorrectly viewed as social isolation or solitude and that some older adults experienced loneliness and its negative effects, despite living with a partner or spouse. Later in my studies, I completed a qualitative, phenomenological research study, "Loneliness in the Older Adult." This research gave me a better understanding of loneliness as a significant human phenomenon: it is more than social isolation; it is experienced differently in the older adult compared to the younger cohort; and, if not addressed, can lead to serious health issues, such as depression, anxiety, addiction, and even suicide. Moreover, older adults' perception of the social relationship was a powerful predictive of whether or not they experienced loneliness. Understanding the nature and importance of social support in older adults is imperative if the nurse is to help prevent or mitigate the factors that lead to loneliness, which is a major mental health problem.

Using the survey data from the Atlantic Seniors Housing Research Alliance, I worked with two other researchers to explore the emotional and informational needs of community-dwelling Atlantic Canadians age 65 years. For our research, social support was understood as the emotional and informational resources that persons perceive to be available or that are provided to them by nonprofessionals in the context of both formal support groups and informal helping relationships. Emotional support consists of the acts of empathy, listening, understanding, reassurance, friendship, intimacy, and attachment (Finfgeld-Connett, 2007; Stewart, Barnfather, Neufeld, et al., 2006). Informational or affirmational support involves acts of advice, assistance with problem-solving, and provision of feedback (Stewart et al., 2006). Our study found that the emotional and informational support needs of older adults in Atlantic Canada were partially met. Moreover, moderate gender and age differences were evident, which in turn placed some of our older adults at increased risk for social isolation and/or loneliness. We found that sufficient support decreased with age. For example, those participants ages 80–84 reported "insufficient" (58%) for the items "someone to do things with" and "with someone to help you get your mind off of things" and (55%) for the item "with someone whose advice you really want." Seventy percent of those age 85 and over reported insufficiencies. Gender differences were noted, with items rated "no support" high for men (none or little support).

The following case scenario highlights the importance of determining what is perceived as sufficient or insufficient social support in an older adult. The case identifies how these needs are influenced by age and gender and how nursing and other health care providers can intervene effectively to assist in addressing these deficiencies.

CASE SCENARIO

Bob Clark is an 85-year-old retired teacher who resides in Atlantic Canada. He has been married to Clara for 60 years, and they still live in the home they built 40 years ago. The Clarks have two adult children: Ben, age 55, and Mitchell, age 52. Both children live in Central Canada and get home once a year, usually for 2 weeks during their summer vacation. The children email and text Bob often; however, communicating with Clara has been more difficult. Clara has been diagnosed with probable Alzheimer's disease for 7 years, and up until 6 months

ago she required little help with her personal care, although she required constant supervision for wandering and other safely issues. Bob has recently hired a home care aide to assist in Clara's personal care and to supervise Clara for one afternoon a week while Bob tends to groceries and other required chores. Over the past 7 years, Bob has devoted most of his time to caring for Clara, which has meant giving up most of his normal hobbies, playing music, golfing, and volunteering at the local school as a senior mentor for students with learning challenges. Clara was always the social person in the family as she would plan all the social activities for her family, especially for the holidays and special family celebrations. As a result, Bob has lost many of his previous social connections.

Over the past 2 years, Bob has noticed that he is experiencing some health changes, such as hesitancy in urinating, difficulty seeing as clearly as he used to despite the help of prescription glasses, and difficulty falling and staying asleep. He does not wish to burden his sons with his concern, yet he knows that the stress of caring for Clara, coupled with his health issues, is becoming too much for him. Feeling more alone than not, Bob is beginning to see little hope in any change in his present life situation and worries more about Clara's future. He begins to question if life is still worth living.

Bob's situation is not new for many Canadians, especially those living in Atlantic Canada. Men and women are living longer, and many of their adult children move

away for better jobs, resulting in less filial support. Also, older adults have less available sibling and/or friend support and often find that their social support needs are not being adequately met. Emotional needs such as affection may no longer be met or seem a priority. However, not having someone in one's life to take an interest or demonstrate concern, not having help with stress and negative private feelings, not having healthy distractions such as something to do with others, not getting one's mind off of negative things, and not receiving information support, especially in a crisis, can all stir up feelings of being alone, loneliness, and abandonment, resulting in a deficiency in social support, as in Bob's case.

In Bob's situation, social support (emotional and informational) intervention should have occurred as soon as the change in Clara's cognitive status was confirmed. The family physician should have referred the Clarks to a support program such as the Alzheimer's Society. If Bob did not respond to the first offer of support, a follow-up reminder should have been considered. Also, the family physician should have ensured that Bob's health was closely monitored. Home care nursing could have provided additional support by assessing both Bob's and Clara's health. Suggestions for Bob to attend a seniors' active living program as a social outlet, along with a friendly visitor program for Clara, would have been a great benefit. Bob has many talents that should have been encouraged. Giving him the time to leave Clara and take up a few of his activities would have added meaning and purpose in his life, which would have decreased the likelihood of experiencing a serious mental health problem. The Clarks' sons should have been involved with the intervention. Knowing their father's situation, they could have encouraged and arranged for social opportunities for the father.

IN SUMMARY

Sufficient social support in the older adult's life is a strong determinant of health and well-being. Moreover, considerations for how gender and age may affect the older adult's social support, networks, preferences, and beliefs must be considered by nurses and other health care providers. Nursing practices that are based on sound research can only enhance the likelihood of positive outcomes in nursing care. ■

REFERENCES

Finfgeld-Connett, D. (2007). Concept comparison of caring and social support. *International Journal of Nursing Terminologies and Classifications*, *18*(2), 58–68.

Mental Health Commission of Canada. (2013). *Issues: Seniors*. Retrieved from http://www.mentalhealthcommission. ca/English/focus-areas/seniors.

Stewart, M., Barnfather, A., Neufeld, A., et al. (2006). Accessible support for family caregivers of seniors with chronic conditions: From isolation to inclusion. *Canadian Journal on Aging*, *25*(2), 179–191.

Honouring Stories: Mi'kmaq Women's Experiences With Pap Screening in Eastern Canada

Catherine MacDonald, Ruth Martin-Misener, Audrey Steenbeek, Annette Browne

Mi'kmaq women are reported to have lower rates of Papanicolaou (Pap) screening and higher rates of cervical cancer than non-Aboriginal women. This qualitative participatory study used postcolonial feminist perspectives and Indigenous principles to explore Mi'kmaq women's experiences with Pap screening within the contexts that shaped their experiences. Community facilitators assisted with the research process. Talking circles and individual in-depth interviews were conducted with 16 Mi'kmaq women. Also, health-care providers were interviewed in 2 Mi'kmaq communities. The findings indicate that historical and social contexts are shaping Mi'kmaq women's screening experiences and that these experiences are diverse, as are their understandings about screening. Some women were accessing regular screening despite challenging personal circumstances. The results highlight the need for nurses and other health-care providers to understand the uniqueness of each woman's experiences with Pap screening. Improvements in screening rates depend on multifaceted nursing approaches developed in partnership with Mi'kmaq women.

KEYWORDS: Aboriginal women, cervical cancer prevention, Pap screening, participatory action research, postcolonial feminist perspectives, health-care access

Résumé

Histoires de dignité: comment le test de Pap est vécu par des Micmaques de l'Est du Canada

Catherine MacDonald, Ruth Martin-Misener, Audrey Steenbeek, Annette Browne

Selon les données, les Micmaques subissent le test de Papanicolaou (Pap) en plus petite proportion que les femmes non autochtones et présentent un taux plus élevé de cancer du col de l'utérus. La présente étude qualitative et participative adopte une approche féministe postcoloniale et s'appuie sur les principes autochtones pour examiner la façon dont les Micmaques vivent le dépistage du cancer du col de l'utérus (test de Pap), et les différents contextes où leur expérience de ce dépistage prend forme. Des animateurs communautaires ont pris part au processus de recherche. Des cercles de discussion et des entrevues individuelles approfondies ont eu lieu auprès de 16 Micmaques. Des fournisseurs de soins de santé ont également fait l'objet d'entrevues dans deux communautés micmaques. Les constatations indiquent que les contextes social et historique contribuent à façonner l'expérience vécue par les Micmaques au moment du test de Pap et que cette expérience varie, de même que la compréhension qu'ont les femmes du dépistage. Certaines femmes participent à un dépistage régulier, malgré une situation personnelle difficile. Les résultats obtenus font ressortir la nécessité pour les infirmières et les autres fournisseurs de soins de santé de comprendre le caractère unique de l'expérience de dépistage vécue par chaque femme. L'amélioration des taux de dépistage est tributaire de la mise en place d'approches à multiples facettes des soins infirmiers élaborées en partenariat avec les Micmaques.

MOTS-CLÉS: femmes autochtones, dépistage du cancer du col de l'utérus, test de Pap, étude participative, approche féministe postcoloniale, soins de santé

The health of Aboriginal[1] women is foundational to the well-being of their families, communities, and Nations (Native Women's Association of Canada, 2007). Despite recent improvements in health status at the population level, and despite the collective efforts of Aboriginal women to foster strength and health within their families and communities, health and social inequities persist in this population in comparison with the general Canadian population (Halseth, 2013).

In this article we explore cervical cancer as one particular health issue that needs attention. Although Papanicolaou (Pap) screening has been effective in decreasing the morbidity and mortality rates of cervical cancer (Canadian Cancer Society, 2012), Aboriginal women continue to have lower rates of screening and higher rates of cervical cancer than other Canadian women (Brassard et al., 2012; Zehbe, Maar, Nahwegahbow, Berst, & Pintar, 2012).

Much of the health-care literature, particularly the epidemiological literature, reports that Aboriginal women have higher rates of cervical cancer than non-Aboriginal women. Often, these rates are reported along with risk factors for cervical cancer, such as certain high-risk behaviours, lower rates of screening, and high rates of sexually transmitted infections (Gerberding, 2004; Johnson, Boyd, & MacIsaac, 2004; Reeves, 2008; Sheets, 2002; UNAIDS & World Health Organization, 2006). When the high rates of cervical cancer among Aboriginal women are attributed to these risk factors, Aboriginal women are frequently labelled as "high risk in terms of their reproductive health" (Browne & Smye, 2002, p. 32). However, research indicates that multiple factors impact the health status of Aboriginal women and shape their access to health services and their health-care experiences. It is therefore imperative to contextualize health status in light of sociopolitical, historical, and economic factors affecting health (Adelson, 2005; Browne, 2007; Browne et al., 2011). It is equally important to recognize that women's health is shaped by various strengths and abilities, including knowledge of local languages and community and cultural practices and ceremonies (Kirmayer, Dandeneau, Marshall, Phillips, & Williamson, 2011).

In many cases the mainstream health-care system is poorly aligned with the health-care needs of Aboriginal people because it tends to conceptualize health and illness as stemming from "lifestyle" or cultural differences and to overlook the contextual factors that shape health and illness (Browne & Dion Stout, 2012). Health-care policies and strategies aimed at helping Aboriginal people but based on Western models of health-care delivery and on individualistic, disease-based discourses can perpetuate racism, social exclusion, marginalization, and inequitable access to care (Barton, 2008; Martin, 2012). Nurses are in key positions to address inequities that affect access to Pap screening for Aboriginal women by incorporating the concept of cultural safety into screening practices, developing respectful relationships prior to screening, tailoring screening approaches to the specific needs of individual women, and adopting relational and collaborative approaches.

---

[1]The word Aboriginal refers to the original peoples of North America and their descendants. The Canadian Constitution recognizes three groups of Aboriginal people: First Nations, Métis, and Inuit. These are three distinct peoples with unique histories, languages, cultural practices, and spiritual beliefs (Aboriginal Affairs and Northern Development Canada, 2013).

The purpose of this article is to report on findings from a community-based participatory study conducted in partnership with two Mi'kmaq communities in eastern Canada focused on cervical cancer screening. This qualitative study explored women's experiences with Pap screening in the two rural Mi'kmaq communities using a broader lens to conceptualize their health-care experiences. This allowed for women's participation in Pap screening to be considered with a fuller understanding of the historical, economic, and sociopolitical contexts that construct these experiences. Storied interviews were conducted with Aboriginal women and health-care providers. The research questions were as follows: 1. *What are Aboriginal women's experiences with Pap screening?* 2. *What are Aboriginal women's awareness of and knowledge about Pap screening?* 3. *What are the perceptions of Aboriginal women and health-care providers regarding the reasons why some Aboriginal women are not participating in Pap screening?* 4. *What are the sociopolitical, economic, and historical factors that shape Aboriginal women's participation in Pap screening?*

THEORETICAL AND METHODOLOGICAL PERSPECTIVES

The study was informed by postcolonial feminist theoretical perspectives (Anderson, 2004; Reimer-Kirkham & Anderson, 2002) and Indigenous principles in a two-eyed seeing approach. The term "two-eyed seeing" (Sesatu'k Etuaptmnkl) refers to the need to learn from one eye the strengths of Aboriginal traditional knowledge and from the other eye the strengths of Western scientific knowledge (Iwama, Marshall, Marshall, & Bartlett, 2009). Postcolonial feminist theory provides an analytic lens for exploring how women's lives and health have been positioned and shaped by politics and history (Browne, Smye, & Varcoe, 2005, 2007). "Postcolonial" does not mean that colonialism is over or completed: "the

post in postcolonial refers to a notion of both working against and beyond colonialism" (McConaghy, 2000, p. 268). The use of postcolonial feminist perspectives allowed for Mi'kmaq women to be viewed not as a gendered group but as individuals with distinct historical, socio-economic, and political experiences (Lewis & Mills, 2003). There was an understanding of how power, privilege, socio-economics, and race have contributed to inequities in access.

Indigenous principles fundamental to conducting respectful research with Aboriginal people provided the foundation for the theoretical development of the study (Martin, 2012; Weber-Pillwax, 2004). Indigenous principles of relationality, respect, reciprocity, relevance, and responsibility were also incorporated into the framework (Loppie, 2007; MacDonald, 2012). Respectful relationships with community members were developed through frequent visits to the health centre and attendance at community events prior to initiating the study. This was vitally important for the acquisition of knowledge about the communities, community members, community norms, and community expectations with regard to the research.

THE STUDY

Qualitative Participatory Action Research Design

The research process was guided by a qualitative research design using participatory action research (PAR) and Indigenous principles. The qualitative nature of the study provided a means for analyzing and interpreting how the colonial past and the current sociopolitical and economic climate impact Aboriginal women's access to Pap screening. PAR principles of equity, social justice, democratic collective decision-making, and reciprocity (Loppie, 2007; MacDonald, 2012; Ortiz, 2003; Vollman, Anderson, & McFarlane, 2004; Vukic, Gregory, & Martin-Misener, 2012) were applied throughout the research. These principles were upheld by enabling the participation of community members, acknowledging that the viewpoints of all participants were valued, using collaborative decision-making regarding the research process and dissemination of findings, developing relationships, and fostering open communication. PAR is grounded in the practical problems and health issues of people in a given community. Thus, the research topic was determined with some community members by developing collaborative relationships while visiting the communities and the community health centre.

Women told stories from their contextualized social, economic, political, and historical realities and were considered co-investigators and active participants in different phases of the research. They provided input into the research questions, participant recruitment, data collection and analysis, modification of the interview guide, and dissemination of findings.

Ethical approval was obtained from the University Health Sciences Human Research Ethics Committee at Dalhousie University, Mi'kmaq Ethics Watch at Cape Breton University, and Mi'kmaq community leaders. The OCAP (ownership, control, access, and procession) principles (1998) and the Canadian Institutes of Health Research (2007) guidelines for health research involving Aboriginal people were also followed. The OCAP principles were respected by informing the women about the entire study prior to their participation, discussing anonymity and confidentiality with them, ensuring that each informed consent form was signed and a copy given to the participant, and engaging participants in discussions about the findings and their dissemination.

Role of community facilitator. Community members, who were recommended (based on interest and willingness to participate) by healthcare providers in each community, were invited and agreed to be the community facilitators. Their role was to organize the talking circles (described below), assist with recruitment, act as liaison between the community and the primary researcher, provide feedback regarding the interview guide and the research process, and review and comment on themes throughout the analysis. Community facilitators expressed an interest in being active throughout the research process and repeatedly affirmed the relevance of the research topic for their community. They communicated the information that there were some women in the community who did not go for Pap screening and that in each community they knew a woman who had a diagnosis of cervical cancer or who had died of cervical cancer.

Recruitment of Mi'kmaq women. Sixteen women were recruited using purposive and snowball sampling. Aboriginal women of diverse ages, socio-economic backgrounds, education, and Pap screening experiences were purposively recruited by community facilitators, who invited 20 to 30 Mi'kmaq women to participate in a talking circle with a health professional, a health centre director, and the primary researcher. The purpose of the talking circle was to facilitate collaboration and promote co-designing of the study.

The primary researcher used talking circles because traditionally a talking circle is structured to permit all voices to be heard (Tompkins, 2002). The talking circles for this study, one in each community, were premised on the PAR principles of respect, shared decision-making, reciprocity, and relationality, allowing for the mutual exchange of information in a comfortable environment with food. Women posed questions, made comments, told stories, and provided suggestions regarding the interview questions and the research process. The first talking circle comprised eight women and a nurse, while the second comprised 10 women, a nurse, and a health centre director. Those who participated in the talking circle informed other women in the community about the study, which resulted in the recruitment of a few other women.

To be included in the study, women had to (1) be a self-identified or status Aboriginal Mi'kmaq; (2) live in one of the two Mi'kmaq communities; (3) be between 21 and 75 years of age; (4) have had a least one Pap screening; (5) be able to provide informed consent; and (6) be able to read, understand, and speak English. A letter of introduction describing the study was distributed.

After consent for participation had been obtained, storytelling interviews using an in-depth guide, developed for the study with input from the community facilitators and women, were arranged at a time and location agreeable to each participant.

In-depth interviews. The women had the choice of taking part in one or two in-depth interviews so that each would have an opportunity to tell her stories about beliefs, attitudes, and experiences with respect to Pap screening. The interviews lasted from 60 to 90 minutes. A total of 16 women participated in the first interview (13 attended the talking circles) and all but one agreed to take part in the follow-up interview. The second interview took place following transcription of the first interview and preliminary analysis of the findings. During the second interview, the women were asked to provide feedback on data interpretation, preliminary findings, and emerging themes. Five health-care providers volunteered to take part in an in-depth interview and four agreed to a follow-up interview. In total, there were 40 interviews.

Data Analysis

After the audiotaped interviews were transcribed verbatim, data were imported into NVivo 8 qualitative software. Women had an opportunity to read and validate their transcribed interviews and provided input about preliminary themes and subthemes. Thematic analysis processes described by Sandelowski (1995) and O'Connor and Gibson (2003) were employed to identify themes elicited from the participants' stories. Although these themes were coded primarily by the researcher, women changed some of the titles of the themes and subthemes and offered explanations from an Indigenous perspective why the titles were or were not appropriate. Women clarified, altered, or confirmed that the data adequately reflected and were consistent with their stories

and their experiences of Pap screening. Community facilitators also reviewed some of the coding processes to ensure validity of themes and subthemes. The trustworthiness of the research was enhanced through member checking, recording of field notes, forming of partnerships with and debriefing with community facilitators, peer review, and debriefing.

FINDINGS AND DISCUSSION

The five themes and subthemes (see Figure A.1) identified in the Mi'kmaq women's stories will be presented by integrating excerpts from interviews. The findings and their interpretation are interwoven with the literature in a relational manner that honours and represents Aboriginal women's stories in an attempt to minimize the fracturing of knowledge passed on in oral form (Brown & Strega, 2005; Smylie, 2001).

Finding Our Way

This theme and its two subthemes reveal how Aboriginal women are finding their way by paying attention to and taking care of their health and the health of their families and communities. Women described being committed to taking care of their health by seeking knowledge, becoming educated, and sharing knowledge with family and community members.

Taking care of our health. Many women described the importance of taking care of their health by taking action to address some of the determinants of health, even though they were confronted with considerable disadvantages and adversity. Some talked about taking care of their health by becoming educated, being employed, and instituting early childhood learning. Others told stories about returning to cultural and traditional ways, revitalizing their language, and passing along parenting skills. For some women, seeking knowledge about health care was a way of taking care of their health.

A few women took care of their health by making sure follow-up appointments were made

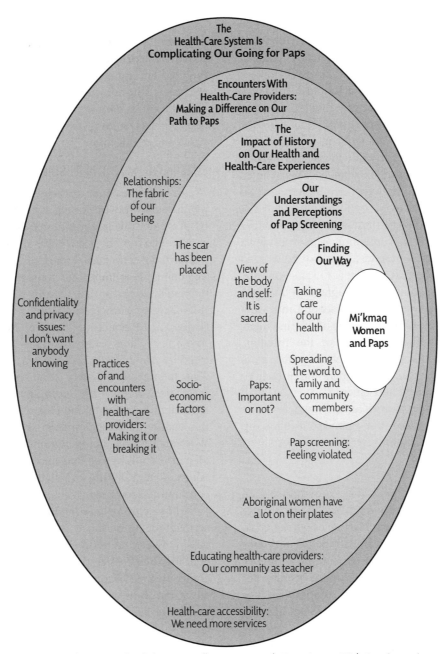

FIG. A.1 Themes and Subthemes: Mi'kmaq Women's Experiences With Pap Screening

for their test results and treatments and keeping track of the dates for these appointments: "I know when my appointments [for Pap screening] are due. Usually I'll remember and I keep track."

These findings offer a counterbalance to much of the epidemiological literature implying that Aboriginal women do not take care of their health nor make personal efforts to do so. Much of the research has focused on women's low rates of Pap screening, high rates of cervical cancer, barriers to accessing health services, strategies to improve Pap screening rates, and reproductive health issues currently confronting Aboriginal women (Black, 2009; Johnson et al., 2004; O'Brien, Mill, & Wilson, 2009; Steven et al., 2004). Epidemiological statistics alone do not convey the current state of Aboriginal health (Graham & Stamler, 2010) and suggest that lifestyle choices are the reason for women not accessing Pap screening. According to Nelson (2012), the burden of responsibility for health and social problems is continually placed on Aboriginal people, who are denied the resources needed to adequately tackle these problems. Epidemiological research needs to be developed with other types of research that consider the contexts of Aboriginal people's lives.

Spreading the word to family and community members. This subtheme concerns the importance that the women placed on sharing their knowledge and wisdom about health and Pap screening with family and community members. While some women said that there has been a loss of some traditional ways and knowledge, they continued to use storytelling with family and community as a path to taking care of their health. The women also spoke of the knowledge and advice they could share with health-care providers and policymakers to make Pap screening a more positive experience. A few viewed sharing words of wisdom about Pap screening to be their personal responsibility as women, mothers, aunts, grandmothers, and friends, as it was traditionally with other aspects of health: "We learned about it [Pap screening] through word of mouth from family."

Some women in the community had taken on more formal educational roles, such as appearing on posters or presenting at health conferences; this was seen as important for raising awareness and recruiting Aboriginal women for Pap screening. One woman spoke of an acquaintance who attended health conferences and appeared on posters to share her knowledge about the importance of Pap screening and prevention of cervical cancer: "She was going to a health conference and they asked her to participate [in it] because she's . . . on the posters and stuff . . . that's probably the first time I really heard of it as cancer prevention, and that would have been . . . 4 years ago."

The interview data show that Aboriginal women are often forced to seek information about health care from Western sources such as pamphlets and other print materials, which are not always representative or reflective of their realities. Several participants indicated that brochures and other educational materials that are reflective of Aboriginal women's lives positively influenced Aboriginal women to access Pap screening: "It would seem important for them to attend [screening], and they could relate to those women in the pamphlets." This demonstrates the importance of having information that is relevant and appropriate for Aboriginal women and that promotes "the empowerment of Aboriginal women to take control of their own health care needs" (Black, 2009, p. 174).

Our Understanding and Perceptions of Pap Screening

The women expressed a multitude of beliefs, experiences, and feelings about Pap screening that often involved cultural ways of thinking about the body and self.

View of the body and self: It is sacred. Several participants explained that an Aboriginal view of the body is holistic and encompasses physical, emotional, mental, and spiritual domains that are not viewed as distinct or separate. Some women described their perceptions of the body and self as holistic, rooted in culture and traditions.

Some women described the perineum as a "sacred area." One woman viewed that part of the body as sacred because "that's where your baby's life comes through, of course it's sacred." In traditional Aboriginal culture, the ability to give birth and raise children positions women in an esteemed, sacred, and respected role (Carroll & Benoit, 2004). Some women referred to the area of the body where Pap screening is conducted as a "private area." A few said that they did not associate this part of the body with Aboriginal culture: "I don't really feel like there's a cultural thing — it's a private area."

Although some of the women expressed the opinion that Aboriginal and Western views of the body and self are different, others did not. One woman said, "Not all First Nations people view the body and self in the same way."

A few women attributed the reluctance to discuss or seek Pap screening to the legacy of residential schooling and abuse. Traditionally in Aboriginal culture, teaching and knowledge acquisition about the body and sexuality were passed on from one generation to the next orally by way of narratives, storytelling, talking circles, and sharing circles (Barnes, Josefowitz, & Cole, 2006). However, due to residential schooling and the fracturing of families, many teachings passed down to children about the body have been lost. Women talked about the loss of children to residential schools and the resultant disruption in traditional parenting and teaching. Children were removed from their family, community, and home environments and placed in a foreign environment where they were abused and forbidden to speak of or follow any traditional teachings. Consequently, children were no longer educated about aspects of the body, health, sexual health, and historical teachings that previously had been passed down and had contributed to their well-being and the strengthening of family ties (Kinnon & Swanson, 2002).

Paps: Important or not? This subtheme describes women's understandings and perceptions regarding the importance of Pap screening and its impact on their accessing of screening services. Many women communicated similar yet at times diverse and conflicting perceptions of the role of Pap screening. Several believed that Pap screening, although uncomfortable and at times embarrassing, is important and continued to regularly access services: "I don't like it, but I know it's important to make sure, health-wise, everything is OK in your female area."

Some of the women accessed Pap screening to remain healthy in order to care for their children, to be able to have children, and, when pregnant, to prevent cervical disease through early detection: "I don't want to find out that I have cervical cancer. I want to make sure that I don't end up with any kind of disease . . . and if so, [that] they can get it early." Others, however, illustrated that not all women view Pap screening as valuable, relevant, or necessary, due to a lack of knowledge and the impact of residential schooling, which is discussed under the next subtheme.

In a few other instances, fear of having cervical cancer was a reason given for *not* being screened. This finding is similar to what others (Black, 2009; Letendre, 2008; O'Brien et al., 2009) have found in studies with Aboriginal women. Fear of cervical cancer prompted some women in the study to access screening and prevented others from doing so.

Pap screening: Feeling violated. This subtheme represents Aboriginal women's accounts of their negative experiences with Pap screening. Some women told explicit personal stories of Pap screening making them feel violated: "Sexual abuse could be a reason for our women [Aboriginal] not to go. It could bring up bad memories from the past."

Some of those who described feeling violated linked it to prior experiences of abuse and a filtering down from residential school experiences; others did not articulate this experience: "Abuse and everything that filters out of residential school . . . there [were] a lot of things that happened that make Paps uncomfortable."

For some women, not accessing Pap screening was a way to protect themselves against reliving experiences of sexual abuse and violation. Pap screening for Aboriginal women can be viewed as an extension of colonization and the pain and suffering from sexual abuse and acts of violence that occurred in residential schools. This abuse and violence has affected not only residential school survivors themselves but also their descendants. A potential additive of historical trauma and sexual abuse is having a Western health-care provider, particularly a male, perform Pap screening.

The literature highlights Aboriginal women's lack of knowledge and information about Pap screening and lack of understanding about what happens to them during the screening experience (Amankwah, Ngwakongnwi, & Quan, 2009; O'Brien et al., 2009; Steven et al., 2004). In the present study, women linked a lack of knowledge about and understanding of Pap screening with being traumatized or violated. A few even revealed that although they were informed about the procedure, they remained terrified and fearful of the results. Many of the women demonstrated courage in moving on from extremely violating experiences of sexual abuse and assault to engage in regular Pap screening, a procedure that itself can be a violating experience.

The Impact of History on Our Health and Our Health-Care Experiences

This theme comprises three subthemes wherein women discuss the historical, social, political, and economic factors that influenced their health, their health care, and particularly their accessing of Pap screening.

The scar has been placed. This subtheme reflects the women's perceptions concerning the impact of historical trauma on their accessing of health services, including Pap screening. Almost every participant described in depth the impact of historical trauma, particularly with reference to residential schooling and/or colonization, on

Aboriginal people's access to health services and Pap screening. Despite the historical trauma, they continued to thrive in less than adequate circumstances and struggled against negative forces that resulted from pain, suffering, and losses inflicted by residential schooling. Two of the women had been in residential schools themselves. Many others shared stories illuminating inequities in health and access to health care and the disempowering impact of residential schooling: "Issues with trusting health-care providers and the health-care system, I think, have been passed on from our history, from our ancestors that attended residential schools . . . They still have power over us, just like they did when we were in residential schools."

One woman spoke of being stereotyped as a First Nation person when accessing health care: "It's just like where you're from or what your background is or what your culture is — right away you're stereotyped just from what other people say." This perspective is supported by the findings of a qualitative study conducted by Tang and Browne (2008) into Aboriginal people's perception that they are treated differently by health professionals when accessing care due to their Aboriginal identity and low socio-economic status. Discrimination, stereotyping, or racism in encounters with health-care providers was influential in shaping their access to Pap screening. Historical trauma as a result of residential schooling has engendered distrust of non-Aboriginal people and affected Aboriginal women's accessing of health services (Dion Stout, 2012; Haskell & Randall, 2009; Waldram, Herring, & Young, 2006).

Socio-economic factors. Socio-economics was a primary factor in the failure to access health services and Pap screening. Participants identified being poor, lacking money for transportation or child care, lacking education, being a young, single parent, and being economically dependent on the government as factors that influenced their accessing of Pap screening. Some alluded to gender and Aboriginal identity as contributing to their socio-economic status and access to care. The women were focused on daily survival and making ends meet. Reasons for not accessing Pap screening are summed up in the comment of one woman: "We never had a lot of money or education. We didn't know it [Pap screening] was important."

Kurtz, Nyberg, Van den Tillaart, and Mills (2008) report that economic and social disadvantage caused by poverty, lack of education, and unemployment are associated with poor health and health outcomes, especially among Aboriginal women. Similarly, Black, Yamada, and Mann (2002) identify poverty, Aboriginal status, and lack of education as reasons for failure to access Pap screening. Essentially, one cannot expect Aboriginal women to access health care when their basic needs are not being met and poverty related to disconnection from lands, traditions, and families due to colonization persists (Dion Stout, 2012).

Several women reported that being pregnant ensured economic stability and being cared for by the community. Being pregnant is not linked to economic security in the literature. The women did not expand on why they were assured access to health services such as Pap screening only when they were pregnant or on why resources to access Pap screening when needed were not provided.

Aboriginal women have a lot on their plates. This subtheme elucidated the issues and multiple and diverse roles and responsibilities of Aboriginal women within their families and their communities that impacted their access to health services and Pap screening. Some participants spoke of not accessing screening due to working outside the home, attending school, keeping house, or having community and childcare responsibilities: "Having a lot on their plates, they do not place themselves at the top of the list for care, particularly when they are single parents or have jobs." However, some made time for Pap screening. One married working mother said that she took time for health care and screening: "I've been really busy, hard to find time, but I go for Paps."

These findings are consistent with those reported in the literature. Women's family and caregiving responsibilities and roles directly affect their health, and in many Aboriginal communities other health-care issues take precedence over women's health (Barnett, White, & Horne, 2002; National Aboriginal Health Organization, 2006). For many participants, it was evident that mothering and family were the most prominent of all traditional roles and values. Some women had been forced to take low-paying jobs outside the home or even outside the community while continuing to be responsible for the care of the family and community, which at times took priority over Pap screening.

Encounters With Health-Care Providers: Making a Difference on Our Path to Paps

This theme described women's perceptions of how health-care providers are making a difference in their access to Pap screening.

Relationships: The fabric of our being. This subtheme concerns the women's perceptions about the impact of relationships with health-care providers on their accessing of Pap screening. The majority detailed the importance of building meaningful, trusting, and respectful relationships with health-care providers, which positively influenced their access to Pap screening. One woman said that fostering relationships was "building a start to increasing Pap testing." Another said, "The way we're treated and looked at by health-care providers plays a big part in how we see ourselves."

Several participants suggested that visiting the community and attending cultural ceremonies and funerals were ways for health-care providers to build relationships in the community. Others expressed the view that not all health-care providers are trusted by community members and that this complicates relationship-building. These viewpoints reflect the diversity of perspectives within Aboriginal communities and among Aboriginal community members as a result of the differences in historical and social experiences and encounters with non-Aboriginal people, including health-care providers. For some of the participants the gender of the health-care provider also had an impact on their ability to form a relationship during Pap screening. A young woman explained: "A female health-care provider understands what it is like to be a woman and knows what it is like to experience Pap smear screening." For a few others, the provider's gender was not considered important for relationship-building during Pap screening. Building and maintaining relationships are considered cornerstones of life, health, and survival in Aboriginal communities (Henderson, 2000; Wilson, 2001). Aboriginal women want relationships with health-care providers that foster the creation of safe and ethical spaces where their voices and their concerns about health and health-care access can be heard (Kurtz et al., 2008). One woman expressed this eloquently: "Relationships are part of the fabric of our being."

Practices of and encounters with health-care providers: Making it or breaking it. The women's perceptions about the practices of and encounters with health-care providers influenced their accessing of health services and Pap screening. Women gave examples of when providers' practices either helped or hindered their accessing of health care. The stories were about their own health-care encounters or those of members of their family or their community. Some women indicated that mainstream health services were not aligned with their needs when accessing Pap screening. Others described negative experiences with providers and gave examples of being discriminated against and not receiving culturally safe and competent care: "They generalize [about] us too much. They think we're drunks. You're hung over or something like that. Or . . . pill poppers."

In some health-care systems, women are receiving culturally unsafe care as a result of the devaluing of Aboriginal knowledge, traditions, and ways. Culturally unsafe nursing care and practices encompass situations in which an action

"diminishes, demeans or disempowers the cultural identity and well-being of any individual" (Nursing Council of New Zealand, 2011, p. 7). The literature reveals instances of Aboriginal women encountering health-care providers whose unsafe practices include stereotyping, discrimination, and racism (Browne et al., 2011; Browne et al., 2012; McGibbon & Etowa, 2009). In the present study, lack of cultural safety was evident in the few Aboriginal pamphlets or teaching tools available or offered in mainstream health-care settings. Not a single participant told of being provided with information about health or health care in her own language.

Although the women seldom used the term "cultural safety" in their stories, they provided examples and expressed a preference for culturally relevant services. A few related positive experiences and described receiving culturally safe care from health-care providers who explained information adequately. For the participants, a key requirement for positive and safe care was relationships built on trust and mutual respect, as well as health-care providers being educated with regard to Aboriginal people and communities.

Educating health-care providers: Our community as teacher. Several participants indicated that health-care providers working in Aboriginal communities need specific knowledge about their culture, history, and language, which can be taught by community members. A few also conveyed the importance of health-care providers being able to talk with community members and listen to their stories as a way of becoming knowledgeable about the community and its members. Thus, health-care providers need to learn to understand nuanced, non-verbal communication and how to address an Elder. They also need to learn how to initiate conversations about sensitive topics like Pap screening and ways to convey information to Aboriginal women. Participants spoke of the need for health-care providers to be educated about the community where they are working, and not just by reading about the community and Aboriginal people: "Get educated and trusted in the community, and learn from the community as opposed to just [from] a book . . . I think that maybe if they [came to] study in here [community] for a bit, they would understand us more." One woman spoke of the need for healthcare providers to be educated not only about the history of Aboriginal people, but also about the family unit, which has changed over time: "I think they should know a little bit about the history. They should also know about family units, [about] how families survive."

Also apparent was the importance of recognizing the diversity that exists among Aboriginal people and not "essentializing" all Aboriginal people or using a "one size fits all" approach to health care in Aboriginal communities. According to the National Aboriginal Health Organization (2010), health-care providers need to become acquainted with and understand cultural beliefs, attitudes, and practices in order to address barriers that Aboriginal people confront when accessing Pap screening. Several women mentioned that Pap screening workshops in their community would be helpful in educating women about the procedure, the results, and the importance of regular screening. Some even suggested that these workshops could be enjoyable social events for women by featuring food, presents, and door prizes. Black (2009) also raises the idea of organizing a day or week dedicated to Pap screening in the community, such as Pap Week or Papalooza, with games and prizes as incentives.

The Health-Care System Is Complicating Our Going for Paps

The women perceived the health-care system as influencing and complicating their access to services such as Pap screening.

Confidentiality and privacy issues: I don't want anybody knowing. Women described issues around confidentiality and privacy that they or others had experienced and also fears about lack of confidentiality around Pap screening. For most participants, confidentiality and privacy were major concerns that affected their comfort in accessing screening services. Confidentiality concerns included being seen by others at the health centre, security issues with records, sharing of information by community members employed at the health centre, and sharing of information by health-care providers who socialized with community members. In both communities, almost half of the women revealed that they did not go to their community health centre for Pap screening for fear of confidentiality and privacy breeches. Instead, they opted to leave their community to access Western health services. One woman stated: "I've never actually been there [community health centre] for a Pap test. . . . The reason is [that] I know my results will come back there. I know my file will be there, everything about me — anybody can look at my file. That's why I won't go there." This woman said that she was uncomfortable with other community members having access to her health file: the community was "so close knit" that everyone knew each other.

According to Bourke et al. (2004), social relations impact confidentiality in rural communities. The lack of anonymity has specific consequences for sensitive health issues such as sexual and reproductive health. Confidentiality is more difficult to maintain in rural and small communities, particularly if the receptionist, patient, and health-care provider have relationships prior to and separate from the health-care encounter (Bourke et al., 2004). In rural communities, people know many of the particulars of each other's lives. Also, community members may have more than one role because of their social position or occupation, which can result in the sharing of personal information about other community members (Bourke, 2001). In a study conducted in British Columbia, confidentiality and privacy concerns were cited as barriers for Aboriginal women obtaining Pap screening (Black, 2009); women residing on reserve did not want to have Pap screening at their community health centre when outside health-care providers came to the reserve, for the reason that other community members would know their business.

A few participants also mentioned that community medical drivers could be related to them and want to know why they were going for a certain appointment. In order to be paid, the drivers had to submit medical forms stating why the person required medical transportation.

Yet not all women had concerns about confidentiality or privacy in their community health centre: "I have [had] Pap smears there [community health centre] and there were no issues around privacy or confidentiality."

Health-care accessibility: We need more services. Some women identified issues within mainstream health-care systems that impact Aboriginal women's access to Pap screening. Several reported a lack of Pap screening services, timely appointments, transportation, and interpreters. Accessibility issues were compounded by the confidentiality concerns discussed above. Even when health services were available, they were not accessible to all Aboriginal women: "We need more services. I like the idea of women's clinics and women's health days that would be accessible for everyone."

For the few who spoke primarily Mi'kmaq, there were literacy issues and a lack of translators available for services provided outside the community. One Elder said, "Each hospital should have an interpreter." The women also viewed mainstream health-care systems as inflexible, unwelcoming, indifferent, and not always considerate of their wishes. These findings indicate that the needs and preferences of Aboriginal women are not always the same in terms of Pap screening. To respond to the differences, health services should be available both within the community and outside it. Barnett et al. (2002) propose that health-care scheduling be not only flexible and convenient for Aboriginal women but also responsive to their diverse needs so that the right

services are being offered to meet their specific needs and life contexts.

Strengths and Limitations of the Study

The use of PAR approaches, Indigenous principles, talking circles, and in-depth interviews enabled respectful and trusting relationships to be developed between researcher and participants. This approach fostered open dialogue and the opportunity to share diverse and rich stories about Pap screening in the context of Mi'kmaq women's lives. Many of the participants said that they had not previously talked about their experiences with Pap screening. Thus, it is evident that this research provided women an opportunity to give voice to their experiences.

Although the sample represented a broad range of ages, having only two women over the age of 60 is a study limitation. Also, the inclusion requirement that women speak, read, and understand English may have been a deterrent to participation. Women under 21 years of age and women who had never had Pap screening were excluded from the study; therefore, the findings may not be transferable to their experiences or perspectives.

Health-Care Practice and Policy Recommendations

It is evident from the results that health-care providers need to take account of the social determinants of health and the contexts of Aboriginal women's lives when considering why they are or are not accessing Pap screening. It is also vital that providers appreciate the impact of historical trauma, interpersonal violence, and trauma-informed care for Aboriginal people while at the same time being aware that Aboriginal people have strengths to counter traumas and violence. A "one size fits all" approach to health care will not be effective; it is essential that Pap screening practices with Aboriginal women be individualized. Health-care providers must acknowledge the limitations of mainstream standards and best practice guidelines and the fact that these may not always apply to Aboriginal people. It is critical that time be invested in building relationships in communities prior to the initiation of screening. Health-care providers should enhance education and knowledge about Pap screening with Aboriginal women in ways that acknowledge the women's realities, needs, and requests and that include opportunities for them to share their stories, perceptions, and experiences with other women. This would raise awareness of the importance of screening and honour storytelling as an authentic method for sharing knowledge. Also, Pap screening should be offered consistently in communities, with extended clinic hours and personal reminders, in order to increase access for Aboriginal women.

We need policies to address the complex determinants of health that contribute to major disparities in access to health care and Pap screening for Aboriginal women. We need to formalize confidentiality and privacy policies with Aboriginal communities and to educate health-care providers and all workers in community health centres about patients' right to privacy and confidentiality. We also need to develop and implement confidentiality policies for medical drivers who transport Aboriginal women to health services, including Pap screening. In addition, we need policies that clarify jurisdictional responsibilities for funding and screening supplies in Aboriginal communities. Finally, Aboriginal women and community members should be consulted on policy development, implementation, and evaluation related to Pap screening.

CONCLUSION

This qualitative study explored Mi'kmaq women's experiences with Pap screening in two First Nation communities in eastern Canada and considered the historical, economic, and sociopolitical contexts that shaped these experiences. It is important to recognize that some Aboriginal women are accessing Pap screening regularly in spite of challenging circumstances. In general,

epidemiological data alone do not provide insight into women's experiences with Pap screening nor identify reasons why women are or are not accessing screening. There are multiple factors, such as history, politics, socio-economics, health-care providers, and health-care systems, that impact women's access. It is critical that nurses and other health-care providers be aware of these diverse factors and how they influence women's access to Pap screening. Health-care providers need to consider the social determinants of health and the contexts of women's lives when considering why they are or are not accessing screening and need to individualize care, while offering consistent and convenient screening services. Building relationships with communities, creating safe spaces for screening, educating women, and providing trauma-informed and culturally safe care are also vital in encouraging Aboriginal women to access Pap screening. Improving Pap screening services for Mi'kmaq women requires multifaceted, culturally safe nursing approaches that are developed in partnership with the women themselves and their communities.

REFERENCES

Aboriginal Affairs and Northern Development Canada. (2013). *Aboriginal peoples and communities*. Ottawa: Author. Retrieved March 2, 2015, from https://www. aadnc aandc.gc.ca/eng/1100100013785/1304467449155.

Adelson, N. (2005). The embodiment of inequity: Health disparities in Aboriginal Canada. *Canadian Journal of Public Health, 96*, S45–S61.

Amankwah, E., Ngwakongnwi, E., & Quan, H. (2009). Why many visible minority women in Canada do not participate in cervical cancer screening. *Ethnicity and Health Journal, 14*(4), 337–349.

Anderson, J. M. (2004). Lessons from a postcolonial-feminist perspective: Suffering and a path to healing. *Nursing Inquiry, 11*(4), 238–246.

Barnes, R., Josefowitz, N., & Cole, E. (2006). Residential schools: Impact on Aboriginal students' academic and cognitive development. *Canadian Journal of School Psychology, 21*(1/2), 18–32.

Barnett, R., White, S., & Horne, T. (2002). *Voices from the front lines: Models of women-centred care in*

Manitoba and Saskatchewan. Winnipeg: Prairie Women's Health Centre of Excellence. Retrieved March 2, 2015, from http://www.pwhce.ca/voicesFrontLines.htm.

Barton, S. (2008). Discovering the literature on Aboriginal diabetes in Canada: A focus on holistic methodologies. *Canadian Journal of Nursing Research, 40*(4), 26–54.

Black, A. T. (2009). Cervical cancer screening strategies for Aboriginal women. *Pimatisiwin: A Journal of Aboriginal and Indigenous Community Health, 7*(2), 157–179.

Black, M. A., Yamada, J., & Mann, V. (2002). A systematic literature review of the effectiveness of community-based strategies to increase cervical cancer screening. *Canadian Journal of Public Health, 93*(5), 386–393.

Bourke L. (2001). One big happy family! Social problems in rural communities. In S. Lockie & L. Bourke (Eds.), *Rurality bites: The social and environmental transformation of rural Australia* (pp. 89–102). Sydney: Pluto.

Bourke, L., Sheridan, C., Russell, U., Jones, G., DeWitt, D., & Liaw, S. T. (2004). Developing a conceptual understanding of rural health practice. *Australia Journal of Rural Health, 12*, 181–186.

Brassard, P., Jiang, Y., Severini, A., Goleski, V., Santos, M., Chatwood, S., & Mao, Y. (2012). Factors associated with human papillomavirus infection among women in the Northwest Territories. *Canadian Journal of Public Health, 103*(4), 282–287.

Brown, L., & Strega, S. (2005). *Research as resistance: Critical, Indigenous, and antioppressive approaches.* Toronto: Canadian Scholars'/Women's Press.

Browne, A. J. (2007). Clinical encounters between nurses and First Nations women in a western Canadian hospital. *Social Science and Medicine, 64*(10), 2165–2176.

Browne, A., & Dion Stout, M. (2012). Moving towards Nahi: Addressing health equity in research involving Indigenous people. *Canadian Journal of Nursing Research, 44*(2), 7–10.

Browne, A., & Smye, V. (2002). A post-colonial analysis of healthcare discourses addressing Aboriginal women. *Nurse Researcher, 9*(3), 28–41.

Browne, A. J., Smye, V. L., Rodney, P., Tang, S. Y., Mussell, B., & O'Neil, J. D. (2011). Access to primary care from the perspective of Aboriginal patients at an urban emergency department. *Qualitative Health Research, 21*(3), 333–348.

Browne, A. J., Smye, V., & Varcoe, C. (2005). The relevance of postcolonial theoretical perspectives to research in Aboriginal health. *Canadian Journal of Nursing Research, 37*(4), 16–37.

Browne, A. J., Smye, V. L., & Varcoe, C. M. (2007). Postcolonial-feminist theoretical perspectives and women's health. In M. H. Morrow, O. Hankivsky, & C. M. Varcoe (Eds.), *Women's health in Canada: Critical perspectives on theory and policy* (pp. 124–142). Toronto: University of Toronto Press.

Browne, A. J., Varcoe, C. M., Wong, S. T., Smye, V. L., Lavoie, J. G., Littlejohn, D., & Lennox, S. (2012). Closing the health equity gap: Evidence-based strategies for primary health care organizations. *International Journal for Equity in Health, 11*(59), 1–15.

Canadian Cancer Society. (2012). *What is cervical cancer?* Toronto: Author. Retrieved March 2, 2915, from https://www.cancer.ca/en/cancer-information/cancer-type/cervical/cervical-cancer/?region=on.

Canadian Institutes of Health Research. (2007). *Guidelines for health research involving Aboriginal people.* Ottawa: Author. Retrieved May 16, 2008, from http://www.cihr-irsc.gc.ca/e/documents/ethics_aboriginal_guidelines_e.pdf.

Carroll, D., & Benoit, C. (2004). Aboriginal midwifery in Canada: Merging traditional practices and modern science. In I. V. Bourgeault, C. Benoit, & R. Davis-Floyd (Eds.), *Reconceiving midwifery* (pp. 263–286). Montreal and Kingston: McGill-Queen's University Press.

Dion Stout, M. (2012). Ascribed health and wellness, *Atikowisi miýw-āyāwin*, to achieved health and wellness, *Kaskitamasowin miýw-āyāwin*: Shifting the paradigm. *Canadian Journal of Nursing Research, 44*(2), 11–14.

Gerberding, J. L. (2004). *Report to Congress: Prevention of genital human papillomavirus infection.* Centers for Disease Control and Prevention. Retrieved March 2, 2015, from http://www.cdc.gov/std/hpv/2004hpv-report.pdf.

Graham, H., & Stamler, L. L. (2010). Contemporary perceptions of health from an Indigenous (Plains Cree) perspective. *Journal of Aboriginal Health, 6*(1), 6–17.

Halseth, R. (2013). *Aboriginal women in Canada: Gender, socio-economic determinants of health, and initiatives to close the wellness gap.* Prince George, BC: National Collaborating Centre for Aboriginal Health.

Haskell, L., & Randall, M. (2009). Disrupted attachments: A social context complex trauma framework and the lives of Aboriginal peoples in Canada. *Journal of Aboriginal Health, 5*(3), 48–99.

Henderson, J. Y. (2000). The context of the state of nature. In M. Battiste (Ed.), *Reclaiming Indigenous voice and vision* (pp. 10–38). Vancouver: UBC Press.

Iwama, M., Marshall, M., Marshall, A., & Bartlett, C. (2009). Two-eyed seeing and the language of healing in community-based research. *Canadian Journal of Native Education, 32*(2), 3–23.

Johnson, G. M., Boyd, C. J., & MacIsaac, M. A. (2004). Community-based cultural predicators of Pap smear screening. *Canadian Journal Public Health, 95*(2), 95–98.

Kinnon, D., & Swanson, S. (2002). *Finding our way: A sexual and reproductive health sourcebook for Aboriginal communities.* Ottawa: Aboriginal Nurses Association of Canada & Planned Parenthood Federation of Canada.

Kirmayer, L. J., Dandeneau, S., Marshall, E., Phillips, M. K., & Williamson, K. (2011). Rethinking resilience from Indigenous perspectives. *Canadian Journal of Psychiatry, 56*(2), 84–91.

Kurtz, D. L. M., Nyberg, J. C., Van den Tillaart, S., & Mills, B. (2008). Silencing of voice: An act of structural violence — Urban Aboriginal women speak out about their experiences with health care. *Journal of Aboriginal Health, 4*(1), 53–63.

Letendre, A. (2008). *Aboriginal female sexual health in a context of cervical cancer and cervical cancer cytology screening with reference to the Cree and Cree-Metis of Northern Alberta.* Unpublished doctoral dissertation, University of Alberta.

Lewis, R., & Mills, S. (2003). *Feminist postcolonial theory: A reader.* New York: Routledge.

Loppie, C. (2007). Learning from the grandmothers: Incorporating Indigenous principles into qualitative research. *Qualitative Health Research, 17*(2), 276–284.

MacDonald, C. (2012). Understanding participatory action research: A qualitative research methodology option. *Canadian Journal of Action Research, 13*(2), 35–40.

Martin, D. H. (2012). Two-eyed seeing: A framework for understanding Indigenous and non-Indigenous approaches to Indigenous health research. *Canadian Journal of Nursing Research, 44*(2), 20–42.

McConaghy, C. (2000). *Rethinking Indigenous education: Culturalism, colonialism and the politics of knowing.* Brisbane: Post Pressed.

McGibbon, E. A., & Etowa, J. B. (2009). *Anti-racist healthcare practice.* Toronto: Canadian Scholars' Press.

National Aboriginal Health Organization. (2006). *Cancer of the cervix in North American Indian women: A literature review.* Ottawa: Author.

National Aboriginal Health Organization. (2010). *Cervical cancer in First Nations women: Information for health care providers.* Ottawa: Author.

Native Women's Association of Canada. (2007, June 20–22). *Aboriginal women and reproductive health, midwifery, and birthing centres: An issue paper.* Paper presented at National Aboriginal Women's Summit, Corner Brook, NL. Retrieved March 2, 2015, from http://www.laa.gov.nl.ca/laa/naws/pdf/nwac-reproductive_health-midwifery-birthing-jun1607.pdf.

Nelson, S. (2012). *Challenging hidden assumptions: Colonial norms as determinants of Aboriginal mental health.* Prince George, BC: National Collaborating Centre for Aboriginal Health. Retrieved March 2, 2015, from http://www.nccah-ccnsa.ca/Publications/Lists/Publications/Attachments/70/colonial_norms_EN_web.pdf.

Nursing Council of New Zealand. (2011). *Guidelines for cultural safety, the Treaty of Waitangi and Maori health in nursing education and practice.* Wellington: Author.

O'Brien, B. A., Mill, J., & Wilson, T. (2009). Cervical cancer screening in Canadian First Nation Cree women. *Journal of Transcultural Nursing, 20*(1), 83–92.

O'Connor, H., & Gibson, N. (2003). A step-by-step guide to qualitative data analysis. *Pimatisiwin: A Journal of Aboriginal and Indigenous Community Health, 1*(1), 64–90.

Ortiz, L. M. (2003). Toward authentic participatory research in health: A critical review. *Pimatisiwin: A Journal of Aboriginal and Indigenous Community Health, 1*(2), 1–26.

Reeves, A. (2008). *Honouring womanhood: Understanding the conceptualization and social construction of young adult First Nation women's sexuality in Atlantic Canada.* Master's thesis, Dalhousie University.

Reimer-Kirkham, S., & Anderson, J. M. (2002). Postcolonial nursing scholarship: From epistemology to method. *Advances in Nursing Science, 25*(1), 1–17.

Sandelowski, M. (2000). Focus on research methods: Whatever happened to qualitative description? *Research in Nursing and Health, 23*, 334–340.

Sheets, E. E. (2002). Cervical cancer and human papillomavirus. In K. J. Carlson, S. A. Eisenstat, F. D. Frigoletto, & I. Schiff (Eds.), *Primary care of women* (pp. 687–691). St Louis: Mosby.

Smylie, J. (2001). SOGC policy statement: A guide for health professionals working with Aboriginal peoples. Health issues affecting Aboriginal peoples. *Journal of Society of Obstetricians and Gynecologists of Canada, 23*(1), 54–68.

Steven, D., Fitch, M., Dhaliwal, H., Kirk-Gardner, R., Sevean, P., Jamieson, J., & Woodbeck, H. (2004). Knowledge, attitudes and beliefs, and practices regarding breast and cervical cancer screening in selected ethnocultural groups in northwestern Ontario. *Oncology Nursing Forum, 1*(2), 305–311.

Tang, S. Y., & Browne, A. J. (2008). "Race" matters: Racialization and egalitarian discourses involving Aboriginal people in the Canadian health care context. *Ethnicity and Health, 13*(2), 109–127.

Tompkins, J. (2002). Learning to see what they can't: Decolonizing perspectives on Indigenous education in the racial context of rural Nova Scotia. *McGill Journal of Education, 37*(3), 405–422.

UNAIDS & World Health Organization. (2006). *Oceania. In 2006 AIDS epidemic update* (p. 61). Geneva: Authors. Retrieved March 2, 2015, from http://www.who.int/hiv/mediacentre/11-Oceania_2006_EpiUpdate_eng.pdf.

Vollman, A. R., Anderson, E. T., & McFarlane, J. (2004). *Canadian community as partner*. Philadelphia: Lippincott Williams & Wilkins.

Vukic, A., Gregory, D., & Martin-Misener, R. (2012). Indigenous health research: Theoretical and methodological perspectives. *Canadian Journal of Nursing Research, 44*(2), 146–161.

Waldram, J. B., Herring, D. A., & Young, T. K. (2006). *Aboriginal health in Canada* (2nd ed.). Toronto: University of Toronto Press.

Weber-Pillwax, C. (2004). Indigenous research and Indigenous research methods: Cultural influences or cultural determinates of research methods. *Pimatisiwin: A Journal of Aboriginal and Indigenous Community Health, 26*(1), 77–90.

Wilson, S. (2001). What is an Indigenous research methodology? *Canadian Journal of Native Education, 25*(2), 175–179.

Zehbe, I., Maar, M., Nahwegahbow, A. J., Berst, K. S. M., & Pintar, J. (2012). Ethical space for a sensitive research topic: Engaging First Nations women in the development of culturally safe human papillomavirus screening. *Journal of Aboriginal Health, 8*(1), 41–50.

ACKNOWLEDGEMENTS

The first author would like to acknowledge the participation of the Mi'kmaq women in this study as well as the input of Dr. Charlotte Loppie-Reading (University of Victoria) and Dr. Marilyn MacDonald (Dalhousie University).

The study received funding from the following: Atlantic Aboriginal Health Research Program (AAHRP); Psychosocial Oncology Research Training (PORT) Fellowship; Electa MacLennan Scholarship, Dalhousie University; AstraZeneca Rural Scholarship, Canadian Nurses Foundation; and Saint Francis Xavier University.

Catherine MacDonald, RN, PhD, is Associate Professor, School of Nursing, Saint Francis Xavier University, Antigonish, Nova Scotia, Canada. Ruth Martin-Misener, RN, PhD, is Associate Professor, School of Nursing, Dalhousie University, Halifax, Nova Scotia. Audrey Steenbeek, RN, PhD, is Associate Professor and Assistant Director of Graduate Programs, Dalhousie University. Annette Browne, RN, PhD, is Professor, School of Nursing, University of British Columbia, Vancouver, Canada.

Impact of Workplace Mistreatment on Patient Safety Risk and Nurse-Assessed Patient Outcomes

Heather K. S. Laschinger, PhD, RN, FAAN, FCAHS

OBJECTIVE: The aim of this study was to investigate the impact of subtle forms of workplace mistreatment (bullying and incivility) on Canadian nurses' perceptions of patient safety risk and, ultimately, nurse-assessed quality and prevalence of adverse events.

BACKGROUND: Workplace mistreatment is known to have detrimental effects on job performance and in nursing may threaten patient care quality.

METHODS: A total of 336 nurses from acute care settings across Ontario responded to a questionnaire that was mailed to their home address in early 2013, with a response rate of 52%.

RESULTS: Bullying and incivility from nurses, physicians, and supervisors have significant direct and indirect effects on nurse-assessed adverse events (R^2 = 0.03-0.06) and perceptions of patient care quality (R^2 = 0.04-0.07), primarily through perceptions of increased patient safety risk.

CONCLUSIONS: Bullying and workplace incivility have unfavorable effects on nurse-assessed patient quality through their effect on perceptions of patient safety risk.

Author Affiliations: Distinguished University Professor and Arthur Labatt Family Nursing Research Chair in Health Human Resources Optimization, The University of Western Ontario, London, Ontario, Canada.
Funding was received from the Ministry of Health and Long-Term Care.
The author declares no conflicts of interest.
Correspondence: Dr Laschinger, Health Sciences Addition, Room H41, 1151 Richmond Street, London, Ontario, Canada N6A 5C1 (*hkl@uwo.ca*).
DOI: 10.1097/NNA.0000000000000068
Heather K. Laschinger, "Impact of Workplace Mistreatment on Patient Safety Risk and NurseAssessed Patient Outcomes," *J Nurs Adm.* 2014 May, 44(5):284-90, http://journals.lww.com/jonajournal/pages/default.aspx

High-quality patient care is a fundamental expectation of an effective healthcare system, and nurses, representing almost one-half of all healthcare workers in Canada,[1] play a critical role in ensuring that patients are provided with comprehensive nursing care. An extensive body of research has shown that nursing work environments that support professional nursing practice and foster high-quality relationships among employees are associated with high-quality nurse and patient outcomes.[2] However, recent studies have shown that nurses are reporting frequent exposure to workplace bullying and incivility,[3-5] which are associated with higher levels of burnout and job turnover intentions.[6] However, little research has linked these subtle forms of workplace violence to patient care quality.

Workplace aggression appears to be on the rise.[7] The World Health Organization[8] recently identified workplace bullying as a serious public health threat in light of evidence that workplace bullying is reaching epidemic levels worldwide. Workplace mistreatment is known to have detrimental effects on job performance and workplace well-being.[9] In the nursing profession, poor performance has serious implications for patient care quality and patient safety.[10,11] However, there are few large-scale studies that have systematically examined the effects of workplace mistreatment on patient safety outcomes.[10]

WORKPLACE MISTREATMENT

Recently, scholars have identified the detrimental effects of seemingly minor forms of workplace violence, such as incivility or bullying.[12]

Workplace bullying consists of "repeated and prolonged exposure to predominantly psychological mistreatment, directed at a target who is typically teased, badgered and insulted, and who perceives himself or herself as not having the opportunity to retaliate 'in kind."[13(p350)] Incivility refers to low-intensity rude or disrespectful behaviors with an ambiguous intent to harm others[14] and differs from bullying in terms of degree, duration, and intentionality.[12] A growing body of knowledge in the management field has linked bullying and workplace incivility to numerous negative work outcomes, including increased turnover intentions, poor mental health, and absenteeism.[15,16] Pearson and Porath[17] found that mistreated employees often missed work to avoid the bully before finally leaving the organization altogether. In a systematic review of studies linking hostile clinician behaviors in nursing work environments to patient care quality, Hutchison and Jackson[10] found that negative interpersonal behaviors among nurses were associated with perceived threats to patient care quality as a result of decreased teamwork and poor morale, which ultimately hindered nurses' ability to provide high-quality patient care. Their review also highlights the effect of negative nurse-physician relations on patient safety outcomes. Bullying and incivility have also been linked to burnout,[18,6] a phenomenon consistently associated with reduced performance and poor patient outcomes.[19] Thus, understanding how these forms of workplace mistreatment influence patient safety and quality is an important area for research.[10] Hutchinson and Jackson[10] concluded from their systematic review that this is an underresearched area that requires attention.

PATIENT SAFETY RISK AND ADVERSE PATIENT OUTCOMES

The patient safety literature has documented the importance of high-quality nursing environments to the provision of safe patient care.[20] A report by the Institute of Medicine[20] emphasized the need for ensuring that nursing work environments be designed to promote honest communication and collaborative teamwork to create a safety culture to reduce patient risk. A positive patient safety culture is characterized by mutual respect among healthcare professionals such that individuals feel free to voice concerns or seek help regarding patient safety concerns without fear of retribution.[21] Negative patient safety cultures have been linked to high medication error rates,[22] increased work-related injuries,[23] and reluctance to report errors.[24] Squires et al[25] found that patient safety climate was significantly related to supportive professional practice environments and, subsequently, fewer medication errors.

Recent research has shown that nurses' assessments of patient care quality on their units are valid indicators of actual quality.[26] Researchers found that nurses' ratings of the quality of care delivered to patients on their units were significant predictors of 30-day patient mortality and failure to rescue, as well as positive patient ratings of their hospital experiences. Clarke et al[23] found that supportive professional practice environments were significantly related to nurse-assessed quality of care, a finding corroborated in numerous studies.[25,26] Lucero et al[27] reported that nurses' reported frequency of adverse events in their practice was significantly related to unmet patient care needs, but also that this effect was weakened when nurses felt that their work environments were supportive.

It is reasonable to expect that work environments in which bullying or incivility are common are not conducive to a positive patient safety climate and may therefore be associated with higher patient safety risk. Indeed, research has linked workplace violence to caregiving errors[28] and unsafe medication practices in nursing settings.[29] However, we could find no studies linking more subtle forms of workplace mistreatment to patient safety risk and nurse-assessed patient care quality and patient adverse events. The purpose of this study was to investigate the impact of subtle forms of workplace mistreatment on Canadian nurses' perceptions of patient safety risk and, ultimately, nurse-assessed quality and prevalence of adverse events.

HYPOTHESIZED MODEL

Guided by the systematic review of Hutchison and Jackson[10] of research linking workplace violence to patient safety outcomes, we used the concept of workplace bullying of Einarsen and Mikkelsen[30] and the construct of workplace incivility of Andersson and Pearson[14] to examine the influence of seemingly minor forms of workplace mistreatment on nurses' assessment of patient safety risk and, ultimately, their ratings of patient care quality and experiences of common adverse events. We argue that higher levels of bullying and incivility from coworkers, physicians, and supervisors will result in concerns about higher risks to patient safety because of poor communication among health team members and hesitancy to raise concerns about patient care. Consequently, nurses will be more likely to rate patient care quality lower and report more frequent experiences of adverse events in their daily practice. We therefore expect that bullying and civility influence nurse-assessed quality outcomes through their effect at nurses' perceptions of patient safety risk in their work settings emanating from negative workplace interactions (Figure B.1).

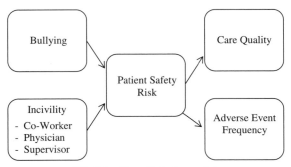

FIG. B.1 Overall study model.

METHODS
Design and Sample

We tested our hypothesized model using data from a larger study of nurses in acute care hospitals across Ontario in the fall of 2012. After ethical approval from the university institutional ethics review board was received, a random sample of nurses working in Ontario hospitals (N = 641) was obtained from the College of Nursing provincial registry list, who were invited to participate in this study. A total of 336 responded to a questionnaire that was mailed to their home address, for a response rate of 52%. The initial survey was followed by a reminder letter 3 weeks later and a replacement package 1 month after the reminder. Most of the nurses were women (88.7%) and baccalaureate prepared (60.7%) and worked full-time (69%) in acute care (78.3%) (Table B.1). With the exception of educational preparation, the demographic profile is similar to that of nurses in the province of Ontario and Canada.[1]

Measures
Bullying Behaviors

Bullying was measured by the Negative Acts Questionnaire-Revised (NAQ-R),[31] which taps perceived exposure to 3 types of bullying at work (work-related, personal, and physical intimidation). The NAQ consists of 22 items rated on a 5-point Likert scale ranging from 1 = never to 5 = daily. Cronbach's α reliability is excellent (>.70), and there is confirmatory factor analysis support for construct and predictive validity.[31]

Workplace Incivility

Cortina's Workplace Incivility Scale[32] was modified slightly to create 3 scales based on specific sources of uncivil behavior: supervisor, coworker, and physician. Nurses responded to 7 items in reference to the frequency of exposure to uncivil behaviors from each source of incivility in the past 6 months using a scale ranging from 1 = never to 5 = daily. Cortina et al[32] has established good

TABLE **B.1**

DEMOGRAPHICS

	M	SD
Age	42.17	13.01
Years as a registered nurse	16.04	13.57
	n	**%**
Gender		
Female	298	88.7
Male	37	11.0
Highest education		
Degree	204	60.7
No degree	123	36.6
Unit specialty		
Medical-surgical	124	36.9
Critical care	65	19.3
Maternal child	42	12.5
Mental health	26	7.7
Other (non-acute care)	73	21.7
Employment status		
Full-time	232	69.0
Part-time	82	24.4
Casual	19	5.7

psychometrics (Cronbach's α reliability of .89 and .81 for supervisor and coworker, respectively) for this tool across studies in nonhealthcare settings.

Patient Safety Risk

Five items were used to tap nurses' perceptions of the effects of negative interpersonal interactions in the work unit related to patient safety. For instance, nurses rated on a 5-point Likert scale the extent to which they agreed with statements such as "negative interpersonal relationships on my unit create a risk to patient safety," "result in failure to report errors in patient care," and "threaten communication about patient care within the healthcare team." These items are consistent with factors identified in the systematic review of Hutchison and Jackson[10] of the impact of hostile clinician behaviors on patient care outcomes.

Nurse-Assessed Adverse Events

We used a scale developed by Sochalski[33] derived from the American Nurses Association Nursing

Quality Indicators[34] consisting of 5 items that assess nurses' perceptions of the frequency of common adverse patient outcomes over the past year (medication errors, nosocomial infections, falls, work-related injury, and patient complaints) on a scale from 1 = never to 4 = frequently. This scale has been used extensively in nursing and has shown acceptable reliability and validity.[35]

Perception of Patient Care Quality

Perception of patient care quality was measured by a single item developed by Aiken et al[2] in Magnet® hospital studies. Nurses are asked to rate on a scale ranging from 1 (poor) to 4 (excellent) the quality of care of their unit. This scale has been widely used in studies of Magnet hospitals in the United States and Canada and shown to be a valid indicator of nurse-assessed quality of care.

Data Analysis

Analyses were conducted using the Statistical Package for Social Sciences (Armonk, New York). Descriptive statistics and a series of mediated multiple regression (ordinary least squares) analyses were conducted to examine the effects of bullying and different sources of workplace incivility on patient outcomes through their effects on nurses' perception of patient safety risk. We used the approach of Baron and Kenny[36] to testing mediation, that is, the extent to which an intervening variable influences the impact of an independent variable on an outcome variable. This approach permits identifying both direct and indirect effects of a focal variable of interest (in this case bullying and incivility) on outcomes (quality of care and frequency of adverse events).

RESULTS

Descriptive Statistics

Exposure to bullying experience, on average, was not high (mean [SD], 1.45 [0.59]) nor was nurses' exposure to incivility in the workplace. Nurses reported relatively high quality of patient care on their units (mean [SD] 3.34 [0.69]), relatively few experiences of adverse events (mean [SD], 2.03 [0.69]), and low workplace violence-related patient safety risk (mean [SD], 2.31 [1.04]). Complaints from patients and families about patient care quality and work-related injuries were highest rated individual adverse events, whereas medication errors were rated the lowest. Bullying and all sources of incivility were significantly related to both nurse-assessed quality of care, adverse events, and perceptions of patient safety risk. Patient/family complaints was the individual adverse event most strongly related to bullying and physician and coworker incivility (Table B.2).

Testing the Mediating Effects of Patient Safety Risk

Eight separate mediation models were tested to examine the direct and indirect effects of bullying and 3 sources of workplace incivility on patient safety outcomes (through patient safety risk). The results are summarized in Tables B.3 and B.4. Regression analyses revealed that all forms of workplace mistreatment had direct effects on both nurse-assessed quality of care and reported frequency of adverse events in their units, supporting the 1st condition for establishing mediating effects of Baron and Kenny,[36] that is, that the independent variable significantly predicts the outcome variable of interest. The magnitude of these effects on patient care quality was similar for all sources of workplace mistreatment, with physician incivility having the strongest effect ($B = -0.234$, $\rho < .05$). Bullying and physician incivility were most strongly related to overall frequency of patient adverse events ($B = 0.241$ and 0.166, respectively; $\rho < .05$), followed by coworker incivility ($B = 0.148$, $\rho < .05$). Supervisor incivility was less strongly (although significantly) related to adverse event frequency. The 2nd condition required for testing mediation models, that the independent variable significantly predicts the proposed mediator (patient safety risk), was supported. All workplace mistreatment variables were significantly related to

patient safety risk, with bullying having the strongest effect ($B = 0.328$), followed by physician incivility ($B = 0.228$). The final condition for establishing full mediation, that is, the effect of the independent variable on the outcome is reduced and nonsignificant after controlling for the mediator, revealed that increased patient safety risk partially mediated the effect of physician incivility on both nurse-assessed quality of care and frequency of adverse events (ie, the effect was reduced but remained significant reflecting direct and indirect effects). The effect of coworker incivility on patient care quality was fully mediated by patient safety risk, which also partially mediated coworker incivility effects on adverse events frequency. The effect of supervisor incivility on quality care was partially mediated by patient safety risk, which also fully mediated its effects on adverse event frequency. On the other hand, patient safety risk did not mediate the effect of workplace bullying on quality outcomes, rather the effects were direct.

DISCUSSION

Our results support the suggestion of Hutchison and Jackson[10] that subtle forms of workplace mistreatment can have detrimental effects on patient safety outcomes. To our knowledge, this is the 1st study to provide empirical support for this proposition. Although previous research has linked workplace violence to lower quality of care, few studies have examined both workplace bullying and different sources of workplace incivility in the analysis. In addition, our results point to a previously unestablished mechanism through which bullying and incivility influence patient outcomes, that is, perceived patient safety risk. The results suggest that negative interpersonal interactions among nurses and other health professionals, such as physicians, may interfere with effective communication about patient care needs and processes, which, in turn, may hinder delivery of high-quality patient care and result in adverse nurse sensitive outcomes. The mediating effects of perceived safety risk were strongest for

TABLE B.2

DESCRIPTIVE STATISTICS

STUDY VARIABLE	MEAN	SD	α	1	2	3	4	5	6	7	8	9	10	11
1. Coworker incivility	1.52	0.70	.93											
2. Physician-workplace incivility	1.45	0.56	.85	0.53										
3. Supervisor incivility	1.32	0.51	.88	0.38	0.30									
4. Bullying	1.45	0.59	.89	0.66	0.48	0.57								
5. Quality of care	3.34	0.69	NA	−0.19	−0.23	−0.20	−0.19							
6. Total adverse events	1.98	0.68	.79	0.14	0.17	0.10	0.23	−0.22[a]						
7. Medication errors	1.64	0.76	NA	0.05	0.11	0.02	0.14	−0.17[a]	0.70[a]					
8. Nosocomial infection	1.97	0.98	NA	0.16	0.12	0.05	0.18	−0.09	0.71[a]	0.48[a]				
9. Patient falls	1.80	0.93	NA	0.04	0.05	0.03	0.09	−0.19[a]	0.73[a]	0.47[a]	0.47[a]			
10. Work-related injuries	2.09	0.93	NA	0.09	0.15	0.14	0.18	−0.12[a]	0.76[a]	0.42[a]	0.38[a]	0.45[a]		
11. Patient/family complaints	2.41	1.03	NA	0.17	0.21	0.12	0.26	−0.22[a]	0.73[a]	0.35[a]	0.38[a]	0.39[a]	0.53[a]	
12. Patient safety risk	2.31	1.04	.94	0.21	0.23	0.20	0.33	−0.18[a]	0.16[a]	0.13[a]	0.06	0.09	0.18	0.20

Abbreviation: NA, not applicable.

TABLE B.3

MEDIATION MODEL RESULTS FOR NURSE-ASSESSED PATIENT CARE QUALITY

MISTREATMENT TYPE	PATHS TESTED IN MEDIATION ANALYSIS	NURSE-ASSESSED QUALITY OF CARE			
		β	SE	R^2	p
Bullying[a]					
Condition 1	Bullying → quality	.187	0.007		
Condition 2	Bullying → safety	.328	0.001		
Condition 3	Bullying + safety → quality			0.04	.007
	Bullying	.133	0.07		
	Safety	.134	0.07		
Incivility					
Physician incivility[b]					
Condition 1	MD incivility → quality	.234	0.001		
Condition 2	MD incivility → safety risk	.228	0.001		
Condition 3	MD incivility + patient safety → quality			0.07	.000
	MD incivility	.215	0.003		
	Patient safety	.130	0.070		
Coworker incivility[c]					
Condition 1	Coworker incivility → quality	.185	0.003		
Condition 2	Coworker incivility → patient safety	.211	0.001		
Condition 3	Coworker incivility + PSR → quality			0.04	.005
	Coworker incivility	.133	0.06		
	Patient safety	.156	0.03		
Supervisor incivility[b]					
Condition 1	Supervisor incivility → quality	.204	0.003		
Condition 2	Supervisor incivility → patient safety	.198	0.001		
Condition 3	Supervisor incivility + patient safety → quality			0.05	.002
	Supervisor incivility	.157	0.026		
	Patient safety	.165	0.019		

[a]Full mediation.
[b]Partial mediation.
[c]No mediation.

coworker and physician incivility, the highest rated source of incivility in this study, highlighting the importance of addressing the need to create more positive relationships among these key members of the healthcare team. Our results showed that although bullying/incivility rates were not high, when present, they were associated with a perceived increase in patient safety risk and poor patient care quality.

Limitations

This study used cross-sectional data and therefore precludes attribution of cause and effect among the study variables. The relatively low return rate and targeted sample of acute care nurses limit the generalizability of the findings to nurses in other settings. In addition, patient outcomes were nurse-assessed outcomes, not institutional data. Future research using institutional patient-related data is needed to provide further evidence linking workplace mistreatment to patient safety outcomes.

Implications for Management

Managers play a key role in creating environments that support professional nursing practice that promote high-quality patient care, and establishing a positive patient safety culture is an important facet of healthcare managers' mandate to ensure positive patient outcomes. Taking concrete actionable steps to prevent negative interpersonal interactions such

TABLE **B.4**

MEDIATION MODEL RESULTS FOR NURSE-ASSESSED ADVERSE EVENTS (NAAEs)

MISTREATMENT TYPE	PATHS TESTED IN MEDIATION ANALYSIS	β	SE	R^2	ρ
	NAAEs				
Bullying[a]					
Condition 1	Bullying → adverse events	.241	0.001		
Condition 2	Bullying → safety risk	.328	0.001		
Condition 3	Bullying + safety risk → adverse events			0.06	.000
	Quality	.212	0.001		
	Safety risk	.097	0.092		
Incivility					
Physician incivility[b]					
Condition 1	Physician incivility → adverse events	.166	0.003		
Condition 2	Physician incivility → safety risk	.228	0.001		
Condition 3	Physician incivility + safety risk → adverse events			0.04	.001
	Physician incivility	.132	0.021		
	Safety risk	.131	0.022		
Coworker incivility[b]					
Condition 1	Coworker incivility → adverse events	.148	0.008		
Condition 2	Coworker incivility → safety risk	.211	0.001		
Condition 3	Coworker incivility + safety risk → adverse events			0.03	.002
	Coworker incivility	.114	0.045		
	Safety risk	.141	0.013		
Supervisor incivility[c]					
Condition 1	Supervisor incivility → adverse events	.109	0.05		
Condition 2	Supervisor incivility → safety risk	.198	0.001		
Condition 3	Supervisor incivility + safety risk → adverse events			0.03	.005
	Supervisor incivility	.084	0.136		
	Safety risk	.149	0.009		

[a]No mediation.
[b]Partial mediation.
[c]Full mediation.

as bullying and incivility is an important 1st step in this process. Establishment and enforcement of zero tolerance bullying/workplace incivility policies have been shown to be effective in troubled organizations. Workplace civility interventions, such as the Civility, Respect, and Engagement in the Workplace project developed by the Veterans Health Administration, have been shown to result in positive employee and patient outcomes.[37,38] This program involves employee-driven strategies to work on building positive interpersonal working relationships on an ongoing basis with the goal of embedding this process as part of the culture of the organization. Research has shown that relational leadership styles, such as authentic leadership, result in reduced bullying and subsequent burnout, highlighting the need for nurse managers to develop these competencies.[6] Leadership is considered critical to the establishment of a positive patient safety culture.[39]

CONCLUSION

The results of this study suggest that seemingly harmless forms of workplace mistreatment can threaten patient safety outcomes by creating a sense of higher patient safety risk in work environments characterized by workplace bullying and incivility among health professionals.

REFERENCES

1. Shields, M. (2005). *Findings From the 2005 National Survey of the Work and Health of Nurses.* Ottawa, Ontario, Canada: Health Canada and Canadian Institute for Health Information.

2. Aiken, L. H., Smith, H. L., & Lake, E. T. (1994). Lower Medicare mortality among a set of hospitals known for good nursing care. *Med Care, 32*(8), 771–787.

3. Laschinger, H. K. S., Grau, A. L., Finegan, J., & Wilk, P. (2010). New graduate nurses' experiences of bullying and burnout in hospital settings. *J Adv Nurs, 66,* 2732–2742.

4. Lewis, P., Malecha, A. (2011). The impact of workplace incivility on the work environment, manager skill, and productivity. *J Nurs Adm, 41*(7/8), S17–S23.

5. Laschinger, H. K. L., Wong, C., Regan, S., Young-Ritchie, C., & Bushell, P. (2013). Workplace incivility and new graduate nurses' mental health: the protective role of resiliency. *J Nurs Adm, 43*(7-8), 415–421.

6. Laschinger, H. K. S., & Fida, R. A. Time-lagged analysis of the effect of authentic leadership on workplace bullying, burnout and occupational turnover intentions [published online ahead of print 2013]. *Eur J Work Organ Psychol.* doi:10.1080/1359432X.2013.804646.

7. Sliter, M. T., Sliter, K. A., & Jex, S. M. (2012). The employee as a punching bag: the effect of multiple sources of incivility on employee withdrawal behavior and sales performance. *J Organ Behav, 33,* 121–139.

8. World Health Organization (WHO). (2010). Prevention of bullying- related morbidity and mortality: a call for public health policies. Prepared by Jorge C. Srabstein & Bennett L. Leventhal. *Bulletin of the World Health Organization, 88,* 403–403.

9. Estes, B., & Wang, J. (2008). Workplace incivility: Impacts on individual and organizational performance. *Hum Res Dev Rev, 7,* 218–240.

10. Hutchison, M., & Jackson, D. (2013). Transformational leadership in nursing: towards a more critical interpretation. *Nurs Inq, 20*(1), 11–22.

11. Vessey, J. A., Demarco, R., & DiFazio, R. (2010). Bullying, harassment, and horizontal violence in the nursing workforce: the state of the science. *Annu Rev Nurs Res, 28,* 133–157.

12. Hershcovis, M. S. (2011). Incivility, social undermining, bullying . . . Oh my! A call to reconcile constructs within workplace aggression research. *J Organ Behav, 32,* 499–519.

13. Hauge, L. J., Skogstad, A., & Einarsen, S. (2009). Individual and situational predictors of workplace bullying: why do perpetrators engage in the bullying of others? *Work Stress, 23*(4), 349–358.

14. Andersson, L. M., Pearson, C. M. (1999). Tit for tat? The spiraling effect of incivility in the workplace. *Acad Manag Rev, 24*(3), 452–471.

15. Berthelsen, M., Skogstad, A., Lau, B., Einarsen, S. (2011). Do they stay or do they go? A longitudinal study of intentions to leave and exclusion from working life among the targets of workplace bullying. *Int J Manpower, 32*(2), 178–193.

16. Einarsen, S., Hoel, H., & Notelaers, G. (2009). Measuring exposure to bullying and harassment at work: validity, factor structure and psychometric properties of the Negative Acts Questionnaire-Revised. *Work Stress, 23*(1), 24–44.

17. Pearson, C. M., & Porath, C. L. (2005). On the nature, consequences, and remedies of workplace incivility: "no time for 'nice'? Think again." *Acad Manag Exec, 19,* 7–18.

18. Chipps, E., Stelmaschuk, S., Albert, N., Bernhard, L., & Holloman, C. (2013). Workplace bullying in the OR: results of a descriptive study. *AORN J, 98*(5), 479–493.

19. Aiken, L. H., Sermeus, W., Van den Heede, K., et al. (2012). Patient safety, satisfaction, and quality of hospital care: cross sectional surveys of nurses and patients in 12 countries in Europe and the United States. *BMJ, 344.*

20. Institute of Medicine (IOM). (2003). *Keeping Patients Safe: Transforming the Work Environment of Nurses.* Washington, DC: National Academy Press.

21. Frankel, A. S., Leonard, M. W., & Denham, C. R. (2006). Fair and just culture, team behavior, and leadership engagement: the tools to achieve high reliability. *Health Res Educ Trust, 41,* 1690–1709.

22. Hofmann, D. A., & Mark, B. (2006). An investigation of the relationship between safety climate and medication errors as well as other nurse and patient outcomes. *Pers Psychol, 59,* 847–869.

23. Clarke, S. P., Sloane, D. M., & Aiken, L. H. (2002). Effects of hospital staffing and organizational climate on needlestick injuries to nurses. *Am J Public Health, 92*(7), 1115–1119.

24. Chiang, H., & Pepper, G. A. (2006). Barriers to nurses reporting of medication administration errors in Taiwan. *J Nurs Scholarsh, 38,* 392–399.

25. Squires, M., Tourangeau, A., Laschinger, H. K. S, & Doran, D. (2010). The link between leadership and safety outcomes in hospitals. *J Nurs Manag, 18,* 914–925.

26. McHugh, M. D., & Witkoski, S. (2012) Nurse reported quality of care: a measure of hospital quality. *Res Nurs Health*, *35*(6), 566–575.

27. Lucero, R. J., Lake, E. T., & Aiken, L. H. (2010). Nursing care quality and adverse events in US hospitals. *J Clin Nurs*, *19*(15-16), 2185–2195.

28. Rowe, M., & Sherlock, H. (2005). Stress and verbal abuse in nursing: do burn out nurses eat their young? *J Nurs Manag*, *13*, 242–248.

29. Institute for Safe Medication Practices. (2004). *Intimidation: Practitioners Speak Up About This Unresolved Problem (Part I). Safety Alert*! Community/Ambulatory Care edition. http://www.ismp.org/Newsletters/acutecare/articles/20040311_2.asp. Published March 11, 2004. Accessed March 19, 2014.

30. Einarsen, S., & Mikkelsen, E. G. (2003). Individual effects of exposure to bullying at work. In S. Einarsen, H. Hoel, D. Zapf, & C. L. Cooper (Eds.), *Bullying and Emotional Abuse in the Workplace: International Perspectives in Research and Practice* (pp. 127–144). London, England: Taylor & Francis.

31. Einarsen, S., & Hoel, H. (2001, May). The Negative Acts Questionnaire: development, validation and revision of a measure of bullying at work. Paper presented at the 10th European Congress on Work and Organisational Psychology, Prague, Czech Republic.

32. Cortina, L. M., Magley, V. J., Williams, J. H., & Langhout, R. D. (2001). Incivility in the workplace: incidence and impact. *J Occup Health Psychol*, *6*(1), 64–80.

33. Sochalski, J. (2001). Quality of care, nurse staffing and patient outcomes. *Policy Polit Nurs Pract*, *2*(1), 9–18.

34. American Nurses Association (ANA). (2000). *Nurse Staffing and Patient Outcomes in the Inpatient Hospital Setting, Report*. Washington, DC: ANA.

35. Sochalski, J. (2004). Is more better? The relationship between nurse staffing and the quality of nursing care in hospitals. *Med Care*, *42*(2), II-67–II-73.

36. Baron, R. M., & Kenny, D. A. (1986). The moderator-mediator variable distinction in social psychological research: conceptual, strategic and statistical considerations. *J Pers Soc Psychol*, *51*, 1173–1182.

37. Osatuke, K., Moore, S. C., Ward, C., Dyrenforth, S. R., & Belton, L. (2009). Civility, Respect, Engagement in the Workforce (CREW): nationwide organization development intervention at Veterans Health Administration. *J Appl Behav Sci*, 45, 384–410.

38. Leiter, M. P., Laschinger, H. K. S., Day, A., & Gilin-Oore, D. (2011). The impact of civility interventions on employee social behavior, distress, and attitudes. *J Appl Psychol*, *96*, 1258–1274.

39. Ruchlin, H. S., Dubbs, N. L., & Callahan, M. A. (2004). The role of leadership in instilling a culture of safety: lessons from the literature. *J Healthc Manag*, *49*(1), 47–58; discussion 58–59.

Toward Cultural Safety: Nurse and Patient Perceptions of Illicit Substance Use in a Hospitalized Setting

Bernadette (Bernie) Pauly, PhD, RN, Jane McCall, MSN, RN, Annette J. Browne, PhD, RN, J. Parker, MA, Ashley Mollison, MA

As a group, people who use illicit drugs and are affected by social disadvantages often experience health inequities and encounter barriers such as stigma and discrimination when accessing health care services. Cultural safety has been proposed as one approach to address health inequities and mitigate stigma in health care. Drawing on a qualitative ethnographic approach within an overarching collaborative framework, we sought to gain an understanding of what constitutes culturally safe care for people who use(d) illicit drugs. The findings illustrate that illicit substance use in hospitals is often negatively constructed as (1) an individual failing, (2) a criminal activity, and (3) a disease of "addiction" with negative impacts on access to care, management of pain, and provision of harm-reduction supplies and services. These constructions of illicit substance use impact patients' feelings of safety in hospital and nurses' capacity to provide culturally safe care. On the basis of these findings, we provide recommendations and guidance for the development of culturally safe nursing practice.

KEY WORDS: *access to health services, addiction, cultural safety, drug use, health equity, harm reduction, homelessness, illicit substance use, marginalization, poverty, stigma*

Author Affiliations: *School of Nursing and Centre for Addictions Research of BC (Dr Pauly) and Society of Living Illicit Drug Users (Ms Mollison), Victoria, British Columbia, Canada; and HIV Program, St. Paul's Hospital, Providence Health Care (Ms McCall), School of Nursing, University of British Columbia (Dr Browne), and Critical Research in Health and Healthcare Inequities, University of British Columbia School of Nursing (Ms Parker), Vancouver, British Columbia V8W 2Y2, Canada.*

We thank Michael Smith Foundation for Health Research For Funding to support the conduct of this research. We also gratefully acknowledge our appreciation for the patients, nurses and members of SOLID (Society of Living Intravenous Drug Users) who contributed to this work.

The authors have disclosed that they have no significant relationships with, or financial interest in, any commercial companies pertaining to this article.

Correspondence: *Bernadette (Bernie) Pauly, PhD, RN, School of Nursing, Centre for Addictions Research of BC, Box 1700 STN CSC, University of Victoria, Victoria, British Columbia V8W2Y2, Canada (bpauly@uvic.ca).*

DOI: 10.1097/ANS.0000000000000070

Bernadette Pauly, Jane McCall, Annette Browne, et al, "Toward Cultural Safety: Nurse and Patient Perceptions of Illicit Substance Use in a Hospitalized Setting," *Advances in Nursing Science*, April/June 2015 - Volume 38 - Issue 2 - p 121–135, http://journals.lww.com/advancesinnursing-science/pages/default.aspx

Social positioning (eg, age, gender, ethnicity, socioeconomic status) dramatically impacts health and access to resources for health.[1-4] When illicit drug use intersects with poverty and homelessness, people who use illicit drugs are particularly vulnerable to health inequities and often experience poorer health than the rest of the population.[5-7] The stigma encountered in daily life and when accessing health care is implicated in the development of health inequities.[8-13] When in need of health care, people who use illicit drugs may mistrust, avoid, or delay seeking health care services or leave hospital early.[14-17] While stigma and discrimination associated with illicit substance use have repeatedly been identified as concerns in health care practice, few models for health care have been developed to address these issues. One proposed model, cultural safety, has been identified as having potential to address inequities in health and access to health care for people experiencing marginalization and discrimination.[18,19]

The primary research question for this project was: What constitutes culturally safe care for people who use(d) illicit drugs and are affected by social disadvantages such as poverty and homelessness? Illicit substance use refers to the use of drugs that are currently considered illegal in the Canadian context, such as marijuana, heroin, cocaine/crack, and methamphetamine. Our goal was to generate knowledge to foster an understanding of the meaning and context of cultural safety in acute care settings for people who use, have used in the past, or are suspected of using illicit substances and are affected by poverty and/or homelessness. In this article, we make explicit the various constructions of illicit substance use that operate in hospitals as a beginning point for critical reflection on how such constructions may be navigated to enhance health care delivery for people who use illicit drugs and are experiencing poverty and/or homelessness.

BACKGROUND

A growing body of evidence shows that people who use, have used, or are suspected of using illicit drugs, particularly when this intersects with visible markers of poverty, homelessness, or mental health issues, experience high rates of discrimination, stigmatization, and social exclusion in the health care sector.[10,11] In particular, nurses and other health care providers have been found to hold negative attitudes toward people who use illicit substances.[8,12,13,20] Stigma can be understood as a difference in power relations in which one group has the power to name differences, label, stereotype, and stigmatize another group on the basis of certain characteristics or behaviors.[21,22] More recently, stigma has been conceptualized as a structural or macro-level process intersecting with broader social discourses, media representations, and public and legal policies that influence and are enacted during micro-level interactions, with serious implications for health and well-being.[23] Structural stigma is defined "as societal-level conditions, cultural norms, and institutional policies that constrain the opportunities, resources, and wellbeing" of people and groups who are stigmatized[24(p2)] Thus, structural stigma can be understood as deeply embedded in health and social system culture and norms and enacted consciously or unconsciously during health care interactions.

Stigma in health care can contribute to delays in access to needed health care services, avoidance of health care, mistrust of the system, and other factors that constrain access to timely health care services.[14-17] To avoid the harmful effects of stigma and stigmatizing processes, people who use(d) illicit drugs may avoid or delay seeking care until they are severely ill, or may leave hospital against medical advice without completion of treatment. Thus, resulting in missed opportunities to reduce and prevent health issues and the need for more intensive treatment and longer periods of hospitalization later.

To address inequities in health outcomes, the notion of cultural safety has been proposed as an approach to care that aims to mitigate the effects of stigma, discrimination, and marginalization in health care contexts.[18,19] Cultural safety was originally developed by Indigenous nurse-scholars and educators as a way of providing more respectful care to Indigenous populations in the New Zealand context.[25-28] Cultural safety has gained traction in Canada as a strategy for extending beyond cultural sensitivity and cultural competence, and focusing attention on power imbalances, institutional discrimination, and the inequitable positioning of certain groups within these dynamics.[18,29-31] Cultural safety has been particularly relevant in the Canadian context in relation to understanding the impact of historical trauma, and ongoing patterns of institutionalized racial discrimination influencing Indigenous peoples' access to health care, health care experiences, and overall health status.[12,30,32,33] In 2005, the New Zealand Nursing Council articulated the clinical relevance of cultural safety as an approach to care that requires health care providers at all levels of organizations to (1) reflect on their own, often unconsciously held, attitudes and beliefs about others; (2) examine the ways in which history, social relations, and politics continue to shape people's responses, needs, access, and health; and (3) demonstrate flexibility in how they relate with others, especially those that differ from themselves.[34] These guidelines provide a useful framework for understanding how cultural safety might be enacted in clinical contexts to mitigate marginalization, stigma, and discrimination.

For people who use illicit drugs and experiencing poverty and homelessness, it is important to consider how structural violence and histories of trauma may be impacting their lives. There is evidence that people who use illicit drugs are much more likely to have experienced adverse childhood events, including neglect or other forms of abuse as children.[35] As adults, people who use illicit drugs often experience stigma, discrimination, and dismissal in daily life, which are ongoing forms of trauma. As a result, it can be difficult for them to form trusting relationships with health care providers and others in positions of power and authority. Nurses working at Insite, a supervised injection site, identified that adopting principles of cultural safety in practice was helpful in establishing respectful and responsive working relationships with all people who use illicit drugs.[19] Thus, cultural safety is proposed as one model to address these issues in health care.

However, little is known about the application and practice of cultural safety for people who use illicit drugs and are experiencing social disadvantages such as poverty and homelessness, particularly when receiving care in hospital settings. In this article, we discuss varying conceptualizations of illicit substance use and people who use illicit drugs that we found to be operating in a hospital setting with impacts on the delivery of

nursing and other health care services. We conclude with recommendations for enhancing culturally safe nursing care.

Research Design and Sample

In this project, we used a qualitative exploratory research design drawing on ethnographic research methods. Ethnographic designs are particularly appropriate for a study of this type where the focus is on gaining an understanding of the context within which a phenomenon occurs.[36] The study was conducted in a large urban hospital on 2 medical units. One of the units was well known for their expertise in the provision of care to people with human immunodeficiency virus (HIV) infection and illicit drug use. Nurse and peer (people who use drugs) advisory groups were established to guide the research. To obtain input from nurses, we presented information about the study and the findings at regular intervals throughout the project to groups of nurses working on the 2 medical units where the study was being conducted during their workday at coffee or lunch times. The peer advisory group consisted of people who use(d) illicit drugs and who were representatives of a regionally based peer-run drug user organization, the Society of Living Illicit Drug Users (SOLID). As with the nurses, we met with peer advisors at regular intervals, obtaining their input on the interview questions, providing updates on progress in data collection and analysis, and eliciting their interpretations of emerging findings. While the peer group consisted of 10 people who consistently participated throughout the project, the nurse advisory was, by necessity, a fluid arrangement, as it was difficult for nurses with families and shift work commitments to participate in meetings outside of work hours. Thus, the composition and the number of nurses on the nurse advisory shifted from meeting to meeting. Both groups were involved in planning a final policy forum and developing recommendations from the findings.[37]

Data collection consisted of in-depth interviews with a purposive sample of nurses and patients, participant observation, and reviewing hospital policy documents. In total, we interviewed 34 people, including 15 patients (8 men, 6 women, and 1 person who identified as transgendered) and 19 nurses (12 front-line staff nurses and 7 nurse managers and educators). Patients ranged in age from 30 to 51 years; 7 participants identified as Aboriginal. All patient participants self-identified as using illicit drugs in the previous 12 months. All were unemployed, living on social assistance and unstably housed. The nurses ranged in age from 27 to 57 years with nursing experience ranging from 4 months to 33 years. Seventeen of the nurses were bachelor's-prepared and 2 had master's degrees. When asked, only a small number of nurses reported having received specific education related to substance use and addiction. All interviews were conducted in a private setting in the hospital and audiorecorded. The interviews focused on participants' experiences in giving and receiving care, understandings of comfort, safety, and how welcome they felt in health care settings, and the various barriers and enablers to providing or receiving care.

We conducted participant observation throughout the study to gain an understanding of the specific contexts in which nursing care was provided to people who use drugs. Two members of the research team (Parker and Pauly) completed approximately 275 hours of participant observation, recording their observations in field notes. Policy documents included in the analysis were related to the organizational mission, vision and values, and organizational policies about substance use and harm reduction. We obtained ethical approval for the project from the University of Victoria and the University of British Columbia, as well as the hospital where the study was conducted. Informed consent was obtained from all participants prior to both in-depth interviews and participant observation.

Interviews and field notes were transcribed verbatim, reviewed for accuracy, and entered into NVivo, a qualitative software package to organize and code qualitative data. We used interpretive description (ID) as our approach to data analysis. Interpretive description is a qualitative method of data analysis that acknowledges the constructed and contextual nature of human experience while allowing for shared realities[38] The emphasis of ID on examining the constructed and contextual nature of everyday practice made it a fitting approach for the focus of this project.

Three members of the research team independently coded the transcribed interviews, field notes, and documents and developed the initial coding framework before entering it into NVIVO. As more data were analyzed, coding categories were refined to reflect multiple understandings of illicit substance use and culturally safe care. The same team members read the transcribed data repeatedly and, together with the whole research team and advisory groups, identified and mapped recurring, converging, and contradictory patterns of interaction, key concepts, and emerging themes from the data. Throughout the process, emerging themes and categories were reviewed and compared and taken to a higher level of conceptualization for the purpose of developing broader analytic insights. One outcome of this process of data analysis was the identification of themes that illustrate the ways in which illicit substance use and culturally safe care within a hospital context were understood and constructed from the perspectives of nurses and patients.

Standards for rigor in qualitative research include credibility, confirmability, and transferability.[39] Credibility was enhanced through transcribing interviews and field notes, immersion of the researchers in the setting through participant observation, triangulation of data from multiple sources, and multiple readings of the data. Confirmability was achieved through involvement of multiple researchers independently reading and coding the data and the inductive development of the coding framework. Furthermore, the research team's experience and the involvement of nurse and peer advisory groups in the interpretation of the data contributed to confirmability. For example, one of our research team members had more than 30 years of experience in nursing and care of people with HIV/AIDS and illicit substance use. Three of our research team members had experience working with peer-run organizations of people who use drugs in 2 different Canadian provinces. Transferability is achieved when others see the applicability or resonance of the findings in other settings and situations. Opportunities to present this work at 3 forums confirmed that our findings were relevant and applicable to other groups of nurses and advocacy groups for people who use illicit substances.

Findings

Based on an analysis of patient and nurse data, 3 different constructions of illicit substance use and people who use illicit drugs emerged. The constructions identified were (1) illicit drug use as an individual failing, (2) illicit drug use as a criminal activity, and (3) illicit drug use as a disease of addiction. These constructions of illicit drug use reflect highly stigmatized constructions of illicit substance use found to be operating systemically in health care.

ILLICIT DRUG USE AS AN INDIVIDUAL FAILING

Patient Perspectives: Being Judged as a "Drug Addict."

Overwhelmingly, patient participants were concerned that they would be seen, judged, and labeled as a "drug addict" when entering the hospital, and worried that such judgments would impact the quality of care that they received. One patient participant highlighted how the attitudes of nurses are different when they suspect someone of using drugs. "But you can tell, you know, just the way they talk to you, snotty attitude toward you. It's like [not respectful]." Another patient participant elaborated,

> It just seems to me that if they had no idea of your prior drug use or anything, the care they give you, how they talk to you, how they treat you, everything

is different. You know, they're more attentive, they'll spend . . . that extra five minutes and let me fluff your pillows for you, or 'let me do this,' 'are you okay that way?' When you're not, it's like [gruffly] 'here's your medicine', [make sounds] get in, they're out of there, gone. (Patient participant)

Numerous participants reflected on stereotypes and judgments they had experienced or witnessed in hospital settings during multiple hospitalizations and how that impacted their care.

> There was only one nurse there that I had a conversation with that we talked outside and stuff like that; every other nurse didn't care to talk about anything and they were always opinionated, they always had an opinion on what I was doing to myself. And I just got a bad feeling when I was there, I didn't like being there at all. (Patient participant)

This participant, and many others, expressed feelings of discomfort about going to or being in hospital that stem in part from experiences and fears of facing opinions and judgments from nurses and others about drug use and a perceived failure to address problems related to substance use.

Patients described how being labeled a "drug addict" meant they were more likely to be judged, discarded, not listened to, or written off. One patient stated,

> . . . I've seen the way they treat people when they, uh, they've had drugs, you're a drug addict, you know, you're considered a drug addict, I don't know, it's like a label, you know, *drug addict*. . . and they just discard you. (Patient participant)

The label of "drug user" or "addict" was associated with feeling of less worth than other patients. Participants worried that nurses and others in the health care system would see them as undeserving of care, wasting their time, or that they would receive second-rate care. The implication being that drug use is an individual failing and there is not much that health care providers can do about that. For example, one patient said, "they kind of labeled me as a drug addict and they pretty much said, 'there's not a lot we can do for you.'" This label and being suspected of illicit drug use was a concern for participants, regardless of their actual drug use patterns. Of particular concern was that they felt their care would be affected by the stigma of illicit substance use contributing to their reluctance to access health care.

Patient concerns about being judged as drug addict' made it difficult for patients to "let their guard down" and led to the feeling of "having to have your game face on all of the time" adding to a lack of trust in health care providers and the already stressful experiences of hospitalization. Importantly, regardless of actual experiences in hospital, patients come to hospital with fears and worries about the care they might receive and did not trust that they would be treated with respect and concern. They characterized the health care system as being unsafe and prone to negative and moralizing judgments that contributed to decisions to delay care and/or leave the hospital early.

Nurse Perspectives: An Individual Problem

All of the nurses we interviewed asserted that the study hospital is a place where people who use illicit drugs are treated well compared with other hospitals. They expressed that it was part of the hospital's philosophy to care for people who use drugs. Regardless, some nurse participants highlighted that ultimately patients have to take responsibility for their drug use. For example,

> I find that so much of our care is based on getting them better, and so we give them so many chances. But at the end of the day, if they don't want to get better, or for whatever reason, they are the ones who have to make it happen. So I think we need to let go a bit more, you know, we have to respect the fact that it's not happening for this person. This person has made poor choices in their life, they continue to make poor choices, and we need to let go and not be so, you know, focused on getting them better.

This quote suggests that the people are making poor choices rather than being in difficult circumstances in which choices are limited. This nurse and others expressed the view that addressing

addiction was a problem that individuals needed to tackle and that there is a limit to what health care providers can do if the person does not take responsibility. This perspective aligns with patient perceptions that illicit substance use is often constructed as an individual problem and that health care providers sometimes discard or give up on you.

Nurses who held views of illicit substance use as an individual problem had difficulty understanding patients' behaviors and decisions about their health care and life priorities, and the context in which such decisions were made. One nurse stated,

> So we need to hone in on a better balance, because at the end of the day why is this person getting so many more chances and so much more care than this [other] person? It's not fair either. Why is the ninety-six-year old Chinese grandma who doesn't speak a stitch of English getting shafted around because we need to accommodate for the really rowdy crew, drug-seeking, you know, drug-dealing crew? So, okay, we'll put her there because the grandma, she's quiet, she's not gonna complain and, you know what I mean, right? Sometimes it is unfair and it's unfair to our other patients too. You know, why is our grandma not getting a bed? And then some other person repeatedly getting beds and AMA-ing [going against medical advice]? Can we not just admit them and treat our people who are diligent and compliant with our care, and who really want to get better?

This quote highlights the way in which viewing illicit substance use as an individual problem can impact decisions around resource allocation.

In contrast, other nurse participants took a view that illicit substance use and addiction were a product of life circumstances over which the individual has had little control, emphasizing their lack of choice in relation to social positioning and circumstances.

> But just to remind ourselves of how, that people don't choose to end up like this. Like this is not, this is not ideal, you know, to have no teeth and to have festering wounds and to be covered in bed bugs. And it, you know, it's gross for us in the immediacy of the moment, but like it's really gross to live, like it

must be really horrible to live like that. So it's not an imposition, they're not trying to impose on us; their life is shitty, you know. (Nurse participant)

This suggests an understanding of social circumstances that have led to the person's situation and, thus, they are not necessarily to blame for making bad choices or failing to take responsibility.

Nurses who viewed illicit substance use as a product of life circumstances understood that people were making decisions and taking action within the constraints of their lives. These nurses were more likely to put patient behaviors into context and recognize that choices and decisions were a product of life circumstances. In such a view, patients who use illicit drugs are judged as being deserving of time and resources because of deficits in their life circumstances. This view is aligned with health equity and social justice thinking in which a structural analysis is applied to understand the conditions in which individuals make choices and enact decisions. While it was clear in this study that some nurses saw patients as having little control over their life circumstances, it was not clear the extent to which nurses who held this view also saw patients as having agency and control over their bodies and health care decision making.

ILLICIT SUBSTANCE USE IS A CRIMINAL ACTIVITY

Patient Perspectives: Feeling Under Surveillance

Closely related to fears of being judged as a "drug addict" were patient descriptions of "feeling under surveillance" in hospital. Patients variously described the hospital environment as alien, foreign, and in one case "like a prison" where all activities are regulated from what time they eat to having to ask permission to take a shower. This perspective impacted their decisions to access and continue treatment. In the following example, a patient relays how this played out in his decision to leave the unit,

Patient: I just left, it was eleven o'clock at night, the guy is demanding a urinalysis from me. And I said "You want a urinalysis test from me?" I said "what for?" He said "because you've been going out on walks a lot." I said "because I'm going out, I'm getting fresh air, that means that you're suspecting me for doing drugs?" . . . You know, what kind of right does he have to ask me for, I'm doing drugs because I go and take walks to relieve stress . . . What's wrong with doing that?

Researcher: And so did he ask you if you had used anything or he . . .?

P: He just straight out said, you know, "We want a urine sample because we think you're doing drugs." And I just said, "Okay, yeah, I'll give you one of them right away." And I put it down, put my clothes on— pshooo—out the door right away.

R: Do you think it would have been different if he had just asked you, instead of skipping right to the test?

P: Well why did he even ask me? I wasn't doing dope. What right would he have to even ask me? I wasn't high.

Second, it was clear from the findings that patients were concerned that they would be labeled as "drug seeking" if they asked for pain medications and thus they were cautious to ask, even if they were in pain.

Researcher: So you asked them to increase your dose or . . .?

Patient: No, no, they actually offered it, I didn't say nothing, I never asked for it. I just, you know, I don't want to be mislabeled. Because if I'm asking for it, they're going to think "well does he really need it?,". If you're in pain and you're asking for pain medication, they'll doubt it. . . Half the time they 'll think "oh, he just wants to get high" instead of "this guy is really hurting, you know, let's give him some pain medication".

A third concern related to feeling under surveillance was the association between illicit substance use and theft. One participant described having his room searched multiple times when another patient's dentures went missing, and feeling it was because he had been labelled as someone who uses illicit drugs.

Patient: Well if they had searched once I could see it. After I had told them I had already cleaned up from the search and, no, they're not here. Searching once

I can see. Twice to me is just a little suspect. Like, you know, what now you figure that since they were there that I moved them or something and changed the location? "Oh, she's gone, I'll switch locations!" Because, you know, whatever. It just sounds pretty hokey to me, that's all, you know, it's kind of insulting. Not even kind of, to me it's highly insulting. As I said, if I was some old man, they wouldn't have questioned me even once. They would have taken a quick look and went, oh, okay, yeah, it's not here.

Researcher: Has that ever happened before in this hospital, that you've had your stuff searched?

P: Yeah, if you've been involved in drugs, or there's drugs on your record, then anything happens, that's wrong, you're always the first one to be looked at. [pause]. That's a given.

Both searches occurred during the course of a research interview. As highlighted in the examples given previously, the feeling of being under surveillance is expressed in relation to concerns about being suspected of drug misuse, drug seeking and/or theft, which aligns with criminalized views of substance use. As a response to these stereotypes, patient participants attempted to distinguish themselves as "good" rather than "bad" drug users, as a way to avoid being labeled as misusing drugs, drug seeking, or being accused of theft. One participant highlighted how he did not associate with other people who use illicit drugs in hospitals so that health care providers would not associate and label him as a "drug user." He describes,

> Like there was a kid in particular on this floor who was borrowing money off older people and he was just a bad person. He was doing drugs and stuff like that while he was here, and rude to the nurses, stuff like that. So, you know, I don't want to be associated as a friend to that person because they're being watched as a bad influence. I don't need to be put in that category.

"Bad" drug users were described as those who victimize others, take advantage of people, and commit crimes in order to feed their need for drugs. In the peer advisory's review of the preliminary findings of this research, the group affirmed that this distancing from stereotypes of bad drug users is a strategy they have used. Thus, patients try to present themselves in ways that establish their identity separately from stereotypes of "bad drug users" that they expect to be operating in health care, and to instead attempt to construct themselves as credible patients who are worthy and deserving of care.

Nurse Perspectives: We don't View People as Criminals, But...

Interestingly, none of the nurses in this study explicitly expressed a view of illicit substance use as criminalization. In fact, some nurses suggested that the current criminal justice approach to drug use might be the reason for drug-related crime. For example,

> I think most of the harm from drugs is from prohibition itself; it's where I think all the crime comes from. You know because drugs are sold by drug dealers who are gangsters and they're getting all the money... Also drugs are illegal, so it makes these people who use drugs criminals just for, you know, doing what they're doing, what they're addicted to.

In a presentation of emerging findings to the nurse advisory, the nurses expressed surprise at the suggestion that nurses might view illicit substance use as a criminal issue. One nurse observed,

> "I guess that some of our patients have committed crimes, they come with guards. But we couldn't give care if we thought of them in that way."

Both of these examples suggest that nurses can and do resist overt societal characterization of people who use drugs as criminals and criminalization as a response to the harms of drug use. The nurse participants described a commitment to serving those who are marginalized by drug use, poverty, and homelessness as an important feature of the organization's culture and values.

> I think we've always been known as the hospital where people can go to and they won't get judged and they won't get bad treatment based on who they are as a person. And by that I mean like, the marginalized population in [our city] or people coming from First Nations reserves as well. We are

first of all told about that in like our general orientation, how that's like the philosophy of care that we have here. But then I do find that like it really shines through with the way that the nurses and like allied health . . . work with the patients as well.

It is difficult to know whether nurses held views related to criminalization, but did not express them because they thought it would be politically incorrect to do so in an organization committed to the care of people who use drugs. Thus, there may be cultural norms operating in the setting that prevented nurses from expressing views of substance use as a criminal problem.

While nurses did not openly express views of illicit substance use as criminalization, observations and examination of policies highlighted the extent to which surveillance and criminalization were evident in the organizational culture. For example, we noted the offering of seminars for staff on the issues of pain management and drug seeking that suggest there is an intention to address this problem among staff. During participant observations and interviews, nurses highlighted their concerns about patients being labeled by others as "drug seeking."

> Drug-seeking, patients are [seen as] drug-seeking when they have pain. There was a patient who was in our hallway and they moved her down to [unit A] and she came back and she was crying at the desk because they wouldn't give her pain medicine. They told her "you've already had enough." And I felt sick because I thought, you know, there's such a power imbalance when a patient comes into a place like [this hospital], you know, the big bad hospital. And our patients are so marginalized, and to have someone like a nurse have all that control over what medication you get, and how much and how often, like that must have been completely terrifying for the patient.

Nurse participants said that the hospital had a harm-reduction philosophy. However, most nurses were unclear as to exactly what the harm-reduction policy said, where it could be found, or what they could or should do when they became aware of illicit drug use. In a review of the hospital policy documents, we did not find a specific harm-reduction policy but did locate policies on substance use. Hospital policies highlighted zero tolerance for all types of substance use and policy guidance directed nurses to call security if and when staff becomes aware of substance use. Both nurse and patient participants mentioned the zero tolerance policy, and signs indicating zero tolerance for substance use were posted on bathroom doors.

> So like I said there's a no tolerance to it, so there's no, there is no using in here. So we don't do what people do in the community, and there's no education really about kind of using clean needles and doing things safely and cleanly and, you know, like [supervised injection facility] does and [residential HIV treatment program] and different places like that. We don't do that because, because we have no tolerance. So I think it's hard, like we don't really give any education to patients around that stuff.

Thus, hospital policies were more clearly aligned with criminalization as a response to illicit substance use given the focus on zero tolerance and organizational policy calling for room searches by security in the event that illicit drug use is suspected. As a consequence, nurses responded in various ways to illicit substance use, such as ignoring drug use, or reporting it to their manager.

> I remember seeing [clean needles] in, like she had a little makeup bag. I didn't take them away. Because to me that's not, that's not harm reduction at all. If I take them away, you know, I might be putting her in a position where she's got to go and share with somebody else.

Some nurses indicated that they could not give sharps containers to patients—which would enhance patients' and nurses' safety— because they believed it was not consistent with hospital policy. Only a few nurses mentioned promoting safer drug use, for example, by providing supplies or education for safer use. Nurses were aware of the substance use policy that explicitly highlighted the option of calling for room searches. However, nurses did not necessarily call on security except when behaviors became dangerous or impeded their work. At the same time, drug alerts (eg, warnings about tainted drugs in the community) were available on the unit and some nurses received education on harm reduction. Hospital policies emphasizing zero tolerance of illicit substance use, the espoused harm-reduction philosophy, and the lack of explicit harm-reduction policies left nurses caught between professional ethical commitments to health promotion and official policies more aligned with criminalization.[14,40]

ILLICIT SUBSTANCE USE AS A DISEASE OF ADDICTION

Patient Perspectives: We're not Just Helpless Victims of Disease

Some patients described how people do not choose to be addicted but that when using, drugs take control of their lives. One patient stated,

> Using sucks. I don't know why the general public thinks we like it; I really don't. Well maybe there's some addicts that do but I know the majority of us don't. We have no control when we're in that zone; it takes over your whole life.

While some patients expressed a view of addiction as a disease, which takes over, others asserted that they were not just helpless out of control victims. Patient participants asserted that they had valuable medical knowledge about their bodies such as where and how to access veins for the taking of blood or starting an intravenous administration. Such assertions can be seen as resistance to the constructions of self as a helpless victim of disease. The patient participants in this study asserted the value and importance of knowing their own bodies and bringing bodily knowledge into their experiences of hospitalization.

> Participants indicated that nurses did not always listen to the knowledge that they had about their bodies and their health. Being a helpless victim reflects stereotypes and constructions of illicit substance use as a disease of addiction. The idea that addiction takes control leaves little room for or recognition of personal agency.

Nurse Perspectives: Addiction Takes Over

Likewise, some nurses in this study expressed the view that addiction is a disease or illness that takes over. For example,

> But when you work here, you know, and you start to understand the nature of addiction, and how it can really happen to anyone and how it does take over someone's life, and it's just that different perspective of when you know the disease process, you know. And, no, it doesn't make it right or good but if you have that, if you're educated and aware of how it happens and why it happens, you know, it's, you know, you don't blame the person or finger point or label, you know.

This nurse highlights addiction's disease-like ability to take over a person's life. Many nurses described patient lives as chaotic and out of control. Like the nurse earlier, some nurses emphasized the importance of understanding someone's life as a consequence of their disease rather than an individual failing. In discourses of addiction related to drug prohibition, addiction is often constructed as a disease that takes hold of the person who is then unable to take control or take responsibility for their behavior leading to drug-induced crime and other problems. The nurse above is careful not to blame the individual for their disease, just as a person with cancer or any other chronic disease would not be blamed or labeled. This, is seen as a more enlightened and compassionate view. However, such views are still reflective of biomedical (disease orientated) and individualized constructions of addiction. In such constructions, people may be viewed as "lost souls" consumed by addiction. It was not clear in this study if viewing patients as "helpless victims" meant writing them off or holding more paternalistic views in which health care providers know what is best for the patient. However, this finding highlights the importance of nurses resisting views of addiction as disease and individuals as helpless victims of disease to value and respect clients' knowledge of their bodies and support personal agency. As well as pointing to the relevance of understanding the broader social circumstances that impact illicit substance use or the social determinants of illicit substance use.

LIMITATIONS OF THE STUDY

This is a qualitative ethnographic study that contributes to in-depth insights into the discursive constructions and stereotypes of illicit substance use held by patients and nurses on 2 medical units in 1 large urban inner-city hospital. This hospital serves a large population of patients who use illicit drugs and are living in poverty and may not be reflective of rural hospital settings or hospitals in less-urbanized environments. The patients interviewed had multiple and lengthy experiences with the study hospital. Thus, participants had a level of comfort with accessing health care that may be different for participants who avoid or delay care. In spite of this, these findings can sensitize us to stigmatizing constructions of illicit substance use and how they operate in hospitalized settings to create unsafe environments in health care for people who use drugs.

DISCUSSION

A key finding of this study is that patients who use illicit drugs characterize the health care system as unsafe due to stigmatizing constructions that individualize, criminalize, and medicalize illicit substance use in hospital settings. For example, fears of being judged as a "drug addict" and "drug seeking" highlight patient worries and concerns about being blamed for their drug use and seen as unworthy of care impacting their decisions to seek health care or pain relief. This is consistent with previous research in which people who use(d) illicit drugs felt judged, ignored, subjected to negative assumptions, and deprived of adequate pain and withdrawal relief by hospital staff.[41,42] What stands out in this study is that patients endured pain rather than ask for relief out of fear of being judged, they did not have evidence-based public health harm-reduction strategies available to them, and in some cases left hospitals early. These findings resonate with

research with Indigenous people in Canada who similarly reported being judged negatively on the basis of their identity as Aboriginal peoples and their presumed (and most often mistaken) propensity to be seeking narcotics when in fact they were seeking help for legitimate pain issues.[12,43]

Understanding the ways in which patients and nurses construct illicit substance use is highly relevant to explorations of cultural safety in nursing and health care. The concept of cultural safety prompts nurses to reflect on the structures, discourses, and assumptions that frame the delivery of health care and what can be done to counteract power differentials in health care.[18] The constructions of illicit substance use expressed by patients and nurses in this study provide insights into the possible negative and stigmatizing constructions of illicit substance use in hospitals and what is needed to foster cultural safety in nursing practice. In the discussion, we highlight key insights for fostering culturally safe nursing practice in relation to illicit drug use for patients who use(d) illicit drugs and are experiencing social disadvantages and hospitalization.

People who use illicit drugs are often distrustful of health care providers and the health care system.[16, 20] On the street, the assumption of trust is a poor survival tactic and people have to be vigilant and constantly alert to potential dangers. In addition, many people may be experiencing past and current trauma. Thus, when coming to hospitals, patients may continue to feel wary and distrustful. A key aspect of cultural safety is the examination of one's own privilege and power in relation to patients, and how one's values, assumptions, and perspectives can impact the development of trusting and therapeutic relationships with patients. As part of fostering cultural safety, it is important for nurses to recognize this gap in trust, especially given that trust is often assumed to be present in health care. The findings of this study reveal the importance of nurses reflecting on how societal stereotypes may be influencing the development of relationships and how stereotypes of "addiction" and "addicts" can and do play out in health care and nursing practice inhibiting the development of trust and creating the need for specific attention to actions that develop trust.[44] In this study, all illicit substance use was primarily understood as "addiction" rather than as encompassing a range of substance use from beneficial to problematic and participants did not acknowledge that substances are widely used for a range of reasons including enhancing mood, performance, and celebration.[45] Nurses would benefit from broader and more nuanced understandings of theories and history of substance use and addiction.

Views of illicit substance use as an individual failing are dominant in Canadian and North American societies reflecting a highly individualized, or neoliberal and moralized perspective on addiction that tends to blame people for their problems.[46, 47] Individualizing the blame for drug use is underpinned by a belief that "drug addicts" are undeserving because they have failed to engage in responsible behavior to stop using or change patterns of illicit drug use.[48] In neoliberal societies where individual responsibility and behavior are highly valued, there is often little consideration or attention to the social conditions that shape drug use and individual behaviors. As a result, people who use drugs are often viewed as failing to take individual responsibility for changing harmful and addictive patterns of illicit substance use. Regardless of the actual attitudes that nurses hold toward illicit substance use, illicit substance use as an individual failing is a common societal view and patients came to hospital expecting to be judged and treated as a "drug addict" who is to blame or at fault for their drug use.

Patients and nurses readily recognized how an individualizing perspective on substance use operated in health care to cast patients as unworthy and undeserving of care. Such perspectives are consistent with the previous research described at the beginning of this article related to the experiences of stigma and discrimination that people who use illicit drugs confront in health care and society. In practice, referring to people as "drug seeking," frequent flyers, "manipulative," "junkies," and "drug addicts"

are highly stigmatized terms that not only convey negative portrayals but personalize and blame people for problems. Such stereotypes and language need to be challenged and shifted in health care to move toward a model of culturally safe care.

The finding that some nurses see drug use as a product of life circumstances is an important one. This is consistent with looking to the "structural roots" of problems and is aligned with social justice and cultural safety in nursing.[49] Such a perspective draws attention to the determinants of harms of substance use and recognition that people make choices and live their lives within particular social, historical, economic, and political contexts. This understanding of substance use as a product of life circumstances is consistent with an understanding of life course perspectives and the development of health inequities that emphasizes how life trajectories position people differently.[50]

"Feeling under surveillance" is reflective of criminalization and prohibition discourses in which people are on alert and fear being criminalized because of real or suspected illicit substance use. "Feeling under surveillance" clearly played a role in decisions to leave before discharge and reluctance to ask for pain medications. Nurses would benefit from additional knowledge and organizational approaches that include better assessment and understandings of substance use and pain management. Patients clearly sought to distinguish between "good" and "bad" drug users to distance themselves from stereotypes related to criminalization, a strategy for managing identity that has been reported in other research.[51] A cultural safety approach would also point to the importance of understanding history and in this case the history of drug policy and criminalization of drugs that has contributed to stereotypes and escalated harms of drug use.[14,40]

A cultural safety lens also prompts us to reflect on organizational policies and societal beliefs that impact the delivery of nursing care. While individual nurses did not openly express views of addiction as criminalization, formal hospital policies were premised on a zero tolerance for substance use and there was a lack of harm-reduction policies. In fact, hospital policies and espoused harm-reduction approaches to care of patients with illicit drug use were conflicting and contradictory. The availability of methadone maintenance for hospitalized patients in the study setting does highlight the organizational acceptability of 1 harm-reduction strategy but one more aligned with addiction as a medical disease that can be fraught with challenges.[8] The lack of organizational harm-reduction policy and a primary focus on methadone maintenance meant that other evidence-based public health harm-reduction strategies, such as provision of clean supplies or education on safer drug use, were not available leaving nurses caught between evidence-based practice and organizational policy.[40] This draws attention to the context in which nursing care is provided and the need for attention to the development of policies that are consistent with current evidence and espoused approaches. We would argue that harm reduction and cultural safety are part of an integrated approach to addressing health inequities.[49]

Addiction as a disease is an individualized and medicalized discourse in which addiction is seen to be a product of genetic make-up or a blameless misfortune in life. While both patients and nurses viewed addiction as a disease, patients were more likely to resist this concept, expressing resistance to the idea that they are helpless victims. An important principle of cultural safety is to acknowledge patients as experts about their health and social needs and what constitutes supportive care.[25] The power relationship is skewed in favor of the health care provider. This points to the importance of nurses recognizing the bodily knowledge that patients have and highly value, as well as the importance of learning from patients about their views and preferences for care. This is a characteristic of good care for all patients but may have particular significance in relation to people who often experience trauma, particularly sexual or physical abuse, discrimination, and stigmatization. Learning from and getting to know patients and their preferences may be particularly valuable in contributing to more accurate assessments and management of pain as well as building trust.

It is interesting to note that neither the patients nor the nurses in this study described illicit substance use as a public health problem. Although the construction of addiction as a disease takes a perspective on substance use as a "health or disease issue," this can be differentiated from substance use as a public health issue and concerns with population health. Framed as a public health issue, the priority is most often to stop the spread of blood-borne pathogens through implementation of harm-reduction strategies. In part, the lack of a public health perspective or failure to implement such a perspective might explain the gap in harm-reduction policies and approaches. However, taking a public health approach to illicit substance use should also be premised more broadly on social justice and the promotion of equity and evidence such as the approach described by the Canadian Public Health Association with implications for drug policy reform and inclusion of people who use drugs in decisions that affect them.[52] A public health perspective provides another lens through which to view substance use that may have particular benefits if appropriately understood and implemented.

CONCLUSION

People who use illicit drugs and are socially marginalized have expressed fears about being patients in acute care hospitals and often delay and avoid care because of real and perceived stigma associated with illicit drug use. As demonstrated by the findings of this study, there are multiple and competing conceptions of illicit substance use that embody stigma in hospital settings and that impact on decisions to ask for pain relief and to leave hospitals before discharge. Furthermore, patients did not have access to a broad range of evidence-based harm-reduction services. This has implications for health outcomes including worsening health conditions, and moralization of illicit substance use with far-reaching public health implications. Cultural safety provides a potential lens for examining the discourses, structures, and assumptions that shape nursing interactions with people who use drugs. It is important for nurses to critically reflect on how substance use is taken up and framed in health care and how that impacts interactions with people who use illicit drugs as part of a culturally safe approach to nursing care.

REFERENCES

1. Braveman, P., Kumanyika, S., Fielding, J., et al. (2011). Health disparities and health equity: the issue is justice. *Am J Public Health*, *101*(S1), S149–S155.
2. Commission on the Social Determinants of Health. (2008). *Closing the Gap in a Generation: Achieving Health Equity Through Action on the Social Determinants of Health*. Geneva, Switzerland: World Health Organization.
3. Starfield, B., Gérvas, J., & Mangin, D. (2012). Clinical care and health disparities. *Ann Rev Public Health*, *33*(1), 89–106.
4. Graham, H. (2004). Social determinants and their unequal distribution: clarifying policy understandings. *Milbank Q*, *82*(1), 101–124.
5. Ahern, J., Stuber, J., & Galea, S. (2007). Stigma, discrimination and the health of illicit drug users. *Drug Alcohol Depend*, *88*, 188–196.
6. Galea, S., & Vlahov, D. (2002). Social determinants and the health of drug users: socioeconomic status, homelessness and incarceration. *Public Health Rep*, *117*(suppl 1), S135–S145.
7. Bird, S. T., Bogart, L., & Delahanty, D. (2004). Health-related correlates of perceived discrimination in HIV care. *AIDS Patient Care STD's*, *18*(1), 19.
8. Smye, V., Browne, A., Varcoe, C., & Josewski, V. (2011). Harm reduction, methadone maintenance treatment and the root causes of health and social inequities: an intersectional lens in the Canadian context. *Harm Reduct J*, *8*, 17.
9. Lang, K., Neil, J., Wright, J., Dell, C., Berenbaum, S., & EL-Aneed, A. (2013). Qualitative investigation of barriers to accessing care by people who inject drugs in Saskatoon, Canada: perspectives of service providers. *Subst Abuse Treat Prev Policy*, *8*(35), 1–11.
10. Lloyd, C., & Lloyd, C. (2013). The stigmatization of problem drug users: a narrative literature review. *Drugs (Abingdon, Engl)*, *20*(2), 85–95.
11. Room, R. (2005). Stigma, social inequality and alcohol and drug use. *Drug Alcohol Rev*, 24(2), 143–155.
12. Browne, A. J., Smye, V. L., Rodney, P., Tang, S. Y., Mussell, B., & O'Neil, J. D. (2011). Access to primary care from the perspective of Aboriginal patients at an urban emergency department. *Qual Health Res*, *21*(3), 333–348.
13. van Boekel, L. C., Brouwers, E. P., van Weeghel, J., & Garretsen, H. F. (2013). Stigma among health professionals towards patients with substance use disorders and its consequences for healthcare delivery: systematic review. *Drug Alcohol Depend*, *131*(1), 23–35.
14. Pauly, B. M., Goldstone, I., McCall, J., Gold, F., & Payne, S. (2007). The ethical, legal and social context of harm reduction. *Can Nurse*, *103*(8), 19–23.
15. McNeil, R., Small, W., Wood, E., & Kerr, T. (2014). Hospitals as a "risk environment": an ethno-epidemiological study of voluntary and involuntary discharge from hospital against medical advice among people who inject drugs. *Soc Sci Med*, *105*, 59–66.
16. Merrill, J., Rhodes, L., Deyo, R., Marlatt, A., & Bradley, K. (2002). Mutual mistrust in the medical care of drug users. *J Gen Intern Med*, *17*, 327–333.
17. Rachlis, B., Kerr, T., Montaner, J., & Wood, E. (2009). Harm reduction in hospitals: is it time? *Harm Reduct J*, *6*, 19.
18. Browne, A. J., Varcoe, C., Smye, V., Reimer Kirkham, S., Lynam, J., & Wong, S. (2009). Cultural safety and the challenges of translating critically oriented knowledge in practice. *Nurs Philos*, *10*, 167–179.
19. Lightfoot, B., Panessa, C., Hayden, S., Thumath, M., Goldstone, I., & Pauly, B. M. (2009). Gaining Insite: harm reduction in nursing practice. *Can Nurse*, *105*(4), 16–22.
20. Pauly, B. M. (2008). Shifting moral values to enhance access to health care: harm reduction as a context for ethical nursing practice. *Int J Drug Policy*, *19*, 195–204.
21. Link, B., & Phelan, J. (2001). Conceptualizing stigma. *Ann Rev Sociol*, *27*, 363–385.
22. Link, B., & Phelan, J. (2006). Stigma and its public health implications. *The Lancet*, *367*, 528–529.
23. Link, B., & Phelan, J. (2014). Stigma power. *Soc Sci Med*, *103*, 24–32.
24. Hatzenbuehler, M., & Link, B. (2014). Introduction to the special issue on structural stigma and health. *Soc Sci Med*, *103*, 1–6.
25. Ramsden, I. (2000). Cultural safety/Kawa Whakaruruhau ten years on: a personal overview. *Nurs Prax N Z*, *15*(1), 4–12.
26. Ramsden, I. (2002). *Cultural Safety and Nursing Education in Aotearoa and Te Waipounamu*. Wellington, New Zealand: University of Wellington.
27. Kearns, R., Dyck, I., & Robinson, Ke. (1996). Cultural safety, biculturalism and nursing education

in Aotearoa/New Zealand. *Health Soc Care Community*, *4*(6), 371–380.

28. Papps, E., & Ramsden, I. (1996). Cultural safety in nursing: the New Zealand experience. *Int J Q Health Care*, *8*(5), 491–497.

29. Varcoe, C., & Browne, A. J. (2014). Culture and cultural safety: beyond cultural inventories. In: D. Gregory, C. Raymond-Seniuk, L. Patrick, & T. C. Stephen (Eds.), *Fundamentals: Perspectives on the Art & Science of Canadian Nursing* (pp. 216–237). Philadelphia, PA: Lippincott Williams & Wilkins.

30. Browne, A. J., Varcoe, C. M., Wong, S. T., et al. (2012). Closing the health equity gap: evidence-based strategies for primary health care organizations. *Int J Equity Health*, *11*(1), 59.

31. Anderson, J. M., Rodney, P., Reimer-Kirkham, S., Browne, A. J., Khan, K. B., & Lynam, M. J. (2009). Inequities in health and healthcare viewed through the ethical lens of critical social justice. Contextual knowledge for the global priorities ahead. *Adv Nurs Sci*, *32*(4), 282–294.

32. Canadian Association of Schools of Nursing, Aboriginal Nurses Association of Canada. (2013). *Educating Nurses to Address Socio-cultural, Historical, and Contextual Determinants of Health Among Aboriginal Peoples*. Ottawa, Ontario, Canada: Canadian Association of Schools of Nursing.

33. Hole, R. D., Evans, M., Berg, L. D., et al. (2015). Visibility and voice aboriginal people experience culturally safe and unsafe health care [published online ahead of print January 12, 2015]. *Qual Health Res*. doi:1049732314566325.

34. Nursing Council of New Zealand. (2005). *Guidelines for Cultural Safety, the Treaty of Waitangi and Maori Health in Nursing Education and Practice*. Wellington, New Zealand: Nursing Council of New Zealand.

35. Dube, S., Felitti, V., Dong, M., Chapman, D., Giles, W., & Anda, R. (2003). Childhood abuse, neglect and household dysfunction and the risk of illicit drug use: the adverse childhood experiences study. *Pediatrics*, *3*(3), 564–572.

36. Hammersley, M., & Atkinson, P. (1995). *Ethnography: Principles in Practice* (2nd ed.). New York: Routledge.

37. Pauly, B. M., McCall, J., Parker, J., McLaren, C., Browne, A., & Mollison, A. (2013). *Creating Culturally Safe Care in Hospital Settings for People Who Use(d) Illicit Drugs*. Victoria, British Columbia, Canada: University of Victoria.

38. Thorne, S. (2008). *Interpretive Description*. Walnut Creek, CA: Left Coast Press Inc.

39. Lincoln, Y. S., & Guba, E. C. (1985). *Naturalistic Inquiry*. Beverly Hills, CA: Sage.

40. Canadian Nurses Association. (2011). *Harm Reduction and Currently Illegal Drugs: Implications for Nursing Policy, Practice, Education and Research*. Ottawa, Ontario, Canada: Canadian Nurses Association.

41. Butters, J., & Erickson P. G. (2003). Meeting the health care needs of female crack users: a Canadian example. *Women Health*, *37*(3), 1.

42. Vandu Women CARE Team. (2009). *Me, I'm Living It: The Primary Health care Experiences of Women Who Use Drugs in Vancouver's Downtown Eastside*. Vancouver, British Columbia, Canada: BC Centre of Excellence for Women's Health.

43. Browne, A. J. (2007). Clinical encounters between nurses and First Nations women in a Western Canadian hospital. *Soc Sci Med*, *64*(10), 2165–2176.

44. Pauly, B. M. (2014). *Close to the Street: Nursing Practice With People Marginalized by Homelessness and Substance use*. Ottawa, Ontario, Canada: University of Ottawa Press.

45. Duff, C. (2008). The pleasure in context. *Int J Drug Policy*, *19*, 384–392.

46. Pauly, B. M., Langlois, A., Perkin, K., et al. (2011, November 7). *Contaminated spaces: the construction of stigma and drug use in the media*. Paper presented at: The Canadian Centre for Substance Abuse Annual Conference. Vancouver, British Columbia, Canada.

47. Keane, H. (2002). *What's Wrong With Addiction?* New York: New York University Press.

48. Moore, D., & Fraser, S. (2006). Putting at risk what we know: reflecting on the drug-using subject in harm reduction and its political implications. *Soc Sci Med*, *62*, 3035–3047.

49. Pauly, B. M. (2012). Challenging health inequities: enacting social justice in nursing practice. In J. L. Storch, P. A. Rodney, & R. C. Starzomski (Eds.), *Toward a Moral Horizon: Nursing Ethics for Leadership and Practice* (2nd ed., pp. 430–447). Toronto, Ontario, Canada: Pearson Canada.

50. Braveman, P. (2013). What is health equity: and how does a life-course approach take us further toward it? *Matern Child Health J*, *10*, 10.

51. Radcliffe, P., & Stevens, A. (2008). Are drug treatment services only for "thieving junkie scumbags"? Drug users and the management of stigmatised identifies. *Soc Sci Med*, *67*, 1065–1073.

52. Canadian Public Health Association. (2014). *A New Approach to Managing Illegal Psychoactive Substances in Canada*. Ottawa, Ontario, Canada: Canadian Public Health Association.

An Intervention to Promote Breast Milk Production in Mothers of Preterm Infants

Marjolaine Héon[1,2], Céline Goulet[1,3], Carole Garofalo[1,4], Anne Monique Nuyt[1,4], Emile Levy[1,4]

ABSTRACT

A pilot study was conducted to estimate the effects of a breast milk expression education and support intervention on breast milk production outcomes in mothers of very and extremely preterm infants. Forty mothers of hospitalized preterm infants (<30 weeks of gestation) were randomized to the experimental intervention or standard care for 6 weeks. Duration and frequency of breast milk expressions and volume of expressed breast milk were measured daily. Samples of breast milk were collected thrice during the study and analyzed for their lipid concentration. Mothers in the experimental group had a statistically significant higher duration of breast milk expression in min/day ($p = .043$). Differences observed between the two groups regarding the frequency of breast milk expression, volume of breast milk, and lipid concentration were not statistically significant. Results suggest that the experimental intervention may promote breast milk production in mothers of very and extremely preterm infants.

[1]Université de Montréal, Québec, Canada
[2]Quebec Nursing Intervention Research Network, Montréal, Québec, Canada
[3]Université de Lausanne, Switzerland
[4]CHU Sainte-Justine Research Center, Montréal, Québec, Canada

Corresponding Author:

Marjolaine Héon, Faculté des sciences infirmières, Université de Montréal, C.P. 6128, succursale Centre-ville, Montréal, Québec, Canada H3C 3J7.
Email: marjolaine.heon@umontreal.ca

Marjolaine Héon, Céline Goulet, Carole Garofalo, et al, *Western Journal of Nursing Research,* Volume: 38 issue: 5, page(s): 529-552, Copyright © 2016, © SAGE Publications. Reprinted by Permission of SAGE Publications, Inc.

KEYWORDS breast milk expression, breastfeeding, milk production, nursing intervention, preterm infants

Breastfeeding, which refers to the provision of human milk (World Health Organization [WHO], 2008), represents the optimal form of nutrition for preterm infants, including very (28 to <32 weeks of gestation; WHO, 2013) and extremely (< 28 weeks of gestation; WHO, 2013) preterm infants. Human milk confers health, nutritional, immunologic, and developmental advantages to them, and health and psychological benefits to their mothers (American Academy of Pediatrics, 2012). However, very and extremely preterm infants are breastfed for a shorter period of time compared with term infants (Flacking, Nyqvist, & Ewald, 2007; Killersreiter, Grimmer, Bührer, Dudenhausen, & Obladen, 2001; Perrella et al., 2012). Their mothers are more likely than mothers of term infants to struggle with the initiation, establishment, and maintenance of a sufficient breast milk production ($\geq$500 mL/day; Hill, Chatterton, & Zinaman, 2005a) and more at risk for breastfeeding failure (Maastrup et al., 2014); approximately half of very and extremely preterm infants are no longer fed breast milk at hospital discharge (Barois, Grognet, Tourneux, & Leke, 2013; Bonet et al., 2011; Lee & Gould, 2009; Pineda, Foss, Richards, & Pane, 2009). An insufficient breast milk production is one of the major barriers that compromise breastfeeding in these preterm infants (Callen, Pinelli, Atkinson, & Saigal, 2005).

Numerous factors, such as suboptimal breast milk expression, may contribute to an insufficient breast milk production in mothers of very and extremely preterm infants (Hill, Aldag, Chatterton, & Zinaman, 2005b). It is recommended that breast milk expression be initiated as soon as possible after birth (Parker, Sullivan, Krueger, Kelechi, & Mueller, 2012) and frequently, at least 7 times daily (Hill et al., 2005b). A frequency higher than 8 times per day would prevent the decline of the concentration of plasma prolactin between expressions (Cox, Owens, & Hartmann, 1996). However, in mothers of very and extremely preterm infants, the initiation of breast milk expression after birth is generally delayed (>6 hr after birth; Alexandre, Bomy, Bourdon, Truffert, & Pierrat, 2007; Furman, Minich, & Hack, 2002; Hill et al., 2005b; Maastrup et al., 2014) and low frequency of breast milk expression (< 6 times per day) in the first weeks postpartum is common (Acuña-Muga et al., 2014; Fewtrell et al., 2001; Hill, Aldag, & Chatterton, 2001; Hill et al., 2005a).

Suboptimal breast milk expression not only impedes breast milk production, it may also have an impact on breast milk composition. The degree of breast emptying explains approximately 70% of the variance of breast milk lipid concentration (Daly, Di Rosso, Owens, & Hartmann, 1993). The latter seems to decrease proportionally to the elapsed time between breast milk expressions (Jackson et al., 1988), but results are inconsistent among studies (Khan et al., 2012). As lipids represent 40% to 50% of breast milk total energy (Koletzko, Agostoni, Bergmann, Ritzenthaler, & Shamir, 2011), suboptimal expression has the potential to reduce the dietary energy supplied by breast milk to preterm infants, and to reduce the intake of essential fatty acids. It is therefore critical to promote breast milk expression and support mothers in the initiation, establishment, and maintenance of a sufficient breast milk production that meets the high caloric needs of their preterm infants.

Few breastfeeding education and support interventions for mothers of preterm infants can be identified in the scientific literature. On the one hand, interventions given by peers aim primarily at raising the rate of breastfeeding initiation (Pereira, Schwartz, Gould, & Grim, 1984), breastfeeding duration (Agrasada, Gustafsson, Kylberg, & Ewald, 2005; Merewood et al., 2006; Pereira et al., 1984), and exclusivity (Agrasada et al., 2005). On the other hand, professional interventions focus mainly on reducing the delay of breast milk expression after birth (Ahmed, 2008), and raising the rate of breastfeeding initiation (Meier, Engstrom, Mingolelli, Miracle, & Kiesling, 2004; Sisk, Lovelady, Dillard, & Gruber, 2006), frequency of breast milk expression (Ahmed, 2008), proportion of breast milk feedings (Meier et al., 2004), number of preterm infants fed with breast milk at hospital discharge (Gonzalez et al., 2003), and breastfeeding duration (Pinelli, Atkinson, & Saigal, 2001) and exclusivity (Ahmed, 2008). None of these interventions specifically target breast milk production as an outcome in terms of frequency and duration of milk expression, breast milk volume, and lipid concentration in breast milk.

A pilot study was conducted to estimate the effects of a breast milk expression education and support intervention on breast milk production in mothers of preterm infants. The objective of this article is to present the estimation of the intervention effects on breast milk production outcomes. The research hypothesis was as follows: Compared with mothers of preterm infants who receive standard care, mothers of preterm infants receiving the breast milk expression education and support intervention over a 6-week period present with a significantly higher (a) frequency of breast milk expression/day, (b) duration of breast milk expression/day, (c) expressed breast milk volume/day, and (d) lipid concentration of breast milk. This pilot study was guided by the Hill-Aldag Lactation Model (Hill et al., 2005b).

THEORETICAL FRAMEWORK

The Hill-Aldag Lactation Model (Hill et al., 2005b) identifies primary and secondary mediators that influence lactation in mothers of very and extremely preterm infants (≤ 31 weeks of gestation at birth) in the first 6 weeks postpartum. Primary mediators are variables that exist prior to and at birth, while secondary mediators are modifiable variables that are present after birth (Hill et al., 2005b). Mother's annual income and level of education, number of weeks of gestation at birth, timing of the decision regarding breastfeeding, intended duration of breastfeeding, previous breastfeeding experience, cohabitation with the father of the preterm infant, and ethnicity are included as primary mediators in the initial model, whereas early frequency of breast milk expression, early volume of expressed breast milk, kangaroo mother care, and time of initiation of breast stimulation following birth are comprised as secondary mediators (Hill et al., 2005b). In mothers of preterm infants, annual income and number of weeks of gestation at birth predict 11% of the variance of breast milk volume at Week 6 postpartum, whereas early frequency of breast milk expression per day and early volume of expressed breast milk per day predict 49% of it. Together, these primary and secondary mediators predict 54% of the variance in breast milk volume 6 weeks after birth in mothers of very and extremely preterm infants.

In the pilot study, the Hill-Aldag Lactation Model (Hill et al., 2005b) served as a basis for the development of the content of the experimental intervention, as it points to some of the variables that can be manipulated (secondary mediators) so as to promote breast milk production in mothers of very and extremely preterm infants. It also identified the main confounding variables (primary mediators) that needed to be considered in the pilot study as those might have an influence on breast milk production in a context of prematurity. Finally, it is worth noting that the initial model also included reactions to stressors in a context of lactation, namely maternal physiological stress and psychological distress. However, as subsequent studies reported that sleep difficulty, fatigue, and perceived stress (Hill, Aldag, Chatterton, & Zinaman, 2005c), as well as dysphoria, anxiety, depression, and hostility

(Hill, Aldag, Demirtas, Zinaman, & Chatterton, 2006), do not seem to have an apparent effect on breast milk production in mothers of preterm infants, physiological stress and psychological distress were not considered in this pilot study.

METHOD

Research Design

A pragmatic pilot randomized controlled trial (RCT) was conducted to estimate the effects of the education and support intervention. Pragmatic RCT evaluate interventions with a wide range of participants (Glasgow, Magid, Beck, Ritzwoller, & Estabrooks, 2005; King, 2008), in a context that illustrates the variability and complexity of clinical settings (Tunis, Stryer, & Clancy, 2003). This approach maximizes the external validity of the study, while maintaining a valid and adequate internal validity (King, 2008). Prior to the start of the study, research ethics board approval was obtained from Sainte-Justine University Hospital Center, Montreal, Canada, where participants were recruited from October 27, 2008 to August 30, 2010.

Setting and Sample

The study was conducted at a 65-bed neonatal intensive care unit in a university teaching hospital in Montreal, Canada. The sample size for this study was 40 mothers of very or extremely preterm infants, as suggested for a pilot study (Kieser & Wassmer, 1996; Melnyk & Cole, 2005). Mothers were eligible to participate if (a) their very or extremely preterm infants were born before 30 weeks of gestation and hospitalized at the neonatal intensive care unit, (b) they were ≥ 18 years, and (c) had decided to breastfeed. Mothers were excluded if they (a) had opted for mixed feeding method (breast milk and formula), (b) had previous breast surgery, and (c) had severe physical or mental health problems impeding their participation in the study. The principal investigator approached eligible mothers within 24 hr after birth, explained the study, and obtained their informed written consent.

Control

Mothers allocated to the control group (CG) received education and support normally provided by staff nurses to mothers of preterm infants with regard to breast milk production. In general, nutritional and immunological benefits of breast milk for preterm infants and psychological advantages for their mothers were discussed with mothers, along with methods for the mechanical expression of breast milk, breast care and prevention of problems related to lactation, breast milk storage, and cleaning and sterilization of breast pump accessories (Lafond, 2003). Mothers were encouraged to express breast milk for 20 min every 2 hr to 3 hr to establish breast milk production, then 20 min 6 to 8 times/24 hr to maintain it (Lafond, 2003). Kangaroo mother care and breast milk expression at the preterm infant's bedside were also encouraged. A Symphony® double electric breast pump (Medela) and accessory sets were loaned for the period of the study. As this model was different from the one used at the neonatal intensive care unit, an education session on how to express breast milk mechanically with the Symphony® breast pump was offered to mothers by the principal investigator. Finally, on Days 5, 10, 15, 20, 28, 35, and 40 of the study, mothers were also contacted by phone by the principal investigator strictly to remind them of the research procedures related to biological specimen and data collection, and ensure the proper functioning of the loaned material; breast milk expression and production or any topics related to lactation were not discussed with mothers.

Experimental Intervention

Mothers allocated to the experimental group (EG), in addition to standard care and the loan of a Symphony® double electric breast pump (Medela) with accessory sets for the period of the study, received the breast milk expression education and support intervention. The secondary mediators of the Hill-Aldag Lactation Model (Hill et al., 2005b) and empirical evidence guided the development of the intervention content. This experimental intervention was delivered individually by an International Board Certified Lactation Consultant nurse and had two components: an education session on breast milk expression and support through a telephone follow-up and a helpline for 6 weeks.

The 2-hr education session was delivered to mothers in their semi-private hospital room during their hospitalization, which usually ranged over a period of 48 to 72 hr after delivery. Nutritional, immunological, gastro-intestinal, and neurodevelopmental benefits of breast milk for preterm infants and physical and psychological health advantages for mothers were discussed with them, and their decision regarding breastfeeding was positively reinforced. Manual expression of colostrum (Jones & Hartmann, 2005; Morton et al., 2009) and mechanical expression (Jones & Hartmann, 2005; Lawrence & Lawrence, 2005) with a Symphony® double electric breast pump (Medela) were taught to mothers. The lactation consultant nurse assisted mothers with breast milk expression until they felt comfortable with the use of the breast pump. Mothers were encouraged to express 5 to 6 times/day minimally (Lawrence & Lawrence, 2005) and 8 to 10 times/day (Hurst & Meier, 2010) optimally. The importance of early frequent expressions for breast milk lipid concentration (Jackson et al., 1988), blood prolactin (Cox et al., 1996), and volume of expressed breast milk in subsequent postpartum weeks (Hill et al., 2001) was emphasized. Mothers were encouraged to express 15 to 20 min/expression (Meier, 2001), for at least 100 min/day (Lawrence & Lawrence, 2005). The lactation consultant nurse also underscored the necessity of expressing until 2 min after breast milk flow has stopped (Meier, 2001) to express an optimal volume of hindmilk (Daly et al., 1993), which has a lipid concentration 2 to 3 times higher than foremilk (Dorea, Horner, Bezerra, & Campanate, 1982; Neville et al., 1984; Saarela, Kokkonen, & Koivisto, 2005), and empty breast from their milk content to promote breast milk production (Daly & Hartmann, 1995). Kangaroo mother care (Hill et al., 2005b; Hurst, Valentine, Renfro, Burns, & Ferlic, 1997), along with breast milk expression at the preterm infant's bedside (Acuña-Muga et al., 2014; Hurst & Meier, 2010; Meier, 2001), looking at a picture of the preterm infant while expressing (Spicer, 2001), smelling a piece of preterm infant's clothing (Spicer), and listening to soft music (Spicer, 2001) or a relaxation/guided imagery audiotape (Feher, Berger, Johnson, & Wilde, 1989; Keith, Weaver, & Vogel, 2012), were identified to mothers as beneficial interventions to stimulate breast milk ejection and production. Finally, breast care and prevention of problems related to lactation were also discussed with mothers, and information on breast milk storage and cleaning and sterilization of breast pump accessories was given or revised with them.

The lactation consultant nurse also provided support through a telephone follow-up on Days 5, 10, 15, 20, 28, 35, and 40 of the study. The telephone follow-up aimed to evaluate mothers' breast milk production, provide personalized support according to their breast milk production to promote and maintain a sufficient breast milk production, address issues and challenges related to their experience, and manage lactation problems. Mothers were invited to call or meet at the neonatal unit if necessary. The helpline was intended to offer support with any urgent or major lactation issues or problems in the most diligent manner.

Data Collection

Mothers of both groups were encouraged to keep a diary on the frequency and duration of their breast milk expressions and volume of expressed breast milk for the 42 days of the study. They were taught to accurately measure the volume of expressed breast milk by using graded sterile containers, according to standard care. Three samples of composite breast milk were collected in both groups on Days 7, 21, and 42 of the study,

at the first breast milk expression in the morning. At the end of complete breast milk expression, mothers were required to pour 2 to 4 mL of breast milk into a graduated sample tube. Breast milk samples were kept frozen at a temperature of $-70°C$ until lab assays. Lipid concentration of breast milk samples was calculated by the sum of triglycerides, total cholesterol, and phospholipids concentrations. Triglycerides GPO-PAP enzymatic kit (Roche/Hitachi), Cholesterol CHOD-PAP enzymatic kit (Roche/Hitachi), and the method of Bartlett (1959) were used for triglyceride, total cholesterol, and phospholipid analyses, respectively.

Mother's sociodemographic characteristics and confounding variables were collected from the medical records and a written questionnaire at the beginning of the study. Confounding variables included the primary mediators of the Hill-Aldag Lactation Model (Hill et al., 2005b): annual income, level of education, number of weeks of gestation at birth, timing of the decision regarding breastfeeding, intended duration of breastfeeding, previous breastfeeding experience, cohabitation with the father of the preterm infant, and ethnicity. Furthermore, data on time elapsed between birth and initiation of breast milk expression, frequency of kangaroo mother care, preterm infants' supplementation with formula, pregnancy, and childbirth were collected. Finally, since cigarette smoking decreases breast milk production (Hopkinson, Schanler, Fraley, & Garza, 1992; Howard & Lawrence, 1999), and significantly reduces lipid concentration in breast milk (Agostoni et al., 2003; Hopkinson et al., 1992), data on smoking status were also collected.

Procedures

During the recruitment period, and according to the availability of the lactation consultant nurse, medical charts of mothers of very and extremely preterm infants admitted to the neonatal intensive care unit were screened for eligibility by the principal investigator. To avoid potential selection bias, mothers were screened on a consecutive format. The principal investigator approached eligible mothers to inform them about the study and enquire if they would like to hear more about it. The study was explained in details to interested mothers and their questions were answered. When their partners were absent, mothers were encouraged to discuss their participation in the study with them before coming to a decision. They were given the time they needed to consent.

After obtaining their written informed consent, mothers were randomly assigned to receive standard care (CG) or the breast milk expression education and support intervention (EG), using computerized blocked randomization and sequentially numbered sealed opaque envelopes prepared by a neutral third party. Blocked randomization ensures a balanced allocation of participants between the groups over time and reduces bias (Efird, 2011; Matthews, Cook, Terada, & Aloia, 2010). Due to the nature of the intervention, both participants and the interventionist were aware of the allocated arm. However, the lab analysts and statistician were kept blinded to the allocation.

Statistical Analyses

An independent professional statistician performed all the statistical analyses with SPSS Version 19. Mothers of both groups (EG and CG) were compared on sociodemographic and confounding variables using with Student's t test, Fisher's exact test, and Pearson's chi-squared test, depending on the types of variables. To estimate differences in evolution between groups over 6 weeks for frequency and duration of breast milk expression and volume of expressed breast milk, and over Days 7, 21, and 42 of the study for lipid concentration, a complete case analysis was conducted using a general linear model repeated-measures analysis of variance (ANOVA) with two factors, a within-subject time factor and intersubject group factor. All analyses were conducted according to the group to which participants were randomized. A significance level of $p < .05$ was used and adjusted by the Bonferroni correction for post hoc tests.

RESULTS

The medical records of 75 potential participants out of 161 were reviewed to assess the eligibility of mothers of preterm infants (Figure D.1). Eighteen mothers had at least one exclusion criterion: formula feeding ($n = 6$), mixed feeding ($n = 4$), severe physical or mental health problems ($n = 3$), speak neither French nor English ($n = 2$), previous breast surgery ($n = 1$), less than 18 years of age ($n = 1$), and death of the preterm infant ($n = 1$). Seventeen mothers refused to participate in the study. The reasons given by mothers who explained their refusal were as follows: lack of time ($n = 2$), expected lack of compliance to keep the breast milk expression diary ($n = 2$), fatigue ($n = 2$), and significant health problems in preterm infant ($n = 1$). Forty mothers of preterm infants were randomly allocated to the CG or EG; 14 mothers in the EG and 19 in the CG completed the study (Figure D.1). Reasons for attrition were death of the preterm infant ($n = 3$), transfer of the preterm infant to a regional hospital ($n = 1$), and cessation of breastfeeding ($n = 2$). Reasons given by mothers who discontinued breastfeeding were personal and not related to their participation in the study.

No statistically significant differences were noted between the two groups relating to their sociodemographic characteristics and confounding variables. Mothers had an average age of 29.3 years ($SD = 5.4$; EG: mean = 28.6 ± 5.7; CG: mean = 30.0 ± 5.1; $p = .419$) and gave birth on average at 27.5 weeks of gestation ($SD = 1.7$; EG: mean = 27.4 ± 1.6; CG: mean = 27.7 ± 1.8; $p = .587$) to a very or extremely preterm infant with an average birth weight of 1,014.4 g ($SD = 292.9$; EG: mean = 973.5 ± 272.2; CG: mean = $1,055.3 \pm 288.5$; $p = .363$). In both groups, mothers were mostly non-smoker (EG: 85%, 17/20; CG: 80%, 16/20; $p = 1.000$), primiparous (EG: 85%, 17/20; CG: 60%, 12/20; $p = .155$), had a singleton birth (EG: 85%, 17/20; 80% 16/20; $p = 1.000$), and delivered

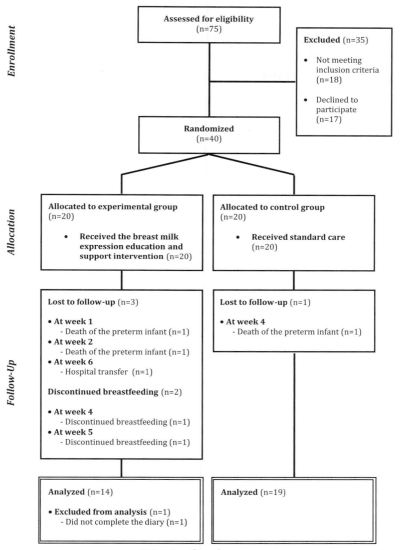

FIG. D.1 Flow diagram.

vaginally (EG: 55%, 11/20; CG: 55%, 11/20; p = .522). No statistically significant differences were found between mothers of both groups regarding the primary mediators of the Hill-Aldag Lactation Model (Table D.1). Thus, mothers had similar ethnicity (p = .597), education level (p = .483), annual income (p = .727), cohabitation status with the father of the preterm infant (p = 1.000), previous breastfeeding experience (p = .058), and timing of decision regarding breastfeeding (p = .210). Also, on average, they intended to breastfeed for a minimum of 8.1 months (SD = 4.5; EG: mean = 8.7 ± 5.3; CG: mean = 7.4 ± 3.4; p = .416) and a maximum of 9.3 months (SD = 4.5; EG: mean = 9.9 ± 5.4; CG: mean = 8.7 ± 3.5; p = .507). Mothers initiated breast milk expression 12.8 hr after birth on average (SD = 6.6; EG: mean = 12.5 ± 6.2; CG: mean = 13.0 ± 7.0; p = .847). There were

TABLE D.1

CONFOUNDING VARIABLES RELATED TO PRIMARY MEDIATORS OF THE HILL-ALDAG LACTATION MODEL FOR ALL PARTICIPANTS

VARIABLES	EXPERIMENTAL GROUP (n = 20)	CONTROL GROUP (n = 20)	P
Ethnicity, n (%)			.597[a]
White	16 (80)	17 (85)	
Hispanic	1 (5)	0 (0)	
Black	3 (15)	3 (15)	
Education level, n (%)			.483[a]
Primary school	1 (5)	1 (5)	
High school	4 (20)	4 (20)	
Professional training	2 (10)	2 (10)	
College	1 (5)	5 (25)	
University	12 (60)	8 (40)	
Annual income, n (%)			.727[a]
Less than $10,000	2 (10)	2 (10)	
$10,000$-29,999	5 (25)	2 (10)	
$30,000$-$49 999	3 (15)	3 (15)	
$50,000-$69,999	3 (15)	5 (25)	
More than $70,000	6 (30)	8 (40)	
Missing data	1 (5)	0 (0)	
Cohabitation with the father of the preterm infants n (%)			1.000[b]
Yes	19 (95)	18 (90)	
No	1 (5)	2 (10)	
Previous breastfeeding experience n (%)			.058[a]
Yes	2 (10)	7 (35)	
No	18 (90)	13 (65)	
Timing of the decision about breastfeeding n (%)			.210[a]
Before pregnancy	15 (75)	13 (65)	
During pregnancy	4 (20)	4 (20)	
Since birth	0 (0)	3 (15)	
Missing data	1 (5)	0 (0)	

[a] Pearson's chi-squared test.
[b] Fisher's exact test.

no statistically significant differences between groups in terms of frequency of kangaroo mother care per day, from Week 1 (EG: mean = 1.6 ± 1.8; CG: mean = 2.7 ± 3.1; $p = .202$) to Week 6 (EG: mean = 1.0 ± 1.7; CG: mean = 0.8 ± 1.7; $p = .783$). Similarly, there were no statistically significant differences between groups with regard to percentage of formula in the preterm infants' diet, from Week 1 (EG: mean = 7.5 ± 11.9; CG: mean = 13.6 ± 25.9; $p = .346$) to Week 6 (EG: mean = 7.4 ± 21.3; CG: mean = 16.5 ± 35.8; $p = .369$).

Frequency of Breast Milk Expression

The weekly overall means of daily breast milk expression frequency for participants who completed the study ranged from 5.6 ± 1.4 to 5.9 ± 0.9 times/day for the EG, and 4.8 ± 1.7 to 5.4 ± 1.4 times/day for the CG (Table D.2). No significant difference was detected between groups, $F(5, 155) = 0.399$, $p = .849$; partial $\eta^2 = .013$ (Table D.3). However, when only Week 1 and Week 6 are compared, a difference of evolution of 0.3 breast milk expression/day with 95%

CI [−0.793, 1.3472] was observed between the groups, in favor of the EG. However, this difference was not statistically significant ($p = .569$).

Duration of Breast Milk Expression

The weekly overall means of daily breast milk expression duration ranged from 112.10 ± 31.22 to 128.33 ± 41.69 min/day for the EG, and 92.72 ± 39.97 to 105.42 ± 29.32 min/day for the CG (Table D.2). A significant difference of evolution was detected between the groups, $F(5, 155) = 2.353, p = .043$; partial $\eta^2 = .071$ (Table D.3). In intent to treat, on complete data only, when the time was set, no significant difference was observed between the groups for Weeks 1 ($p = .502$), 2 ($p = .225$), and 3 ($p = .082$) of the study. However, a statistically significant difference was observed between the two groups for Week 4 ($p = .016$), Week 5 ($p = .025$), and Week 6 ($p = .019$). Thus, the durations of breast milk expression/day for mothers in the EG at Weeks 4, 5, and 6 were significantly higher than those of mothers in the CG. When only Weeks 1 and 6 are considered, a difference of evolution of 27.9 min/day with 95% CI [−1.395, 57.193] was observed between the groups, in favor of the EG. This difference was not statistically significant ($p = .061$).

Volume of Expressed Breast Milk

The weekly overall means of daily expressed breast milk volume for mothers in the EG ranged from 237.56 ± 124.56 to 705.57 ± 436.48 mL/day, and from 308.69 ± 219.81 to 658.19 ± 432.63 mL/day for the mothers of the CG (Table D.2). No significant difference was detected between both groups for the volume of expressed breast milk/day, $F(5,155) = 0.802, p = .550$; partial $\eta^2 = 0.025$ (Table D.3). When only Weeks 1 and 6 are considered, a difference of evolution of 113.6 mL/day with a 95% [174.237, 401.501] was observed between both groups, in favor of the EG. This difference was not statistically significant ($p = .427$).

Lipid Concentration of Breast Milk

The overall means of breast milk lipid concentration for the three samples for participants who collected all samples ranged from 24.40 ± 7.30 to 37.14 ± 10.72 mg/mL for mothers of the EG, and from 27.14 ± 7.43 to 35.12 ± 10.25 mg/mL for mothers assigned to the CG (Table D.2). No significant difference was detected between both groups, $F (2, 54) = 1.399, p = .256$; partial $\eta^2 = .049$ (Table D.3). When the Days 7 (Week 1) and 42 (Week 6) are considered, regardless of Day 21 (week 3), a difference of evolution ($p = .123$) of 4.8 mg/ mL with 95% CI [−11.088, 1.389] was observed between both groups, in favor of the CG. This difference was not statistically significant ($p = .123$).

DISCUSSION

To enlighten the conduct of a larger scale trial, a pilot RCT aimed at estimating the effects of a breast milk expression education and support intervention on breast milk production in mothers of preterm infants was undertaken to evaluate if the results are oriented in the direction hypothesized (Sidani & Braden, 2011) and to determine an adequate sample size for a full RCT (Conn, Algase, Rawl, Zerwic, & Wyman, 2010). The discussion will then focus on the relevance of the research hypothesis and the unique features of the procedures.

It was anticipated that the research hypothesis could not be supported, due to the low statistical power that increases the probability of a Type II error (Burns & Grove, 2009). Nonetheless, it is encouraging to observe that the results are oriented in the same direction as the research hypothesis, with the exception of breast milk lipid concentration. Mothers of preterm infants could potentially benefit from this education and support intervention in terms of frequency and duration of breast milk expression and volume of expressed breast milk. Thus, these promising results support the relevance of the first three parts of the research hypothesis for a larger scale trial.

TABLE D.2

MEANS OF BME, DURATION OF BME, VOLUME OF EBM AND BREAST MILK LIPID CONCENTRATION FOR EXPERIMENTAL AND CONTROL GROUP PARTICIPANTS

VARIABLES	EXPERIMENTAL						CONTROL					
	WEEK 1 M (SD)	WEEK 2 M (SD)	WEEK 3 M (SD)	WEEK 4 M (SD)	WEEK 5 M (SD)	WEEK 6 M (SD)	WEEK 1 M (SD)	WEEK 2 M (SD)	WEEK 3 M (SD)	WEEK 4 M (SD)	WEEK 5 M (SD)	WEEK 6 M (SD)
Frequency of BME per day[a]	5.6	6.0	5.7	5.9	5.7	5.9	5.0	5.4	4.9	4.8	5.0	5.0
	(1.4)	(1.5)	(1.1)	(0.0)	(1.0)	(0.9)	(1.3)	(1.4)	(1.8)	(1.7)	(1.6)	(2.0)
Duration of BME in min per day[a]	112.1	117.7	119.7	126.7	123.1	128.3	104.4	105.4	96.7	95.4	95.1	92.7
	(31.2)	(26.3)	(36.8)	(35.8)	(35.3)	(41.7)	(32.9)	(29.3)	(35.9)	(34.0)	(32.8)	(40.0)
Volume of EBM in mL per day[a]	237.6	536.8	646.6	670.7	705.6	672.2	308.7	575.7	595.6	628.0	658.2	629.7
	(124.6)	(299.8)	(361.7)	(384.1)	(436.5)	(489.0)	(219.8)	(350.9)	(359.4)	(383.3)	(432.6)	(417.1)
EBM lipid concentration in mg/mL[b]	39.3		28.6			25.3	36.4		27.8			27.6
	(10.0)		(6.5)			(6.8)	(10.0)		(7.1)			(8.9)

Note. BME = breast milk expression; EBM = expressed breast milk.
[a] Experimental group: n = 14; Control group: n = 19.
[b] Experimental group: n = 12; Control group: n = 17.

TABLE **D.3**

RESULTS OF THE GENERAL LINEAR MODEL REPEATED-MEASURES ANALYSIS OF VARIANCE (GROUP × TIME)

VARIABLES	WITHIN PARTICIPANTS EFFECT			BETWEEN-PARTICIPANTS EFFECT			INTERACTION EFFECT		
	F	df	η_p^2	F	df	η_p^2	F	df	η_p^2
Frequency of BME per day[a]	1.083	5,155	0.034	2.995	1,31	0.088	0.399	5,155	0.013
Duration of BME in min per day[a]	0.167	5,155	0.005	5.017	1,31	0.139	2.353*	5,155	0.071
Volume of EBM in mL per day[a]	25.557**[c]	5,155	0.452	0.100	1,31	0.000	0.802	5,155	0.025
EMB lipid concentration in mg/mL[b]	30.412**[c]	2,54	0.530	0.037	1,27	0.001	1.399	2,54	0.049

Note. η_p^2 = Partial eta-squared; BME = breast milk expression; EBM = expressed breast milk.
a. Experimental group: $n = 14$; Control group: $n = 19$.
b. Experimental group: $n = 12$; Control group: $n = 17$.
c. Adjustment for multiple comparisons: Bonferroni.
*$p = .043$. **$p < .001$.

In the light of the interpretation of the confidence intervals related to the first three parts of the hypothesis, the sample size of an adequately powered RCT would be of 40 participants per group, taking into account an attrition rate similar to this pilot study (17.5%). This sample size would be sufficient to detect a difference of evolution of 1 breast milk expression/day, 30 min of breast milk expression/day, and 300 mL of expressed breast milk/day between the two groups. A more conservative difference of evolution of 200 mL of expressed breast milk/day between the two groups would require 78 participants per group, with an attrition rate of 17.5%. This second scenario would definitely require more than one recruitment site.

The success of the breast milk expression education and support intervention and the study lies in several aspects related to its applicability to the health care setting. The pragmatic approach of the study represents an undeniable strength of the study. By getting as close as possible to the real conditions of clinical practice (Oxman et al., 2009; Zwarenstein & Treweek, 2009a, 2009b), pragmatic clinical trials wittingly inform clinical decisions in a real context of practice (Zwarenstein & Treweek, 2009a, 2009b), which is why they are relevant (Thorpe et al., 2009). Consequently, the implementation of the intervention

in actual clinical nursing practice, with mothers of very and extremely preterm infants who were representative of the target population, strengthens the external validity of the pilot study.

The novelty of the dependent variables is also a distinctive characteristic of this pilot study. None of the previous studies have evaluated the effects of an intervention on the frequency and duration of breast milk expressions as well as on the volume of breast milk expressed by mothers of preterm infants. Hence, the selection of these dependent variables, based on the Hill-Aldag Lactation Model (Hill et al., 2005b), is both innovative and relevant as they are closely related to breast milk production in mothers of very and extremely preterm infants.

Another strength is the loan of a Symphony® double electric breast pump (Medela) to all the mothers. As breast pump suction patterns differ in their efficiency (Meier, Engstrom, Janes, Jegier, & Loera, 2012), the loan of the same model neutralized an important confounding variable that could have affected breast milk production. By controlling this non-negligible confounding variable, it contributes to solidify the internal validity of the study.

On the other hand, our pilot study also has serious limitations. It was sometimes laborious for the lactation consultant nurse to reach participants by telephone, which endangered the fidelity and dose while attenuating the effects of the intervention. Obtaining a second phone number with voicemail or a mobile phone number with short message service (SMS) for each participant as well as an established protocol to return phone calls are unavoidable aspects of a telephone follow-up in a larger scale trial. The telephone follow-up in the CG, which aimed to remind participants about the study procedures and reinforce the observance of the diary, has also potentially mitigated the differences between the two groups. Some mothers allocated to the CG reported perceiving these regular contacts with the principal investigator as a form of support. Thus, they should be limited to the timing of collecting breast milk samples.

During this 6-week long pilot study, data on mothers' adherence to recommended interventions that stimulate breast milk production, such as breast milk expression at the preterm infant's bedside, were not collected apart from frequency of kangaroo mother care. Similarly, data related to mothers' use of co-interventions, for example support from other health care professionals, community breastfeeding resources, family members or peers, were not rigorously gathered. As these interventions might influence volume of expressed breast milk, and thus threaten the internal validity of a study, they should be carefully appraised in a larger scale trial.

In addition, as both mothers' and preterm infants' hospital rooms were semi-private, participants in the CG might have heard the content of the education session or shared information with participants allocated to the EG. Close proximity of participants increases the risk of contamination (Feeley & Cossette, 2016). However, no data relating to this threat to internal validity were gathered in the pilot study. As contamination attenuates the magnitude of the effects of an intervention (Keogh-Brown et al., 2007), strategies should be implemented to control this bias (Sussman & Hayward, 2010), and clinical trials of educational interventions should report the nature, extent, and effects of contamination (Keogh-Brown et al., 2007).

Another major limitation concerns the measurement of breast milk volume. As part of the clinical practice at the neonatal unit, at-breast feedings were gradually introduced during the period of the study. Data on the duration and frequency of these feedings were gathered by mothers of both groups and were included in statistical analyses. However, data relating to breast milk intake during theses feeding were not collected, thus limiting the statistical conclusion validity of the study with regard to breast milk volume. Reliable data on breast milk intake during at breast feedings could have been collected through test weighing. Weighing very and extremely preterm infants before and after at breast feedings, under strictly controlled conditions, and conversion of weight gain in gram to volume of intake in milliliters provide an objective and accurate estimate of breast milk volume (Haase, Barreira, Murphy, Mueller, & Rhodes, 2009; Meier & Engstrom, 2007; Meier, Lysakowski, Engstrom, Kavanaugh, & Mangurten, 1990). Researchers conducting clinical trials on breast milk production with breast pump-dependent mothers of non-nursing preterm infants should consider this procedure when at-breast feedings are introduced.

Data on confounding variables that may have affected the activation of lactogenesis, such as fatigue, maternal obesity, alcohol, opioids, and Depo-Provera (Hartmann & Ramsay, 2005), as well as confounding variables that may have affected breast milk production, like galactogogues (Campbell-Yeo et al., 2010; Zuppa et al., 2010) and stress (Ueda, Yokoyama, Irahara, & Aono, 1994), were not collected in this pilot study but should be considered in a full-scale trial. Finally, efforts should be made to include mothers of preterm infants with low socioeconomic status in clinical trials, as they are more at risk for early breastfeeding cessation (Flacking, Nyqvist, & Ewald, 2007; Flacking, Wallin, & Ewald, 2007; Zachariassen et al., 2010).

In conclusion, this pilot study has offered the first evidence that a breast milk expression education and support intervention may be beneficial for the establishment and maintenance of an adequate breast milk production in mothers of preterm infants, in terms of the frequency and duration of breast milk expression and volume of expressed breast milk. Our results underscore the importance of educating and supporting mothers of preterm infants with regard to breast milk expression in early postpartum. A pragmatic RCT will determine the beneficial effects of this innovative intervention on breast milk production outcomes.

ACKNOWLEDGEMENTS

The authors would like to thank mothers of preterm infants who participated in this study, Marie-Claude Perreault who delivered the experimental intervention, Émilie Grenier and Alain Montoudis who performed the laboratory analyses, and Miguel Chagnon who conducted the statistical analyses.

DECLARATION OF CONFLICTING INTERESTS

The author(s) declared no potential conflicts of interest with respect to the research, authorship, and/or publication of this article.

FUNDING

The author(s) disclosed receipt of the following financial support for the research, authorship, and/or publication of this article: Funding for this pilot study was provided by AWHONN Canada, Canadian Institutes of Health Research (CIHR), Canadian Nurses Foundation, and Groupe de recherche interuniversitaire en interventions en sciences infirmières du Québec (GRIISIQ). Financial support was provided to the principal investigator during her doctoral studies by the CIHR, Faculté des études supérieures et postdoctorales de l'Université de Montréal, Faculté des sciences infirmières de l'Université de Montréal, Fondation CHU Sainte-Justine, Fondation de recherche en sciences infirmières du Québec (FRESIQ), GRIISIQ, Ministère de l'Éducation, du Loisir et du Sport du Québec, and Ordre des infirmières et infirmiers du Québec (OIIQ). Medela Canada offered complimentary breast pump accessory sets.

REFERENCES

Acuña-Muga, J., Ureta-Velasco, N., de la Cruz-Bértolo, J., Balleseros-López, R., Sánchez-Martínez, R., Miranda-Casabona, E, & Pallás-Alonso, C. (2014). Volume of milk obtained in relation to location and circumstances of expression in mothers of very low birth weight infants. *Journal of Human Lactation, 30,* 41–46. doi:10.1177/0890334413509140.

Agostoni, C., Marangoni, F., Grandi, F., Lammardo, A. M., Giovannini, M., Riva, E., & Galli, C. (2003). Earlier smoking habits are associated with higher serum lipids and lower milk fat and polyunsaturated fatty acid content in the first 6 months of lactation. *European Journal of Clinical Nutrition, 57,* 1466–1472. doi:10.1038/sj.ejcn.1601711.

Agrasada, G. V., Gustafsson, J., Kylberg, E., & Ewald, E. (2005). Postnatal peer counselling on exclusive breast-feeding of low-birthweight infants: A randomized, controlled trial. *Acta Paediatrica, 94,* 1109–1115. doi:10.1111/j.1651-2227.2005. tb02053.x.

Ahmed, A. H. (2008). Breastfeeding preterm infants: An educational program to support mothers of preterm infants in Cairo, Egypt. *Pediatric Nursing, 34,* 125–138.

Alexandre, C., Bomy, H., Bourdon, E., Truffert, P., & Pierrat, V. (2007). Accompagnement des mères de nouveau-nés prématurés dans leur projet d'allaitement maternel. Évaluation d'un programme de formation dans une unité périnatale de niveau III. [Lactation counselling support provided to mothers of preterm babies who intend to breastfeed. Evaluation of an educational intervention in a level III perinatal unit]. *Archives de Pédiatrie, 14,* 1413–1419. doi:10.1016/j.arcped.2007.08.017.

American Academy of Pediatrics. (2012). Breastfeeding and the use of human milk. Section on breastfeeding. *Pediatrics, 129,* e827–ee841. doi:10.1542/peds.2011-3552.

Barois, J., Grognet, S., Tourneux, P., & Leke, A. (2013). Facteurs maternels et néonatals associés au succès de l'allaitement maternel à la sortie d'un service de néonatalogie chez les grands prématurés [Maternal and neonatal factors associated with successful breastfeeding in very preterm infants]. *Archives de Pédiatrie, 20,* 969–973. doi:10.1016.j.arcped. 2013.06.018.

Bartlett, G. R. (1959). Colorimetric assay methods for free and phosphorylated glyceric acids. *Journal of Biochemistry*, *243*, 469–471.

Bonet, M., Blondel, B., Agostino, R., Combier, E., Maier, R. F., Cuttini, M., & MOSAIC Research Group. (2011). Variations in breastfeeding rates for very preterm infants between regions and neonatal units in Europe: Results from the MOSAIC cohort. *Archives of Diseases in Childhood Fetal and Neonatal Edition*, *96*, F450–F452. doi:10.1136/adc.2009.179564.

Burns, N., & Grove, S. K. (2009). *The practice of nursing research: Appraisal, synthesis, and generation of evidence* (6th ed.). St. Louis, MO: Saunders.

Callen, J., Pinelli, J., Atkinson, S., & Saigal, S. (2005). Qualitative analysis of barriers to breastfeeding in very-low-birthweight infants in the hospital and postdischarge. *Advances in Neonatal Care*, *5*, 93–103. doi:10.1016/j.adnc.2004.12.005.

Campbell-Yeo, M. L., Allen, A. C., Joseph, K. S., Ledwidge, J. M., Caddell, K., Allen, V. M., & Dooley, K. C. (2010). Effect of domperidone on the composition of preterm human breast milk. *Pediatrics*, *125*, e107–e114. doi:10.1542/peds.2008-3441.

Conn, V. S., Algase, D. L., Rawl, S. M., Zerwic, J. J., & Wyman, J. F. (2010). Publishing pilot intervention work. *Western Journal of Nursing Research*, *32*, 994–1010. doi:10.1177/019394591036722.

Cox, D. B., Owens, R. A., & Hartmann, P. E. (1996). Blood and milk prolactin and the rate of milk synthesis in women. *Experimental Physiology*, *81*, 1007–1020.

Daly, S. E. J., Di Rosso, A., Owens, R. A., & Hartmann, P. E. (1993). Degree of breast emptying explains changes in the fat content, but not fatty acid composition, of human milk. *Experimental Physiology*, *78*, 741–755.

Daly, S. E. J., & Hartmann, P. E. (1995). Infant demand and milk supply. Part 1: Infant demand and milk production in lactating women. *Journal of Human Lactation*, *11*, 21–26.

Dorea, J. G., Horner, M. R., Bezerra, V. L., & Campanate, M. L. (1982). Variation in major constituents of fore-and hindmilk of Brazilian women. *Journal of Tropical Pediatrics*, *28*, 303–305.

Efird, J. (2011). Blocked randomization with randomly selected block sizes. *International Journal of Environmental Research and Public Health*, *8*, 15–20. doi:10.3390/ijerph8010015.

Feeley, N., & Cossette, S. (2016). Pilot studies. In S. J. Henly (Ed.), *The Routledge international handbook of advanced quantitative methods in nursing research*. New York, NY: Routledge.

Feher, S. D., Berger, L. R., Johnson, J. D., & Wilde, J. B. (1989). Increasing breast milk production for premature infants with a relaxation/imagery audiotape. *Pediatrics*, *83*, 57–60.

Fewtrell, M. S., Lucas, P., Collier, S., Shinghal, A., Ahluwalia, J. S., & Lucas, A. (2001). Randomized trial comparing the efficacy of a novel manual breast pump with a standard electric breast pump in mothers who delivered preterm infants. *Pediatrics*, *107*, 1291–1297. doi:10.1542/peds.107.6.1291.

Flacking, R., Nyqvist, K. H., & Ewald, U. (2007). Effects of socioeconomic status on breastfeeding duration in mothers of preterm and term infants. *European Journal of Public Health*, *17*, 579–584. doi:10.1093/eurpub/ckm019.

Flacking, R., Wallin, L., & Ewald, U. (2007). Perinatal and socioeconomic determinants of breastfeeding duration in very preterm infants. *Acta Paediatrica*, *96*, 1126–1130. doi:10.111/j.1651-2227.2007.00386.x.

Furman, L., Minich, N., & Hack, M. (2002). Correlates of lactation in mothers of very low birth weight infants. *Pediatrics*, *109*, e57. doi:10.1542/peds.109.4.e57.

Glasgow, R. E., Magid, D. J., Beck, A., Ritzwoller, D., & Estabrooks, P. A. (2005). Practical clinical trials for translating research to practice. Design and measurement recommendations. *Medical Care*, *43*, 551–557.

Gonzalez, K. A., Meinzen-Derr, J., Burke, B. L., Hibler, A. J., Kavinsky, B., Hess, S., & Morrow, A. L. (2003). Evaluation of a lactation support service in a children's hospital neonatal intensive care unit. *Journal of Human Lactation*, *19*, 286–292. doi:10.1177/0890334403255344.

Haase, B. A. L., Barreira, J., Murphy, P. K., Mueller, M., & Rhodes, J. (2009). The development of an accurate test weighing technique for preterm and high-risk hospitalized infants. *Breastfeeding Medicine*, *4*, 151–156. doi:10.1089/bfm.2008.0125.

Hartmann, P. E., & Ramsay, D. T. (2005). Mammary anatomy and physiology. In E. Jones & C. King (Eds.), *Feeding and nutrition in the preterm infant* (pp. 53–68). New York, NY: Elsevier Churchill Livingstone.

Hill, P. D., Aldag, J. C., & Chatterton, R. T. (2001). Initiation and frequency of pumping and milk production in mothers of non-nursing preterm infants. *Journal of Human Lactation*, *17*, 9–13. doi:10.1177/089033440101700103.

Hill, P. D., Aldag, J. C., Chatterton, R. T., & Zinaman, M. (2005a). Comparison of milk output between mothers of preterm and term infants: The first

6 weeks after birth. *Journal of Human Lactation, 21*, 22–30. doi:10.1177/0890334404272407.

Hill, P. D., Aldag, J. C., Chatterton, R. T., & Zinaman, M. (2005b). Primary and secondary mediators' influence on milk output in lactating mothers of preterm and term infants. *Journal of Human Lactation, 21*, 138–150. doi:10.1177/0890334405275403.

Hill, P. D., Aldag, J. C., Chatterton, R. T., & Zinaman, M. (2005c). Psychological distress and milk volume in lactating mothers. *Western Journal of Nursing Research, 27*, 676–693. doi:10.1177/0193945905277154.

Hill, P. D., Aldag, J. C., Demirtas, H., Zinaman, M., & Chatterton, R. T. (2006). Mood states and milk output in lactating mothers of preterm and term infants. *Journal of Human Lactation, 22*, 305–314. doi:10.1177/0890334406290003.

Hopkinson, J. M., Schanler, R. J., Fraley, J. K., & Garza, C. (1992). Milk production by mothers of premature infants: Influence of cigarette smoking. *Pediatrics, 90*, 934–938.

Howard, C. R., & Lawrence, R. A. (1999). Drugs and breastfeeding. *Clinics in Perinatology, 26*, 447–478.

Hurst, N. M., & Meier, P. P. (2010). Breastfeeding the preterm infant. In J. Riordan & K. Wamback (Eds.), *Breastfeeding and human lactation* (4th ed., pp. 425–470). Sudbury, MA: Jones and Bartlett.

Hurst, N. M., Valentine, C. J., Renfro, L., Burns, P., & Ferlic, L. (1997). Skin-to-skin holding in the neonatal intensive care unit influences maternal milk volume. *Journal of Perinatology, 17*, 213–217.

Jackson, D. A., Imong, S. M., Silprasert, A., Ruckphaopunt, S., Woolridge, M. W., Baum, J. D., & Amatayakul, K. (1988). Circadian variation in fat concentration of breast-milk in a rural northern Thai population. *British Journal of Nutrition, 59*, 349–363.

Jones, E., & Hartmann, P. E. (2005). Milk expression. In E. Jones & C. King (Eds.), *Feeding and nutrition in the preterm infant* (pp. 69–85). New York, NY: Elsevier Churchill Livingstone.

Keith, D. R., Weaver, B. S., & Vogel, R. L. (2012). The effect of music-based listening interventions on the volume, fat content, and caloric content of breast milk-produced by mothers of premature and critically ill infants. *Advances in Neonatal Care, 12*, 112–119. doi:10.1097/ANC.0b013e31824d9842.

Keogh-Brown, M. R., Bachmann, M. O., Shepstone, L., Hewitt, C., Howe, A., Ramsay, C. R., & Campbell, M. J. (2007). Contamination in trials of educational interventions. *Health Technology Assessment, 11*(43), ix–107.

Khan, S., Hepworth, A. R., Prime, D. K., Lai, C. T., Trengove, N. J., & Hartmann, P. E. (2012). Variation in fat, lactose, and protein composition in breast milk over 24 hr: Association with infant feeding patterns. *Journal of Human Lactation, 29*, 81–89. doi:10.1177/0890334412448841.

Kieser, M., & Wassmer, G. (1996). On the use of the upper confidence limit for the variance from a pilot sample for sample size determination. *Biometrical Journal, 38*, 941–949. doi:10.1002/bimj.4710380806.

Killersreiter, B., Grimmer, I., Buhrer, C., Dudenhausen, J. W., & Obladen, M. (2001). Early cessation of milk feeding in very low birthweight infants. *Early Human Development, 60*, 193–205. doi:10.1016/S0378-3782(00)00116-x.

King, K. M. (2008). Pragmatic trials: Is this a useful method in nursing research? *Journal of Clinical Nursing, 17*, 1401–1402. doi:10.1111/j.1365-2702.2008.02297.x.

Koletzko, B., Agostoni, C., Bergmann, R., Ritzenhaler, K., & Shamir, R. (2011). Physiological aspects of human milk lipids and implications for infant feeding: A workshop report. *Acta Paediatrica, 100*, 1405–1415. doi:10.1111/j.1651-2227.2011.02343.x.

Lafond, L. (2003). *L'allaitement maternel à l'unité néonatale* [Breastfeeding at the neonatal unit; booklet]. Montreal, Quebec, Canada: Hôpital Sainte-Justine.

Lawrence, R. A., & Lawrence, R. M. (2005). *Breastfeeding: A guide for the medical profession* (6th ed.). St. Louis, MO: Elsevier Mosby.

Lee, H. C., & Gould, J. B. (2009). Factors influencing milk versus formula feeding at discharge for very low birth weight infants in California. *Journal of Pediatrics, 155*, 657–662. doi:10.1016/j.jpeds.2009.04.064.

Maastrup, R., Hansen, B. M., Kronborg, H., Bojesen, S. N., Hallum, K., Frandsen, A., & Hallström, I. (2014). Factors associated with exclusive breastfeeding of preterm infants. Results from a prospective national cohort study. *PLoS ONE, 9*(2), e89077. doi:10.1371/journal.pone.0089077.

Matthews, E. E., Cook, P. F., Terada, M., & Aloia, M. S. (2010). Randomizing research participants: Promoting balance and concealment in small samples. *Research in Nursing & Health, 33*, 243–253. doi:10.1002/nur.20375.

Meier, P. P. (2001). Breastfeeding in the special care nursery: Prematures and infants with medical problems. *Pediatric Clinics of North America, 48*, 425–442.

Meier, P. P., & Engstrom, J. L. (2007). Test weighing for term and premature infants is an accurate procedure. *Archives of Disease in Childhood Fetal & Neonatal Edition, 92*, F155–F156. doi:10.1136/dc.2006.113480.

Meier, P. P., Engstrom, J. L., Janes, J. E., Jegier, B. J., & Loera, F. (2012). Breast pump suction patterns that mimic the human infant during breastfeeding: Greater milk output in less time spent pumping for breast pump-dependent mothers with premature infants. *Journal of Perinatology, 32*, 103–110. doi:10.1038/jp.2011.64.

Meier, P. P., Engstrom, J., Mingolelli, S. S. L., Miracle, D. J., & Kiesling, S. (2004). The Rush Mothers' Milk Club: Breastfeeding interventions for mothers with very-low-birth-weight infants. *Journal of Obstetric, Gynecologic, and Neonatal Nursing, 33*, 164–174. doi:10.1177/0884217504263280.

Meier, P. P., Lysakowski, T. Y., Engstrom, J. L., Kavanaugh, K. L., & Mangurten, H. H. (1990). The accuracy of test weighing for preterm infants. *Journal of Pediatric Gastroenterology & Nutrition, 10*, 62–65.

Melnyk, B. M., & Cole, R. (2005). Generating evidence through quantitative research. In B. E. Melnyk & E. Fineout-Overholt (Eds.), *Evidence-based practice in nursing & healthcare: A guide to best practice* (pp. 239–281). Philadelphia, PA: Lippincott Williams & Wilkins.

Merewood, A., Chamberlain, L. B., Cook, J. T., Philipp, B. L., Malone, K., & Bauchner, H. (2006). The effect of peer counselors on breastfeeding rates in the neonatal intensive care unit. Results of a randomized controlled trial. *Archives of Pediatrics & Adolescent Medicine, 160*, 681–685.

Morton, J., Hall, J. Y., Wong, R. J., Thairu, L., Benitz, W. E., & Rhine, W. D. (2009). Combining hand techniques with electric pumping increases milk production in mothers of preterm infants. *Journal of Perinatology, 29*, 757–764. doi:10.1038/jp.2009.87.

Neville, M. C., Keller, R. P., Seacat, J., Casey, C. E., Allen, J. C., & Archer, P. (1984). Studies on human lactation. I. Within-feed and between-breast variation in selected components of human milk. *American Journal of Clinical Nutrition, 40*, 635–646.

Oxman, A. D., Lombard, C., Treweek, S., Gagnier, J. J., Maclure, M., & Zwarenstein, M. (2009). Why we will remain pragmatists: Four problems with the impractical mechanistic framework and a better solution. *Journal of Clinical Epidemiology, 62*, 485–488. doi:10.1016/j.jclinepi.2008.08.015.

Parker, L. A., Sullivan, S., Krueger, C., Kelechi, T., & Mueller, M. (2012). Effect of early breast milk expression on milk volume and timing of lactogenesis stage II among mothers of very low birth weight infants: A pilot study. *Journal of Perinatology, 32*, 205–209. doi:10.1038/jp.2011.78.

Pereira, G. R., Schwartz, D., Gould, P., & Grim, N. (1984). Breastfeeding in neonatal intensive care. Beneficial effects of maternal counseling. *Perinatology-Neonatology, 8*, 35–42.

Perrella, S. L., Williams, J., Nathan, E. A., Fenwick, J., Hartmann, P. E., & Geddes, D. T. (2012). Influences on breastfeeding outcomes for healthy term and preterm/sick infants. *Breastfeeding Medicine, 7*, 255–261. doi:10.1089/bmf.20n.0118.

Pineda, R. G., Foss, J., Richards, L., & Pane, C. A. (2009). Breastfeeding changes for VLBW infants in the NICU following staff education. *Neonatal Network, 28*, 311–319.

Pinelli, J., Atkinson, S. A., & Saigal, S. (2001). Randomized trial of breastfeeding support in very low-birth-weight infants. *Archives of Pediatrics & Adolescent Medicine, 155*, 548–553.

Saarela, T., Kokkonen, J., & Koivisto, M. (2005). Macronutrient and energy contents of human milk fractions during the first six months of lactation. *Acta Paediatrica, 94*, 1176–1181. doi:10.1080/08035250510036499.

Sidani, S., & Braden, C. J. (2011). *Design, evaluation, and translation of nursing interventions*. West Sussex, UK: Willey-Blackwell.

Sisk, P. M., Lovelady, C. A., Dillard, R. G., & Gruber, K. J. (2006). Lactation counseling for mothers of very low birth weight infants: Effect on maternal anxiety and infant intake of human milk. *Pediatrics, 117*, e67–e75. doi:10.1542/peds.2005-0267.

Spicer, K. (2001). What every nurse needs to know about breast pumping: Instructing and supporting mothers of premature infants in the NICU. *Neonatal Network, 20*(4), 35–41.

Sussman, J. B., & Hayward, R. A. (2010). An IV for the RCT: Using instrumental variables to adjust for treatment contamination in randomised controlled trials. *British Medical Journal, 340*, c2073. doi:10.1136/bmj.c2073.

Thorpe, K. E., Zwarenstein, M., Oxman, A. D., Treweek, S., Furberg, C. D., Altman, D. G., & Chalkidou, K. (2009). A pragmatic-explanatory continuum indicator summary (PRECIS): A tool to help trial designers. *Canadian Medical Association Journal, 180*(10), E47–E57. doi:10.1503/cmaj.090523.

Tunis, S. R., Stryer, D. B., & Clancy, C. M. (2003). Practical clinical trials. Increasing the value of clinical research for decision making in clinical and health policy. *Journal of American Medical Association, 290*, 1624–1632. doi:10.1001/jama. 290.12.1624.

Ueda, T., Yokoyama, Y., Irahara, M., & Aono, T. (1994). Influence of psychological stress on suckling-induced pulsatile oxytocin release. *Obstetrics & Gynecology, 84*, 259–262.

World Health Organization. (2008). *Indicators for assessing infant and young child feeding practices. Part 1 Definitions.* Retrieved from http://www.who.int/mater-nal_child_adolescent/documents/9789241596664/en/.

World Health Organization. (2013, November). *Preterm birth.* Retrieved from http://www.who.int/mediacentre/factsheets/fs363/en/.

Zachariassen, G., Faerk, J., Grytter, C., Esberg, B. H., Juvonen, P., & Halken, S. (2010). Factors associated with successful establishment of breastfeeding in very preterm infants. *Acta Paediatrica, 99*, 1000–1004. doi:10.1111./j.1651-2227.2010.01721.x.

Zuppa, A. A., Sindico, P., Orchi, C., Carducci, C., Cardiello, V., Romagnoli, C., & Catenazzi, P. (2010). Safety and efficacy of galactogogues: Substances that induce, maintain and increases breast milk production. *Journal of Pharmacy & Pharmaceutical Sciences, 13*, 162–174.

Zwarenstein, M., & Treweek, S. (2009a). What kind of randomised trials do patients and clinicians need? *Evidence-Based Medicine, 14*, 101–103. doi:10.1016/j. jclinepi.2009.01.011.

Zwarenstein, M., & Treweek, S. (2009b). What kind of randomized trials do we need? *Canadian Medical Association Journal, 180*, 998–1000. doi:10.1503/cmaj.082007.

Follow-up for Improving Psychological Well Being for Women After a Miscarriage (Review)

Fiona A. Murphy[1], Allyson Lipp[2], Diane L. Powles[2]

This is a reprint of a Cochrane review, prepared and maintained by The Cochrane Collaboration and published in *The Cochrane Library* 2012, Issue 3.

ABSTRACT

BACKGROUND. Miscarriage is the premature expulsion of an embryo or fetus from the uterus up to 23 weeks of pregnancy and weighing up to 500 grams. International studies using diagnostic tools have identified that some women suffer from anxiety, depression and grief after miscarriage. Psychological follow-up might detect those women who are at risk of psychological complications following miscarriage. This review is necessary as the evidence is equivocal on the benefits of psychological follow-up after miscarriage.

OBJECTIVES. Whether follow-up affects the psychological well being of women following miscarriage.

[1]College of Human & Health Science, Swansea University, Swansea, UK.
[2]Faculty of Health, Sport and Science, Department of Care Sciences, University of Glamorgan, Pontypridd, UK.
Contact address: Fiona A Murphy, College of Human & Health Science, Swansea University, Singleton Park, Swansea, West Glamorgan, SA2 8PP, UK. f.murphy@swan.ac.uk.

Editorial group: Cochrane Pregnancy and Childbirth Group.
Publication status and date: New, published in Issue 3, 2012.
Review content assessed as up-to-date: 31 December 2011.
Citation: Murphy FA, Lipp A, Powles DL. Follow-up for improving psychological well being for women after a miscarriage. *Cochrane Database of Systematic Reviews* 2012, Issue 3. Art. No.: CD008679. DOI: 10.1002/14651858. CD008679.pub2.

SEARCH METHODS. We searched the Cochrane Pregnancy and Childbirth Group's Trials Register (31 December 2011), reference lists of all retrieved papers and contacted professional and lay organisations to obtain any ongoing trials or unpublished data.

SELECTION CRITERIA. Randomised controlled trials only.

DATA COLLECTION AND ANALYSIS. All potential trials for eligibility according to the criteria specified in the protocol by screening the titles and abstracts, retrieving full reports of potentially relevant trials for assessment. All review authors extracted data and checked for accuracy. No studies were published in duplicate. When data were missing and only the abstract was available, we attempted to contact the trial authors. We resolved any disagreement through discussion.

MAIN RESULTS. Six studies involving 1001 women were included. Three trials compared one counselling session with no counselling. There was no significant difference in psychological well being including anxiety, grief, depression avoidance and self-blame. One trial compared three one-hour counselling sessions with no counselling at four and 12 months. Some subscales showed statistical significance in favour of counselling and some in favour of no counselling. The results for two trials were given in narrative form as data were unavailable for meta-analyses. One trial compared multiple interventions. The other trial compared two counselling sessions with no counselling. Neither study favoured counselling.

AUTHORS' CONCLUSIONS. Evidence is insufficient to demonstrate that psychological support such as counselling is effective post-miscarriage. Further trials should be good quality, adequately-powered using standardised interventions and outcome measures at specific time points. The economic implications and women's satisfaction with psychological follow-up should also be explored in any future study.

PLAIN LANGUAGE SUMMARY

Follow-up for Improving Psychological Well Being for Women After a Miscarriage

Miscarriage is the premature, or loss of a fetus, up to 23 weeks of pregnancy. Some women suffer from anxiety and depression after miscarriage which may be part of their grief following the loss. Psychological follow-up might detect those women who are at risk of psychological complications following miscarriage. This review of six studies, involving 1001 women, found that there is insufficient evidence from randomised controlled trials to recommend any method of psychological follow-up. Timing of the counselling interventions varied from one week following miscarriage up to 11 weeks. In all studies the interventions were delivered by different professional groups including a midwife, psychologists and nurses. Measurements of the outcomes were made from one month to 12 months after miscarriage in the different studies, which highlights the uncertainty surrounding the rate of psychological recovery following miscarriage. The two larger studies included a complex combination of interventions and outcome measures so that any potentially significant effects may have been diluted.

Further robust research is needed to determine if any recognised psychological follow-up is effective is hastening psychological recovery following miscarriage.

BACKGROUND

Description of the Condition

Although definitions of miscarriage vary internationally, it is defined by the World Health Organization (WHO) as the premature expulsion of an embryo or fetus from the uterus up to 23 weeks of pregnancy and weighing up to 500 grams (WHO 2001). Early pregnancy loss is defined as a confirmed empty sac or sac with fetus but with no fetal heart activity at less than 12 weeks' gestation (Farquharson 2005; RCOG 2006). It is difficult to quantify Blohm precisely how many women will have a miscarriage but in a longitudinal Swedish study, 2008 found that clinical miscarriage constituted 12% of all pregnancies, and 25% of women who had been pregnant by 39 years of age had experienced at least one miscarriage.

This review will focus on spontaneous miscarriage and will not include elective termination of pregnancy, ectopic pregnancy, stillbirth and neonatal death.

There are various categorisations of miscarriage, in that a miscarriage may be complete with all the products of conception passed or incomplete in which some of the products are retained within the uterus. There is an additional category of 'silent' miscarriage or early fetal demise in which the fetus may have been dead for some weeks but has not yet been expelled from the uterus (Trinder 2006). The characteristic symptoms of miscarriage are vaginal blood loss which may be accompanied by pain.

Physical management of women with miscarriage in the UK optimally involves rapid referral to an early pregnancy unit with ultrasound confirmation that the pregnancy is not viable. Management will depend on the category of miscarriage and the woman's clinical condition; women may be offered the option of expectant management where there is no active medical intervention with the miscarriage proceeding of its own accord. Other options are surgical management, in which the retained products of conception are evacuated usually under general anaesthetic; and medical intervention, in which medications are given to induce uterine contractions and evacuation of retained products usually without the need for surgical intervention (RCOG 2006). Systematic reviews by Nanda 2006 and Neilson 2010 suggest that all of these treatments are acceptable and women should be supported to make the choice of treatment which is most suitable for them.

Unlike physical management of women following miscarriage, the evidence on psychological management is less well developed and is the focus of this review. There has been increased awareness of the psychological consequences of miscarriage for women and their partners. International studies using diagnostic tools identified that some women suffer from anxiety and depression after miscarriage (Neugebauer 1997; Nikcevic 1999; Stirtzinger 1999). These and other feelings that women describe have been conceptualised by many as being part of a pattern of grief in response to the loss of a baby (Frost 2007; Malacrida 1998; Mander 1997). Accounts from women about their hospital experiences in one study were critical of how health professionals cared for them with little awareness of their feelings of distress and no effective interventions to support them (Stratton 2008).

Description of the Intervention

Strategies to provide some kind of psychological follow-up after miscarriage have been proposed. However, these are characterised by their diversity both in terms of the type of follow-up and who provides it. They range from telephone counselling provided by women who have already had a miscarriage to more formal counselling programmes. The mode of intervention could be passive, such as written or electronic information, or active, via telephone, clinic appointment or one-to-one or group support.

How the Intervention Might Work

Follow-up might detect those women who are at risk of developing or who actually have psychological complications following miscarriage such as anxiety, distress and depression. The United Kingdom RCOG guidelines (RCOG 2006) on the management of women after early pregnancy loss state that support and counselling for women after miscarriage can have significant positive effects on psychological well being. However, a Cochrane review of support after perinatal death, concluded that there is insufficient evidence that such interventions are beneficial (Flenady 2008). Similarly, Stratton 2008 in a review of hospital-based interventions, found little evidence to suggest that follow-up after miscarriage has positive outcomes. It is possible that psychological follow-up

could reduce any adverse effects on women such as on their employment, relationships with their partners and other close family members.

Why It Is Important to Do This Review

Currently once any complications are detected via follow-up, women can be referred to specific agencies which will provide interventions to manage these complications and reduce any adverse psychological outcomes following miscarriage. There is a need to systematically review the evidence on follow-up after miscarriage as it is not known which interventions are effective.

OBJECTIVES

Primary

To identify whether follow-up by healthcare professionals or lay organisations at any time affects the psychological well being of women following miscarriage.

Secondary

To compare the effects of different types of interventions on the psychological well being of women following miscarriage.

METHODS

Criteria for Considering Studies for This Review

Types of Studies

All published and unpublished randomised controlled trials including cluster trials that compare different methods of follow-up after miscarriage. We did not include quasi-randomised trials (e.g. trials that allocate treatment by sequential record number, sequential admitting number, by day of the week).

Types of Participants

Females of child-bearing age experiencing miscarriage defined as premature expulsion of an embryo or fetus from the uterus up to 23 weeks of pregnancy and weighing up to 500 grams (WHO 2001).

Types of Interventions

We considered trials if they compared interventions following miscarriage.

1. Psychological intervention versus no intervention.
2. Psychological intervention versus usual care.
3. Psychological intervention versus another psychological intervention.

Types of Outcome Measures

PRIMARY OUTCOMES

1. Psychological well being as defined by the trial authors.
2. Patient satisfaction as defined by the trial authors.

SECONDARY OUTCOMES

1. Adverse reaction to follow-up.
2. Referral to primary healthcare services.
3. Admission to hospital.
4. Costs associated with follow-up.

Search Methods for Identification of Studies

Electronic Searches

We contacted the Trials Search Co-ordinator to search the Cochrane Pregnancy and Childbirth Group's Trials Register (31 December 2011). The Cochrane Pregnancy and Childbirth Group's Trials Register is maintained by the Trials Search Co-ordinator and contains trials identified from:

1. quarterly searches of the Cochrane Central Register of Controlled Trials (CENTRAL);
2. weekly searches of MEDLINE;
3. weekly searches of EMBASE;
4. handsearches of 30 journals and the proceedings of major conferences;
5. weekly current awareness alerts for a further 44 journals plus monthly BioMed Central email alerts.

Details of the search strategies for CENTRAL, MEDLINE and EMBASE, the list of hand-searched journals and conference proceedings, and the list of journals reviewed via the current awareness service can be found in the 'Specialized Register' section within the editorial information about the Cochrane Pregnancy and Childbirth Group.

Trials identified through the searching activities described above are each assigned to a review topic (or topics). The Trials Search Co-ordinator searches the register for each review using the topic list rather than keywords.

Searching Other Resources

We searched reference lists of all retrieved papers for additional studies and contacted professional and lay organisations in order to obtain any ongoing trials or unpublished data. We did not apply any language restrictions.

Data Collection and Analysis

We assessed all potential trials for eligibility according to the criteria specified in the protocol by screening the titles and abstracts. We retrieved full reports of potentially relevant trials for assessment of eligibility based on the inclusion criteria. All review authors extracted the data and checked for accuracy, and we resolved discrepancies by discussion. No studies were published in duplicate. When data were missing, or if only the abstract was available, we attempted to contact the trial authors to obtain the missing information. We resolved any disagreement through discussion or we consulted the Pregnancy and Childbirth Review Group.

Selection of Studies

All review authors independently assessed for inclusion all the potential studies we identified as a result of the search strategy.

Data Extraction and Management

We designed a form to extract data. For eligible studies, all review authors extracted the data using the agreed form. We entered data into review manager software (Revman 2011) and checked for accuracy.

When information regarding any of the above was unclear, we attempted to contact authors of the original reports to provide further details.

Assessment of Risk of Bias in Included Studies

All review authors independently assessed risk of bias for each study using the criteria outlined in the *Cochrane Handbook for Systematic Reviews of Interventions* (Higgins 2011).

(1) RANDOM SEQUENCE GENERATION (CHECKING FOR POSSIBLE SELECTION BIAS). We described for each included study the method used to generate the allocation sequence in sufficient detail to allow an assessment of whether it should produce comparable groups. We assessed the method as:

- low risk of bias (any truly random process, e.g. random number table; computer random number generator);
- high risk of bias (any non-random process, e.g. odd or even date of birth; hospital or clinic record number);
- unclear risk of bias.

(2) ALLOCATION CONCEALMENT (CHECKING FOR POSSIBLE SELECTION BIAS). We described for each included study the method used to conceal allocation to interventions prior to assignment and assessed whether intervention allocation could have been foreseen in advance of, or during recruitment, or changed after assignment. We assessed the methods as:

- low risk of bias (e.g. telephone or central randomisation; consecutively numbered sealed opaque envelopes);
- high risk of bias (open random allocation; unsealed or nonopaque envelopes, alternation; date of birth);
- unclear risk of bias.

(3.1) *BLINDING OF PARTICIPANTS AND PERSONNEL (CHECKING FOR POSSIBLE PERFORMANCE BIAS).* We described for each included study the methods used, if any, to blind study participants and personnel from knowledge of which intervention a participant received. We consider that studies are at low risk of bias if they were blinded, or if we judge that the lack of blinding would be unlikely to affect results. We assess blinding separately for different outcomes or classes of outcomes. We assessed the methods as:

- low, high or unclear risk of bias for participants;
- low, high or unclear risk of bias for personnel.

(3.2) BLINDING OF OUTCOME ASSESSMENT (CHECKING FOR POSSIBLE DETECTION BIAS). We described for each included study the methods used, if any, to blind outcome assessors from knowledge of which intervention a participant received. We assessed blinding separately for different outcomes or classes of outcomes. We assessed methods used to blind outcome assessment as:

- low, high or unclear risk of bias.

(4) INCOMPLETE OUTCOME DATA (CHECKING FOR POSSIBLE ATTRITION BIAS DUE TO THE AMOUNT, NATURE AND HANDLING OF INCOMPLETE OUTCOME DATA). We described for each included study, and for each outcome or class of outcomes, the completeness of data including attrition and exclusions from the analysis. We stated whether attrition and exclusions were reported and the numbers included in the analysis at each stage (compared with the total randomised participants), reasons for attrition or exclusion where reported, and whether missing data were balanced across groups or were related to outcomes. Where sufficient information was reported, or could be supplied by the trial authors, we re-included missing data in the analyses which we undertook.

We assessed methods as:

- low risk of bias (e.g. no missing outcome data; missing outcome data balanced across groups);
- high risk of bias (e.g. numbers or reasons for missing data imbalanced across groups; 'as treated' analysis done with substantial departure of intervention received from that assigned at randomisation);
- unclear risk of bias.

(5) SELECTIVE REPORTING (CHECKING FOR REPORTING BIAS). We described for each included study how we investigated the possibility of selective outcome reporting bias and what we found. We assessed the methods as:

- low risk of bias (where it is clear that all of the study's prespecified outcomes and all expected outcomes of interest to the review have been reported);
- high risk of bias (where not all the study's prespecified outcomes have been reported; one or more reported primary outcomes were not prespecified; outcomes of interest are reported incompletely and so cannot be used; study fails to include results of a key outcome that would have been expected to have been reported);
- unclear risk of bias.

(6) OTHER BIAS (CHECKING FOR BIAS DUE TO PROBLEMS NOT COVERED BY (1) TO (5) ABOVE). We described for each included study any important concerns we may have had about other possible sources of bias.

Was the trial stopped early due to some data-dependent process? Was there extreme baseline imbalance?

We assessed whether each study was free of other problems that could put it at risk of bias:

- low risk of other bias;
- high risk of other bias;
- unclear whether there is risk of other bias.

(7) OVERALL RISK OF BIAS. We made explicit judgements about whether studies were at high risk of bias, according to the criteria given in the *Cochrane Handbook for Systematic Reviews of Interventions* (Higgins 2011). With reference to (1) to (6) above, we assessed the likely magnitude and direction of the bias and whether we considered it was likely to impact on the findings. We explored the impact of the level of bias through undertaking sensitivity analyses - *see* Sensitivity analysis.

Measures of Treatment Effect

DICHOTOMOUS DATA. For dichotomous data, we planned to present results as summary risk ratio with 95% confidence intervals.

CONTINUOUS DATA. For continuous data, we intended to use the mean difference if outcomes were measured in the same way between trials. We used the standardised mean difference to combine trials that measured the same outcome, but used different methods.

Unit of Analysis Issues

CLUSTER-RANDOMISED TRIALS. If identified, we would have included cluster-randomised trials in the analyses along with individually randomised trials. We would have adjusted their sample sizes using the methods described in the *Cochrane Handbook for Systematic Reviews of Interventions* using an estimate of the intracluster correlation co-efficient (ICC) derived from the trial (if possible), or from another source. If ICCs from other sources had been used, we would have reported this and conducted sensitivity analyses to investigate the effect of variation in the ICC. If we had identified both cluster-randomised trials and individually-randomised trials, we planned to synthesise the relevant information. We considered it reasonable to combine the results from both if there was little heterogeneity between the study designs and the interaction between the effect of intervention and the choice of randomisation unit was considered to be unlikely. We also acknowledged heterogeneity in the randomisation unit and would have performed a separate sensitivity analysis to investigate the effects of the randomisation unit.

Dealing with Missing Data

For included studies, we noted levels of attrition. We explored the impact of including studies with high levels of missing data in the overall assessment of treatment effect by using Sensitivity analysis. For all outcomes we carried out analyses, as far as possible, on an intention-to-treat basis, i.e. we attempted to include all participants randomised to each group in the analyses and all participants would have been analysed in the group to which they were allocated, regardless of whether or not they received the allocated intervention. The denominator for each outcome in each trial was the number randomised minus any participants whose outcomes were known to be missing.

Assessment of Heterogeneity

We assessed statistical heterogeneity in each meta-analysis using the T^2, I^2 and Chi^2 statistics. We regarded heterogeneity as substantial if T^2 is greater than zero and either I^2 is greater than 30% or there is a low P value (less than 0.10) in the Chi^2 test for heterogeneity.

Assessment of Reporting Biases

If there were 10 or more studies in the meta-analysis, we planned to investigate reporting biases (such as publication bias) using funnel plots. We would have assessed funnel plot asymmetry visually, and used formal tests for funnel plot asymmetry. For continuous outcomes, we would have used the test proposed by Egger 1997, and for dichotomous outcomes, we planned to use the test proposed by Harbord 2006. If we had detected asymmetry in any of these tests or by a visual assessment, we would have performed exploratory analyses to investigate it.

Data Synthesis

We carried out statistical analysis using the Review Manager software (RevMan 2011). We planned to use fixed-effect meta-analysis for combining data where it was reasonable to assume that studies were estimating the same underlying treatment effect: i.e. where trials are examining the same intervention, and the trials' populations and methods were judged sufficiently similar. Where there was clinical heterogeneity sufficient to expect that the underlying treatment effects differed between trials, or if substantial statistical heterogeneity was detected, we used random-effects meta-analysis to produce an overall summary if an average treatment effect across trials was considered clinically meaningful. The random-effects summary was treated as the average range of possible treatment effects and we discussed the clinical implications of treatment effects differing between trials. If the average treatment effect was not clinically meaningful, we did not combine trials. Using random-effects analyses, the results were presented as the average treatment effect with 95% confidence intervals, and the estimates of T^2 and I^2.

Subgroup Analysis and Investigation of Heterogeneity

If we had identified substantial heterogeneity, we would have investigated it using subgroup analyses and sensitivity analyses. We would have considered whether an overall summary was meaningful, and if it was, we would have used random-effects analysis to produce it.

We planned to carry out the following subgroup analyses.

1. Recurrent miscarriage versus sporadic miscarriage.
2. Early versus late miscarriage.
3. Pre-existing psychological condition versus no psychological condition.

We planned to use the following outcome in subgroup analysis.

- Psychological well being.

For fixed-effect meta-analyses, we planned to conduct subgroup analyses classifying whole trials by interaction tests as described by Deeks 2001. For random-effects and fixed-effect meta-analyses using methods other than inverse variance, we intended to assess differences between subgroups by inspection of the subgroups' confidence intervals; nonoverlapping confidence intervals indicate a statistically significant difference in treatment effect between the subgroups.

Sensitivity Analysis

We planned to carried out sensitivity analyses to explore the effect of trial quality separating using the 'Risk of bias' table to distinguish high-quality from low-quality trials, for example, in allocation concealment and blinding of outcome assessors.

RESULTS

Description of Studies

See Evolve ⊖: Characteristics of included studies; Characteristics of excluded studies.

Results of the Search

Nineteen papers were identified in the search which covered psychological support for women

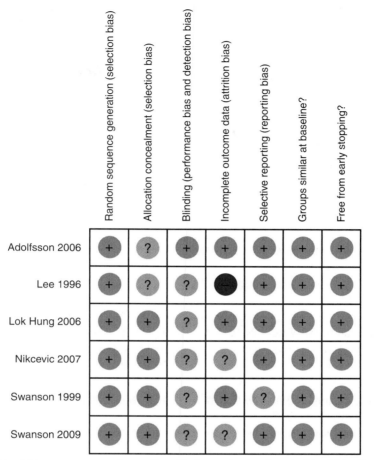

FIG. E.1 Risk of bias summary: review authors' judgements about each risk of bias item for each included study.

who have had a miscarriage up to 23 weeks' gestation. We included six studies involving 1001 women (Adolfsson 2006; Lee 1996; Lok Hung 2006; Nikcevic 2007; Swanson 1999; Swanson 2009). We excluded the remaining 13 papers as they were either not randomised controlled trials or were not within gestation limits. Some excluded trials did not provide interventions (*see* Characteristics of excluded studies).

Risk of Bias in Included Studies

Overall, the quality of the studies was moderate to good. Some studies were unclear regarding blinding. *See* Figure E.1; 'Risk of bias' summary

and Figure E.2 'Risk of bias' graph and Characteristics of included studies.

Sequence Generation

Randomisation was adequate in all studies. We contacted one author to confirm that randomisation was by an independent person pulling one of four cards blindly from a box (Swanson 1999).

Allocation Concealment

This was low risk in the majority of studies and clear in only one study where allocation concealment was described in personal correspondence from the author (Swanson 1999).

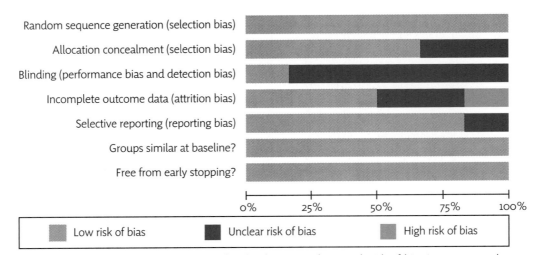

FIG. E.2 Risk of bias graph: review authors' judgements about each risk of bias item presented as percentages across all included studies.

Blinding

Following personal communication, blinding was considered adequate in one study (Adolfsson 2006) and for the remainder it was not clear that the participants, clinicians or outcome assessors were blinded. Because of the nature of the interventions, blinding was not considered crucial for the participants or clinicians.

Incomplete Outcome Data

Loss to follow-up, withdrawals and exclusions after randomisation were not excessive and explained in all studies. An intention-to-treat analysis was performed in one study (Lok Hung 2006).

Selective Outcome Reporting

We were only able to access one study protocol to be assured that there was no selective outcome reporting (Lok Hung 2006). One study reported that two subscales measured were dropped from the analysis because they were confounded by alterations due to the women's pregnancy loss (Swanson 1999).

Other Potential Sources of Bias

The participants in all studies were similar at baseline except for percentage of women with children

(Lee 1996) and history of infertility (Lok Hung 2006) and were judged by the review authors to be at low risk of bias for this issue. As far as could be ascertained, no studies were stopped early for any reason.

Effects of Interventions

1. One Counselling Session Versus No Counselling (Three Studies 236 Women) (Analysis 1.1–See Evolve ⓔ)

PRIMARY OUTCOMES

Psychological Well Being. This analysis included three studies with 236 women and compared one counselling session with no counselling (Adolfsson 2006; Lee 1996; Nikcevic 2007). The counselling sessions were based on recognised counselling techniques and lasted 50 minutes (Nikcevic 2007) or one hour (Adolfsson 2006; Lee 1996). All three studies used a number of measures to assess psychological well being at four months after miscarriage (Analysis 1.1). For the purpose of analysis, components of the tools used to measure psychological well being are displayed separately. Two studies used the Hospital Anxiety and Depression (HADs) scale (Lee 1996; Nikcevic 2007). Both studies recognised greater than 11 as the threshold for 'caseness' with HADs. When compared with no counselling, one counselling session did not result in a statistically significant reduction in anxiety with the standardised mean difference (SMD) -0.24 (95% confidence interval (CI) -0.62 to 0.15) (Analysis 1.1.1) or depression SMD -0.25 (95% CI -0.63 to 0.14) (Analysis 1.1.2).

When combined, grief as measured on the modified Texas Grief Inventory (Nikcevic 2007) and the Perinatal Grief Scale (Swedish version) (Adolfsson 2006) showed no statistically significant reduction in grief in the counselling group (SMD -0.12; 95% CI - 0.43 to 0.20) (Analysis 1.1.3).

In addition to HADs, Lee 1996 employed the Impact of Events scale and neither of the two components measured were statistically significantly reduced in the counselling group for avoidance (SMD 0.18; 95% CI -0.45 to 0.81) (Analysis 1.1.4) and intrusion (SMD -0.42; 95% CI -1.06 to 0.22) (Analysis 1.1.5). The Perinatal grief Scale (Adolfsson 2006) measured difficulty in coping (SMD -0.08; 95% CI -0.50 to 0.34) (Analysis 1.1.6) as well as grief (see above) and despair (SMD 0.01; 95% CI -0.41 to 0.43) (Analysis 1.1.7). Neither component was statistically significantly reduced by one-hour counselling. In addition to HADs, Nikcevic 2007 used the Texas Grief Inventory which measured grief (see above), self-blame (SMD 0.03; 95% CI -0.45 to 0.51) (Analysis 1.1.8) and worry (SMD -0.42; 95% CI -0.91 to 0.06) (Analysis 1.1.9). Neither analysis showed statistically significant reduction in self-blame or worry as a result of one 50-minute counselling session.

The other primary outcome of patient satisfaction was not assessed in any of the studies.

SECONDARY OUTCOMES. The other prespecified secondary outcomes were not assessed.

2. Three One-Hour Counselling Sessions Versus No Counselling (At Four Months) (One Study 242 Women) (Analysis 2.1–See Evolve ⓔ)

PRIMARY OUTCOMES
Psychological Well Being. One study compared three one-hour counselling sessions with no counselling

based on a technique devised by the main author of the study (Swanson 1999). The sessions were conducted at one, five and 11 weeks. A Solomon four group randomised design was used in this study. Instead of omitting the pretest in two of the four groups, as recommended by Solomon, the study authors delayed it. This modification was justified by the study author to reduce the risk of early focused attention on loss serving as a form of treatment.

Outcome measures comprised self-esteem measured on the 10-item Rosenberg scale. Mood states were measured by the Profile of Mood States (POMS) as 'overall mood disturbance' and six subscales of anxiety-tension, depression-dejection, anger-hostility, vigour-fatigue, confusion-bewilderment. The outcome measures of vigour-fatigue were omitted by the author. In addition, the Impact of Miscarriage Scale (IMS) was developed by the author to measure 'overall impact of miscarriage' and four subscales of 'devastating event', 'lost baby' (this refers to whether the woman views the loss as a fetus or a baby), 'personal significance' and 'feeling isolated.'

Of the scores on any of the three scales and eight subscales of all outcome measures (early and delayed measure) (22 in total), only three showed statistical significance for any intervention, either early or delayed at four months. The subscales which identified a significant result were in the measurement tool developed by Swanson 1999. These were Lost baby (early measure) which showed that those women who did not have counselling had improved psychological well being than those who had counselling (SMD 3.99; 95% CI 3.27 to 4.72) (Analysis 2.1.15) (P = 0.00001). However, those women who undertook counselling (early measure) were statistically significantly less likely to view the miscarriage as a Devastating event (SMD -2.52; 95% CI -3.08 to -1.95) (Analysis 2.1.19) (P = 0.00001). Women who undertook counselling (delayed measure) stated that they felt less isolated than women who did not (SMD -0.42; 95% CI -0.84 to -0.01) (Analysis 2.1.22) (P = 0.04).

Only two of the three statistically significant results favour counselling. All three significant results were from subscales of the instrument developed by the author (IMS).

Although another study used three counselling sessions as one of the interventions measured at three and five months, data were not available for this analysis despite contact with the author (Swanson 2009).

Patient satisfaction was not assessed in this study.

SECONDARY OUTCOMES. The other prespecified secondary outcomes were not assessed.

3. Three One-Hour Counselling Sessions Versus No Counselling (At 12 Months) (One Study 242 Women) (Analysis 3.1–See Evolve ⓔ)

One study compared three one-hour counselling sessions with no counselling based on a technique devised by the main author of the study (Swanson 1999). The sessions were conducted at one, five and 11 weeks. To counter the potential effect of data gathering unwittingly producing a beneficial effect Solomon four group randomised design was implemented where measurements were delayed on half of the treated and half of the control group. Outcome measures comprised self-esteem measured on the 10-item Rosenberg scale. Mood states were measured by the POMS as 'overall mood disturbance' and six subscales of anxiety-tension, depression-dejection, anger-hostility, vigour-fatigue, confusion-bewilderment. The outcome measures of vigour-fatigue were omitted by the author. In addition, the IMS was developed by the author to measure 'overall impact of miscarriage' and four subscales of 'devastating event', 'lost baby', 'personal significance' and 'feeling isolated'.

Of the scores on any of the three scales and eight subscales of all outcome measures (early and delayed measure) (22 in total), only three showed statistical significance for any intervention, either early or delayed at four months. The subscales which measured a significant result were in the measurement tool (IMS) developed by Swanson 1999. At 12 months, the overall impact of miscarriage (delayed measurement) (SMD -0.43; 95% CI -0.85 to -0.01) showed a statistically significant effect (P = 0.05) (Analysis 3.1.14) towards three one-hour counselling sessions compared with no counselling. Lost baby (delayed measurement) showed a statistically significant effect (SMD 2.15; 95% CI 1.48 to 2.82) (Analysis 3.1.16) for no counselling compared with three one-hour counselling sessions. Personal significance (delayed measurement) (SMD -0.66; 95% CI -1.09 to -0.24) (Analysis 3.1.18) and devastating event (delayed measurement) showed a statistically significant effect (SMD -0.45; 95% CI -0.87 to -0.04) (Analysis 3.1.20) towards three one-hour counselling sessions compared with no counselling. Three of the four significant results favoured counselling over no counselling. All the significant results were from a subscale of an instrument developed by the author (IMS). Significant findings at 12 months differed in that the subscale of isolation at four months was replaced by that of personal significance at 12 months.

Although another study used three counselling sessions as one of the interventions measured at 12 months, data were not available for this analysis despite contact with the author (Swanson 2009).

SECONDARY OUTCOMES. The other prespecified secondary outcomes were not assessed.

4. Two Counselling Sessions Versus No Counselling (One Study 280 Women) (Analysis 4.1)

PRIMARY OUTCOMES

Psychological Well Being. One study compared two nurse-led counselling sessions with no counselling (Lok Hung 2006). The first session was 60 minutes face-to-face counselling by a nurse counsellor before discharge. The second session was 30 minutes telephone counselling two weeks after discharge. Outcome measures were the 12-item General Health Questionnaire (GHQ-12) (caseness greater than four), the Beck Depression Inventory (BDI) (caseness greater than 12) and the Dyadic Adjustment Scale (DAS) completed at six weeks, three months and six months after miscarriage.

Medians were used to express data in this study and we were unable to extract the means or obtain them despite attempts to contact the author, therefore, the results are in narrative form.

At six weeks post-miscarriage 56/132 (33.3%) women scored at least four on GHQ (median three, interquartile range (IQR) zero to six) in the counselling group compared with 60/136 (44.1%) (median three, IQR zero to seven) in the no-counselling group. Thirty-three women/132 (25%) scored at least 12 on BDI (median four, IQR two to 12) in the counselling group compared with 41/136 (30.1%) (median seven, IQR two to 13) in the no-counselling group. No significant differences were found between the counselling and control groups using an intention-to-treat analysis.

At three months post-miscarriage 32/132 (24.2%) women scored at least four on GHQ (median one, IQR 0 to three) in the counselling group compared with 42/136 (30.9%) (median one, IQR 0 to 4.75) in the no-counselling group. Twenty-four/132 (18.2%) scored at least 12 on BDI (median three, IQR 0 to seven) in the counselling group compared with 27/136 (19.9%) (median four, IQR one to 10) in the no-counselling group. No significant differences were found between the counselling and control groups using an intention-to-treat analysis.

At six months post-miscarriage, 30/132 (22.7%) women scored at least four on GHQ (median 0, IQR zero to three) in the counselling group compared with 27/136 (19.9%) (median one, IQR zero to three) in the no-counselling group. Twenty women/132 (15.2%) scored at least 12 on BDI (median two, IQR zero to seven) in the counselling group compared with 23/136 (16.9%) (median seven, IQR zero to 8.75) in the no-counselling group. No significant differences were found between the counselling and control groups using an intention-to-treat analysis.

Patient satisfaction was not assessed in this study.

SECONDARY OUTCOMES. The other prespecified secondary outcomes were not assessed.

5. Combined Caring (CC), Nurse Caring (NC), Self Caring (SC) and No Treatment (NT) (One Study 341 Women)

One study compared four interventions based on a counselling technique, videos and a workbook devised by the author (Swanson 2009). The comparisons were combined care (CC) comprising one counselling session by nurse counsellors based on the author's postmiscarriage counselling model, three 18-minute videos of the author coaching couples on ways to practice self and partner caring, plus one workbook; nurse caring (NC) comprising three one hour counselling sessions; self-care (SC) comprising three videos plus workbook; and no treatment (NT) (Swanson 2009).

Primary outcomes were measured as depression (CES-D). Women scoring 16 were associated with a higher risk of clinical depression. The secondary outcome of grief was measured by two subscales of the Miscarriage Grief Inventory; (MGI) pure grief (PG) and grief related emotions (GRE) which is adapted from the Texas Grief Inventory (TGI).

Women in all three treatment groups showed a faster rate of recovery from depression (CES-D) compared with women receiving no treatment. However, only three one-hour counselling sessions (NC) met the author's criterion for substantial evidence favouring NC over SC, CC and no treatment for accelerating resolution of depression (Bayesian Odds Ratio 7.9 median -0.7 P = 0.89).

Relative to no treatment there was, according to the author, substantial evidence that all three interventions (NC, SC, CC) hastened women's resolution of pure grief (PG) (Bayesian odds ratio 3.1 median -0.2 P = 0.76). The evidence favoured the impact of SC in hastening women's resolution of GRE (Bayesian odds ratio 3.2 median -0.2 P = 0.76).

According to Swanson 2009, there was no substantial evidence that no treatment was preferable to NC, SC or CC in accelerating women's resolution of pure grief, grief-related emotion or depression.

Patient satisfaction was not assessed in this study.

SECONDARY OUTCOMES. The other prespecified secondary outcomes were not assessed.

DISCUSSION

Summary of Main Results

There is an assumption that miscarriage is an adverse event distressing all affected women to a greater or lesser degree. Until now the extent to which psychological follow-up is necessary to reverse this state has not been examined in a Cochrane systematic review. Given the international nature of systematic reviews, the WHO definition of miscarriage was used with the limit of 23 weeks' gestation in contrast to the UK definition of 24 weeks' gestation (RCOG 2006). It is possible that a very small number of women were between 23 and 24 weeks' gestation in one study (Lok Hung 2006) although this was calculated as unlikely by the review authors, although two other studies (Neugebauer 2006; Rajan 1993) were sufficiently at risk of including women up to 28 weeks that they were excluded. Planned sensitivity analyses were not possible as no studies examined recurrent miscarriages as a specific event, differentiated between early and late miscarriages or between women with a pre-existing psychological condition and those without.

The interventions following miscarriage mainly consisted of one or a number of counselling sessions using recognised counselling techniques. Timing of the interventions varied from one week following miscarriage (Swanson 1999; Swanson 2009), up to 11 weeks (Swanson 1999; Swanson 2009). It was not possible to compare different types of psychological follow-up via a meta-analysis given the heterogeneity between studies.

In all studies the interventions were delivered by different professional groups including a midwife (Adolfsson 2006), psychologists (Lee 1996; Nikcevic 2007) and nurses (Lok Hung 2006; Swanson 1999; Swanson 2009), which may have had an impact on the way in which the intervention was delivered. No study compared professionals delivering the intervention. The time span of the studies covered more than a decade and so it is possible that psychological interventions may have changed during that period.

The major primary outcome was psychological well being. We were unable to report the majority of the studies as meta-analyses but were able to report them as forest plots with narrative. Under the primary outcome of psychological well being, a wide range of outcomes were measured from those more commonly anticipated such as grief, anxiety and depression to emotional disturbance, self-esteem and isolation. Outcome measures used included validated tools, some of which had been modified, for example, a Swedish version of the Perinatal grief Scale (Adolfsson 2006) and others which had been developed by the study authors (Impact of Miscarriage Scale Swanson 1999) (Miscarriage Grief Inventory Swanson 2009). The tools also varied in that some were generic such as the Hospital Anxiety and Depression Scale (Lee 1996; Nikcevic 2007) and others were miscarriage specific (Swanson 1999; Swanson 2009). Caseness, or the level at which women were judged to benefit from psychological follow-up using a specific tool, was not made clear in all studies. Some studies did not state whether a high score indicated psychological ill health or well being (Nikcevic 2007; Swanson 2009). All of these issues made it challenging to pool the results and compare findings.

Timing of outcome measurements differed markedly between studies from one month (Lok Hung 2006) to 12 months (Swanson 1999) highlighting the uncertainty surrounding the rate of psychological recovery following miscarriage. One study noted that anxiety, depression and grief reduced significantly in all three groups with time (Nikcevic 2007). Psychological well being was measured and improved with time which may or may not have been influenced by the intervention in four other studies (Lee 1996; Lok Hung 2006; Swanson 1999; Swanson 2009).

The possibility that the measurement of grief, depression and other associated symptoms act as part of the healing process by allowing the woman to talk about her feelings was explored in one study. The author attempted to manage this possibility by organising early or delayed measurement, but this did not make a difference to the overall results (Swanson 1999).

Generally the studies have shown that women's reactions to miscarriage vary and the extent of depression, grief and anxiety differ. Only one study showed some significant outcomes. However, they were unlikely to be of significance overall as they represented differences between delayed and early measures as well as individual subscales on a complex tool developed by the study author (Swanson 2009). No significant results were found in this study on the widely used, standardised scales.

Three studies, two of which were combined in a forest plot, measured the generic outcomes of anxiety, depression and grief. Although the results favoured counselling none were significant. The other primary outcome of patient satisfaction was not measured in any of the trials. We maintain that this is an important outcome as evidence of satisfaction alone is not a reason to provide a service. In addition, none of the secondary outcomes identified by the review authors as important were reported. They included adverse reaction to follow-up, referral to primary healthcare services, admission to hospital and costs associated with follow-up. It is possible that an adverse reaction, referral or admission to hospital following psychological follow-up is unlikely and therefore these outcomes may not be a priority outcome measure for primary studies.

Overall Completeness and Applicability of Evidence

Our published protocol described our plan to analyse a series of major and minor outcomes. We were able to analyse one of the primary outcomes but none of the secondary outcomes were included in any studies. All eligible randomised controlled trials were included up to April 2011. The majority of studies lacked power. The two larger studies (Swanson 1999; Swanson 2009)

included such a complex combination of interventions and outcome measures that any potentially significant effects may have been diluted.

Quality of the Evidence

This review examined psychological follow-up for 1001 women after miscarriage in six randomised controlled trials. The studies were single centre, from a range of countries, over a decade and a half. Overall, the risk of bias was judged to be low, although allocation concealment and blinding was unclear as it was not stated in the majority of studies. It was recognised that given the nature of the trials, blinding of the participants and clinicians would not be possible.

Potential Biases in the Review Process

There are a number of limitations to this review. Surprisingly, most of the studies published in the last decade did not have a published protocol and to our knowledge, had not registered their study in one of the many trial registries, indicating that a broad search strategy was still necessary. Lay organisations providing psychological follow-up were included in the search strategy, but none were found.

Strengths of this review include the methodological rigour applied, including a published protocol, data analysis and narrative, which allowed us to make the findings explicit.

Agreements and Disagreements with other Studies or Reviews

A Cochrane review on perinatal death (Flenady 2008), has indicated that there is insufficient evidence to show that psychological follow-up improves the well being of women following perinatal death. Similarly, this review has found a lack of evidence to show that psychological follow-up is beneficial for women following miscarriage. However, some women may benefit from psychological follow-up and the review authors recommend that any service already in place should continue taking into account women's preference pending further evidence.

AUTHORS' CONCLUSIONS

Implications for Practice

Evidence is insufficient to demonstrate the superiority of either psychological support such as counselling or no intervention postmiscarriage. Given the equivocal evidence, women's preference should play a large role in the decision-making process.

Implications for Research

Further evaluation of the effectiveness of psychological follow-up for women following miscarriage should be based on good quality, adequately-powered randomised trials. Future trials should use standardised interventions, standardised outcome measures at specified time points.

Women's satisfaction with psychological follow-up should be explored in future studies. Given the costs of these interventions, the economic implications for this service should also be integrated into any future study.

ACKNOWLEDGMENTS

All authors would like to acknowledge Swansea University and the University of Glamorgan for allowing them the time to undertake the protocol and the full review. As part of the pre-publication editorial process, this review has been commented on by three peers (an editor and two referees who are external to the editorial team) and the Group's Statistical Adviser.

REFERENCES

References to Studies Included in this Review
Adolfsson 2006 (published data only)
Adolfsson, A. (2006, June). *The effect of structured second visit to midwifes in women with early miscarriages, a randomized study*. Lund, Sweden: 10th International Conference of Maternity Care Researchers.
*Adolfsson, A., Bertero, C., & Larsson, P. G. (2006). Effect of a structured follow-up visit to a midwife on women with early miscarriage: a randomized

study. *Acta Obstetricia et Gynecologica Scandinavica, 85*, 330–335.
Lee 1996 (published data only)
Lee, C., Slade, P., & Lygo, V. (1996). The influence of psychological debriefing on emotional adaptation in women following early miscarriage: a preliminary study. *British Journal of Medical Psychology, 69*(Pt 1), 47–58.
Lok Hung 2006 (published and unpublished data)
Lok, I. H. (2006). *Psychological morbidity after miscarriage* [thesis]. University of Hong Kong.
Nikcevic 2007 (published data only)
Nikcevic, A. V., Kuczmierczyk, A. R., & Nicolaides, K. H. (2007). The influence of medical and psychological interventions on women's distress after miscarriage. *Journal of Psychosomatic Research, 63*(3), 283–290.
Swanson 1999 (published data only)
Swanson, K. M. (1999). Effects of caring, measurement, and time on miscarriage impact and women's wellbeing. *Nursing Research, 48*(6), 288–298.
Swanson 2009 (published data only)
Swanson, K. M., Chen, H. T., Graham, C. J., Wojnar, D. M., & Petras, A. (2009). Resolution of depression and grief during the first year after miscarriage: a randomized controlled clinical trial of couples-focused interventions. *Journal of Women's Health, 18*(8), 1245–1257.
References to Studies Excluded from this Review
Broen 2004 (published data only)
Broen, A. N., Moum, T. R., Bødtker, A. S., & Ekeberg, O. (2004). Psychological impact on women of miscarriage versus induced abortion: a 2-year follow-up study. *Psychosomatic Medicine, 66*(2), 265–271.
Broen 2005 (published data only)
Broen, A. N., Moum, T. R., Bødtker, A. S., & Ekeberg, O. (2005). The course of mental health after miscarriage and induced abortion: a longitudinal, five-year follow-up study. *BMC Medicine, 3,* 265-71.
Cordle 1994 (published data only)
Cordle, C. J., & Prettyman, R. J. (1994). A 2-year follow-up of women who have experienced early miscarriage. *Journal of Reproductive and Infant Psychology, 12*, 37–43.
Jacobs 2000 (published data only)
Jacobs, J., & Harvey, J. (2009). Evaluation of an Australian miscarriage support programme. *British Journal of Nursing, 9*(1), 2–6.
Lefkof 2002 (published data only)
Lefkof, J., & Glazer, G. (2002). Grief after miscarriage: practical interventions can assist with far-reaching loss. *Advance for Nurse Practitioners, 10*(10), 79–82.

---

*Indicates the major publication for the study

Luise 2002 (published data only)

Luise, C., Jermy, K., Collons, W. P., & Bourne, T. H. (2002). Expectant management of incomplete, spontaneous first-trimester miscarriage: outcome according to initial ultrasound criteria and value of follow-up visits. *Ultrasound in Obstetrics & Gynecology, 19*(6), 580–582.

Neugebauer 2006 (published data only)

Neugebauer, R., Kline, J., Markowitz, J. C., et al. (2006). Pilot randomized controlled trial of interpersonal counseling for subsyndromal depression following miscarriage. *Journal of Clinical Psychiatry, 67*(8), 1299–1304.

Neugebauer 2007 (published data only)

Neugebauer, R., Kline, J., Bleiberg, K., et al. (2007). Preliminary open trial of interpersonal counselling for subsyndromal depression following miscarriage. *Depression and Anxiety, 24*(3), 219–222.

Nikcevic 1998 (published data only)

Nikcevic, A. V., Tunkel, S. A., & Nicolaides, K. H. (1998). Psychological outcomes following missed abortions and provision of follow-up care. *Ultrasound in Obstetrics and Gynecology, 11*(2), 123–128.

Nikcevic 2003 (published data only)

Nikcevic, A. V. (2003). Development and evaluation of a miscarriage follow up clinic. *Journal of Reproductive & Infant Psychology, 21*(3), 207–217.

Rajan 1993 (published data only)

Rajan, L., & Oakley, A. (1993). No pills for heartache: the importance of social support for women who suffer pregnancy loss. *Journal of Reproductive and Infant Psychology, 11*, 75–87.

Sejourne 2011 (published data only)

Sejourne, N., Callahan, S., & Chabrol, H. (2011). The efficiency of a brief support intervention for anxiety, depression and stress after miscarriage [French]. *Journal de Gynecologie, Obstetrique et Biologie de la Reproduction, 40*(5), 437–443.

Thaper 1992 (published data only)

Thapar, A. K., & Thapar, A. (1992). Psychological sequelae of miscarriage: a controlled study using the General Health Questionnaire and the Hospital Anxiety and Depression scale. *British Journal of General Practice, 42*(356), 94–96.

Additional References

Blohm 2008

Blohm, F., Friden, B., & Milsom, I. (2008). A prospective longitudinal population-based study of clinical miscarriage in an urban Swedish population. *BJOG: An International Journal of Obstetrics & Gynaecology, 115*(2), 176–183.

Deeks 2001

Deeks, J. J., Altman, D. G., & Bradburn, M. J. (2001). Statistical methods for examining heterogeneity and combining results from several studies in meta-analysis. In M. Egger, G. Davey Smith, & D. G. Altman (Eds.), *Systematic reviews in health care: meta-analysis in context*. London: BMJ Books.

Egger 1997

Egger, M., Smith, G. D., Schneider, M., & Minder, C. (1997). Bias in meta-analysis detected by a simple, graphical test. *British Medical Journal, 315*, 629–634.

Farquharson 2005

Farquharson, R. G., Jauniaux, E., & Exalto, N. (2005). Updated and revised nomenclature for description of early pregnancy events. *Human Reproduction, 20*, 3008–3011.

Flenady 2008

Flenady, V., & Wilson, T. (2008). Support for mothers, fathers and families after perinatal death. *Cochrane Database of Systematic Reviews, 2008*(1), CD000452. doi:10.1002/14651858.CD000452.pub2.

Frost 2007

Frost, J., Bradley, H., Levitas, R., Smith, L., & Garcia, J. (2007). The loss of possibility: scientisation of death and the special case of early miscarriage. *Sociology of Health and Illness, 29*(7), 1003–1022.

Harbord 2006

Harbord, R. M., Egger, M., & Sterne, J. A. (2006). A modified test for small-study effects in meta-analyses of controlled trials with binary endpoints. *Statistics in Medicine, 25*, 3443–3457.

Higgins 2011

Higgins, J. P. T., & Green, S. (Eds.), (2011). *Cochrane Handbook for Systematic Reviews of Interventions Version 5.1.0* [updated March, 2011]. The Cochrane Collaboration. Available from www.cochrane-hand book.org.

Malacrida 1998

Malacrida, C. (1998). *Mourning the dreams*. Alberta Canada: Qual Institute Press.

Mander 1997

Mander, R. (1997). Perinatal grief: understanding the bereaved and their careers. In J. Alexander, C. Roth, & V. Levy (Eds.), *Midwifery practice* (pp. 29–50). Basingstoke, England: Macmillan.

Nanda 2006

Nanda, K., Peloggia, A., Grimes, D. A., Lopez, L. M., & Nanda, G. (2006). Expectant care versus surgical treatment for miscarriage. *Cochrane Database of Systematic Reviews, 2006*(2), CD003518. doi:10. 1002/14651858.CD003518.pub2.

Neilson 2010

Neilson, J. P., Gyte, G. M. L., Hickey, M., Vazquez, J. C., & Dou, L. (2010). Medical treatments for incomplete miscarriage (less than 24 weeks). *Cochrane Database of Systematic Reviews*, *2010*(1), CD007223. doi:10.1002/14651858.CD007223.pub2.

Neugebauer 1997

Neugebauer, R., Kline, J., Shrout, P., et al. (1997). Major depressive disorder in the 6 months after miscarriage. *Journal of the American Medical Association*, *277*(5), 383–388.

Nikcevic 1999

Nikcevic, A., Tunkel, S., & Kuczmierczyk, A. (1999). Investigation of the cause of miscarriage and its influence on women's psychological distress. *British Journal of Obstetrics and Gynaecology*, *106*(8), 808–813.

RCOG 2006

Royal College of Obstetricians and Gynaecologists (RCOG). (2006). *Management of early pregnancy loss*. London: Royal College of Obstetricians and Gynaecologists.

RevMan 2011

The Nordic Cochrane Centre, & The Cochrane Collaboration. (2011). *Review manager (RevMan). 5.1*. Copenhagen: The Nordic Cochrane Centre, & The Cochrane Collaboration.

Stirtzinger 1999

Stirtzinger, R. M., Robinson, D. E., Stewart, D. E., & Ralevski, E. (1999). Parameters of grieving in spontaneous abortion. *International Journal of Psychiatry in Medicine*, *29*, 235–249.

Stratton 2008

Stratton, K., & Lloyd, L. (2008). Hospital-based interventions at and following miscarriage: literature to inform a research-practice initiative. *Australian and New Zealand Journal of Obstetrics and Gynaecology*, *48*, 5–11.

Trinder 2006

Trinder, J., Brocklehurst, P., Porter, R., Read, M., Vyas, S., & Smith, L. (2006). Management of miscarriage: expectant, medical, or surgical? results of randomised controlled trial (miscarriage treatment (MIST) trial). *British Medical Journal*, *332*, 1235–1240.

WHO 2001

World Health Organization (WHO). (2001). *Definitions and indicators in family planning, maternal & child health and reproductive health: WHO regional strategy on sexual and reproductive health*. Geneva: World Health Organization.

ⓔ Go to Evolve at http://evolve.elsevier.com/ Canada/LoBiondo/Research for the tables contained within this article.

Index